2002
YEAR BOOK OF
VASCULAR SURGERY®

The 2002 Year Book Series

Year Book of Allergy, Asthma, and Clinical Immunology™: Drs Rosenwasser, Boguniewicz, Milgrom, Routes, and Spahn

Year Book of Anesthesiology and Pain Management™: Drs Chestnut, Abram, Black, Lang, Roizen, Trankina, and Wood

Year Book of Cardiology®: Drs Schlant, Gersh, Graham, Kaplan, and Waldo

Year Book of Critical Care Medicine®: Drs Dellinger, Parrillo, Balk, Bleck, Carcillo, and Royster

Year Book of Dentistry®: Drs Zakariasen, Boghosian, Dederich, Hatcher, Horswell, and McIntyre

Year Book of Dermatology and Dermatologic Surgery™: Drs Thiers and Lang

Year Book of Diagnostic Radiology®: Drs Osborn, Birdwell, Dalinka, Groskin, Maynard, Oestreich, Pentecost, and Ros

Year Book of Emergency Medicine®: Drs Burdick, Cone, Cydulka, Hamilton, Loiselle, and Niemann

Year Book of Endocrinology®: Drs Mazzaferri, Fitzpatrick, Horton, Kannan, Kennedy, Kreisberg, Meikle, Molitch, Morley, Osei, Poehlman, and Rogol

Year Book of Family Practice®: Drs Bowman, Dexter, Gilchrist, Morrison, Neill, and Scherger

Year Book of Gastroenterology™: Drs Lichtenstein, Ginsberg, Katzka, Kochman, Morris, Nunes, Rosato, and Stein

Year Book of Hand Surgery®: Drs Berger and Ladd

Year Book of Medicine®: Drs Barkin, Frishman, Jett, Klahr, Loehrer, and Mazzaferri

Year Book of Neonatal and Perinatal Medicine®: Drs Fanaroff, Maisels, and Stevenson

Year Book of Neurology and Neurosurgery®: Drs Bradley, Gibbs, and Verma

Year Book of Nuclear Medicine®: Drs Gottschalk, Blaufox, Coleman, Strauss, and Zubal

Year Book of Obstetrics, Gynecology, and Women's Health®: Drs Mishell, Kirschbaum, and Miller

Year Book of Oncology®: Drs Loehrer, Eisenberg, Glatstein, Gordon, Johnson, Pratt, and Thigpen

Year Book of Ophthalmology®: Drs Wilson, Cohen, Eagle, Grossman, Laibson, Maguire, Nelson, Penne, Rapuano, Sergott, Shields, Spaeth, Steinmann, Tipperman, Ms Gosfield, and Ms Salmon

Year Book of Orthopedics®: Drs Morrey, Beauchamp, Peterson, Swiontkowski, Trigg, and Yaszemski

Year Book of Otolaryngology-Head and Neck Surgery®: Drs Paparella, Holt, Keefe, and Otto

2002

The Year Book of VASCULAR SURGERY®

Editor

John M. Porter, MD
Professor of Surgery, Division of Vascular Surgery, Oregon Health and Science University, Portland

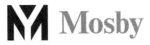 Mosby

St. Louis Baltimore Boston Carlsbad Naples New York Philadelphia Portland London
Madrid Mexico City Singapore Sydney Tokyo Toronto Wiesbaden

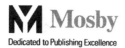

Mosby
Dedicated to Publishing Excellence

Executive Publisher: Cynthia Baudendistel
Associate Publisher: Colleen Cook
Manager, Continuity Production: Idelle L. Winer
Supervisor, Continuity Production: Joy Moore
Senior Production Editor: Pat Costigan
Composition Specialist: Betty Dockins
Illustrations and Permissions Specialist: Steve Ramay

2002 EDITION

Printed in the United States of America
Composition by Thomas Technology Solutions, Inc.
Printing/binding by Maple-Vail

Editorial Office:
Mosby, Inc.
11830 Westline Industrial Drive
St. Louis, MO 63146
Customer Service: hhspcs@harcourt.com

International Standard Serial Number: 0749-4041
International Standard Book Number: 0-323-01575-1

Contributors

Ahmed M. Abou-Zamzam, Jr, MD
Assistant Professor, Division of Vascular Surgery, Loma Linda University Medical Center, Loma Linda, Calif

Elliot L. Chaikof, MD, PhD
Associate Professor, Emory University School of Medicine, Emory University Hospital, Atlanta, Ga

Ronald L. Dalman, MD
Associate Professor of Surgery, Division of Vascular Surgery, Stanford University School of Medicine; Chief, Vascular Section, VA Palo Alto Health Care System, Stanford University Medical Center, Stanford and Palo Alto, Calif

James Edwards, MD
Associate Professor, Oregon Health and Science University; Acting Chief of Surgery, Portland VA Medical Center

Michael A. Golden, MD
Associate Professor of Surgery, University of Pennsylvania, University of Pennsylvania Medical Center, Philadelphia

E. John Harris, Jr, MD
Associate Professor of Surgery, Stanford University, Stanford, Calif

Gregory J. Landry, MD
Assistant Professor of Surgery, Division of Vascular Surgery, Oregon Health and Science University, Portland

Robert B. McLafferty, MD
Assistant Professor of Surgery, Division of Vascular Surgery, Southern Illinois University School of Medicine, Memorial Medical Center and St John's Hospital, Springfield, Ill

James O. Menzoian, MD
Professor of Surgery, Boston University School of Medicine; Chief, Section of Vascular Surgery, Boston Medical Center

Joseph L. Mills, Sr, MD
Professor of Surgery, University of Arizona; Chief, Vascular Surgery, University Medical Center, Tucson, Ariz

Gregory L. Moneta, MD
Professor of Surgery, Chief of Vascular Surgery, Oregon Health Sciences University, Oregon Health and Science University Hospital, Portland VA Medical Center

Mark R. Nehler MD
Assistant Professor of Surgery, University of Colorado Health Sciences Center, Denver

Lloyd Taylor, MD
Professor of Surgery, Oregon Health and Science University, Portland

W. Kent Williamson, MD

Fellow, Vascular Surgery, Oregon Health Sciences University, Portland

Richard A. Yeager, MD

Associate Professor of Surgery, Oregon Health and Science University, Portland VA Medical Center

Table of Contents

Journals Represented

Mosby and its editors survey approximately 500 journals for its abstract and commentary publications. From these journals, the editors select the articles to be abstracted. Journals represented in this YEAR BOOK are listed below.

American Heart Journal
American Journal of Gastroenterology
American Journal of Medicine
American Journal of Neuroradiology
American Journal of Perinatology
American Journal of Physiology
American Journal of Roentgenology
American Journal of Surgery
American Surgeon
Annals of Internal Medicine
Annals of Plastic Surgery
Annals of Surgery
Annals of Thoracic Surgery
Annals of Vascular Surgery
Annals of the Royal College of Surgeons of England
Archives of Dermatology
Archives of Disease in Childhood
Archives of Internal Medicine
Archives of Otolaryngology-Head and Neck Surgery
Archives of Surgery
Blood
Brain
British Journal of Surgery
Cardiovascular Surgery
Circulation
Clinical Orthopaedics and Related Research
European Journal of Vascular Surgery
European Journal of Vascular and Endovascular Surgery
Heart
International Journal of Epidemiology
International Journal of Radiation, Oncology, Biology, and Physics
Journal of Cardiothoracic and Vascular Anesthesia
Journal of Clinical Investigation
Journal of Pediatric Surgery
Journal of Surgical Research
Journal of Ultrasound in Medicine
Journal of Vascular Surgery
Journal of the American College of Dermatology
Lancet
Mayo Clinic Proceedings
Neurology
Neurosurgery
New England Journal of Medicine
Proceedings of the National Academy of Sciences
Radiology
Stroke
Surgery

Thrombosis Research
Thrombosis and Haemostatis
Vascular Surgery

STANDARD ABBREVIATIONS

The following terms are abbreviated in this edition: acquired immunodeficiency syndrome (AIDS), cardiopulmonary resuscitation (CPR), central nervous system (CNS), cerebrospinal fluid (CSF), computed tomography (CT), deoxyribonucleic acid (DNA), electrocardiography (ECG), health maintenance organization (HMO), human immunodeficiency virus (HIV), intensive care unit (ICU), intramuscular (IM), intravenous (IV), magnetic resonance (MR) imaging (MRI), ribonucleic acid (RNA), and ultrasound (US).

NOTE

The YEAR BOOK OF VASCULAR SURGERY® is a literature survey service providing abstracts of articles published in the professional literature. Every effort is made to assure the accuracy of the information presented in these pages. Neither the editors nor the publisher of the YEAR BOOK OF VASCULAR SURGERY® can be responsible for errors in the original materials. The editors' comments are their own opinions. Mention of specific products within this publication does not constitute endorsement.

To facilitate the use of the YEAR BOOK OF VASCULAR SURGERY® as a reference tool, all illustrations and tables included in this publication are now identified as they appear in the original article. This change is meant to help the reader recognize that any illustration or table appearing in the YEAR BOOK OF VASCULAR SURGERY® may be only one of many in the original article. For this reason, figure and table numbers will often appear to be out of sequence within the YEAR BOOK OF VASCULAR SURGERY®.

In Memoriam

JOHN M. PORTER
1938-2001

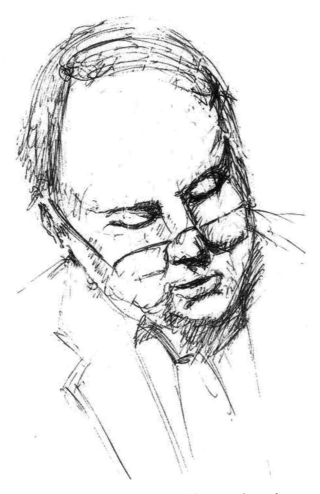

Dr John Wolfe sketched Dr Porter while attending the presidential address at the International Society of Cardiovascular Surgery (ISCVS) meeting in Toronto at the close of Dr Porter's year as president.

Introduction

As most of you are aware, Dr John Porter, Editor of the YEAR BOOK OF VASCULAR SURGERY since 1991, passed away on June 1, 2001, following an operation for a disrupted quadriceps tendon. A number of tributes to Dr Porter have been published in both the electronic and print media since his death. These contain details of the professional and personal life of my friend and partner. Out of respect to Dr Porter's abhorrence of dual publication, I will not repeat the specifics of these eulogies.

Whereas Dr Porter's physical health had been failing for a number of years, his mental acuity and wit remained sharp and incisive. This was clearly evident in his illustrative, probing, occasionally caustic, but always insightful comments in the YEAR BOOK OF VASCULAR SURGERY. For Dr Porter, the YEAR BOOK OF VASCULAR SURGERY was truly a labor of love that grew more pronounced with each new edition. When he assumed the Editorship in 1992, it was to be for only a few years. However, each year Dr Porter would agree to another year as Editor. He constantly complained about the work, but in reality relished the grasp of the vascular surgical literature that the Editorship required and fostered.

Most readers of the YEAR BOOK are probably unaware of the mechanics of its production. Papers considered for the YEAR BOOK OF VASCULAR SURGERY are provided by Mosby to the Editor. Characteristic of his fiercely independent thinking, and therefore not unexpectedly, Dr Porter would reject many of Mosby's suggestions, and replace them with his own selections culled from his personal exhaustive and ongoing perusal of all the medical literature even remotely related to vascular disease. The YEAR BOOK allowed Dr Porter to do what he enjoyed the most in academic medicine: continue to learn and communicate his thoughts to an appreciative and intelligent audience that shared his enthusiasm for vascular surgery.

Dr Porter had selected all the articles to be presented in the 2002 edition of the YEAR BOOK OF VASCULAR SURGERY before his death, and he had completed about half the commentaries accompanying the selected articles. In conjunction with Mosby, the Division of Vascular Surgery at the Oregon Health Sciences University agreed to orchestrate the completion of the 2002 edition of the YEAR BOOK OF VASCULAR SURGERY. After some discussion, it was decided an appropriate tribute to Dr Porter would be to have his fellow faculty members and former trainees contribute their thoughts in the 2002 edition. In this edition, therefore, you will find articles selected by Dr Porter, many with his comments, and those of his guest editors. The remaining commentaries come from his fellow faculty and former vascular surgical residents. While such comments are not "John Porter," they hopefully reflect some of the insight, humor, and love of vascular surgery he imparted to his faculty partners and residents over his long and successful career as surgeon, administrator, educator, and most of all, professor.

Gregory L. Moneta, MD

1 Basic Considerations

Alcohol

Type of Alcohol Consumed and Mortality From All Causes, Coronary Heart Disease, and Cancer
Grønbæk M, Becker U, Johansen D, et al (Univ of Copenhagen)
Ann Intern Med 133:411-419, 2000   1–1

Objective.—Studies have shown that alcohol intake and mortality have a J-shaped relationship. Studies showing that different types of alcohol have different effects are typically based on populations that consume 1 type of alcohol. The effects of intake of different types of alcohol on mortality from all causes, coronary heart disease, and cancer were investigated in several large Danish cohort studies.

Methods.—Cohorts from 3 Danish studies were combined to assess the effects of beer, wine, spirits, and lifestyle-related variables on 13,064 men and 11,459 women, aged 20 to 98 years. Participants' status was followed until death, loss to follow-up, or study end.

Results.—There were 4275 women and 1635 men who drank less than 1 drink/wk, and 64 women and 1032 men who drank 35 or more drinks/wk. Wine was consumed by 69% of the drinkers. During 257,859 person-years of follow-up, 4833 participants died, 1075 of coronary heart disease and 1552 of cancer. Total alcohol intake and mortality had a J-shaped relationship, with drinkers of 1 to 7 drinks/wk having a relative risk (RR) = 0.82 and drinkers of more than 35 drinks/wk having an RR = 1.10. Alcohol intake and death from coronary heart disease were negatively related. Alcohol intake and death from cancer were positively related. Light to moderate consumption of beer and spirits had a small effect on all-cause mortality, but consumption of 8 to 12 glasses of wine per week lowered the risk of all-cause mortality (RR = 0.76). Consumption of fewer than 22 drinks/wk of beer and wine but not spirits reduced all-cause mortality significantly. Light to moderate wine drinkers, but not beer and spirits drinkers, had a lower risk of death from cancer. There was a J-shaped relationship between alcohol intake and mortality adjusted for age, sex, smoking status, educational level, physical activity, and body mass index (Fig 1). Compared with nondrinkers, light drinkers who avoided wine had an RR of 0.76 for death from coronary heart disease, and those who drank wine had an RR = 0.58. The dose-dependent

1

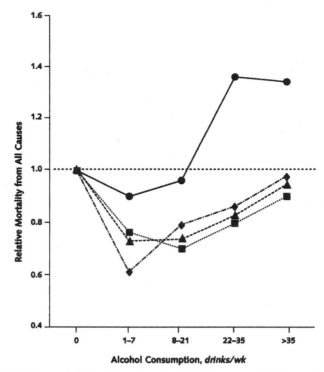

FIGURE 1.—Relative risk for death from all causes in relation to total alcohol intake. Data pertain to nonwine drinkers (*circles*), wine drinkers (*triangles*), drinkers for whom wine made up 1% to 30% of their total alcohol intake (*diamonds*), and drinkers for whom wine made up more than 30% of their total alcohol intake (*squares*). Relative risk is set at 1.00 among nondrinkers (<1 drink/wk). Estimates were adjusted for age, sex, educational level, smoking status, physical activity, and body mass index. (Courtesy of Grønbæk M, Becker U, Johansen D, et al: Type of alcohol consumed and mortality from all causes, coronary heart disease, and cancer. *Ann Intern Med* 133:411-419, 2000.)

association between drinking and cancer began at a higher intake among wine drinkers and was significant only among heavy drinkers. Neither sex nor educational level had an effect on the relationship of all-cause mortality and drinking.

Conclusion.—Light to moderate consumption of wine appears to lower the RR of all-cause mortality and of cancer.

▶ Few principles appear better established in the field of cardiovascular pathophysiology than the observation that alcohol consumption of some type, and in some quantity has a beneficial effect on all-cause mortality. A J-shaped relationship between the intake of alcohol and mortality from all causes has been observed in numerous large cohort studies. In other words, a moderate amount is helpful, but a large amount is clearly harmful. The question remains, however, as to whether the beneficial effects are limited entirely to wine or extend to distilled spirits and beer. A very large cohort of study subjects in Copenhagen were interviewed concerning their alcohol intake. This study found that wine drinkers had a significantly lower mortality rate from both coronary heart disease and cancer than did non–wine drinkers, and that heavy drinkers who avoided wine were at high risk for death from all causes.

The conclusion of this study appears inescapable, namely, that moderate wine drinking produces a lower mortality rate from both coronary heart disease and cancer, compared with individuals who do not drink. Of course, the possibility remains that there may be an unrecognized lifestyle factor distinguishing wine drinkers from non–wine drinkers. Overall, non–wine alcohol consumption appeared to affect things very little in low amounts, but appeared clearly harmful in high amounts.

The current demographic evidence thus suggests that the benefits of wine drinking regarding all-cause mortality may be related to some substance in wine other than alcohol or may be more related to the types of people who choose to drink wine. I suspect this will make an interesting topic for study for generations to come. (See also Abstracts 1–2 and 1–3.)

Alcohol Consumption Raises HDL Cholesterol Levels by Increasing the Transport Rate of Apolipoproteins A-I and A-II

De Oliveira e Silva ER, Foster D, McGee Harper M, et al (Rockefeller Univ, New York; Univ of Washington, Seattle; City Univ of New York; et al)
Circulation 102:2347-2352, 2000   1–2

Objective.—Alcohol appears to increase the concentration of high-density lipoprotein cholesterol (HDL-C). The increase in plasma HDL-C with moderate alcohol consumption was associated with an increase in the transport rate (TR) of apolipoproteins apoA-I and -II without a significant change in the fraction catabolic rate in a controlled, 2-treatment, 2-period crossover trial.

Methods.—Fourteen individuals (9 men), aged 21 to 70, who drank alcohol regularly but had no history of alcoholism in their families consumed a Western-type diet without alcohol (control) or with alcohol (EtOH) for 2 2-week periods. Kinetic studies were performed using radio-iodinated apoA-I and -II. Fasting plasma samples were drawn on days 1, 3, 7, 10, and 14 after isotope injection to determine lipid and lipoprotein concentrations. Postheparin lipase activity was measured, and lipoprotein size was determined. Outcome measures were correlations between the dose of EtOH and the EtOH diet-induced changes in HDL and related parameters.

Results.—HDL-C levels were 18% higher in those on the EtOH diet than in those on the control diet, but HDL size did not change. Total cholesterol, triglyceride, very-low-density lipoprotein cholesterol, and low-density lipoprotein cholesterol levels were essentially unchanged. ApoA-I and -II concentrations were 10% and 17% higher, respectively, for those on the EtOH diet than for those on the control diet. These increases corresponded with 21% and 19% increases in apoA-II TR compared with those on the control diet. There were no significant corresponding changes in apoA-I fraction catabolic rate. Lowering the activity of endothelial lipases appears to lower atherosclerosis risk. There was a dose-response relationship between alcohol intake and HDL-C, apoA-I, apoA-II, and apoA-I TR.

Conclusion.—Alcohol intake increases HDL-C, apoA-I, apoA-II, and apoA-I TR in a dose-dependent manner.

► Perhaps the most interesting observation in this study is that the benefits detected appeared to be results of the intake of vodka, clearly a substance with little or no relationship to wine. The alcohol intake in this study significantly increased HDL-C, and also increased the apoA-I, the major HDL apolipoproteins. The authors speculate the beneficial effect may have resulted from hepatic stimulation by alcohol. Whatever the mechanism, there seems to be little argument that moderate alcohol intake decreases all-cause mortality. I remain concerned how this may interact with Baptist theology.

Genetic Variation in Alcohol Dehydrogenase and the Beneficial Effect of Moderate Alcohol Consumption on Myocardial Infarction
Hines LM, Stampfer MJ, Ma J, et al (Harvard School of Public Health, Boston; Harvard Med School, Boston; Boston Healthcare System)
N Engl J Med 344:549-555, 2001   1–3

Background.—The mechanism by which moderate alcohol intake reduces the risk of myocardial infarction remains unclear. The rate of alcohol metabolism is affected by a polymorphism of the alcohol dehydrogenase type 3 (ADH3) gene. The effect of alcohol intake on risk of myocardial infarction for subjects in different ADH3 genotype groups was assessed.

Methods.—The study included 396 men from the Physicians' Health Study with newly diagnosed myocardial infarction. These patients were matched to 770 randomly selected controls. For each subject, the ADH3 genotype was $\gamma_1\gamma_1$, $\gamma_1\gamma_2$, or $\gamma_2\gamma_2$ determined. Associations among alcohol intake, ADH3 genotype, and plasma high-density lipoprotein level were assessed for the male physicians, as well as in subjects from an independent study of postmenopausal women.

Results.—Men with the $\gamma_2\gamma_2$ genotype—which is associated with a slow rate of ethanol oxidation—were at reduced risk for myocardial infarction, compared with those with the $\gamma_1\gamma_1$ genotype, which is associated with a fast rate of ethanol oxidation. The relative risk was 0.65; 95% confidence interval, 0.43 to 0.99. All 3 groups showed a reduced risk of myocardial infarction with moderate alcohol intake, although the ADH3 genotype had a significant modifying effect. Men homozygous for the γ_1 allele who had 1 or more drinks per day had a relative risk of 0.62 (95% confidence interval, 0.34-1.13), compared with men of similar genotype with a lower alcohol intake. The lowest relative risk (0.14; 95% confidence interval, 0.04-0.45) was observed for men who had 1 or more drinks per day and were homozygous for the γ_2 allele (Fig 1). The same group had the highest

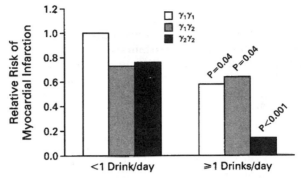

FIGURE 1.—Multivariate relative risk of myocardial infarction according to the ADH3 genotype and the level of daily alcohol consumption. In addition to adjustment for the matching factors of age, smoking status, and time since randomization (in 6-month intervals), the analyses were adjusted for body-mass index (≤23.01, >23.01-24.40, >24.40-26.40, or >26.40), frequency of vigorous physical activity (<1, 1-4, or ≥5 times per week), presence or absence of a family history of myocardial infarction, presence or absence of random assignment to aspirin use, and presence or absence of a history of hypertension, diabetes, and angina at enrollment. The P values are for the comparison with the values in men who consumed less than 1 drink per day and who were homzygous for the γ_1 allele (the reference group); the lowest relative risk of myocardial infarction (0.14; 95% confidence interval, 0.04-0.42) was for the group of men who drank daily and who were homozygous for the γ_2 allele (P = .02 for the interaction between the genotype and the level of alcohol consumption). (Reprinted by permission of *The New England Journal of Medicine* from Hines LM, Stampfer MJ, Ma J, et al: Genetic variation in alcohol dehydrogenase and the beneficial effect of moderate alcohol consumption on myocardial infarction. *N Engl J Med* 344:549-555, 2001. Copyright 2001, Massachusetts Medical Society. All rights reserved.)

measured plasma high-density lipoprotein cholesterol levels. A similar pattern of interactions was noted in the sample of postmenopausal women.

Conclusion.—The genotype of the ADH3 gene has a significant modifying effect on the relationship between alcohol intake and myocardial infarction risk. Subjects who have the slow-oxidizing $\gamma_2\gamma_2$ genotype and a moderate alcohol intake have higher high-density lipoprotein cholesterol levels and a lower risk of myocardial infarction.

▶ I am amazed by this study. Polymorphism in the gene for ADH3 alters the rate of alcohol metabolism. There is apparently a slow gene and a fast gene, and the good gene is the slow gene. If you are homozygous for the slow gene and have moderate alcohol intake you have a remarkable risk reduction to 0.14 for myocardial infarction compared with a risk of 0.62 for those who are homozygous for the fast gene and consume alcohol moderately. The slow gene people also had higher high-density lipoprotein levels, which may have been the mechanism of benefit. On balance, this article presents a remarkable molecular insight into the relationship between moderate alcohol consumption in ADH3 polymorphism. It is noteworthy that this study grouped all alcohol intake together and did not discriminate for 1 type versus another.

Atherosclerosis

Pravastatin Treatment Increases Collagen Content and Decreases Lipid Content, Inflammation, Metalloproteinases, and Cell Death in Human Carotid Plaques: Implications for Plaque Stabilization

Crisby M, Nordin-Fredriksson G, Shah PK, et al (Huddinge Univ, Stockholm; Malmö Univ Hosp, Sweden; Univ of California Los Angeles)
Circulation 103:926-933, 2001   1–4

Background.—The concept of plaque stabilization with lipid-lowering therapy is based on the principle that a reduction in lipid content and inflammatory activity—which are 2 of the major determinants of plaque instability—would result in a reduction in the risk of plaque disruption and prevention of adverse clinical events. This hypothesis has been supported by animal studies, but data in humans have been lacking. The effect of 3 months of pravastatin treatment on composition of human carotid plaques removed during carotid endarterectomy was evaluated in consecutive patients with symptomatic carotid artery stenosis.

Methods.—Eleven consecutive patients with symptomatic carotid artery stenosis received 40 mg/d pravastatin for 3 months before scheduled carotid endarterectomy, while a control group of 13 subjects received no lipid-lowering therapy. Special stains and immunocytochemistry with quantitative image analysis were used for the assessment of plaque composition.

Results.—There was less lipid by oil red O staining in plaques from the pravastatin group (8.2% ± 8.4% of the plaque area) compared with the control group (23.9% ± 21.1% of the plaque area). The pravastatin group also demonstrated less oxidized low-density lipoprotein cholesterol immunoreactivity, fewer macrophages, fewer T cells, less matrix metalloproteinase 2 (MMP-2) immunoreactivity, and fewer macrophages and T cells. In addition, the pravastatin group demonstrated greater tissue inhibitor of metalloproteinase 1 (TIMP-1) immunoreactivity and a higher collagen content by Sirius red staining. The pravastatin group also showed reduced cell death by TUNEL staining compared with the control group.

Conclusion.—The plaque-stabilizing effects of pravastatin in humans were confirmed by these findings, which included decreased lipids, lipid oxidation, inflammation, MMP-2, and cell death along with increased TIMP-1 and collagen content in carotid plaques.

▶ This study examines the novel hypothesis that lipid-lowering statin therapy may reduce clinical events more by plaque stabilization against disruption than by alterations in severity of stenosis. The remarkable results found herein are modestly interpreted by the authors as providing the first strong evidence in support of the plaque-stabilizing effects of statins in humans. On balance, I am impressed. As has been noted increasingly in recent YEAR BOOKS, the stability of the atherosclerotic plaque appears to be the critical element in determining the occurrence of adverse events. We are on the doorstep of beginning to learn what makes a plaque rupture, and we are also beginning to develop imaging techniques that may allow us to determine the rupture potential of an individual plaque before it occurs. Medical or surgical therapy directed toward a critically located unstable plaque may become a clinical reality.

Long-term Effects of Cholesterol Lowering and Angiotensin-Converting Enzyme Inhibition on Coronary Atherosclerosis: The Simvastatin/ Enalapril Coronary Atherosclerosis Trial (SCAT)
Teo KK, for the SCAT Investigators (Univ of Alberta Hosps, Edmonton; et al)
Circulation 102:1748-1754, 2000   1–5

Objective.—Because most patients with coronary atherosclerotic disease (CAD) have normal cholesterol levels, it is not clear how cholesterol lowering will affect CAD progression. Whether angiotensin-converting enzyme inhibition and cholesterol lowering therapy are synergistic also is not known. Results of a randomized, double-blind, placebo-controlled, multicenter, 2 × 2 factorial, clinical trial, testing whether simvastatin and enalapril, alone or in combination, affect CAD progression in normocholesterolemic patients over a 3- to 5-year period, are presented.

Methods.—From June 1991 to July 1995, CAD patients (89% men) were randomly allocated to receive simvastatin (n = 230) or placebo (n = 230) and enalapril (n = 229) or placebo (n = 231) in 4 Canadian centers. Some patients received both drugs, and some perceived a double placebo. Total serum cholesterol levels ranged from 4.1 to 6.2 mmol/L, triglyceride levels were less than 4 mmol/L, and high-density lipoprotein cholesterol levels were less than 2.2 mmol/L. Lipid levels and degree of stenosis were tested monthly for 6 months and then at 9 and 12 months and every 6 months thereafter for an average of 48 months.

Results.—Angiography was performed in 194 simvastatin patients and in 200 placebo patients. During treatment, the mean absolute diameter decreased significantly less in simvastatin patients than in placebo patients (0.07 vs 0.14 mm). Similar results were seen with minimum absolute diameters (0.09 vs 0.16 mm). The mean percentage of stenosis increased significantly more in patients receiving placebo than in patients receiving simvastatin (1.67% vs 3.83%). Paired angiograms in enalapril and placebo patients showed no quantitative differences. Systolic and diastolic blood pressures were significantly lower in enalapril patients than in placebo patients. The effects of enalapril and simvastatin were not additive. Compared with placebo patients, simvastatin patients had fewer revascularization procedures (6% vs 12%) and fewer angioplasties (3% vs 9%). Compared with placebo patients, enalapril patients had a decrease in the combined end point of death/myocardial infarction/stroke (7% vs 13%).

Conclusion.—Lipid-lowering therapy benefits normocholesterolemic CAD patients. Angiotensin-converting enzyme inhibitors exert a neutral angiographic effect on these patients.

▶ As the authors point out, a significant majority of patients with symptomatic CAD have cholesterol levels that are average or normal for the population at large. While the clinical benefits of further reduction in cholesterol have been shown, this study was the first to examine the effect of such cholesterol lowering on angiographic changes in the coronary arteries. The authors also evaluated angiotensin-converting enzyme (ACE) inhibition. The finding that the statin drug has a favorable effect on coronary anatomy is about as predicted. The failure of the ACE inhibitor to have any effect on coronary anatomy is interesting. It is noted that the ACE inhibitor patients had a significantly reduced end point of death, myocardial infarction, or stroke compared with placebo patients. Studies such as this continue to clarify the relationships between lipid and blood pressure lowering and changes in coronary anatomy and clinical outcome.

Multiple Complex Coronary Plaques in Patients With Acute Myocardial Infarction
Goldstein JA, Demetriou D, Grines CL, et al (William Beaumont Hosp, Royal Oak, Mich)
N Engl J Med 343:915-922, 2000   1–6

Introduction.—It is possible that acute myocardial infarction (MI) is caused by rupture of an unstable coronary artery plaque. This plaque appears on angiography as a single lesion. The plaque instability may be the result of pathophysiologic processes, including inflammation, that have adverse effects throughout the coronary vasculature and may therefore result in multiple unstable lesions. The incidence of multiple complex plaques was assessed in patients with acute transmural MI to ascertain their influence on clinical outcome.

Methods.—Angiograms from 253 consecutive patients with acute transmural MI were examined for complex coronary plaques characterized by thrombus, ulceration, plaque irregularity, and impaired flow. Medical records and the hospital database were reviewed to assess clinical variables, in-hospital outcomes, and the clinical course over the 12 months after MI. Patients were grouped according to whether they had single or multiple complex coronary plaques.

Results.—Single complex coronary plaques were observed in 153 patients (60.5%); the remaining 100 patients (39.5%) had multiple complex plaques. Compared with patients who had single complex plaques, those with multiple complex plaques were less likely to require primary angioplasty (86.0% vs 94.8%; $P = .03$) and required urgent bypass surgery more frequently (27.0% vs 5.2%; $P \leq .001$). In the year after MI, the presence of multiple complex plaques was correlated with increased inci-

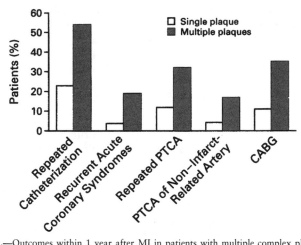

FIGURE 3.—Outcomes within 1 year after MI in patients with multiple complex plaques or single complex plaques. *Abbreviations*: PTCA, Percutaneous transluminal angioplasty; CABG, coronary artery bypass grafting. $P \leq 0.001$ for all comparisons between groups. (Reprinted by permission of *The New England Journal of Medicine* from Goldstein JA, Demetriou D, Grines CL, et al: Multiple complex coronary plaques in patients with acute myocardial infarction. *N Engl J Med* 343:915-922. Copyright 2000, Massachusetts Medical Society. All rights reserved.)

dence of recurrent acute coronary syndromes (19.0% vs 2.6%; $P \leq .001$), especially of non–infarct-related lesions (17.0% vs 2.6%; $P \leq .001$) and of coronary artery bypass graft surgery (35.0% vs 11.1%; $P \leq .001$) (Fig 3).

Conclusion.—Patients with acute MI may have multiple complex coronary plaques that are related to adverse clinical outcomes. Plaque instability may be caused by a widespread process throughout the coronary vessels, which may have an impact on the management of acute ischemic heart disease.

▶ Unfortunately, this article harbors a little bit of data, and a great deal of speculation. In the experience of these investigators, 60% of patients undergoing an acute MI had a single index complex plaque that apparently was the cause of the symptoms. Forty percent of patients had multiple complex plaques. Patients who had multiple complex plaques had an inferior clinical outcome, assessed in multiple ways, compared with those who had a single complex plaque. The authors then speculate that unidentified systemic factors may result in the destabilization of multiple plaques simultaneously. Perhaps one day we shall have some information in this area and, when that occurs, we may be able to develop a reasonable strategy to favorably affect plaque stability. As noted, interest in unstable plaque causation, detection, and prevention is attracting about as much interest presently as any other field in atherosclerosis.

Hyperfibrinogenemia Is Associated With Specific Histocytological Composition and Complications of Atherosclerotic Carotid Plaques in Patients Affected by Transient Ischemic Attacks

Mauriello A, Sangiorgi G, Palmieri G, et al (Universitá di Roma Tor Vergata, Rome; Armed Forces Inst of Pathology, Washington, DC; Mayo Clinic and Mayo Found, Rochester, Minn)
Circulation 101:744-750, 2000   1–7

Background.—Limited data are available on the relationships between risk factors for atherosclerosis and the histologic composition of the plaques. Hyperfibrinogenemia is an independent risk factor for cerebrovascular atherosclerosis, but the mechanism of this association is unknown. The potential effects of hyperfibrinogenemia on the histologic composition of atherosclerotic plaques and thus on the likelihood of carotid thrombosis resulting from plaque rupture were assessed.

Methods.—The study included 71 carotid plaques from patients undergoing endarterectomy after their initial episode of transient ischemic attacks. The histologic findings of the plaques were analyzed, and correlated with the patients' relative plasma fibrinogen levels. Other variables analyzed included cholesterol level, triglyceride level, blood pressure, diabetes, and smoking.

Results.—Patients in the highest tertile of fibrinogen had levels greater than 407 mg/dL. The incidence of thrombosis within this group was 67%, compared with 22% for patients in the lower tertile and 29% for those in the middle tertile. Hyperfibrinogenemia was also associated with a 54% incidence of plaque rupture. On multivariate analysis, hyperfibrinogenemia was independently associated with decreased cap thickness, macrophage foam cell infiltration of the cap, and thrombosis. It remained an independent predictor of carotid thrombosis after adjustment for other risk factors (odds ratio, 5.83) compared with the other risk factors.

Conclusions.—Patients with high plasma fibrinogen levels are predisposed to have carotid atherosclerotic plaques of a composition associated with high rates of rupture and thrombosis. Thus hyperfibrinogenemia is an independent risk factor for carotid thrombosis. Fibrinogen level identifies a group of patients at high risk of rapidly progressive carotid atherosclerosis.

▶ In recent years, serum fibrinogen has come to be firmly established as a risk factor for cerebrovascular atherosclerosis/stroke. I never really understood the mechanism of this association. Fibrinogen, of course, is an acute phase reactant, but by itself that did not appear to be enough. The investigators reporting in this interesting study of excised carotid plaques found that patients who had a high serum fibrinogen had the highest incidence of thrombosis on the plaque, and a much higher incidence of plaque rupture and a decrease in cap thickness than those that were not ruptured. Macrophage foam cell infiltration was increased also in the patients with the highest fibrinogen. Thus, this study suggests that serum fibrinogen level affects plaque behavior. This may indeed be the explanation for the observation that serum fibrinogen constitutes a potent risk factor. This is new information and, indeed, quite interesting.

Markers of Myocardial Damage and Inflammation in Relation to Long-term Mortality in Unstable Coronary Artery Disease
Lindahl B, for the FRISC Study Group (Univ of Uppsala, Sweden)
N Engl J Med 343:1139-1147, 2000   1–8

Background.—Many studies have shown that the elevated levels of troponin T or I are associated with an increased risk of cardiac events after an episode of unstable coronary artery disease. Elevated levels of markers of inflammation in the blood—such as the acute-phase proteins, C-reactive protein, and fibrinogen—are associated with an increased risk of cardiac events in apparently healthy persons who have had an episode of unstable coronary artery disease. Information obtained during an extension of the follow-up period in the Fragmin during Instability in Coronary Artery Disease trial was used in the evaluation of the usefulness of troponin T, C-reactive protein, and fibrinogen levels plus several other risk indicators as predictors of long-term mortality risk from cardiac causes.

Methods.—The cohort consisted of 917 patients included in a clinical trial of low–molecular-weight heparin in unstable coronary artery disease. The levels of C-reactive protein and fibrinogen at enrollment and the maximal level of troponin T during the first 24 hours were measured. Follow-up was for a mean of 37 months.

Results.—One hundred and seventy-three patients had maximal blood troponin T levels of less than 0.06 µg/L, and 1.2% of these patients died of cardiac causes during follow-up. In comparison, 8.7% of the 367 patients with blood troponin T levels of 0.06 µg to 0.59 µg/L and 15.4% of the 377 patients whose blood levels were at least 0.60 µg/L died of cardiac causes during follow-up. Among the 314 patients with C-reactive protein levels of less than 2 mg/L, the mortality rate was 5.7%. The 294 patients with levels of 2 to 10 mg/L had a mortality rate of 7.8%, and among the 309 patients with levels above 10 µg/L, the mortality rate was 16.5%. For blood fibrinogen levels, the mortality rate was 5.4% for the 314 patients with less than 3.4 g/L, 12% for 300 patients with levels of 3.4 to 3.9 g/L, and 12.9% for 303 patients with levels of at least 4.0 g/L (Fig 1). Multivariate analysis revealed that the levels of troponin T and C-reactive protein were independent predictors of risk of death from cardiac diseases.

Conclusion.—Elevated levels of troponin T and C-reactive protein are strongly associated with the long-term risk of death from cardiac causes in patients with unstable coronary artery disease. These markers were shown

FIGURE 1

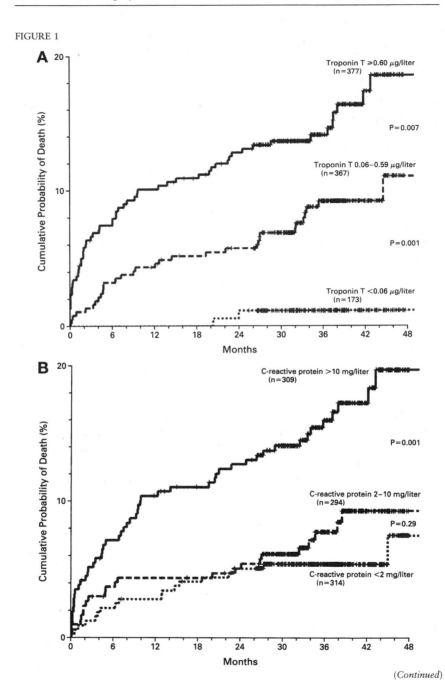

(Continued)

FIGURE 1 (cont.)

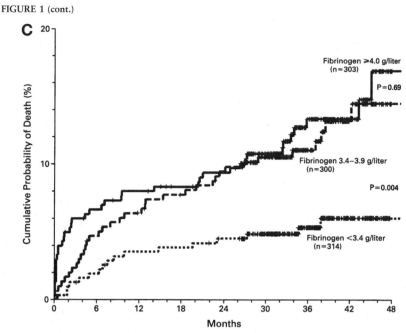

FIGURE 1.—Cumulative probability of death from cardiac causes in relation to maximal troponin T levels during the first 24 hours after enrollment (**A**) and to C-reactive protein levels (**B**) and fibrinogen levels (**C**) at enrollment. The number of patients in each group at the beginning of the study is given in *parentheses. Tick marks* indicate censored patients. (Reprinted by permission of *The New England Journal of Medicine* from Lindahl B, for the FRISC Study Group: Markers of myocardial damage and inflammation in relation to long-term mortality in unstable coronary artery disease. *N Engl J Med* 343:1139-1147, 2000. Copyright 2000, Massachusetts Medical Society. All rights reserved.)

to be independent risk factors with additive effects with respect to each other an in relation to other clinical indicators of risk.

▶ While it seems intuitive that the admitting level of troponin T in patients with unstable coronary artery disease will predict the risk for long-term death from coronary disease, I find it a bit surprising that C-reactive protein behaves in a similar fashion. Interestingly, multivariate analysis indicated that the fibrinogen level was not an independent predictor of risk of death from cardiac causes. Thus, in patients who have unstable coronary artery symptoms, the amount of troponin T and C-reactive protein in the serum upon admission to the care facility seems to accurately predict the patient's risk for future cardiac death. While these authors speculate that an inflammatory condition as evidenced by C-reactive protein may be associated with coronary plaque instability, they have no direct proof of this. The take-away message clearly seems to be that both troponin T and C-reactive protein are important predictors of clinical behavior in patients with unstable coronary syndrome. (See Abstract 1–9.)

Rapid Reduction in C-Reactive Protein With Cerivastatin Among 785 Patients With Primary Hypercholesterolemia

Ridker PM, Rifai N, Lowenthal SP (Brigham and Women's Hosp, Boston; Children's Hosp Med Ctr, Boston; Bayer Pharmaceuticals, Westhaven, Conn)
Circulation 103:1191-1193, 2001   1–9

Background.—C-reactive protein (CRP) levels can be used as an independent predictor of future myocardial infarction and stroke in apparently healthy men and women. The addition of CRP testing to standard lipid screening seems to have provided an improved method for determination of vascular risk. Long-term therapy with hydroxymethylglutaryl coenzyme A reductase inhibitors (statins) has been found to reduce levels of CRP. However, the time course of this effect is unknown, and there are no dose-response data available. These issues were evaluated in a randomized trial of cerivastatin in a cohort of patients with primary hypercholesterolemia.

Methods.—CRP, low-density lipoprotein cholesterol (LDL-C), and high-density lipoproteins cholesterol (HDL-C) levels were measured in 785 patients with primary hypercholesterolemia at baseline and again after 8 weeks of therapy with either 0.4 of 0.8 mg of cerivastatin.

Results.—Treatment with cerivastatin resulted in a reduction of 13.3% in median CRP levels and a reduction of 24.5% in mean CRP levels (Fig 1). There was a prompt decline in LDL-C in a dose-dependent fashion, with a mean reduction in LDL-C of 37.3% at 0.4 mg and 42.2% for 0.8 mg, but there was no clear evidence of a dose-response effect of cerivastatin on CRP. In addition, there was no significant correlation observed between the degree of change in CRP and the magnitude of change in LDL-C or the magnitude of change in HDL-C. Thus, less than 2% of the variance in the change in CRP over the course of the study was attributable

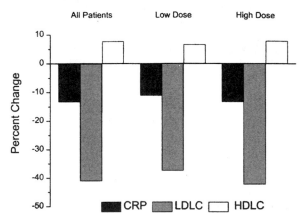

FIGURE 1.—Short-term effects of cerivastatin on C-reactive protein, low-density lipoprotein cholesterol, and high-density lipoprotein cholesterol among 785 patients with primary hypercholesterolemia. (Courtesy of Ridker PM, Rifai N, Lowenthal SP: Rapid reduction in C-reactive protein with cerivastatin among 785 patients with primary hypercholesterolemia. *Circulation* 103:1191-1193, 2001.)

to the percentage change in either of these lipid parameters. There was no evidence of a correlation between baseline levels of CRP and baseline lipid levels or between the CRP levels at the conclusion of the study and the lipid levels at the study's end.

Conclusion.—Among a group of patients with primary hypercholesterolemia, the use of cerivastatin therapy in a lipid-independent manner resulted in a significant reduction in CRP levels within 8 weeks of the initiation of therapy.

▶ It seems established beyond a reasonable doubt that CRP levels are an independent predictor of future myocardial infarction and stroke in both men and women. The evolving complex relationship between statin drugs and the inflammatory state is manifested by CRP, and atherosclerotic plaque destabilization has been mentioned in prior commentaries in this issue of YEAR BOOK. Prior studies have shown that pravastatin does reduce CRP and that this CRP reduction may be part of the favorable effects of this drug on cardiovascular events. In this study, these investigators now show that another statin, cerivastatin, independently reduced CRP levels. Interestingly, the CRP reductions appear to be independent of statin-induced changes in LDL-C. I think it quite likely that a complex interrelationship of CRP and plaque instability is just as prevalent in the peripheral circulation as in the coronary circulation. I wonder if one or more of the statins may have a favorable effect on either the reduction of plaque instability in the peripheral circulation or the reduction in symptoms associated with such plaque instability and rupture.

Lipoprotein-Associated Phospholipase A$_2$ as an Independent Predictor of Coronary Heart Disease

Packard CJ, for the West of Scotland Coronary Prevention Study Group (Glasgow Royal Infirmary, Scotland; et al)
N Engl J Med 343:1148-1155, 2000   1–10

Objective.—Inflammatory cells in atherosclerotic plaques are suspected to lead to plaque rupture. Expression of lipoprotein-associated phospholipase A$_2$, a possible predictor risk of coronary heart disease, is regulated by mediators of inflammation. The extent to which levels of lipoprotein-associated phospholipase A$_2$, C-reactive protein, and other markers of inflammation predicted the risk of a coronary event was investigated, in a nested case-control study, in the West of Scotland Coronary Prevention Study evaluating the effect of pravastatin therapy on the incidence of coronary events and death from cardiac causes.

Methods.—In the study, 6595 men with LDL cholesterol levels between 174 and 232 mg/dL and no history of myocardial infarction were randomly assigned to received 40 mg pravastatin or placebo daily. There were 580 men with a coronary event. Each patient was age- and smoking status–matched with 2 controls from the original cohort. The association between lipoprotein-associated phospholipase A₂, C-reactive protein, fibrinogen levels, white blood cell count, and risk of a coronary event was analyzed.

Results.—Patients who had a coronary event were older, had higher blood pressure and LDL cholesterol levels, and lower HLD cholesterol levels and were more likely to be smokers than patients who did not have a coronary event. All inflammatory markers were significantly associated with coronary events in the highest quintile. White blood cell count was not associated with a significant risk after adjusting for age, systolic blood pressure, and lipoprotein concentrations.

Conclusion.—Markers of chronic inflammation were significantly associated with risk for coronary heart disease and may be useful for risk stratification.

▶ This study is similar to the preceding abstracts just reported, but it reaches slightly different conclusions. The level of C-reactive protein, while predictive, was less impressive when age, systolic blood pressure, and lipoprotein levels were included in a multivariate model. However, the level of lipoprotein-associated phospholipase A₂ (also known as platelet-activating factor acetylhydrolase) had a positive strong association with risk that was not affected by other factors. It is presently unknown whether the increased cardiac risk associated with lipoprotein-associated phospholipase A₂ is related to its platelet-activating activities or contribution to a general inflammatory state. These authors suggest that this substance itself may become a future pharmacologic target for reduction in an effort to reduce cardiac risk. It will be interesting to follow this saga.

Plasma Concentration of Interleukin-6 and the Risk of Future Myocardial Infarction Among Apparently Healthy Men
Ridker PM, Rifai N, Stampfer MJ, et al (Harvard Med School, Boston)
Circulation 101:1767-1772, 2000   1–11

Introduction.—Interleukin-6 (IL-6) plays an important role in inflammation and tissue injury. Epidemiologic data regarding the role of IL-6 in atherogenesis are lacking. A prospective, nested case-control trial of IL-6 as a potential marker for future myocardial infarction (MI) was conducted among participants in the Physicians' Health Study, which was a randomized, double-blind, placebo-controlled trial of aspirin and β-carotene in the primary prevention of cardiovascular disease and cancer.

Methods.—Of 14,916 healthy men, baseline plasma concentration of IL-6 was measured in 202 participants who subsequently developed MI and 202 participants matched for age and smoking status who did not report vascular disease during a 6-year follow-up.

Results.—The median concentrations of IL-6 at baseline were significantly higher among men who subsequently had an MI than those who did not have an MI (1.81 vs 1.46 pg/mL). The median levels of IL-6 rose with

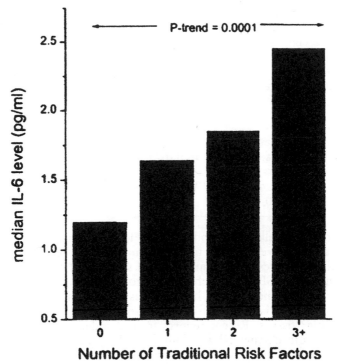

FIGURE 3.—Median baseline IL-6 levels according to number of traditional risk factors present (hypertension, hyperlipidemia, smoking, diabetes, age > 60 years, family history, and body mass index > 27.3 kg/m²). (Courtesy of Ridker PM, Rifai N, Stampfer MJ, et al: Plasma concentration of interleukin-6 and the risk of future myocardial infarction among apparently healthy men. *Circulation* 101:1767-1772, 2000.)

increasing number of traditional risk factors (Fig 3). The risk of a future MI rose significantly with increasing quartiles of baseline IL-6 concentration, such that men in the highest quartile at entry had a significant relative risk 2.3 times higher than those in the lower quartile; for each quartile rise in IL-6, there was a significant 38% increase in risk. This relationship continued to be significant after adjustment for other cardiovascular risk factors, was stable during long periods of follow-up, and was present in all low-risk subgroups, including nonsmokers. The strongest significant correlate of IL-6 was C-reactive protein ($r = .43$), but the relationship of IL-6 with subsequent risk continued significantly after control for this factor.

Conclusion.—Elevated levels of IL-6 are correlated with increased risk of future MI in apparently healthy men. Cytokine-mediated inflammation may play a role in the early stages of atherogenesis.

▶ IL-6 appears to have a central role in acute phase response, as well as determination of the hepatic production of C-reactive protein. It is produced in response to a number of factors, including TNF, interferon, and infection. To date, limited data relate IL-6 to atherosclerosis. This rather weak retrospective study finds that IL-6 in patients who eventually had a myocardial infarction develop was statistically higher than in patients who did not. I suppose we can interpret this as another soft piece of evidence relating inflammation to atherosclerotic, specifically, coronary events. Once again, cumulative data may point the way to a day when we have potent anti-inflammatory medications to specifically counteract these inflammatory-inducing substances in the serum. Stay tuned.

Serum Soluble Heat Shock Protein 60 Is Elevated in Subjects With Atherosclerosis in a General Population

Xu Q, Schett G, Perschinka H, et al (Inst for Biomedical Aging Research, Innsbruck, Austria; Univ Hosp of Vienna; Univ of Innsbruck, Austria; et al)
Circulation 102:14-20, 2000   1–12

Background.—Cells will produce high levels of heat shock protein (HSP) as a protective response to stress stimuli, including high temperature, mechanical stress, infections, surgical stress, and oxidant and cytokine stimulation. HSPs are members of a group of about 2 dozen proteins and cognates that show highly homologous sequences between different species, from bacteria to humans. These proteins are highly expressed in cardiovascular tissues. Recent reports from 2 independent groups have shown that both chlamydial and human HSP60 possess a cytokine-like activity and have the capacity for induction of tumor necrosis factor-α and matrix metalloproteinase production in human and mouse macrophages. It has also been found that both chlamydial and human HSP60 induced E-selectin, intercellular adhesion molecule–1, and vascular adhesion molecule-1 expression and interleukin-6 production in endothelial cells. The suggestion is that HSP60 directly stimulates endothelial cells, which leads to an inflammatory response that contributes to the pathophysiology of atherosclerosis. The possibility that HSP60 is present in the circulation, and thus able to exert its functions, was evaluated.

Methods.—In a population-based study, 826 subjects aged 40 to 79 years were evaluated for serum soluble HSP60 (sHSP60), anti-*Escherichia coli* lipopolysaccharide, anti-HSP65, and anti-*Chlamydia* and anti-*Helicobacter* antibodies, as well as a variety of acute phase reactants and markers of systemic inflammation. Carotid atherosclerosis was assessed twice (in 1990 and 1995), and 15 other risk factors were also evaluated.

Results.—Levels of sHSP60 were significantly higher in subjects who had prevalent/incident carotid atherosclerosis (Fig 1). These higher levels of sHSP60 were correlated with common carotid artery intima/media thickness. Multiple logistic regression analysis revealed that these associations were independent of age, sex, and other risk factors. sHSP60 was also found to be correlated with antilipopolysaccharide, anti-*Chlamydia* and anti-HSP60 antibodies, several markers of inflammation, and the presence of chronic infections. The risk of atherosclerosis associated with

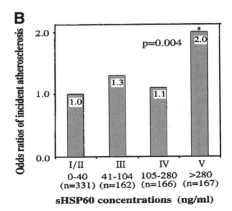

FIGURE 1.—B, Association of serum heat shock protein–60 (*sHSP60*) with incident carotid atherosclerosis. Odds ratios were derived from logistic regression analysis of incident carotid atherosclerosis on quintiles of sHSP60 concentrations, age, sex, and baseline atherosclerosis (reference category, sHSP ≤ 104 ng/mL). (Courtesy of Xu Q, Schett G, Perschinka H, et al: Serum soluble heat shock protein 60 is elevated in subjects with atherosclerosis in a general population. *Circulation* 102:14-20, 2000.)

high sHSP60 levels was even higher in subjects who had clinical or laboratory evidence of chronic infections.

Conclusion.—The first evidence of a strong correlation between sHSP60 and atherosclerosis was provided by these data. An important role for sHSP60 is suggested in the activation of vascular cells and the immune system during the development of atherosclerosis.

▶ HSPs are a highly conserved group of proteins found in almost all organisms, and they appear to serve a chaperone function, ensuring that newly synthesized polypeptides proceed correctly through folding and unfolding to achieve their proper functional conformation. The HSPs also clearly appear to have a protective function against a number of unfavorable conditions. Increasing evidence in recent years has suggested a relationship between the various HSPs and atherosclerosis. This study provides the first evidence of a strong correlation between soluble HSP 60 and atherosclerosis, leading these authors to conclude that HSPs may play an important role in activating vascular cells and the immune system in the development of atherosclerosis.[1] (See also Abstract 1–13.)

Reference

1. 2001 YEAR BOOK OF VASCULAR SURGERY, pp 42 and 44.

The Macromolecular Associations of Heat Shock Protein-27 in Vascular Smooth Muscle

Brophy CM, Molinaro JR, Dickinson M (Med College of Georgia, Augusta; Augusta Veterans Administration Med Ctr, Ga)
Surgery 128:320-326, 2000   1–13

Background.—Vasomotor tone is ultimately modulated by the intrinsic tone of the vascular smooth muscle; increases in vasomotor tone are contributing factors to pathologic conditions such as vasospasm and hypertension. Numerous investigations have demonstrated that behavioral stress is a significant risk factor for both hypertension and atherosclerosis. It has been shown that stress is a factor in the increased expression and phosphorylation of heat shock proteins (HSPs) in vascular smooth muscle. Two of these proteins, HSP27 and HSP20, have been implicated in the regulation of smooth muscle contraction and relaxation. The hypothesis that stress-induced changes in the phosphorylation of HSP27 would affect the macromolecular associations of the small HSPs was tested.

Methods.—Bovine carotid artery smooth muscle was used for this study. The muscle was treated with buffer alone or with arsenite, a chemical stressor. Isoelectric focusing was then used to determine HSP27 phosphorylation, and macromolecular interactions were assayed by means of subcellular fractionation, molecular sieving, and gluteraldehyde cross-linking and immunoblotting.

Results.—Increases were observed in the phosphorylation of HSP27 in the arsenite-treated muscle. Arsenite treatment also led to increases in a redistribution of some HSP27 from a cytosolic to a particulate fraction, as well as the formation of larger macromolecular aggregates of HSP27. HSP27 was shown to exist in monomeric and dimeric forms on gluteraldehyde cross-linking and immunoblotting, which suggested that the large aggregates were not aggregates of HSP27 but instead contained other proteins.

Conclusion.—In intact vascular smooth muscle, cellular stress results in increases in the phosphorylation of HSP27 and in changes in the macromolecular associations of HSP27. In vascular smooth muscle, the functions of the small HSPs may depend on both phosphorylation and macromolecular associations.

▶ This is a very preliminary study that attempts to relate the behavior of an intracellular HSP to chemical stress. Chemical stress, as defined in this study, increased the phosphorylation of HSP 27 and resulted in a type of redistribution of some of the substance from a cytosolic to a particulate fraction and to the formation of larger macromolecular aggregates. This preliminary information suggests that the function of small HSPs in vascular smooth muscle may require both phosphorylation and macromolecular association. Perhaps. I do believe the take-away message is that inflammation is being recognized as having an ever bigger role in atherosclerosis, and HSPs probably are involved somewhere in the process.

Effects of Estrogen Replacement on the Progression of Coronary-Artery Atherosclerosis

Herrington DM, Reboussin DM, Brosnihan KB, et al (Wake Forest Univ, Winston-Salem, NC; Carolinas Med Ctr, Charlotte, NC; LeBauer Cardiovascular Associates, Greensboro, NC; et al)
N Engl J Med 343:522-529, 2000   1–14

Introduction.—Estrogen replacement therapy is commonly recommended for secondary prevention of heart disease in postmenopausal women. However, 1 recent study showed no significant reduction in the risk of cardiac events and death among women taking estrogen. This finding underscores the need for further information about how estrogen affects coronary atherosclerosis, including the possible modifying effects of concomitant progestin. The Estrogen Replacement and Atherosclerosis trial evaluated the effects of hormone replacement therapy on the progression of coronary atherosclerosis in postmenopausal women.

Methods.—The randomized double-blind trial included 309 postmenopausal women with coronary disease, as confirmed by angiography. The patients were assigned to receive 0.625 mg/d conjugated estrogen, with or without 2.5 mg/d medroxyprogesterone acetate (MPA), or placebo. Follow-up continued for a mean of 3.2 years, including quantitative coronary angiography to assess the progression of coronary atherosclerosis.

Results.—In both estrogen-treated groups, the low-density lipoprotein cholesterol levels decreased significantly compared with the placebo group (by 9.4% in the estrogen-only group and by 16.5% in the estrogen-plus-MPA group). Both treatments significantly increased high-density lipoprotein cholesterol levels, by 18.8% in the estrogen-only group and by 14.2% in the estrogen-plus-MPA group. However, the progression of coronary atherosclerosis was similar among groups. With adjustment for baseline measurements, the mean minimal coronary artery diameter at follow-up was 1.87 mm in the estrogen-only group, 1.84 mm in the estrogen-plus-MPA group, and 1.87 mm in the placebo group. Other angiographic outcomes were also similar among the groups, as were the clinical cardiovascular event rates.

Conclusion.—For postmenopausal women with coronary atherosclerosis, estrogen replacement therapy, with or without MPA, does not appear to influence the rate of atherosclerotic progression. Such patients should not expect a cardiovascular benefit from the use of estrogen therapy. Estrogen replacement may still be effective in primary prevention of coronary disease, but this remains to be confirmed.

▶ Postmenopausal estrogen replacement has been recommended for almost every woman on the planet for a variety of reasons, including, but not limited to, the secondary prevention of heart disease. These investigators performed quantitative coronary arteriography in 309 women over the course of 3 years, during which time they received estrogen, estrogen plus medroxyprogesterone, or placebo. Neither estrogen alone nor estrogen plus medroxyprogesterone affected the progression of coronary atherosclerosis in women who had established heart disease at study entry. Sadly, this leads to the conclusion that postmenopausal women using estrogen replacement should not expect a coronary benefit. Too bad.

The Iron (Fe) and Atherosclerosis Study (FeAST): A Pilot Study of Reduction of Body Iron Stores in Atherosclerotic Peripheral Vascular Disease

Zacharski LR, Chow B, Lavori PW, et al (Dept of Veterans Assoc Med Ctrs, White River Junction, Vt; Dept of Veterans Assoc Med Ctrs, Palo Alto, Calif; Dept of Veterans Assoc Med Ctrs, Pittsburgh, Pa; et al)
Am Heart J 139:337-345, 2000   1–15

Background.—Levels of body iron stores increase with age after adolescence in men and after menopause in women but are not elevated in premenopausal women. Some investigators have proposed that these lower body iron stores may explain the reduced risk of myocardial infarction in premenopausal women. Higher levels of body iron are associated with an increased risk of coronary disease in men and with carotid atherosclerosis in both men and women. The release of stored iron from ferritin generates oxygen free radicals, and iron-induced oxidative stress seems to play a role in the pathogenesis of atherosclerosis. Thus, there is much evidence to suggest that reducing iron stores by phlebotomy might improve outcomes in patients with atherosclerosis. In preparation for a clinical trial to examine this possibility, the feasibility and safety of calibrated reductions in iron stores via phlebotomy were examined in patients with advanced peripheral vascular disease in a pilot study.

Methods.—The participants were 48 patients with advanced peripheral vascular disease (47 men and 1 postmenopausal woman; mean age, 66 years). All patients had either current intermittent claudication and a resting ankle–arm supine blood pressure ratio of 0.85 or less in either leg or had histories of intermittent claudication and prior reconstructive surgery or angioplasty of at least 1 leg for atherosclerotic disease. Also, all patients had values in the reference range for hematocrit and red blood cell indexes and no abnormalities in iron balance and renal function. Any patients with a disease that causes bleeding (eg, peptic ulcer disease) had been free of symptoms for 6 months or more. None of the patients had neoplasms (other than nonmelanoma skin cancer), an associated inflammatory disorder (eg, infection) that could elevate ferritin levels, or a comorbid condition that was expected to be fatal within 1 year. Furthermore, the use of vitamins and iron supplements during the study was prohibited. Patients were randomly assigned to the control group (n = 19) or to the iron reduction group (n = 29). The goal of iron reduction was to reduce body iron stores to an equivalent serum ferritin level of about 25 ng/mL, which is the level characteristic of premenopausal women and conditioned athletes. The formula used to calculate the volume of blood to be withdrawn (in milliliters) was (initial serum ferritin level − 25) × 10. Patients were followed up for 3 months for determinination of the feasibility and safety of the protocol.

Results.—None of the patients experienced any adverse laboratory or clinical effects during the 3-month study. The mean number of visits required to remove the targeted volume of blood was 2.62 (range, 1-6 visits), and a mean of 311.2 mL (range, 0-700 mL) of blood was removed at each visit. Follow-up data were complete for 18 control subjects and 26 patients in the iron reduction group. Serum ferritin levels did not change significantly in the control subjects but decreased significantly in the iron reduction group, from 124.5 ng/mL at baseline to 51.54 ng/mL at 3 months.

Conclusions.—The reduction of body iron stores to a predetermined level is, indeed, feasible and can be achieved in a reasonable period of time (3 months). Even though some patients required up to 6 visits to require the targeted volume of blood, compliance was excellent. Clinical trials to test the effects of a targeted reduction of body iron stores via phlebotomy on outcomes in patients with significant atherosclerosis may be conducted successfully.

▶ It has been recognized in recent years that an elevated level of serum iron may be a potent risk factor for coronary disease.[1] While the adverse mechanism of action of iron is not known with certainty, it may involve a process of iron-induced lipid oxidation. This study examines a rather mundane method of reducing serum iron by controlled phlebotomy. The authors have validated a formula for calculating the volume of blood to be removed to achieve a predetermined decrease in serum iron concentration and conclude that their method is accurate and that phlebotomy is not associated with any adverse laboratory or clinical effect. This is actually important information in the therapy of iron overload, once we identify afflicted patients.

Reference

1. 2001 YEAR BOOK OF VASCULAR SURGERY, p 45.

Initial and 6-Month Results of Biodegradable Poly-*l*-Lactic Acid Coronary Stents in Humans

Tamai H, Igaki K, Kyo E, et al (Shiga Med Ctr for Adults, Japan; Igaki Med Planning Co Ltd, Kyoto, Japan)
Circulation 102:399-404, 2000   1–16

Background.—Percutaneous transluminal coronary angioplasty is an acceptable alternative to coronary artery bypass grafting for the treatment of selected patients with coronary artery disease. The success of percutaneous transluminal coronary angioplasty is limited, however, by acute occlusion of the vessel and late stenosis. Stents were developed in response

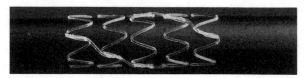

FIGURE 1.—The Igaki-Tamai stent is a premounted, balloon-expandable poly-*l*-lactic acid stent that also has the ability to self-expand. (Courtesy of Tamai H, Igaki K, Kyo E, et al.: Initial and 6-month results of biodegradable poly-*l*-lactic acid coronary stents in humans. *Circulation* 102:399-404, 2000.)

to these issues, and the first clinical use of a metallic stent took place in 1986. Technological advances over the past 13 years have led to the development of new stents. Intravascular stents promise to address the problems of both acute occlusion and late restenosis, but there are many concerns regarding the long-term safety of these stents.

All of the currently available stents are metallic, which means that they induce thrombogenesis to varying degrees, as well as significant intimal hyperplasia. Another potential risk is late thrombosis, particularly after stent implantation followed by brachytherapy. The long-term effects of metallic stents in human coronary arteries are unknown, and these stents can become obstacles to additional treatments. Stents constructed of poly-*l*-lactic acid (PLLA) have recently been developed. PLLA stents are biodegradable and facilitate the local delivery of medication. The feasibility, safety, and efficacy of the PLLA stent were evaluated.

Methods.—Implantation of the PLLA Igaki-Tamai stent for coronary stenoses was performed in 15 patients. The Igaki-Tamai stent is composed of a PLLA monopolymer with a thickness of 0.17 mm and a zigzag helical coil pattern (Fig 1). A balloon-expandable covered sheath system was used in the procedure. The stent self-expanded to its original size with an adequate temperature. A total of 25 stents were implanted successfully in 19 lesions in the 15 patients.

Results.—Angiographic success was achieved in all procedures in all patients, and there were no stent thromboses or major cardiac events in any patient within 30 days. Coronary angiography performed at 1 day, 3 months, and 6 months after the procedure showed both the restenosis rate and target lesion revascularization rate per lesion to be 10.5%. At 6 months, the rates per patient were 6.7%. Intravascular US findings showed no significant stent recoil at 1 day, with stent expansion at follow-up. There were no major cardiac events, with the exception of repeat angioplasty, within 6 months.

Conclusion.—The results of this preliminary experience suggest that the use of coronary PLLA biodegradable stents is feasible, safe, and effective in humans. These findings must be validated with long-term studies of their efficacy.

▶ I have always been concerned about leaving metallic foreign bodies within the vascular system. This certainly includes such devices as vena caval filters and various arterial stents. This remarkable study examines the role of biodegradable stents, specifically studying poly-*l*-lactic acid stents, in patients. A total of 25 stents were successfully implanted in the coronary arteries of 15 patients. Excellent clinical results were achieved, including coronary angiography and intravascular US through 6 months after the procedure. This is the first study to demonstrate the feasibility and safety of coronary biodegradable polymer stents. No major clinical events related to stent implantation occurred in these patients, and the 6-month follow-up showed satisfactory results. These authors conclude, and I believe accurately, that this preliminary experience supports the feasibility, safety, and efficacy of these stents, at least within 6 months. Details of stent resorption cannot be deduced from this study. Unfortunately. I wonder if we will have a bright new future where biodegradable stents are routinely implanted?

Arterial Infection

Detection of *Helicobacter pylori* in Human Carotid Atherosclerotic Plaques
Ameriso SF, Fridman EA, Leiguarda RC, et al (Inst for Neurological Research, Buenos Aires, Argentina)
Stroke 32:385-391, 2001   1–17

Introduction.—Several trials have established a relationship between infectious and inflammatory processes and the occurrence of vascular disease. Transient alterations in coagulation and direct arterial invasion by certain microorganisms have been observed. *Helicobacter pylori* infection is the primary cause of peptic ulcer disease and seems to be a risk factor for ischemic cerebrovascular disease. In contrast to other chronic infectious organisms, *H pylori* has not consistently been isolated from atherosclerotic lesions. The presence of *H pylori* in atherosclerotic plaques was assessed in patients undergoing carotid endarterectomy.

Methods.—The presence of *H pylori* was investigated in 38 atherosclerotic plaques acquired at carotid endarterectomy by morphological and immunohistochemical methods and a sensitive polymerase chain reaction method. Immunohistochemical detection of intercellular adhesion molecule-1, a marker associated with inflammatory cell response, was also undertaken. Seven carotid arteries obtained at autopsy from research subjects without carotid atherosclerosis were also evaluated.

Results.—*H pylori* DNA was detected in 20 of the 38 atherosclerotic plaques. Ten of the *H pylori* DNA-positive plaques also showed morphological and immunohistochemical evidence of *H pylori* infection. None of the 7 normal carotid arteries was *H pylori*-positive. Intercellular adhesion molecule-1 was expressed in 75% and 22%, respectively, of *H pylori*-positive and *H pylori*-negative plaques. The presence of the microorganism was correlated with male gender and was independent of age, vascular risk factor profile, and prior neurologic symptoms.

Conclusion.—*H pylori* is present in many carotid atherosclerotic lesions and is associated with many characteristics of inflammatory cell response.

These data offer additional support for the association between *H pylori* infection and atherosclerotic disease.

▶ In addition to *Chlamydia*, we now have to accept the fact that *H pylori*, or at least *H pylori* DNA, is present in a significant number of atherosclerotic plaques. The viruses that have in general been associated with atherosclerosis include *Chlamydia*, cytomegalovirus, *Helicobacter*, herpes simplex types I and II, and hepatitis A. To me, the critical question remains determining whether these organisms have a causative relationship to the production of the atheromata or whether they are merely fellow travelers settling out in an area of preexisting atherosclerosis. At any rate, to the list of proven organisms in atherosclerotic plaques we need to add *H pylori*.

Detection of Viable *Chlamydia pneumoniae* in Abdominal Aortic Aneurysms

Karlsson L, Gnarpe J, Nääs J, et al (Gävle-Sandviken Central Hosp, Sweden; Karolinska Inst, Stockholm; Univ of Gothenburg, Sweden; et al)
Eur J Vasc Endovasc Surg 19:630-635, 2000   1–18

Background.—It has been suggested that *Chlamydia pneumoniae* might play a role in the complex pathogenesis of abdominal aortic aneurysm (AAA). The presence of *C pneumoniae* in the aortic walls of patients with AAA in comparison with control subjects without cardiovascular disease was investigated.

Methods.—The study comprised 2 groups consisting of 26 consecutive patients undergoing surgical repair of AAA and 17 autopsy control subjects without a history of cardiovascular disease. Evidence of *C pneumoniae* was determined by immunohistochemistry and culture. In addition, throat swabs from 16 AAA patients underwent a polymerase chain reaction assay for *C pneumoniae*. Serologic analysis by microimmunofluorescence was performed in 24 of the patients and in a group of 178 men, aged 70 years.

Results.—Specimens from 20 (77%) of 26 AAA patients tested positive for *C pneumoniae* by immunohistochemistry. Ten of these 20 patients were also culture positive for *C pneumoniae*. In contrast, only 1 (6%) of 17 control subjects had a positive immunohistochemistry result. Five (36%) of 14 patients had a positive result on polymerase chain reaction. The serologic studies found higher titers of *C pneumoniae*-specific antibodies in AAA patients than in the control group.

Conclusions.—This study finds viable *C pneumoniae* in the majority of surgical specimens from patients with AAA. Although further study is needed, the findings support the possible involvement of this organism in the pathogenesis of AAA.

▶ While 80% of aortic samples were positive for *Chlamydia* by immunohistochemical methods, a remarkable 40% were actually culture positive. A fascinating speculation is that one or more of the organisms detected in aneurysm tissue may actually induce enhanced biochemical activity in a number of elements, including perhaps elastase and matrix metalloproteinase, which may in turn be the agents proximally responsible for aneurysm formation. (See also the comments in Abstract 1–17). Clearly, at the present time, we have recognized an impressive presence of infectious organisms within atherosclerotic lesions, as well as within AAA. The more difficult task, of course, will be to determine whether this is a casual or a random association.

Randomized Secondary Prevention Trial of Azithromycin in Patients With Coronary Artery Disease: Primary Clinical Results of the ACADEMIC Study

Muhlestein JB, Anderson JL, Carlquist JF, et al (Univ of Utah, Salt Lake City)
Circulation 102:1755-1760, 2000   1–19

Background.—There appears to be a pathogenic role for local inflammation in atherosclerotic plaque and systemic inflammation in coronary artery disease (CAD). The stimuli for the inflammatory response are unknown, but they are thought to include modified low density lipoproteins and mechanical and toxic factors. Some researchers have also speculated on the possibility that infectious agents may stimulate vascular inflammation. The cytomegalovirus *Chlamydia pneumoniae* has been identified within atherosclerotic plaque, but whether its role is causal or that of innocent commensal in atherogenesis is unknown. However, the response of peptic ulcer disease to antibiotics directed at *Helicobacter pylori* is a dramatic example of the possibility that chronic diseases thought to be noninfectious may in fact have an infectious component that would be amenable to antibiotic therapy.

In a small preliminary study, a reduction of more than 50% in ischemic events was achieved with the use of azithromycin in seropositive patients with CAD. Azithromycin is effective against *C pneumoniae*. These results were tested in a larger, randomized, double-blind study.

Methods.—A group of 302 patients with CAD who were seropositive to *C pneumoniae* were randomly assigned to either placebo or azithromycin, 500 mg/d for 3 days and then 500 mg/wk for 3 months. The primary clinical end point was a cardiovascular event, including death, resuscitated cardiac arrest, nonfatal infarction, unstable angina, stroke, or unplanned coronary revascularization at 2 years.

Results.—The drug was generally well tolerated. Forty-seven first primary events occurred during the trial, including 9 cardiovascular deaths, 1 resuscitated cardiac arrest, 11 myocardial infarctions, 3 strokes, 4 incidents of unstable angina, and 19 unplanned coronary revascularizations. Of these 47 events, 22 occurred in the azithromycin group and 25 occurred in the placebo group. No significant differences were observed in the primary end point between the two groups.

Conclusion.—The results suggest that there is no association between azithromycin and significant early reductions (50% or more) in ischemic events, as was suggested in an initial report. However, a benefit of 20% to 30%, which is considered clinically worthwhile, is possible, although it may be delayed. These results indicate a need for a larger long-term study.

▶ This study impresses me as a first-effort stab in the dark. I would have been absolutely amazed had this small short-term study showed a positive effect of antibiotics, as assessed by a reduction in clinical ischemic events. The numbers are too small and the time is too short. The fact that this study is negative simply indicates that we are not going to get a free lunch in attempting to evaluate the complex relationship of atherosclerosis and infectious organisms. A proper trial, I suspect, will take years.

Demonstration of an Association Between *Chlamydia pneumoniae* Infection and Venous Thromboembolic Disease
Lozinguez O, Arnaud E, Belec L, et al (Hôpital Broussais, Paris)
Thromb Haemost 83:887-891, 2000   1–20

Objective.—Venous thromboembolic disease (VTE) is linked to a genetic risk factor and may also be associated with *Chlamydia pneumoniae*, which is implicated in atherosclerosis. Circulating antibodies to *C pneumoniae* were measured in 176 patients with VTE and 197 age- and sex-matched healthy control subjects to determine retrospectively whether a link exists between *C pneumoniae* infection and venous thrombosis.

Methods.—Anti-*C pneumoniae* IgG antibodies were collected from venous blood of 176 patients and 197 control subjects. DNA samples from the patients and the control group were analyzed for the factor V arg 506 Gln mutation and the prothrombin gene G 20210 A transition. Rates of *C pneumoniae* seropositivity were compared with incidence of first versus recurrent thrombosis, absence vs presence of associated risk factors, and first thrombosis at age of 40 years or younger.

Results.—The prevalence of the factor V arg 506 Gln mutation was 21.9% in patients and 5.1% in the control group. Factor II G 20210 A mutation was 10.2% and 4.1% in patients and the control group, respectively. IgG titers, specific for *C pneumoniae*, were higher in the patient group than in the control group.

Conclusion.—A serological link apparently exists between *C pneumoniae* and VTE.

▶ Retrospective studies such as this are always difficult to interpret. However, the odds ratio for VTE with increasing IgM anti-Chlamydial antibody titers is most impressive. The mechanistic association between Chlamydial infection and thrombosis induction is purely speculative, with no evidence whatsoever in that area. It is noteworthy that the clinical samples obtained in this case were taken from a thrombosis study in which this Chlamydial antibody determination was assuredly not the endpoint. Thus, by its very definition this study is a post hoc analysis (also known as data dredging) and can really only be used properly as an hypothesis-generating exercise. Nonetheless, it does raise an interesting possibility, which certainly would appear to warrant further clinical investigation.

Chlamydia pneumoniae Activates Nuclear Factor κB and Activator Protein 1 in Human Vascular Smooth Muscle and Induces Cellular Proliferation

Miller SA, Selzman CH, Shames BD, et al (Univ of Colorado, Denver)
J Surg Res 90:76-81, 2000   1–21

Background.—Over the past 2 decades, observational data have strongly suggested an association between *Chlamydia pneumoniae* and atherosclerotic cardiovascular disease. *C pneumoniae* has been detected in coronary, aortic, lower extremity, and carotid atheromatous lesions. However, it is not clear whether *C pneumoniae* is a pathophysiologic mediator of atherogenesis or an "innocent bystander." The mechanistic relationship between *C pneumoniae* and human vascular smooth muscle cell (VSMC) physiology was investigated. The influence of human VSMC infection by *C pneumoniae* on VSMC proliferation and activation of the proinflammatory and proliferative transcription factors nuclear factor κB (NF-κB) and activator protein 1 (AP-1) was also evaluated.

Methods.—*C pneumoniae* was grown and isolated from Hep 2 cells, then introduced into human aortic VSMCs in the presence and absence of azithromycin. Direct cell counting was used in assaying cell proliferation 48 hours after infection. Nuclear extracts were isolated 2 hours after infection, and activation of NF-κB and AP-1 was assessed by electrophoretic mobility shift assay.

Results.—In comparison with control cells, VSMC proliferation and DNA binding activity of both NF-κB and AP-1 were stimulated by *C pneumoniae* infection. Concurrent treatment with azithromycin eliminated VSMC proliferation and DNA binding activity of NF-κB and AP-1.

Conclusions.—Proliferative intracellular signals were activated by VSMC infection with *C pneumoniae*, which also stimulated cell growth. The implication from these findings is that *C pneumoniae* is a pathogenic mediator and thus a potential target for therapy aimed at preventing atherosclerotic disease.

▶ While in this study *Chlamydia* appeared to activate 2 important substances that might facilitate smooth muscle proliferation, it is important to note that this was a highly artificial in vitro culture system, and any relationship between this and the actual organism is mere speculation. This does, however, indicate that *Chlamydia pneumoniae* in cell culture at least has the possibility to activate substances that may in turn stimulate smooth muscle proliferation, an essential component of the early lesion in atherosclerosis, as far as we know. This is at least a glimmer of possible insight into the molecular mechanisms of these intralesional infectious agents. As noted repeatedly, we have a desperate need to determine whether the infectious organisms so frequently found in atherosclerotic lesions are causative or fellow travelers.

Coagulation

Venous Thrombotic Risk in Family Members of Unselected Individuals With Factor V Leiden

Lensen RPM, Bertina RM, de Ronde H, et al (Leiden Univ, The Netherlands)
Thromb Haemost 83:817-821, 2000   1–22

Introduction.—The factor V Leiden mutation (FVL) produces a 7-fold increased risk of venous thromboembolism (VTE). In thrombophiliac families, 25% of carriers encounter thrombosis before the age of 40 years. The correlation between FVL and VTE in first-degree family members of unselected symptomatic and asymptomatic carriers of FVL was assessed.

Methods.—Of 56 probands with FVL, 233 eligible first-degree family members (91%) were evaluated. Risk factor status and carrier status was assessed. Participants were tested for the FVL mutation. Incidence rates were determined for both those who were symptomatic and those who were asymptomatic.

Results.—The annual incidence rate of VTE for both symptomatic and asymptomatic affected propositi was 0.34% (18 events in 5294 person-years). For noncarriers, the annual incidence rate was 0.10% (5 events in 5090 person-years). The overall risk ratio for venous thrombus, both deep

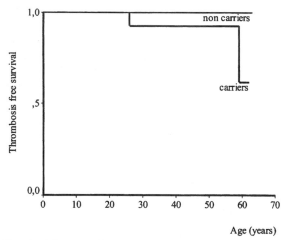

FIGURE 1.—Thrombosis free survival curves in carriers (*lower line,* probandi excluded) and noncarriers (*upper line*) among relatives of asymptomatic propositi. (Courtesy of Lensen RPM, Bertina RM, de Ronde H, et al: Venous thrombotic risk in family members of unselected individuals with factor V Leiden. *Thromb Haemost* 83:817-821, 2000.)

thrombosis and superficial thrombophlebitis, in carriers versus noncarriers was 3.4%. Kaplan-Meier analysis in relatives of symptomatic propositi revealed that at the age of 58 years, thrombosis-free survival rates were significantly decreased to 75% in carriers and 93% in noncarriers (Fig 1). Carriers of FVL had a 3 times greater thrombotic risk, compared with noncarriers. Combined with environmental risk factors, FVL adds to the risk of VTE. The thrombotic incidence rate in unselected relatives with FVL is notably less than what was observed in carriers in thrombophilic families (1.7%/y).

Conclusion.—Patients with a positive family history of venous thromboembolism who are at risk need to be observed closely.

▶ Factor V mutation is present in about 5% of healthy white persons, and has been observed in up to 20% of unselected consecutive patients with deep vein thrombosis. Physicians are constantly questioned about the optimal prophylactic policy both for patients and the relatives of patients. This interesting study examined a significant number of relatives of patients with FVL who suffered venous thrombosis. Carriers of FVL had a 3 times higher thrombotic risk compared with noncarriers. These authors suggest, and I do believe reasonably, that the actual occurrence of venous thrombosis is a multifactorial disease, but in this milieu, FVL mutation may have a significant role. This, however, does appear to justify a policy of anticoagulation treatment for carriers only during exposure to conditions known to cause venous thrombosis, such as postsurgical.

Increased Lipoprotein (a) Levels as an Independent Risk Factor for Venous Thromboembolism
von Depka M, Nowak-Göttl U, Eisert R, et al (Hannover Med School, Germany; Wilhelms-Univ, Münster, Germany; Univ Hosp Frankfurt, Germany)
Blood 96:3364-3368, 2000   1–23

Objective.—A high serum lipoprotein (a) (Lp[a]) level is a risk factor for coronary heart disease, ischemic cerebrovascular disease, and chronic thromboembolic pulmonary hypertension. Not much is known about the part that Lp(a) plays in the development of venous thromboembolism (VTE). Lp(a) was evaluated as a single defect and in combination with established prothrombotic abnormalities of blood coagulation factors in patients with VTE, and its impact on clinical manifestation of VTE was assessed.

Methods.—Serum-activated protein C resistance, protein C, protein S, Lp(a) and antithrombin deficiency were determined in 685 consecutive VTE patients (60.4% women), aged 11 to 77 years, and in 266 healthy age- and sex-matched white control subjects. Blood samples were collected at least 3 months after the last acute thrombotic event. The FV G1691A mutation, prothrombin (PT) G20210A variant, and the MTHFR C677T variant were determined using DNA-based assays.

Results.—Lp(a) levels were significantly higher in patients than in control subjects (21.6 mg/dL vs 11.9 mg/dL). Elevated Lp(a) levels higher than 30mg/dL were found in 135 patients (20%) and 19 control subjects (7%). The odds ratio (OR) of VTE in patients with elevated Lp(a) levels was 3.2. Women using oral contraceptives had a 4.0 OR, similar to that of patients with several exogenous risk factors. Patients with recurrent VTE had a 2.9 OR, significantly higher than that of control subjects. The prevalence of the PT G20210A gene was significantly higher in patients than in control subjects (45 vs 6). Elevated Lp(a) and FV G1691A were found in 49 patients (7%) but only 2 control subjects (0.8%). According to multivariate analysis, Lp(a) higher than 30 mg/dL, presence of the FV G1691A mutation, and of the PT G20210A mutation were independent risk factors for VTE. VTE risk was also increased for Lp(a) levels higher than 20 mg/dL (OR, 2.0) and for Lp(a) of more than 10 mg/dL (OR, 1.5).

Conclusion.—Elevated serum or plasma Lp(a) levels significantly increased the risk for VTE especially in the presence of the gene mutation FV G1691A or other exogenous risks.

▶ Apolipoprotein (a) is the major protein component of Lp(a) and has a high structural homology to plasminogen. Consequently, investigators have speculated that Lp(a) competes with plasminogen for fibrin binding and at high serum concentrations leads to impaired fibrinolysis. Current clinical evidence suggests that Lp(a) is an independent risk factor for atherosclerotic vascular disease, including coronary artery disease and stroke, but its role as a risk factor for VTE has not been well defined.

This report demonstrates that factor V Leiden or resistance to activated protein C is the most common risk factor for VTE, but the presence of an elevated Lp(a) is a close second. Further, while the risk was greatest at Lp(a) levels greater than 30 mg/dL, some risk was noted even at levels greater than 10 mg/dL. While having this information before an operative procedure would certainly identify those patients at increased risk for VTE, it remains uncertain how best to use this information after the fact. I would certainly consider long-term coumadin therapy for patients with a history of VTE and persistently elevated Lp(a), but more guidance on this matter would be helpful.

E. L. Chaikof, MD

Argatroban Anticoagulant Therapy in Patients With Heparin-Induced Thrombocytopenia
Lewis BE, for the ARG-911 Study Investigators (Loyola Univ, Maywood, Ill; et al)
Circulation 103:1838-1843, 2001   1–24

Objective.—Heparin-induced thrombocytopenia (HIT) can result in thrombotic events. More than half of patients with HIT risk having thrombosis develop. Argatroban, a direct thrombin inhibitor, may be of

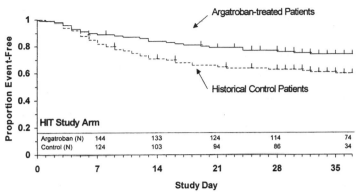

FIGURE 1.—Time to first event for composite end point: heparin-induced thrombocytopenia study arm. Data are presented for argatroban-treated patients (*solid line*; 160 patients, 119 censored) and historical control subjects (*dashed line*; 147 patients, 90 censored) ($P = 0.10$; hazard ratio = 0.60; 95% confidence interval, 0.40-0.89), with *tick marks* indicating days that patients were censored. Number of patients at risk is presented for days 7, 14, 21, 28, and 37. (Courtesy of Lewis BE, for the ARG-911 Study Investigators: Argatroban anticoagulant therapy in patients with heparin-induced thrombocytopenia. *Circulation* 103:1838-1843, 2001.)

use in patients with HIT. The efficacy and safety of argatroban as an anticoagulant was prospectively evaluated in a multicenter, nonrandomized, open-label, historically-controlled trial of patients with HIT or HIT with thrombosis syndrome (HITTS).

Methods.—Patients, aged 18 to 80 years, with HIT (160 patients) or HITTS (144 patients) were treated with escalating IV argatroban (2-10 µg/kg/min) to maintain an activated partial thromboplastin time (aPTT) at 1.5 to 3.0 times the baseline aPTT value. The aPTT was measured daily and 2 hours after each dosage escalation. Patients were treated until their condition resolved, anticoagulation was established with another agent, or treatment had been provided for 14 days. Patients were followed up for 30 days after therapy ended. Results were compared with those of historical controls with HIT (147 patients) or HITTS (46 patients). Outcome measures included the primary efficacy end point: all-cause mortality, all-cause amputation, or new thrombosis.

Results.—The incidence of composite end point was significantly reduced in argatroban-treated patients with HIT compared with historical controls (25.6% vs 38.8%) (Fig 1). The respective composite end point incidences for patients with HITTS and historical controls were 43.8% versus 56.5%. The differences were significant in both comparisons. Both groups of argatroban-treated patients had significantly reduced death rates from thrombosis compared with the historical control group. Amputation incidence was similar for both groups. Thrombocytopenia was resolved in at least 69% of argatroban patients compared with less than 50% of historical controls. Argatroban achieved adequate anticoagulation in 83% of patients with HIT and 94% of patients with HITTS. The incidence of major bleeding was similar for both argatroban patients and historical controls. Diarrhea (11%) and pain (9%) were the most common adverse events in the argatroban group.

Conclusion.—Argatroban anticoagulation therapy is safe and effective for patients with HIT and HITTS.

▶ The authors address a complication, dreaded by all vascular surgeons. HIT is associated with significant morbidity and mortality and has not been well controlled by conventional therapy. The authors demonstrate better results with heparin discontinuation and treatment with argatroban compared with results for historical controls. The authors state that "Control subjects were treated according to the local standard of practice at the time of HIT diagnosis, with typical treatments being heparin discontinuation and/or oral anticoagulation." This is very promising for patients with HIT. However, more studies will need to be done with better controls to more clearly assess the advantages of the different treatment modalities, which include not only argatroban but also coumadin, ancrod, low molecular weight heparin, danaparoid, and recombinant hirudin (Lepirudin).

M. A. Golden, MD

Orally Administered Unfractionated Heparin With Carrier Agent Is Therapeutic for Deep Venous Thrombosis
Gonze MD, Salartash K, Sternbergh WC III, et al (Ochsner Med Institutions, New Orleans, La; Emisphere Technologies, Tarrytown, NY)
Circulation 101:2658-2661, 2000   1–25

Background.—Deep vein thrombosis (DVT) is a significant cause of morbidity and mortality in hospitalized patients. Traditional treatment of DVT utilizes initial therapy with continuous IV (unfractionated) heparin. However, long-term use of continuous IV heparin is not practical, so long-term treatment involves oral agents such as warfarin. Individual response to warfarin treatment varies among patients, unfortunately, so the dosage must be monitored closely during treatment. Orally administered heparin (OHEP) would offer several advantages over warfarin therapy: heparin has no teratogenic effects, and its short half-life (less than 4 hours) allows reversal of anticoagulation should it become necessary. In addition, the pain that is associated with IV or subcutaneous administration could be avoided.

Outpatient treatment of DVT would be facilitated by OHEP. Unfortunately, the poor absorption of OHEP makes it unreliable. An amido acid, sodium-N-(8[2-hydroxybenzoyl]amino) caprylate (SNAC) has been found to facilitate the gastrointestinal absorption of heparin. The effectiveness of OHEP combined with SNAC was evaluated in the treatment of DVT.

Methods.—In 54 male Sprague-Dawley rats, an internal jugular DVT was produced. The animals were randomly assigned to 1 of 6 different groups for 7 days of treatment: untreated control, subcutaneous heparin, SNAC only, OHEP only, low molecular weight heparin, and OHEP/

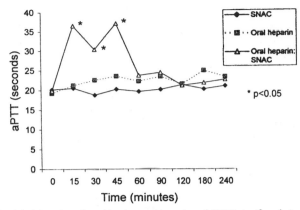

FIGURE 3.—Administration of combination oral heparin and SNAC significantly increased activated partial thromboplastin time (*aPTT*) levels, whereas SNAC alone or oral heparin alone caused no significant changes in aPTT. (Courtesy of Gonze MD, Salartash K, Sternbergh WC III, et al.: Orally administered unfractionated heparin with carrier agent is therapeutic for deep venous thrombosis. *Circulation* 101:2658-2661, 2000.)

SNAC. Levels of activated partial thromboplastin time and anti–factor X were measured.

Results.—After 1 week of treatment, the incidence of residual DVT in the control group was 100%, compared with 10% in the OHEP/SNAC group and 10% in the low molecular weight group. A significant reduction in clot weights was also seen in these groups. There were no significant differences in residual DVT between the SNAC-only or subcutaneous heparin groups compared with the control groups. The activated partial thromboplastin time levels in the OHEP/SNAC group peaked at 30 minutes and were significantly higher than in all other groups (Fig 3). In the OHEP/SNAC group, anti–factor X levels were elevated at 15 minutes after dosing and continued to be significantly elevated at 4 hours.

Conclusion.—Combination OHEP/SNAC was as effective as low molecular weight heparin in resolution of the clot and reduction of clot weight in this rat model. OHEP combined with a novel carrier agent, SNAC, was a successful treatment for DVT.

▶ Conventional therapy of deep vein thrombosis has involved continuous IV unfractionated heparin, followed by warfarin, as the long-term IV administration of heparin is not practical. Oral heparin would have a distinct advantage over warfarin and would certainly be more convenient than low molecular weight heparin. In recent years, an amino acid compound named SNAC has been detected that facilitates the gastrointestinal absorption of heparin. Investigators have shown previously in the rat model that this oral heparin-SNAC combination appeared to reduce the incidence of DVT in the rat model. In this study, the investigators examined the potential role of oral heparin-SNAC in facilitating the resolution of an established venous thrombosis. While the substance appeared to be as effective as IV heparin, it is a bit of a stretch to equate subcutaneous thrombus resolution in a rat model with clinical benefit. Nonetheless, they may well be onto something and perhaps in the next few years, we are going to actually have an oral heparin preparation. Perhaps with only a little extra work we can have an oral low molecular weight heparin preparation. I suspect, on balance, we shall hear a great deal more about this in the future.

Incidence of Cancer After Prophylaxis With Warfarin Against Recurrent Venous Thromboembolism
Schulman S, for the Duration of Anticoagulation Trial (Karolinska Hosp, Stockholm)
N Engl J Med 342:1953-1958, 2000   1–26

Introduction.—The risk of subsequent cancer may be higher among patients with idiopathic deep-vein thrombosis, compared to those with an identified triggering factor. The length of time after a thromboembolic event during which the incidence of cancer is increased was investigated in a retrospective analysis of prospectively collected information.

Methods.—The study included patients who had a first episode of venous thromboembolism and were randomly assigned to either 6 weeks or 6 months of treatment with oral anticoagulation. These patients were questioned annually about any newly diagnosed cancer. In this cohort, the Swedish Cancer Registry was used to identify all persons diagnosed with cancer and their causes of death. The observed number of patients with cancer were compared with the numbers expected on the basis of national incidence rates. Standardized incidence ratios were determined.

Results.—During follow-up, 111 of 854 (13.0%) patients evaluated were diagnosed with first cancer. The standardized incidence ratio for newly diagnosed cancer was 3.4 during the first year after the thromboembolic event and remained between 1.3 and 2.2 for the next 5 years. The rate of cancer diagnosis was 15.8% (66/149) for patients treated with oral anticoagulants for 6 weeks, compared with 10.3% (45/435) for patients treated for 6 months (odds ratio 1.6). The difference was primarily caused by the occurrence of new urogenital cancers, of which there were 28 (6.7%) and 12 (2.8%) patients in the 6-week and 6-month groups, respectively (odds ratio, 2.5). The between-group difference in the rate of cancer became obvious only after 2 years of follow-up and remained significant after adjusting for gender, age, and whether the thromboembolism was idiopathic or nonidiopathic (Fig 2). Older age at the time of the venous thrombosis and an idiopathic thromboembolism were independent risk factors for the diagnosis of cancer. No difference in the rate of cancer-related deaths was observed.

Conclusion.—The risk of newly diagnosed cancer after a first episode of venous thromboembolism was increased during at least 2 years of follow-up. The risk appeared to be lower among patients treated for 6 months versus those treated for 6 weeks.

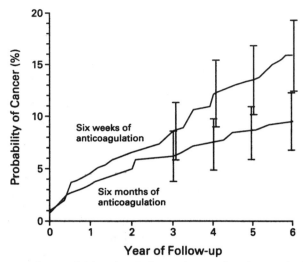

FIGURE 2.—Cumulative probability of newly diagnosed cancer after a first episode of venous thromboembolism. *I bars* represent 95% CI. (Courtesy of Schulman S, for the Duration of Anticoagulation Trial. N *Engl J Med* 342:1953-1958, 2000. Reprinted by permission of *The New England Journal of Medicine*, copyright 2000, Massachusetts Medical Society. All rights reserved.)

▶ The relationship between cancer and venous thromboembolism (VTE) is real, but of uncertain significance. The incidence of cancer is certainly increased during the first year after the diagnosis of VTE, and it may be increased to some extent for at least 10 years. Cancer appears more likely in patients who have idiopathic deep vein thrombosis than among those with an identified triggering factor. The interesting study reported here randomly assigned patients with newly diagnosed VTE to receive treatment with vitamin K antagonist for 6 weeks or 6 months, and the incidence of newly diagnosed cancer was determined. At a mean follow-up of 8.1 years, 13% of patients had a first diagnosis of cancer, including 15.8% among patients treated with 6 weeks of warfarin and 10.3% in those treated for 6 months. The conclusions of this fascinating epidemiologic study are that the risk of newly diagnosed cancer after a first episode of VTE is elevated during at least the next 2 years, and appears to be lower among patients treated with oral anticoagulants for 6 months compared with those treated for 6 weeks. This is absolutely fascinating information. While a biochemical explanation for the association is not forthcoming as yet, the association itself appears to be well established.

High Plasma Levels of Factor VIII and the Risk of Recurrent Venous Thromboembolism

Kyrle PA, Minar E, Hirschl M, et al (Vienna Univ; Hanuschkrankenhaus, Vienna; Wilhelminenspital, Vienna)
N Engl J Med 343:457-462, 2000   1–27

Background.—Elevated plasma levels of factor VIII have been found to be associated with an increased risk of venous thrombosis. Studies have confirmed a significantly higher risk of venous thrombosis among patients with plasma levels of factor VIII above 150 IU/dL. Among patients with venous thrombosis, elevated factor VIII has a prevalence of about 20%. Prevention of recurrent venous thrombosis can be accomplished by the use of prophylactic oral antibiotics, but severe or fatal bleeding can result from the use of these drugs. The optimal duration of prophylaxis depends on the balancing of the risk of recurrent thrombosis after discontinuation of therapy against the risk of hemorrhage. The risk of recurrence of thrombosis after an initial episode of spontaneous venous thromboembolism was investigated in patients with high plasma levels of factor VIII.

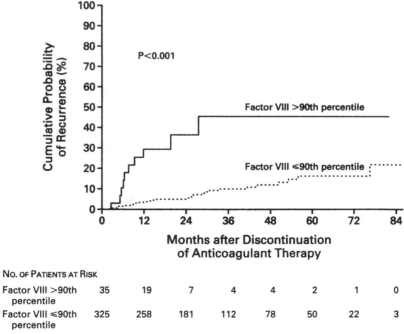

No. of Patients at Risk								
Factor VIII >90th percentile	35	19	7	4	4	2	1	0
Factor VIII ≤90th percentile	325	258	181	112	78	50	22	3

FIGURE 1.—Kaplan-Meier estimates of the risk of recurrent venous thromboembolism according to the plasma level of factor VIII. The probability of recurrent thrombosis was greater among patients with factor VIII levels above the 90th percentile than among patients with factor VIII levels at or below the 90th percentile (*P* < .001 by the Wilcoxon test and by the log-rank test). (Reprinted by permission of *The New England Journal of Medicine* from Kyrle PA, Minar E, Hirschl M, et al: High plasma levels of factor VIII and the risk of recurrent venous thromboembolism. *N Engl J Med* 343:457-462, 2000. Copyright 2000, Massachusetts Medical Society. All rights reserved.)

Methods.—The study group comprised 360 patients who were followed up for an average of 30 months after a first episode of venous thromboembolism and discontinuance of oral anticoagulant therapy. The study's end point was defined as symptomatic recurrent venous thromboembolism.

Results.—In 38 of 360 patients (10.6%), recurrent venous thromboembolism developed. Patients who experienced a recurrence had higher mean plasma levels of factor VIII compared with patients who did not experience recurrence (Fig 1). The relative risk of recurrent venous thrombosis was determined to be 1.08 for each 10 IU/dL increase in the plasma level of factor VIII. For patients with a level of factor VIII above the 90th percentile, the likelihood of recurrence was 37% at 2 years; this compares with a likelihood of 5% among patients with lower factor VIII levels. The overall relative risk of recurrence was 6.7 (after adjustment for age, sex, presence or absence of factor V Leiden or the G20210A prothrombin mutation, and duration of oral anticoagulation) for patients with plasma factor VIII levels above the 90th percentile, compared with patients with lower levels.

Conclusion.—There is an increased risk of recurrent venous thromboembolism among patients with a high plasma level of factor VIII.

▶ This study design appears reasonable and purports to determine that a high plasma level of factor VIII represents an increased risk factor for recurrent venous thromboembolism after an initial episode. While I do not doubt the accuracy of their conclusions, I have significant problems with their study design in that only symptomatic recurrent venous thromboses were investigated and detected. It certainly seems to me that screening of the entire at risk population with duplex regardless of symptomatic status would yield a much more creditable number to allow us to appreciate the real incidence of recurrent venous thromboembolism. I suspect in all reality these authors have only scratched the surface, as they confined their study to symptomatic patients only. These authors speculate as to the desirable duration of anticoagulation in venous thromboembolism patients who have elevated levels of factor VIII. They conclude that extended prophylaxis is the better choice presently.

Treatment of Proximal Deep Vein Thrombosis With a Novel Synthetic Compound (SR90107A/ORG31540) With Pure Anti-Factor Xa Activity: A Phase II Evaluation
Büller HR, for The Rembrandt Investigators (Academic Med Centre, Amsterdam; et al)
Circulation 102:2726-2731, 2000   1–28

Background.—An immediate-acting anticoagulant is needed in the treatment of patients with venous thromboembolism. Currently, unfractionated heparin or low–molecular-weight heparin is used, and there is definitive evidence of their effectiveness. A new synthetic compound,

SR90107a/ORG31540, has been found to have the potential to be effective not only in preventing thrombus extension but also in the treatment of venous thromboembolism. Unlike heparin, the factor Xa inhibitor has shown no cross-reactivity with antibodies associated with heparin-induced thrombocytopenia. The results of a phase II trial of this synthetic agent were reported.

Methods.—The efficacy and safety of SR90107a/ORG31540 at 5, 7.5, and 10 mg once daily were assessed in a randomized, parallel-group phase II trial in relation to low–molecular-weight heparin (dalteparin, 100 IU/kg twice daily) in the treatment of symptomatic proximal deep vein thrombosis. Change in thrombus mass was the primary outcome measure and was assessed by US of the leg veins and perfusion lung scintigraphy performed at baseline and again at day 7 ± 1. A positive outcome was determined to be improvement in the result of a US or perfusion scan without deterioration of either test. Other outcome measures assessed were symptomatic, recurrent venous thromboembolism and major bleeding for a period of 3 months. The observer was unaware of the treatment allocation of the patient during interpretation of all outcomes.

Results.—In patients given SR90107a/ORG31540, positive primary outcomes were observed in 46% of patients given 5 mg, 48% of patients given 7.5 mg, and 42% of patients given 10 mg of the compound, compared with a positive outcome in 49% of patients given dalteparin. In the 334 patients treated with SR90107a/ORG31540, there were 8 recurrent thromboembolic complications (2.4%), compared with 6 such complications among the 119 (5%) patients who received dalteparin. The incidence of bleeding was low and similar for both groups.

Conclusion.—SR90107a/ORG31540, a novel factor Xa inhibitor, appear to be safe and effective in the treatment of deep venous thrombosis across a wide range of doses. Phase III studies are recommended for this synthetic compound.

▶ Synthetic pentasaccharide antifactor Xa compounds represent a new class of anticoagulant drugs. They have already been shown in 4 major prospective randomized trials to be as, or more effective, than low molecular weight heparins in the prevention of deep venous thrombosis and pulmonary embolism in patients undergoing lower extremity orthopedic procedures. The 18-hour half-life of the compound tested in this study, along with its lack of cross reactivity with antibodies associated with heparin-induced thrombocytopenia make it potentially a very attractive anticoagulant. These advantages, along with its apparent efficacy, could lead to the replacement by pentasaccharides of low molecular weight heparins as the drug of choice in both the prevention and treatment of deep venous thrombosis.

G. L. Moneta, MD

Safety of Withholding Heparin in Pregnant Women With a History of Venous Thromboembolism

Ginsberg JS, for the Recurrence of Clot in This Pregnancy Study Group (McMaster Univ, Hamilton, Ont, Canada; Monash Med Ctr, Clayton, Australia; Sunnybrook Health Science Centre, Toronto; et al)
N Engl J Med 343:1439-1444, 2000   1–29

Background.—The risk of pregnancy-related venous thromboembolism (VTE) appears to be increased among women with a past history of such events. There is ongoing debate about whether these women should continue to receive heparin during the antepartum period. The situation is complicated by the lack of accurate data on the risk of recurrent thromboembolism in women not receiving heparin. The safety of withholding heparin during the antepartum period for women with a history of VTE was assessed prospectively.

Methods.—The multicenter, prospective cohort study included 125 consecutive pregnant women with one previous episode of VTE. During the antepartum period, heparin therapy was withheld. Anticoagulant therapy was then resumed, continuing through 4 to 6 weeks postpartum. The rate of recurrent VTE during the antepartum period was analyzed. In addition, 95 patients underwent laboratory studies to assess the incidence of thrombophilia.

Results.—Three women had recurrent VTE during the antepartum period, an incidence of 2.4%. No recurrences developed in a subgroup of 44 patients who had no evidence of thrombophilia and whose previous thrombotic episode was related to a temporary risk factor. Abnormal laboratory results, a previous episode of idiopathic thrombosis, or both were present in 51 women. For this group, the incidence of antepartum recurrence of venous thromboembolism was 5.9%.

Conclusions.—Pregnant women with a single previous episode of VTE are at low risk of recurrent episodes during the antepartum period. Antepartum heparin therapy does not appear to be indicated on a routine basis for such patients. Postpartum anticoagulant therapy is still recommended.

▶ It is widely accepted that a prior episode of venous thromboembolism (VTE) is a risk factor for a recurrent episode. The role of heparin prophylaxis during pregnancy in women who have had a prior episode of VTE is controversial. These authors conclude that women with a prior episode of VTE who do not have identified thrombophilia and who did have a temporary risk factor with the prior episode do not require any anticoagulation. Women who either have thrombophilia or did not have a temporary risk factor during a prior episode may be given a choice of antepartum heparin, but even in them it does not appear essential.

Effects of Fixed Low-Dose Warfarin, Aspirin-Warfarin Combination Therapy, and Dose-adjusted Warfarin on Thrombogenesis in Chronic Atrial Fibrillation

Li-Saw-Hee FL, Blann AD, Lip GYH (City Hosp, Birmingham, England)
Stroke 31:828-833, 2000   1–30

Introduction.—Clinical trials have shown that for patients with nonvalvular atrial fibrillation (AF), adjustment of warfarin dosage to achieve an international normalized ratio of 2:3 reduces the risk of ischemic stroke. However, anticoagulation is associated with bleeding and other complications, and the need for frequent monitoring adds to expense and inconvenience. A strategy of fixed low-dose warfarin, alone or in combination with aspirin, was evaluated for its effects on hemostatic markers.

Methods.—The prospective randomized trial included 61 patients with AF (44 men and 17 women; mean age, 64 years) who had received no previous antithrombotic therapy. They were assigned to one of 3 groups. Patients in group 1 received warfarin, 2 mg; those in group 2 received warfarin, 1 mg, plus aspirin, 300 mg; and those in group 3 received warfarin, 2 mg, plus aspirin, 300 mg. The 3 groups were similar in terms of age, sex, and blood pressure. Hemostatic markers, including plasma fibrin D-dimer, plasminogen activator inhibitor-1 (PAI-1), fibrinogen, and von Willebrand factor (vWF), were measured at baseline and at 2 and 8 weeks after randomization. In a second phase, the same measurements were repeated after 6 weeks of adjusted-dose warfarin.

Results.—Compared with healthy control subjects, the patients with AF had significantly elevated levels of fibrinogen, vWF, and fibrin D-dimer at baseline. The PAI-1 level increased significantly during treatment; this was the only significant change in the first phase of the study. In the second phase, 6 weeks of adjusted-dose warfarin yielded significant reductions in

TABLE 5.—Effect of Dose-Adjusted Warfarin (Achieving Target INR of 2.0-3.0) on Hemostatic Markers in Patients With Chronic AF

	Before Treatment	INR 2.0-3.0	P
Fibrinogen, g/L	2.9±0.9	2.4±0.7	0.023
von Willebrand factor, IU/dL	143±37	134±34	0.33
Plasminogen activator inhibitor-1, IU/dL	6.3 (3.9-10.4)	7.4 (5.9-14.5)	0.198
Fibrin D-dimer, ng/mL	212 (98-515)	130 (61-175)	0.0067
INR	1.05 (1.125)	2.48 (2.1-2.7)	<0.00001

Data are mean ± SD (analyzed with paired *t* test) for fibrinogen and von Willebrand factor; median (interquartile range) (analyzed with paired Wilcoxon test) is given for plasminogen activator inhibitor-1, fibrin D-dimer, and INR.

Abbreviations: INR, International normalized ratio; AF, atrial fibrillation.

(Courtesy of Li-Saw-Hee FL, Biann AD, Lip GYH: Effects of fixed low-dose warfarin, aspirin-warfarin combination therapy, and dose-adjusted warfarin on thrombogenesis in chronic atrial fibrillation. *Stroke* 31:828-833. Copyright 2000, American Heart Association. Reproduced with permission.)

plasma fibrinogen and fibrin D-dimer levels, with no change in PAI-1 or vWF levels (Table 5).

Conclusions.—Patients with AF have elevated levels of vWF, fibrinogen, and fibrin D-dimer, compared with controls. Low-dose warfarin, with or without aspirin, does not significantly reduce any of these markers. However, full adjusted-dose warfarin produces significant reductions in fibrin D-dimer and fibrinogen. As in previous trials, low-dose warfarin and aspirin-warfarin combinations do not compare well with conventional, adjusted-dose warfarin therapy.

▶ I suppose on occasion it is of modest value to confirm what everyone already knew. These authors remarkably conclude that adjusted dose warfarin with an international normalized ratio between 2 and 3 is highly effective in the treatment of patients with nonvalvular chronic atrial fibrillation. Ultra low-dose warfarin with or without aspirin appears ineffectual, at least as assessed by a variety of substances in the blood associated with clotting, such as D-dimer and vWF factor. It appears to me the authors worked very hard to develop a straw man that they could subsequently destroy with great gusto. For repeating what everyone already knew, I hereby convey to these authors an Honorable Mention Camel Dung Award. A similar award goes to the editors of *Stroke* for their willingness to republish what everyone already knew.

Low Molecular Weight Heparin (Enoxaparin) in the Management of Unstable Angina: The ESSENCE Study

Fox KAA, on behalf of the ESSENCE Study Investigators (Univ of Edinburgh, Scotland)
Heart 82:I12-I14, 1999   1–31

Introduction.—The current standard treatment of patients with acute coronary syndromes includes a combination of oral aspirin and intravenous unfractionated heparin (UFH). This regimen does not prevent further ischemic events in many patients. Low molecular weight heparins (LMWHs) have advantages over UFH that may provide greater efficiency and safety, together with the additional advantages of subcutaneous administration and a predictable anticoagulant effect that eliminates the need for activated partial thromboplastin time (aPTT) monitoring. LMWHs also reduce binding to plasma proteins, give greater resistance to inhibition by platelet factor IV, and provide a longer plasma half life than UFH. The ESSENCE trial was a double-blind, prospective, randomized trial of 3171 patients from 176 centers. It compared the safety and efficacy of an LMWH drug enoxaparin with UFH in patients with unstable angina and non-Q-wave myocardial infarction (MI).

Methods.—Patients were randomly assigned to treatment with either enoxaparin 1 mg/kg subcutaneously every 12 hours plus placebo and bolus infusion or UFH (bolus and infusion, dose-adjusted according to

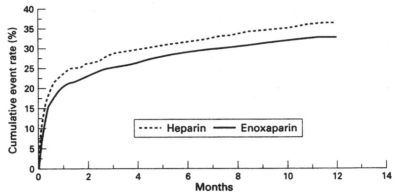

FIGURE 2.—Cumulative event rates for triple end point for enoxaparin and unfractionated heparin at one year follow-up. (Courtesy of Fox KAA, on behalf of the ESSENCE Study Investigators: Low molecular weight heparin (enoxaparin) in the management of unstable angina: The ESSENCE study. *Heart* 82:112-114, 1999, with permission from the BMJ Publishing Group.)

aPTT) and subcutaneous placebo injections. Patients received anticoagulant treatment for a minimum of 48 hours and a maximum of 8 days. Oral aspirin was administered to all patients. The major end point was a composite of the incidence of death, MI, or recurrent angina at 14 days. Secondary end points were the incidence of the same composite end points at 30 days and 1 year.

Results.—Ninety-eight percent of patients received at least 1 dose of study drugs. Mean duration of treatment was 2.6 days in both groups. At 48 hours, a relative risk reduction of 16% was noted that was sustained at 14 and 30 days in patients treated with enoxaparin. The difference in the 2 treatment arms was highly significant at the 14- and 30-day time points. The risk reduction was spread evenly across all individual end points. For the triple end point, the relative difference between enoxaparin and UFH

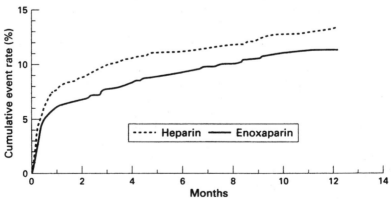

FIGURE 3.—Cumulative event rates for double end point of death or myocardial infarction for enoxaparin and unfractionated heparin at one year follow-up. (Courtesy of Fox KAA, on behalf of the ESSENCE Study Investigators: Low molecular weight heparin (enoxaparin) in the management of unstable angina: The ESSENCE study. *Heart* 82:112-114, 1999, with permission from the BMJ Publishing Group.)

observed at 30 days (19.8% vs 23.3%) was significantly maintained at 1 year (32% vs 35.7%, respectively) (Fig 2). For the double end point of death or MI, the between-group difference at 30 days (6.2% vs 7.7%) was fully maintained at 1 year (11.5% vs 13.5%) (Fig 3). This difference was not significant, but it meant there were about 20 patients per 1000 less who experienced death or MI in the enoxaparin treatment arm.

Conclusion.—The ESSENCE trial is the first large-scale investigation to demonstrate that short-term treatment with an LMWH provides long-term benefits for patients with acute coronary syndromes. For patients with unstable angina or non-Q wave infarction judged to be at increased risk of further events, the recommended treatment may include subcutaneous LMWH in preference to UFH.

▶ Many believe that LMWHs are merely a more convenient dosage administration form of heparin. In fact, LMWH and UFH are really different drugs. LMWHs are more effective than UFH in the prevention and treatment of acute deep venous thrombosis. In this study, it appears that LMWH also offers advantages over UFH in terms of both long-term benefits, as well as short-term benefits in patients with acute coronary syndromes. It is truly progress when a safer and easier to use drug offers real advantage over traditional therapies.

G. L. Moneta, MD

External Pneumatic Compression and Fibrinolysis in Abdominal Surgery

Cahan MA, Hanna DJ, Wiley LA, et al (Univ of Maryland, Baltimore; Univ of Texas, Galveston)
J Vasc Surg 32:537-543, 2000   1–32

Objective.—External pneumatic compression (EPC) prevents deep vein thrombosis (DVT) by reducing lower-extremity venous stasis. EPC may also enhance endogenous fibrinolysis. Whether EPC improves fibrolytic activity or prevents postoperative shutdown was investigated in a randomized study of individuals undergoing major intra-abdominal surgical procedures.

Methods.—The study included 48 patients (1 female; mean age, 67 years) undergoing 12 aortic reconstructions, 24 resections for malignancy, and 12 miscellaneous laparotomies, who were randomly allocated to receive either subcutaneous heparin injections (HEP group, 5000 U twice daily), a thigh-length sequential pneumatic compression device (EPC group), or both (HEP + EPC group). Those with preexisting venous disease were excluded from the study. Antecubital venous blood samples were drawn to measure systemic fibrinolytic activity the day before surgery, after induction of anesthesia, and on postoperative days 1, 3, and 5. Plasminogen activator inhibitor-1 (PAI-1) and tissue plasminogen activator (t-PA) activity levels were measured at each time point. Values were compared with those of age- and sex-matched control subjects.

Results.—The mean t-PA activity was unchanged in all groups during the study, but the mean PAI-1 levels were increased in all treatment groups compared with levels found in the control group. The mean PAI-1 activity increased after induction of anesthesia and on postoperative days 1 (28.5 AU/mL) and 3 (25.1 AU/mL) in the HEP group, and returned to baseline levels by day 5. PAI-1 increased insignificantly in the EPC group after surgery. PAI-1 increased significantly in the HEP + EPC group on postoperative day 1 and returned to baseline levels on day 3. There were no significant differences in PAI-1 activity decreases in the EPC groups compared with the HEP group at any specified point. Patients with cancer had a significantly lower mean preoperative t-PA activity level (1.1 IU/mL) than patients without cancer. The mean preoperative PAI-1 level was 20.6 AU/mL in patients without cancer.

Conclusion.—PAI-1 activity increased in patients after abdominal surgery. Because EPC did not improve postoperative systemic fibrinolysis, these devices do not appear to be effective as prophylactic treatment for DVT unless prevention involves a reduction of stasis.

▶ I am sorry to note that external pneumatic compression as used in venous thrombosis prophylaxis does not appear to enhance fibrinolytic activity. Thus, these authors were unable to confirm a hypothesis concerning the benefits of compression therapy, which has been around for almost 20 years. Too bad.

Local Delivery of Enoxaparin to Decrease Restenosis After Stenting: Results of Initial Multicenter Trial: Polish-American Local Lovenox NIR Assessment Study (The POLONIA Study)

Kiesz RS, Buszman P, Martin JL, et al (Univ of Texas, San Antonio; Silesian Med School, Katowice, Poland; Jefferson Health System-Main Line, Radnor, Pa; et al)
Circulation 103:26-31, 2001   1–33

Objective.—Restenosis remains a problem, even after stenting. Modulation of the stimuli for neointimal hyperplasia could prevent an exaggerated, obstructive proliferative response after stent placement. Enoxaparin inhibits smooth muscle cell proliferation at high tissue concentrations, but systemic enoxaparin has not reduced the incidence of angiographic restenosis or clinical events after coronary angioplasty. A microporous, local drug delivery/angioplasty catheter method was developed to deliver the drug before stenting. Stenting after local delivery of enoxaparin was compared with reduced systemic heparinization and traditional stenting using full systemic heparinization in a multicenter, prospective, randomized study.

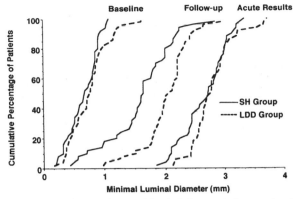

FIGURE.—Cumulative distribution of minimal luminal diameter before stenting, immediately after stenting, and at 6 months of angiographic follow-up. *Solid lines* represent patients randomly allocated to systemic heparinization (SH); *dotted lines* represent patients randomly chosen for local drug delivery (LDD) and reduced systemic heparinization. (Courtesy of Kiesz RS, Buszman P, Martin JL, et al: Local delivery of enoxaparin to decrease restenosis after stenting: Results of initial multicenter trial: Polish-American local Lovenox NIR assessment study (The POLONIA) Study). *Circulation* 103:26-31, 2001.)

Methods.—From February 1996 to April 1998, 100 patients were randomly allocated to receive 2500 U heparin through an arterial sheath and 10 mg enoxaparin during predilation (n = 50, 74% men) or full systemic heparinization with 10,000 U heparin through the arterial sheath (n = 50, 68% men) to obtain a target activated clotting time of 300 seconds. All patients received the same type of stent. The primary end point was late luminal loss at 6 months. Major adverse events, emergency coronary artery bypass grafts, repeat balloon angioplasty, and angiographic restenosis at 6 months were recorded.

Results.—Activated clotting time was significantly lower in the local drug delivery (LDD) group compared with the systemic heparin (SH) group (146 vs 381 s). At 6 months, the LDD group had a significantly lower target lesion revascularization rate than the SH group did (8% vs 22%) and had significantly reduced late luminal loss (0.76 vs 1.07) and loss index (0.38 vs 0.55) (Figure). The mean luminal diameter was significantly larger in the LDD group than in the SH group (2.02 vs 1.59). The restenosis rate was significantly lower in the LDD group than in the SH group (10.0% vs 24.0%).

Conclusion.—Local delivery of enoxaparin significantly decreased late lumen loss and angiographic restenosis.

▶ This interesting article indicates that the local administration of enoxaparin at a site of coronary artery stenting in humans significantly reduced intimal hyperplasia at follow-up and that this trial was the first prospective randomized trial in which the local delivery of enoxaparin has resulted in significant reduction in late luminal loss. This is interesting material. Benefits from enoxaparin in this setting may, of course, have resulted either from its potent effect as an antithrombotic agent from the well-known effects of heparin in decreasing smooth-muscle cell proliferation. I suspect we are on the threshold of seeing the administration of a large number of substances directly to the arterial site of stenting in an effort to reduce subsequent late luminal loss.

Local Treatment With Recombinant Tissue Factor Pathway Inhibitor Reduces the Development of Intimal Hyperplasia in Experimental Vein Grafts

Huynh TTT, Davies MG, Thompson MA, et al (Duke Univ, Durham, NC; Yale Univ, New Haven, Conn)
J Vasc Surg 33:400-407, 2001   1–34

Background.—The development of intimal hyperplasia is a serious deterrent to a good long-term outcome for vein grafts. The development of intimal hyperplasia has been linked to tissue factor (TF)–initiated thrombin generation, and an increase in the expression has preceded the development of intimal hyperplasia. The effectiveness of recombinant human tissue factor pathway inhibitor (rTFPI) in enhancing experimental vein grafts was determined.

Methods.—Bypass carotid artery grafts were done in 36 male New Zealand white rabbits using the reversed ipsilateral jugular vein. Four groups were formed: 10 animals had ex vivo incubation with rTFPI treatment, 10 had incubation with placebo, 8 had both ex vivo incubation and in vivo gel treatment with rTFPI, and 8 had this protocol with placebo. Immunohistochemical and Western blot analyses were done on vein grafts harvested 3 days after surgery; a histomorphological study was done on 28-day vein grafts.

Results.—With rTFPI treatment, TF protein expression was reduced 6.2-fold over no rTFPI treatment. A reduction in CD-18 leukocyte staining also occurred, but Tie-2 endothelial staining increased in all vein grafts treated with rTFPI compared with those in the control or gel-control groups. Ex vivo rTFPI treatment reduced intimal thickness by nearly one

TABLE 2.—Morphometric Analysis of Ex Vivo rTFPI Treatment

	rTFPI (n = 6)	Control (n = 6)	P Value
Luminal area (mm²)	26.7 ± 1.9	29.8 ± 2.8	.40
Intimal area (mm²)	1.24 ± 0.09	1.75 ± 0.18	< .05
Medial area (mm²)	1.30 ± 0.08	1.87 ± 0.16	< .05
Intimal ratio	0.47 ± 0.01	0.49 ± 0.01	.91
Luminal index	38.9 ± 2.1	33.4 ± 1.5	< .05

Note: Wall dimensions of 28-day vein grafts treated with local ex vivo rTFPI incubation or placebo (control). Values are the mean ± SEM. Statistical differences between the 2 groups were compared by use of the Mann-Whitney rank sum test. *Intimal ratio,* Intimal area/(intimal + medial areas); *luminal index,* luminal diameter/(intimal + medial thickness).

Abbreviation: rTFPI, Recombinant human tissue factor pathway inhibitor.

(Courtesy of Huynh TTT, Davies MG, Thompson MA, et al: Local treatment with recombinant tissue factor pathway inhibitor reduces the development of intimal hyperplasia in experimental vein grafts. *J Vasc Surg* 33:400-407, 2001.)

fourth over placebo; in vivo rTFPI treatment reduced it by nearly a third compared with the gel-control group (Table 2).

Conclusions.—The administration of rTFPI locally had early benefits for the endothelium. In addition, the hyperplastic response in vein grafts was significantly reduced. By blocking the initiation of TF-mediated pathways with the use of rTFPI, it may help improve vein graft success.

▶ Alas, does the rabbit have anything to do with human intimal hyperplasia? I secretly suspect it does not. However, with that small limitation, these authors have shown with moderate persuasiveness that the inhibition of TF limits the development of intimal hyperplasia in rabbits. Thus, for all rabbits in whom we perform vein grafts, perhaps we should consider use of this substance. Seriously, it is clear that the promotion of coagulation is a very complex activity which involves the activation of many vascular biological moderators, which may in turn independently induce smooth-muscle proliferation. It is entirely possible that TF may play a role and that rTFPI may prove beneficial. Perhaps.

Association Between Anticardiolipin Antibodies and Mortality in Patients With Peripheral Arterial Disease

Puisieux F, de Groote P, Masy E, et al (Centre Hospitalier et Universitaire de Lille, France)

Am J Med 109:635-641, 2000   1–35

Objective.—Antiphospholipid antibodies and thrombosis are linked, but the pathophysiology of thromboembolic events is not understood. The prevalence of anticardiolipin antibodies in patients with peripheral arterial disease was prospectively investigated, and their association with subsequent mortality was analyzed.

Methods.—Between February 1993 and September 1994, the presence of cardiolipin antibodies was investigated in 100 controls and in 232 symptomatic patients (23 women). The patients had an average age of 59 years and had been given a diagnosis of peripheral arterial disease by means of enzyme-linked immunosorbent assay. Immunoglobulin (Ig)G and IgM fractions were quantified. Demographic information and cardiovascular mortality and thromboembolic event data were collected.

Results.—Elevated titers of anticardiolipin were detected in 41 (18%) patients and 9 (9%) controls ($P = .03$). IgG antibodies were elevated in 36 patients, and IgM antibodies were elevated in 8. Patients with IgG anticardiolipin antibodies were more likely to have a history of deep vein thrombosis and a history of cancer than patients without IgG anticardiolipin antibodies. During an average follow-up of 38 months, 3 patients were lost to follow-up; 12 of 14 patients with vital statistics information only died. Antiplatelet therapy was administered to 203 of the remaining 215 patients. An additional 7 patients received long-term anticoagulation therapy. There were 56 (24%) deaths as a result of cardiovascular disease.

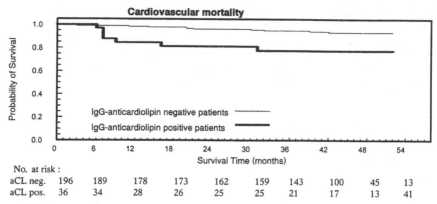

No. at risk :

	0	6	12	18	24	30	36	42	48	54
aCL neg.	196	189	178	173	162	159	143	100	45	13
aCL pos.	36	34	28	26	25	25	21	17	13	41

FIGURE 3.—Cardiovascular mortality in patients with and without immunoglobulin G anticardiolipin (*aCL*) antibodies (P = .001 by log-rank test). (Reprinted from the *American Journal of Medicine* courtesy of Puisieux F, de Groote P, Masy E, et al: Association between anticardiolipin antibodies and mortality in patients with peripheral arterial disease. *Am J Med* 109:635-641, 2000. Copyright 2000, with permission from Excerpta Medica Inc.)

These patients were significantly older (64 vs 58 years), had more severe peripheral arterial disease (stage 2.6 vs stage 2.2), were significantly more likely to have a history of cancer (14% vs 0%), and were significantly more likely to have IgG anticardiolipin antibodies (28% vs 11%). Cumulative survival at 3.5 years was significantly higher for those without IgG anti-cardiolipin antibodies than those with the antibodies (79% vs 55%). Age, severity of disease, history of cancer, and IgG anticardiolipin antibodies were independent predictors of mortality. IgG anticardiolipin antibodies were significantly associated with cardiovascular mortality (Fig 3). Age, history of cancer, and IgG were independent multivariate predictors of cardiovascular mortality. Only age was a predictor of future thromboembolic events.

Conclusion.—Many patients with peripheral arterial disease have elevated levels of anticardiolipin antibodies. These antibodies are independently associated with overall mortality and cardiovascular mortality.

▶ The clinical significance of anticardiolipin antibodies remains elusive. These evanescent antibodies are prone to coming and going at the drop of a hat and are related to dozens and dozens of agents. I have never been able to ascertain with certainty the significance of anticardiolipin antibodies in our patients. However, these authors do present a rather convincing study showing that intermediate-term mortality was twice as high in patients with peripheral vascular disease with anticardiolipin antibodies compared with those without such antibodies. This is potentially important, as 16% of their patients with peripheral vascular disease proved to have the antibodies to start with. The real question is how to determine whether anticoagulant therapy can reduce the impressive death rate in the anticardiolipin patients. I assume there will be more to follow.

Abdominal Thrombotic and Ischemic Manifestations of the Antiphospholipid Antibody Syndrome: CT Findings in 42 Patients

Kaushik S, Federle MP, Schur PH, et al (Univ of Pittsburgh, Pa; Harvard Med School, Boston)
Radiology 218:768-771, 2001   1–36

Objective.—Anticardiolipid antibody and lupus anticoagulant are found in 2% of the general population and in 30% to 40% of patients with systemic lupus erythematosus. Patients with antiphospholipid antibody syndrome (APS) sometimes experience unanticipated and catastrophic abdominal ischemic events. These complications have not been well studied. The abdominal CT findings in patients with APS were retrospectively reviewed.

Methods.—Records of all 1218 patients with circulating antiphospholipid antibodies who underwent testing between 1994 and 1997 were reviewed.

Results.—Patients with conditions known to predispose them to hypercoagulable states and those older than 65 years were excluded from the analysis. Of the remaining patients, 215 had a diagnosis of APS, and 42 (19.5%), aged 32 to 65 years, had evidence of abdominal organ ischemia or thrombosis (Table). Twelve had occluded vessels. In some patients, multiple abdominal sites were involved.

Conclusion.—Major abdominal vascular thromboses and visceral infarctions are common in patients with APS. Multiple abdominal sites may be affected. CT is a useful diagnostic tool in these patients.

▶ A remarkable 20% of 215 patients with APS on abdominal CT scanning had venous or arterial thrombotic disorders, with a preponderance being

TABLE.—Distribution of Abdominal Thrombosis and Ischemia in 42 Patients With Antiphospholipid Antibody Syndrome

Findings	No. of Patients
Vascular thrombosis	22
Inferior vena cava	10
Portal and superior mesenteric veins	7
Splenic vein	4
Aorta	1
Abdominal visceral ischemia	36
Kidney	22
Bowel	13
Spleen	6
Pancreas	3
Liver	2*

Note: In some patients, more than 1 abdominal organ and/or vessel was involved.
*One case of hepatic infarction and 1 case of hepatic veno-occlusive disease and liver failure.
(Courtesy of Kaushik S, Federle MP, Schur PH, et al: Abdominal thrombotic and ischemic manifestations of the antiphospholipid antibody syndrome: CT findings in 42 patients. *Radiology* 218:768-771, 2001. Radiological Society of North America.)

large vein. This is amazing information, although the study is complicated by the fact that certain of these patients did have abdominal symptoms directing the study to be done. Nonetheless, to find this proportion of major visceral thrombotic abnormalities in patients with antiphospholipid antibodies was completely unsuspected. We are only beginning to realize the complex spectrum of antiphospholipid antibody causation. I must say that, as time passes, antiphospholipid antibodies confuse me more and more.

Heparin Induces Synthesis and Secretion of Tissue Factor Pathway Inhibitor From Endothelial Cells In Vitro

Hansen J-B, Svensson B, Olsen R, et al (Univ of Tromsø, Norway; Novo Nordisk AS, Maalov, Denmark)
Thromb Haemost 83:937-943, 2000   1–37

Background.—Tissue factor pathway inhibitor (TFPI) is a serine protease inhibitor that is believed to be the major regulator of tissue factor (TF)-induced blood coagulation. It is constitutively synthesized by and stored in association with endothelial cells. In vivo administration of unfractionated heparin (UFH) is followed promptly by release of TFPI into the circulation. An in vitro model was created to explore the effects of UFH on the synthesis, secretion, and potency of TFPI in endothelial cells.

Methods.—Experiments were performed using the spontaneously transformed immortal endothelial cell line EVC304.

Results.—When the cells were treated with UFH, release of TFPI into the culture medium increased in a dose-dependent fashion (Fig 2). However, immunocytochemical analysis showed no difference in TFPI at the surface membrane. A 1.4-kilobase (kb) and a 4.4-kb mRNA transcript for TFPI was found on Northern blotting. In response to 24 hours of stimulation with UFH, ECV304 cells increased the release of TFPI in a dose-dependent fashion, including expression of both TFPI mRNA species.

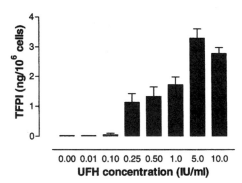

FIGURE 2.—Graph showing the dose-dependent release of tissue factor pathway inhibitor (TFPI) from ECV304 cells to supernatants by exposure to unfractionated heparin (UFH) for 15 minutes (n = 6). Values are means plus or minus 1 SD. (Courtesy of Hansen J-B, Svensson B, Olsen R, et al: Heparin induces synthesis and secretion of tissue factor pathway inhibitor from endothelial cells in vitro. *Thromb Haemost* 83:937-943, 2000.)

When the cells were incubated with UFH at a concentration of 5.0 IU/mL for 48 hours, the TFPI concentration in the medium increased 5-fold to 10-fold during that time. Expression of TFPI mRNA increased within 10 minutes, peaking within 2 to 4 hours. This increase occurred 2 to 4 hours before the synthesis-dependent increase in TFPI release and was sustained throughout the exposure period. Exposure to UFH was associated with a 36% downregulation of cell procoagulant activity. Twenty-four hours of heparin stimulation was associated with a moderate increase in the effect of TFPI on the anticoagulant potency of ECV304 cells.

Conclusions.—These in vitro findings support the importance of TFPI in the anticoagulant activity of heparins. In response to therapeutic levels of UFH, endothelial cells show a sharp rise in the synthesis and release of TFPI, and no effect on antithrombotic potency is seen. The authors call for further exploration of these mechanisms.

▶ This remarkable study concludes that unfractionated heparin greatly augments the endothelial secretion of tissue factor pathway inhibitor, and that this indeed may be of major importance for the anticoagulant function of heparin. It appears actually that heparin upregulates the tissue factor mRNA in the endothelial cells. I find this fascinating new information. The number of clues in recent years are beginning to suggest that the tissue factor participation in coagulation is not limited to the rare mechanical injury formerly suspected, but may indeed play an integral role in coagulant activities. I wonder how low molecular weight heparin affects this substance? Presently, I have no idea at all.

Hirudin Monitoring Using the TAS Ecarin Clotting Time in Patients With Heparin-Induced Thrombocytopenia Type II
Koster A, Hansen R, Grauhan O, et al (Univ of Hamburg, Germany)
J Cardiothorac Vasc Anesth 14:249-252, 2000   1–38

Background.—The anticoagulant effect of the polypeptide hirudin is achieved by direct antithrombin III-independent inhibition of thrombin and the thrombin-dependent reactions in the plasmatic coagulation cascade and platelet aggregation. While heparin inhibits only free plasmatic coagulation factors, hirudin also inhibits platelet-bound thrombin. As hirudin migrates into the forming thrombus, the clot is further polymerized, and this effectively supports lytic therapy. The use of recombinant hirudin (r-hirudin) for anticoagulation of patients with heparin-induced thrombocytopenia type II (HIT II) has been shown to be safe and effective because of its immediate strong anticoagulant effect and rapid renal elimination. Because the individual response to r-hirudin is quite variable, its use for high-dose anticoagulation requires close and precise monitoring. The urgency of precise monitoring of these patients is underscored by the fact that there is no antidote for r-hirudin overdose. Measurement of the whole-blood ecarin clotting time (ECT) has been shown to be a reliable

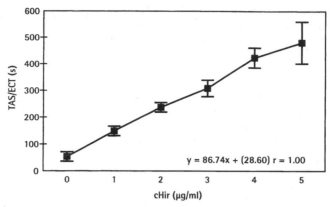

FIGURE 1.—Calibration curve for the TAS/ecarin clotting time (ECT) assay using 6 different concentrations of r-hirudin (cHir). (Courtesy of Koster A, Hansen R, Grauhan O, et al: Hirudin monitoring using the TAS ecarin clotting time in patients with heparin-induced thrombocytopenia type II. *J Cardiothorac Vasc Anesth* 14:249-252, 2000.)

assay for anticoagulation during cardiopulmonary bypass. The only ready-to-use point-of-care test for ECT measurement is the ECT card for the Thrombolytic Assessment System (TAS) analyzer. This test has been used during cardiopulmonary bypass with r-hirudin in patients with HIT II but has not previously been validated in a clinical study.

Methods.—Five healthy volunteers and 11 patients undergoing cardiovascular surgery were enrolled in the study. In the healthy volunteers, blood samples were obtained and spiked with 6 defined concentrations of r-hirudin (Fig 1). Measurements were performed in duplicate and in parallel with 2 TAS analyzers. A calibration curve was constructed. Of the 11 patients, 8 underwent surgery with cardiopulmonary bypass (CPB) (Group I), and 3 underwent surgery without CPB. In both groups, r-hirudin was monitored with the TAS/ECT analyzer and compared with the standard reference laboratory method for measuring the antithrombin IIa-based chromogenic assay.

Results.—Linearity and reliability to an r-hirudin concentration of 5 μg/mL was demonstrated by the TAS/ECT analyzer and was not influenced by the varying conditions of the concentrations of r-hirudin in samples from healthy volunteers. For the patient group, the correlation to the laboratory method was 0.74 for the CPB group and 0.87 for the non-CPB group.

Conclusions.—TAS/ECT demonstrated reliability as an assay for monitoring r-hirudin levels at the point of care. The use of the TAS/ECT test should result in safer and more efficacious use of r-hirudin during surgery or angioplasty.

▶ As the use of hirudin creeps into our clinical practice, we are going to need some measure of hirudin blood level and activity. These authors convinced me that the PAS/ECT method for online monitoring of hirudin is an accurate and reproducible method. Of course, this method seems to accurately correlate with the micrograms of hirudin present in the blood. It is noteworthy that there seems to be considerable variation in the initial bolus necessary to achieve a target concentration in the blood. This certainly indicates that the individual response to recombinant hirudin differs markedly among individuals, thus emphasizing the need for online monitoring.

Homocysteine

High Prevalence of Mild Hyperhomocysteinemia in Patients With Abdominal Aortic Aneurysm

Brunelli T, Prisco D, Fedi S, et al (Univ of Florence, Italy; Univ of Rome)
J Vasc Surg 32:531-536, 2000   1–39

Background.—Homocysteine has been recently shown to interact in vitro with the aortic wall by inducing both elastolysis and endothelial perturbation. Homocysteine plasma levels and their relationship with aortic diameter and endothelial damage in patients with abdominal aortic aneurysm (AAA) were studied.

Methods.—The study included 58 consecutive men patients, aged 49 to 78 years, undergoing AAA surgery. Twenty-two patients had no clinical or instrumental evidence of atherosclerosis. The patient group was compared with a control group of 60 age-matched men. Total homocysteine and thrombomodulin plasma levels and the distribution of the C677T methylenetetrahydrofolate reductase gene mutation were measured in all subjects.

Findings.—Forty-eight percent of the patient group had hyperhomocystinemia. Mean homocysteine plasma concentrations were significantly greater in patients than in the control group (15.7 vs 9.6 µmol/L) (Figure). In addition, the patients with AAA but with no evidence of

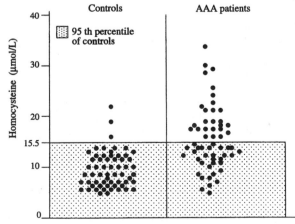

FIGURE.—Distribution of homocysteine plasma levels in patients with AAA and controls. (Courtesy of Brunelli T, Prisco D, Fedi S, et al: High prevalence of mild hyperhomocysteinemia in patients with abdominal aortic aneurysm. *J Vasc Surg* 32:531-536, 2000.)

atherosclerosis had significantly greater mean homocysteine plasma levels than men in the control group (14.8 vs 9.6 µmol/L). Hyperhomocystinemic patients had larger aneurysms than patients with normal homocysteine plasma concentrations. In the patient group, homocysteine plasma concentrations and 677TT methylenetetrahydrofolate reductase genotype were significantly correlated. Thrombomodulin plasma levels were significantly greater in patients than in control subjects. Thrombomodulin concentrations were significantly higher in hyperhomocystinemic patients than in normohomocystinemic patients. In the patient group, homocysteine was directly, significantly associated with thrombomodulin concentrations.

Conclusions.—The presence of AAA in these patients was associated with increased homocysteine plasma levels. Homocysteine may induce endothelial perturbation and stimulation in such patients.

▶ It is interesting to note that both AAA patients with and AAA patients without obvious atherosclerotic disease elsewhere showed similar elevations of serum homocysteine. I have no idea what to make of this, but because only 48% of the AAA patients had hyperhomocystinemia, the whole thing may be an artifact. Stay tuned. I am sure we shall find an ever-increasing list of things associated with hyperhomocystinemia.

Effect of Plasma Homocysteine Concentration on Early and Late Events in Patients With Acute Coronary Syndromes

Stubbs PJ, Al-Obaidi MK, Conroy RM, et al (Watford Gen Hosp, England; St George's Hosp, London; Royal College of Surgeons in Ireland, Dublin)
Circulation 102:605-610, 2000   1–40

Background.—In epidemiological studies, moderately elevated levels of homocysteine have been identified as a potentially modifiable risk factor for coronary disease. Homocysteine is a nonessential amino acid that is produced by the demethylation of methionine. Very high levels of homocysteine are found in genetically inherited enzyme defects of homocysteine metabolism, and these defects are known to be associated with aggressive and premature vascular disease. It is not known whether an elevated plasma cysteine level is associated with adverse cardiac outcome in patients admitted with acute coronary syndromes. The relation between plasma homocysteine levels and short-term and long-term prognosis in acute coronary syndromes was evaluated.

Methods.—In 440 consecutive patients, the relation of quintiles of homocysteine to fatal and nonfatal early (28 days) and late (29 days to a median of 2.5 years) events was evaluated. The study group was composed of 204 patients with unstable angina and 236 patients with myocardial infarction. End points for the study were cardiac death and/or myocardial (re)infarction. With the use of Cox regression and logistic regression, the relation of homocysteine to coronary events was estimated.

Results.—Cardiac death occurred in 67 patients, and myocardial (re) infarction occurred in 30 patients. Within the first 28 days the event rate, which included 22 cardiac deaths and 5 nonfatal infarctions, was not related to homocysteine level on admission. Among the 203 patients with unstable angina and the 214 patients with myocardial infarction who survived, a threshold effect was apparent on long-term follow-up, with a significant step-up in event frequency between the lowest 3 quintiles (14 cardiac deaths and 11 nonfatal infarctions) and the upper 2 quintiles (31 fatal events and 12 nonfatal events). Patients who were within the upper 2 quintiles had a 2.6-fold increased risk for cardiac events.

Conclusions.—Elevated total homocysteine levels on admission are strongly predictive of late cardiac events in patients with acute coronary syndromes.

▶ This study appears to have shown a rather weak correlation between homocysteine level and the late occurrence of myocardial infarction and coronary death in patients who initially presented with unstable angina. Perhaps reducing the serum homocysteine with appropriate drug therapy may reduce the long-term incidence of cardiovascular death and myocardial infarction. Clearly, a prospective randomized study is needed to resolve this conundrum.

Association Between High Homocyst(e)ine and Ischemic Stroke Due to Large- and Small-Artery Disease but Not Other Etiologic Subtypes of Ischemic Stroke
Eikelboom JW, Hankey GJ, Anand SS, et al (McMaster Univ, Hamilton, Canada; Royal Perth Hosp, Australia)
Stroke 31:1069-1075, 2000   1–41

Background.—Increased plasma homocyst(e)ine may be a causal, modifiable risk factor for ischemic stroke. However, previous research has yielded conflicting findings, possibly because homocyst(e)ine may be associated only with certain pathophysiologic subtypes of such stroke.

Methods.—Two hundred nineteen patients hospitalized for a first-ever stroke and 205 persons selected randomly from the community were included in a case-control study. The control group was stratified by age, sex, and postal code. Stroke cases were classified by etiologic subtype.

Findings.—Increasing homocyst(e)ine was a strong, independent risk factor for ischemic stroke, with an adjusted odds ratio (OR) of 2.7 for a 5-μmol/L increase in fasting homocyst(e)ine from 10 to 15 μmol/L (Fig 1). The highest quartile of homocyst(e)ine, compared with the lowest quartile, was associated with an adjusted ischemic stroke OR of 2.2. The mean plasma homocyst(e)ine was significantly greater in patients with ischemic stroke from large-artery and small-artery disease compared with control subjects but not in cardioembolic or other ischemic stroke subtypes. Compared with the lowest quartile of homocyst(e)ine, the second, third, and

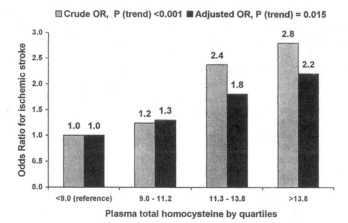

FIGURE 1.—Association between quartiles of homocyst(e)ine and risk of ischemic stroke. *Abbreviation*: OR, odds ratio. (Courtesy of Eikelboom JW, Hankey GJ, Anand SS, et al: Association between high homocyst(e)ine and ischemic stroke due to large- and small-artery disease but not other etiologic subtypes of ischemic stroke. *Stroke* 31:1069-1075, 2000. Reproduced with permission of *Stroke*. Copyright 2000, American Heart Association.)

fourth quartiles were correlated with an adjusted OR of 3.0, 5.6, and 8.7, respectively, for ischemic stroke from large-artery disease. The TT MTHFR genotype was clearly associated with increased fasting plasma homocyst(e)ine, but the MTHFR genotype was not correlated with ischemic stroke or a subtype of ischemic stroke.

Conclusion.—A strong, graded association exists between increasing plasma homocyst(e)ine and ischemic stroke caused by large-artery atherosclerosis. To a lesser degree, it is also associated with ischemic stroke from small-artery disease. Increasing plasma homocyst(e)ine is not associated with cardioembolic or other etiologic subtypes of ischemic stroke. The data are consistent with the notion that the negative effect of high homocyst(e)ine is mediated primarily by a proatherogenic mechanism.

▶ At least in this study, increasing homocysteine was a strong and independent risk factor for ischemic stroke with an odds ratio of 2.7. Interestingly, the positive correlation to serum homocysteine occurred only for large artery and small artery stroke, not for cardioembolic or other etiologic subtypes of ischemic stroke. The authors appropriately interpret these results as consistent with the hypothesis that the adverse effects of elevated homocysteine are mediated primarily through a proatherogenic effect. Hopefully, this relationship will be clarified by several large clinical trials currently in progress designed to determine whether reducing homocysteine will result in a reduced risk of stroke.

Hyperhomocysteinemia Increases Risk of Death, Especially in Type 2 Diabetes: 5-Year Follow-up of the Hoorn Study

Hoogeveen EK, Kostense PJ, Jakobs C, et al (Vrije Universiteit, Amsterdam)
Circulation 101:1506-1511, 2000   1–42

Background.—Both diabetes and hyperhomocysteinemia are independent risk factors for the development of cardiovascular disease. Type 2 diabetes is also associated with increased mortality from cardiovascular disease. A combination of type 2 diabetes and hyperhomocysteinemia may produce an interaction that significantly increases the risk of death of cardiovascular disease.

Methods.—Serum samples were obtained from 2484 patients (men and women) aged 50 to 75 years. Fasting serum total homocysteine levels were measured in the samples from 171 patients who died and in those from 640 survivors who served as a control group. The follow-up extended for 5 years, with the mortality risk calculated by logistic regression.

Results.—Among all samples, the prevalence of hyperhomocysteinemia was 25.8%. With adjustments for several factors, the overall odds ratio for 5-year mortality was 1.56 for those with hyperhomocysteinemia and 1.26 for each 5-μmol/L increase of serum total homocysteine. Among nondiabetic patients, the odds ratio for 5-year mortality for hyperhomocystenemia was 1.34; among diabetics it was 2.51.

Conclusions.—Hyperhomocysteinemia appears to be a risk factor for mortality in patients with type 2 diabetes independent of cardiovascular disease risk factors and of serum albumin levels, which normally are interpreted to indicate health. The presence of hyperhomocysteinemia increases the risk of death among patients with diabetes above that found in nondiabetic subjects.

▶ It seems hardly surprising to learn that hyperhomocystinemia is a greater factor for death in diabetics than in nondiabetics, as is almost everything else. The odds ratio for 5-year mortality associated with hyperhomocystinemia was 1.34 in nondiabetics, which is not a very strong relationship, but 2.51 in diabetics, which gets your attention. Overall, 47.5% of patients dying did so of cardiovascular disease, with the remainder of the deaths being due to a variety of malignant neoplasms and other causes. Large cohort studies such as this are always interesting, but by themselves prove nothing, because we cannot be certain that the hyperhomocystinemia is not simply a fellow traveler accompanying a more important risk factor. Long-term, high-volume, placebo-controlled treatment studies will be essential to sort out these problems.

Serum Folate and Cardiovascular Disease Mortality Among US Men and Women

Loria CM, Ingram DD, Feldman JJ, et al (Ctrs for Disease Control and Prevention, Hyattsville, Md)
Arch Intern Med 160:3258-3262, 2000   1–43

Objective.—Low serum folate is associated with carotid artery stenosis, but the link between serum folate and cardiovascular disease (CVD) has not been incontrovertibly established. Serum folate levels were measured in a representative sample of US adults (National Health and Nutrition Examination Survey II Mortality Study) whose status was followed prospectively for 12 to 16 years to determine whether folate levels were associated with risk of CVD and whether age, alcohol consumption, and diabetes mellitus modified the relationship.

Methods.—Folate levels were determined in blood drawn from 689 adults, aged 30 to 75, with no CVD at baseline in the years from 1976 to 1980. Cox proportional hazards models were used to estimate relative risks of CVD and total mortality by folate level tertile.

Results.—At the end of the follow-up period, 25 participants with diabetes had died, 12 of them of CVD. Among the other participants, 122 died, 49 of CVD. Participants without diabetes in the lowest tertile had a relative risk of CVD mortality of 2.64 compared with counterparts in the highest tertile after adjusting for age and sex. Serum folate levels were not related to total mortality, although age- and sex-related risks were increased for those in the lowest tertile compared with those in the highest tertile.

Conclusion.—Folate levels do not appear to be related to mortality for those with diabetes, but there is an increased risk of CVD in adults without diabetes who have low folate levels.

▶ I am hardly surprised to find that low serum folate concentrations are associated with increased risk for CVD mortality among nondiabetic adults. On balance, the interesting information contained herein suggests that a considerable proportion of the adult US population—at least between the years 1976 and 1980—had serum folate concentrations that may well have increased their risk of dying of CVD. The need for a placebo-controlled clinical trial in this area is patently obvious. Recent efforts to fortify the US food supply with folic acid have certainly increased the folate intake and serum concentrations of our citizens, but it is unknown whether the increase has been sufficient to decrease the proportional risk of CVD.

Improved Vascular Endothelial Function After Oral B Vitamins: An Effect Mediated Through Reduced Concentrations of Free Plasma Homocysteine

Chambers JC, Ueland PM, Obeid OA, et al (Hammersmith Hosp, London; Univ of Bergen, Norway; Queen Mary and Westfield College, London; et al)
Circulation 102:2479-2483, 2000   1-44

Objective.—Hyperhomocysteinemia is a known risk factor for coronary heart disease (CHD), but little is known about the beneficial effects of lowering homocysteine levels in patients with CHD. Folate supplementation reduces plasma homocysteine levels. The effects of dietary folate and vitamin B_{12} supplementation on vascular endothelial function and the relation between vascular endothelial function and concentrations of total, protein-bound, and free plasma homocysteine were examined in patients with CHD in a randomized, double-blind study.

Methods.—Brachial artery flow-mediated dilatation and nitroglycerine-induced dilatation were measured in 89 men with CHD, aged 39 to 67 years, before and 8 weeks after placebo (n = 30) or daily folic acid (5 mg) and vitamin B_{12} (1 mg) (n = 59). Fasting total and free plasma homocysteine, serum folate, vitamin B_{12}, glucose, total and HDL cholesterol, and triglycerides were measured at baseline and at 8 weeks.

Results.—Flow-mediated dilatation improved significantly from baseline to 8 weeks in the vitamin group (2.5% to 4.0%) both in the 13 patients with elevated homocysteine (>15 µmol/L) and in the 46 patients with normal homocysteine levels but not in the placebo group. Compared with baseline values, there were significant changes in 8-week levels of free plasma homocysteine (4.3 to 3.0 µmol/L), protein-bound homocysteine (8.7 to 6.2 µmol/L), total plasma homocysteine (13.0 to 9.3 µmol/L), serum folate (10.3 to 31.2 ng/mL), and serum vitamin B_{12} (314 to 661 pg/mL). There was a significant inverse relation between flow-mediated dilatation and free homocysteine, according to multivariate analysis after adjustment for the other variables and for age and blood pressure. When adjusted for free plasma homocysteine concentration, relation between flow-mediated dilatation and protein-bound homocysteine, folate, and vitamin B_{12} were no longer significant, according to univariate analysis.

Conclusion.—Folic acid and vitamin B_{12} supplementation improved brachial artery endothelium-dependent dilatation in patients with CHD. Such supplementation may reduce cardiovascular risk in these patients.

▶ It is an article of faith in vascular medical circles that endothelial function can be assessed by ultrasonic vascular wall tracking to determine brachial artery flow-mediated dilatation. This technique is well standardized in vascular medical laboratories. Flow-mediated dilatation improved after treatment with B vitamins, which lowered concentrations of serum homocysteine. This leads these investigators to conclude that folic acid and vitamin B_{12} supplementation improves vascular endothelial function in patients with coronary heart disease. I am sure it does, and I certainly hope that the changes they are measuring in the brachial artery are relevant to the entire field of endothelial function, as they seem convinced that it is. Cumulatively, the results of this and the preceding abstracts indicate that we had best get busy with dietary reduction of homocysteine levels.

The Effect of Elevated Homocysteine Levels on Adrenergic Vasoconstriction of Human Resistance Arteries: The Role of the Endothelium and Reactive Oxygen Species

Cipolla MJ, Williamson WK, Nehler ML, et al (Univ of Vermont, Burlington; Oregon Health Sciences Univ, Portland)
J Vasc Surg 31:751-759, 2000   1–45

Background.—Mild to moderate elevations in homocysteine (HC) levels are a risk factor for arterial occlusive disease. These deleterious vascular effects are believed to occur through oxidative damage caused by reactive oxygen species. However, some studies have also found that elevated HC levels decrease the endothelium's production of vasoactive factors. The effects of elevated HC levels both on adrenergic vasoconstriction in isolated and pressurized human resistance arteries and on the endothelial modulation of this vasoconstriction were examined. Also examined was whether treatment with superoxide dismutase (SOD) or catalase (which eliminate reactive oxygen species) could prevent the alterations induced by elevated HC levels.

Methods.—Skin and subcutaneous fat specimens (1.0 cm³) were obtained from 18 patients undergoing lower extremity vascular surgery who did not have renal failure. From each specimen, 30 small arteries (inner diameter, less than 200 μm) were isolated under a dissecting microscope. For each study, control and experimental vessels were taken from the same specimen to ensure that any changes noted were caused by experimental conditions rather than by patient-related confounders. Each paired sample was placed in an arteriograph chamber that allowed precise control of intraluminal pressure. The first set of experiments tested vascular reactivity to adrenergic stimulation. Paired specimens from 6 patients were perfused and superfused with physiologic saline solution (controls) or with physiologic saline solution plus 200 μmol/L of HC. Then varying doses of norepinephrine (NE), acetylcholine, and sodium nitroprusside (SNP) were individually added to the arteriograph bath (with washout periods in between) and lumen diameter was recorded.

In the second set of experiments, another group of 6 paired specimens was incubated in 200 μmol/L HC either alone or in combination with 1200 U/mL catalase and 120 U/mL SOD. NE was added and a concentration-response curve was obtained. The last set of experiments assessed whether HC affects the endothelial production of vasoactive factors. Six paired specimens of either intact or denuded arteries were precontracted with an intermediate concentration of NE. Then either physiologic saline

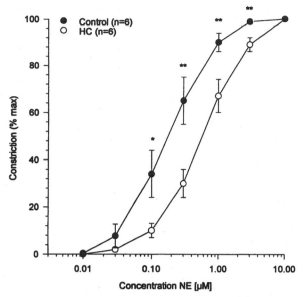

FIGURE 1.—Graph showing the concentration-response to norepinephrine (*NE*) of arteries in physiologic saline solution (*control* indicated by *solid circles*) and exposed to 200 μmol/L homocysteine (*HC*; indicated by *open circles*). *asterisk* indicates $P < .05$; *Double asterisk* indicates $P < .01$. (Courtesy of Cipolla MJ, Williamson WK, Nehler ML, et al: The effect of elevated homocysteine levels on adrenergic vasoconstriction of human resistance arteries: The role of the endothelium and reactive oxygen species. *J Vasc Surg* 31:751-759, 2000.)

solution or increasing concentrations of HC (20-200 μmol/L) were added to the bath and lumen diameter was continuously recorded.

Results.—In the first set of tests, the median effective NE concentration needed to contract arteries by 50% of maximum (EC_{50}) was significantly higher in the HC arteries compared with control (0.65 vs 0.24 μmol/L) (Fig 1). Arterial sensitivities to acetylcholine or SNP did not differ between control and HC conditions. In the second set of tests, adding SOD and catalase to the bath also reduced arterial sensitivity to NE, to a similar degree as in the first set of tests (NE EC_{50}, 0.55 μmol/L). In the third set of tests, HC caused significant vasodilation in both intact and denuded precontracted arteries, although the HC EC_{50} in denuded arteries was significantly higher than that in intact arteries (90 vs 61 μmol/L).

Conclusion.—In vitro testing of human resistance arteries indicates that high levels of HC significantly reduce arterial sensitivity to adrenergic contraction. This effect does not appear to be mediated by reactive oxygen species, as the addition of catalase and SOD did not improve NE sensitivity in the HC arteries. The vasodilatory response to NE is more sensitive in arteries with intact endothelium, but both intact and denuded arteries had decreased adrenergic responsiveness in the presence of HC. Thus, HC affects both endothelial and smooth muscle cells. Thus, elevations in HC levels have 2 effects in human resistance arteries: HC reduces arterial sensitivity to NE, and it also promotes vasodilation of arteries precontracted by NE.

▶ The production of nitric acid appears to be impaired in patients with hyperhomocystinemia. As shown by this study, elevated HC affects arterial reactivity to adrenergic stimulation by affecting both the sensitivity to NE and promoting vasodilatation of arteries contracted with NE. This study appears to be the first to demonstrate a vasoactive effect of HC on the function of the vascular smooth muscle and endothelium. I am certain we shall hear more about the pathophysiologic effects of hyperhomocystinemia in the future.

Homocysteine Stimulates MAP Kinase in Bovine Aortic Smooth Muscle Cells

Woo DK, Dudrick SJ, Sumpio BE (Yale Univ, New Haven, Conn)
Surgery 128:59-66, 2000   1–46

Background.—Elevated homocysteine levels have been associated with atherosclerotic disease, and hyperhomocysteinemia has been implicated in the development of premature atherosclerosis and thromboembolic events in susceptible persons with a deficiency in the enzymes that convert homocysteine to cysteine or methionine. Homocysteinuria has also been recognized as a risk factor for cardiovascular, peripheral vascular, and cerebrovascular diseases in the general population.

The association of homocysteine with vascular disease appears to be independent of other risk factors, including smoking, hypercholesterolemia, diabetes mellitus, and hypertension. One study found that a level of homocysteine only 12% above the upper limit of normal was associated with a greater than threefold increase in the risk of myocardial infarction. A hallmark of atherosclerosis is smooth muscle cell proliferation; the effects of homocysteine on smooth muscle cell proliferation were investigated. The mitogen-activated protein (MAP) kinases and extracellular signal-regulation protein kinase 1 and 2, which are known to play a role in cell proliferation, were also studied.

Methods.—Bovine aortic smooth muscle cells (BASMCs) were used for the proliferation study. The cells were allowed to grow for 2 days before the addition of 2 mmol/L of D,L-homocysteine for 2, 4, 6, and 8 days to simulate a clinical condition of hyperhomocysteinemia. In the MAP kinase study, quiescent BASMCs were exposed to 2 mmol/L of D,L-homocysteine for 1.5, 5, 10, 20, 30 and 60 minutes. Western immunoblotting was used for detection of the active forms of MAP kinase, and densitometry was used for determination of the degree of phosphorylation of MAP kinase.

Results.—BASMC proliferation was stimulated by 20% by D,L-homocysteine at day 8. Activation of MAP kinase phosphorylation was increased by as much as sixfold by D,L-homocysteine, peaking at 30 minutes. An inhibitor of MAP kinase phosphorylation, PD98059, inhibited the homocysteine-induced phosphorylation of MAP kinase and attenuated the increase in BASMC proliferation.

Conclusion.—The hypothesis that MAP kinase activation is involved in the D,L-homocysteine stimulation of BASMC proliferation was supported by these findings.

▶ These are interesting basic investigations into possible mechanisms of adverse action of hyperhomocystinemia on the vascular wall. If these authors are correct, hyperhomocystinemia facilitates MAP kinase phosphorylation, which in turn stimulates vascular smooth muscle cell proliferation. This appears to be an important insight into the molecular mechanisms of homocysteine stimulation of vascular smooth muscle cell proliferation. Undoubtedly, in the final analysis this will be only one of many actions of homocysteine on the vascular wall.

Controlled Comparison of L-5-Methyltetrahydrofolate Versus Folic Acid for the Treatment of Hyperhomocysteinemia in Hemodialysis Patients
Bostom AG, Shemin D, Bagley P, et al (Mem Hosp of Rhode Island, Pawtucket; Rhode Island Hosp, Providence; Jean Mayer Human Nutrition Research Ctr, Boston; et al)
Circulation 101:2829-2832, 2000   1–47

Introduction.—The hyperhomocystinemia frequently observed in patients on hemodialysis is often refractory to combined oral B-vitamin supplementation, including supraphysiologic doses of folic acid. The ability of a high-dose L-5-methyltetrahydrofolate-based regimen to decrease total homocysteine (tHcy)-levels for patients undergoing chronic hemodialysis was assessed.

Methods.—The study included 50 patients with stable hemodialysis who were block-randomized on the basis of their screening predialysis tHcy levels, gender, and dialysis center to treatment with either oral folic acid at 15 mg/d (FA group) or an equimolar amount (17 mg/d) of oral L-5-methyltetrahydrofolate (MTHF group). All patients also received 50 mg/d oral vitamin B_6 and 1.0 mg/d oral vitamin B_{12}.

Results.—The mean percentage decreases in predialysis tHcy were similar between the 2 groups: 17.0% (MTHF) and 14.8% (FA) by matched ANCOVA adjusted for pretreatment tHcy (Table 2). The final on-treatment values were 20.0 µmol/L and 19.5 µmol/L for the MTHF group and FA group, respectively. Neither treatment caused "normalization" of tHcy levels among a significantly different or clinically meaningful number of patients: 1 of 25 (8%) for the MTHF group and 0 of 25 (0%) for the FA group.

Conclusion.—Relative to high-dose folic acid, high-dose oral L-5-methyltetrahydrofolate-based supplementation does not provide decreased tHcy levels in patients on long-term hemodialysis. The treatment refrac-

TABLE 2.—Treatment Effects on Predialysis tHcy Levels

Group	Percent Reduction in Predialysis tHcy	Final On-Treatment Predialysis tHcy Levels, μmol/L
MTHF	17.0*	(12.0%-22.0%)
	20.0*	(18.8-21.2)
FA	14.8%*	(9.6%-20.1%)
	19.5*	(18.3-20.7)
Between-groups comparison of percent reduction in predialysis tHcy, MTHF vs FA		$P=0.444†$

*Mean (95% CI).
†P based on "matched" ANCOVA adjusted for baseline tHcy.
Abbreviations: MTHF, 17 mg L-5-methyltetrahydrofolate, 50.0-mg B_6, and 1.0-mg B_{12}; *FA*, 15-mg folic acid 50-mg B_6 and 1.0-mg B_{12}.
(Courtesy of Bostom AG, Shemin D, Bagley P, et al: Controlled comparison of L-5-methyltetrahydrofolate versus folic acid for the treatment of hyperhomocysteinemia in hemodialysis patients. *Circulation* 101:2829-2832, 2000.)

toriness is not associated with folate absorption or circulating plasma and tissue distribution.

▶ About 90% of patients with end-stage renal disease (ESRD) who were on hemodialysis have elevated homocysteine. These patients are notoriously liable to have advanced atherosclerosis, and it certainly would appear reasonable to attempt to control their hyperhomocystinemia. Remarkably, as shown by this study and others, patients with ESRD on hemodialysis show refractoriness to treatment of hyperhomocystinemia. This is not due to malabsorption, as oral treatment does distinctly elevate the serum folate and MTHF blood levels. Of a special interest is the observation that after successful kidney transplantation the hyperhomocysteine levels invariably decline, and the mild hyperhomocystinemia that persists in that condition appears to be consistently normalizable with standard high-dose FA and B vitamin supplementation. This certainly points to a specific biochemical abnormality associated with hemodialysis, for which we presently have no explanation.

Does Folic Acid Decrease Plasma Homocysteine and Improve Endothelial Function in Patients With Predialysis Renal Failure?

Thambyrajah J, Landray MJ, McGlynn FJ, et al (Univ of Birmingham, England; Queen Elizabeth Hosp, Birmingham, England)
Circulation 102:871-875, 2000   1–48

Background.—An increased plasma concentration of homocysteine has been shown to be an independent risk factor for atherosclerosis development. The mode of action appears to be the induction of endothelial dysfunction. Hyperhomocystinemia can be reduced by folic acid, but untoward effects may result. Both hyperhomocystinemia and atherosclerosis may accompany chronic renal failure, so folic acid treatment may be appropriate for improving endothelial function.

Methods.—The study population included 67 men and 34 women (mean age, 62 years) who had predialysis chronic renal failure. They were randomly assigned to receive either 5 mg folic acid or placebo each day for 12 weeks, and endothelial function was evaluated by measurement of endothelium-dependent brachial artery dilation, serum nitrite/nitrate concentration, and plasma concentration of von Willebrand factor.

Results.—The group receiving folic acid had higher concentrations of folate in both serum (39.0 µg/L) and red blood cells (739 µg/L) than the group receiving placebo (serum, 7.7 µg/L; red blood cells, 220 µg/L). Hyperhomocystinemia was reduced in those receiving folic acid, but no significant difference was noted in endothelium-dependent dilation, serum nitrite/nitrate concentration, or plasma concentration of von Willebrand factor between the groups.

Conclusions.—Among patients with predialysis chronic renal failure, high doses of folic acid can lower but cannot normalize hyperhomocystinemia. Endothelial function does not improve, so vascular disease may remain unchanged in patients with uremia.

▶ The investigators failed to show that a decrease in plasma homocysteine level from 20.1 µmol/L (in the control group) to 15.1 µmol/L (in the treatment group) would improve brachial artery vasoactivity in predialysis patients. They only measured brachial artery diameter and found no significant difference with folic acid treatment. There is still a distinct possibility if the investigators measured brachial artery blood flow in addition to its diameter they could have found a significant increase in blood flow that would suggest improvement in vasoactivity.

A. N. Sidawy, MD

Imaging

Visualization of Fibrous Cap Thickness and Rupture in Human Atherosclerotic Carotid Plaque In Vivo With High-Resolution Magnetic Resonance Imaging

Hatsukami TS, Ross R, Polissar NL, et al (VA Puget Sound Health Care System, Seattle, Wash; The Mountain-Whisper-Light Statistical Consulting, Seattle; Univ of Washington, Seattle)
Circulation 102:959-964, 2000   1–49

Introduction.—The results of studies examining advanced lesions of atherosclerosis indicate that the thickness of the fibrous cap that overlies the necrotic core distinguishes the stable lesion from one that is at high risk for rupture and thromboembolic events. A high-resolution MRI approach has been developed that can distinguish the fine structure of the lesion, including the thickness of the fibrous cap in vivo. The correlation between in-vivo MRI and actual lesion architecture in determining the fibrous cap thickness and its potential to rupture, as observed on histologic and gross tissue examination, was assessed.

Methods.—Twenty-two patients scheduled for carotid endarterectomy underwent MRI with the use of a 3-dimensional multiple overlapping thin slab angiography protocol. The appearance of the fibrous cap was identified as either intact, thick; intact, thin; or ruptured on MRI and gross and histologic sections.

Results.—Thirty-six sites were accessible for comparison between MRI and histologic examination. A high level (89%) of agreement was observed between MRI and histologic findings. The level of agreement for distinguishing intact from ruptured fibrous caps was similarly high.

Conclusion.—High-resolution MRI with a 3-dimensional overlapping thin slab angiography protocol can distinguish between intact, thick fibrous caps and intact thin and disrupted caps in atherosclerotic human carotid arteries in vivo. This noninvasive approach has the potential to allow investigations that evaluate the relationship between fibrous cap changes and clinical outcomes and to permit trials that assess therapy intended to "stabilize" the fibrous cap.

▶ It is always worth recalling that the 5-year risk of stroke in the ACAS trial was 11% among patients with asymptomatic carotid artery occlusive disease treated solely with medical therapy. Thus, the ability to better characterize the risk of a neurologic event would certainly be of benefit, particularly in the older patient with associated comorbid conditions. While this study was not designed to determine whether plaque morphology has predictive value, it certainly demonstrates that technical advances have been able to significantly improve the detailed structure that can be resolved with MR imaging. The ever-improving ability of MR and duplex imaging, for that matter, to define plaque morphology, along with the magnitude of local shear stress and wall tension, has created powerful research tools to determine whether any of these parameters carry prognostic significance above and beyond lumen stenosis alone.

E. L. Chaikof, MD

Magnetic Resonance Techniques for the Identification of Patients With Symptomatic Carotid Artery Occlusion at High Risk of Cerebral Ischemic Events
Klijn CJM, Kappelle LJ, van der Grond J, et al (Univ Med Ctr Utrecht, The Netherlands)
Stroke 31:3001-3007, 2000   1–50

Background.—The surgical management of patients with carotid artery occlusion (CAO) remains controversial. Noninvasive MR studies have assumed an important role in evaluation of cerebral ischemia, including MRI to determine the presence and extent of infarcts, MR angiography to measure arterial flow, and ¹H MR spectroscopy to study metabolic alter-

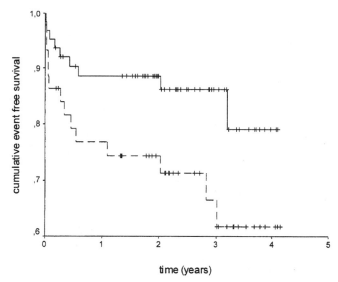

FIGURE 1.—Cumulative recurrent cerebral ischemic event-free survival in patients (n = 44) with a low (*dashed line*) and patients (n = 63) with a normal (*continuous line*) NAA/choline ratio; + indicates that a patient was censored. In 8 patients, the NAA/choline ratio could not be calculated. *Abbreviation: NAA, N*-Acetyl aspartate. (Courtesy of Klijn CJM, Kappelle LJ, van der Grond J, et al: Magnetic resonance techniques for the identification of patients with symptomatic carotid artery occlusion at high risk of cerebral ischemic events. *Stroke* 31:3001-3007, 2000. Reproduced with permission, Stroke Copyright 2000 American Heart Association.)

ations. The capability of these MR techniques to assess the risk of recurrent ischemic events in patients with symptomatic CAO was evaluated.

Methods.—The study included 115 patients with angiographically confirmed CAO causing transient or moderately disabling retinal or cerebral ischemia. Three MR findings were evaluated for their prognostic significance: the presence of a border-zone infarct on MRI; middle cerebral artery (MCA) flow ipsilateral to the CAO, as quantified by MR angiography; and metabolic ratios in the centrum semiovale ipsilateral to the CAO, as assessed by ^{1}H MR spectroscopy.

Results.—The MRI finding of a border-zone infarct and the flow rate in the MCA had no effect on the risk of recurrent cerebral ischemia. However, risk was significantly associated with the ratio of N-acetyl aspartate (NAA) to choline: the annual risk of recurrent, ipsilateral ischemic events was 16.0% for patients with a low NAA/choline ratio compared with 4.2% in those with a normal ratio; hazard ratio, 0.43 (Figs 1 and 2). The average NAA/choline ratio was higher by a mean of 0.25 for patients with retinal symptoms only compared with those with cerebral symptoms, and their recurrence risk was lower.

Conclusions.—In patients with symptomatic CAO, the risk of recurrent cerebral ischemic events is higher for patients with a low NAA/choline ratio, as assessed by ^{1}H MR spectroscopy. Recurrence risk is not predicted by the MRI finding of a border-zone infarct nor the MR angiographic measurement of MCA flow.

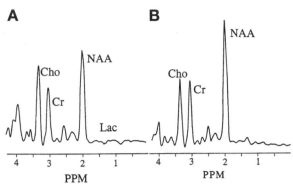

FIGURE 2.—¹H MR spectrum of the centrum semiovale ipsilateral to the carotid occlusion in a 62-year-old man with a low NAA/choline ratio who had a recurrent ipsilateral ischemic stroke 1 week after inclusion in the study (**A**) and in a 76-year-old man with a high NAA/choline ratio who did not have any recurrent cerebral ischemic events but had a fatal myocardial infarct 6 months after inclusion (**B**). *Abbreviations: Cho,* Choline; *Cr,* creatine; *La,* lactate. (Courtesy of Klijn CJM, Kappelle LJ, van der Grond J, et al: Magnetic resonance techniques for the identification of patients with symptomatic carotid artery occlusion at high risk of cerebral ischemic events. *Stroke* 31:3001-3007, 2000. Reproduced with permission, Stroke Copyright 2000 American Heart Association.)

▶ In providing biochemical information along with morphologic data, functional MR studies have generated a great deal of excitement in clinical medicine, particularly in the neurosciences. Functional MRI and spectroscopy has been used to define stroke recovery mechanisms with an aim of developing targeted therapies and to characterize the potential cause of schizophrenia, affective disorders, dementia, and anorexia nervosa. It is therefore of some interest to note that the risk of recurrent cerebral ischemic events among patients with symptomatic CAO is associated with a low NAA/choline ratio as determined by MR spectroscopy. NAA is considered a marker of neuron integrity and a low NAA level may be reflective of neuronal dysfunction due to limited cerebral perfusion. Likewise, increased choline levels may reflect membrane breakdown or a change in acetylcholine metabolism. Nevertheless, as this study serves to emphasize, the risk of recurrent cerebral ischemic events is quite high among patients who present with symptomatic CAO, even among those with a normal NAA/choline ratio. Thus, the use of MR to stratify symptomatic patients for intervention is limited. However, there may be an occasional patient with bilateral disease or with an atypical symptom complex where this information might be of some benefit.

E. L. Chaikof, MD

Determination of Wall Shear Rate in the Human Carotid Artery by Magnetic Resonance Techniques

Stokholm R, Oyre S, Ringgaard S, et al (Aarhus Univ, Denmark)
Eur J Vasc Endovasc Surg 20:427-433, 2000   1–51

Introduction.—In vitro evaluations of averaged geometrical flow models of the carotid artery bifurcation have revealed that low and oscillating wall shear stress occurs in those parts of the vessel circumference where atherosclerosis is likely to develop in humans. The precise geometry of the bifurcation demonstrates major individual variation with subsequent diverse hemodynamic and biomechanical characteristics. It is of theoretical and clinical importance to develop methods for noninvasive and precise determinations of the factors operating in vivo in that specific region. Wall shear rates around the circumference of the human carotid bifurcation were measured throughout the heart cycle in a prospective open trial.

Methods.—Wall shear rates were measured at the carotid bifurcation in 8 healthy volunteers using MR techniques with high resolution and individually adjusted velocity encoding for imaging and hemodynamic mapping. Wall shear stresses were determined assuming a constant value of 4 centiPoise.

Results.—Data relevant for postprocessing were obtained for all research subjects (Fig 4). The primary findings were: unidirectional wall shear rate waveforms and high wall shear rate (mean, $775s^{-1}$) at the flow divider; low wall shear rate (mean, $60s^{-1}$) and a high oscillation index with huge interindividual variation (mean, 85) at the lateral wall.

Conclusion.—Reported for the first time are in vivo data describing in detail the forces of the blood acting on the wall of the carotid bifurcation. These findings do not conflict with theories associating low and oscillating wall shear stress with the development of atherosclerosis.

▶ Cleverly applied, MR techniques can be used to obtain precise information on blood flow velocities in multiple tiny segments of the entire vascular lumen and to perform complex analyses leading to the in vivo determination of wall shear rates. This technique is vividly demonstrated in this article. Significant evidence suggests that there is a definite association between the precise site of atherosclerotic development and diminished shear stress in arterial systems. These authors speculate that the specific geometries of the carotid bifurcation may predispose to the development of atherosclerosis, again alerting the clinician to patients who may be at a particular risk for symptoms. As the authors modestly acknowledge, these are the first in vivo data on wall shear stress determination in the internal carotid artery in humans.

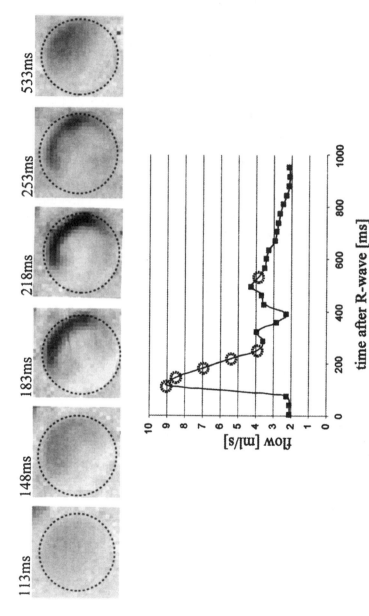

FIGURE 4.—Example of MR-velocity raw data in the internal carotid artery. Phase velocity images from different time points relative to the R-wave of the ECG, as visualized on the flow curve. Gray indicates zero velocity, darker is higher forward velocities, and brighter is higher backward (retrograde) velocities. (Courtesy of Stokholm R, Oyre S, Ringgaard S, et al: Determination of wall shear rate in the human carotid artery by magnetic resonance techniques. *Eur J Vasc Endovasc Surg* 20:427-433, copyright 2000 by permission of the publisher WB Saunders Company Limited London.)

Phosphorus 31 Nuclear Magnetic Resonance Spectroscopy Suggests a Mitochondrial Defect in Claudicating Skeletal Muscle

Pipinos II, Shepard AD, Anagnostopoulos PV, et al (Henry Ford Hosp, Detroit; Univ of Crete, Greece)
J Vasc Surg 31:944-952, 2000   1–52

Background.—Muscle bioenergetics has not been well characterized in patients with peripheral arterial occlusive disease (PAOD). It is believed that the primary cause of muscle dysfunction in claudication is an imbalance between oxygen supply and demand in the affected limb. The normal increase in blood flow needed by skeletal muscle during exercise is restricted by arterial occlusive disease, causing muscle ischemia and symptoms of tightness, cramping, and fatigue. However, there is growing evidence that impaired energy utilization may also contribute to the pathophysiology of PAOD. Studies have described morphologic defects, including hyperplasia, proliferation and ballooning of the cristae, and paracrystalline inclusions in the mitochondria of claudicating skeletal muscle. Recent studies have also demonstrated extensive damage to mitochondrial DNA in muscle biopsies taken from patients with claudication. It is possible that these changes in the structure and genetic fabric of mitochondria result in defects in mitochondrial function and are suggestive of the possibility of impaired energy utilization as a secondary cause of the muscle dysfunction that accompanies intermittent claudication. The investigation of muscle bioenergetics in vivo and noninvasively has been made possible by recent advances in nuclear MR spectroscopy (MRS). MRS was used in the measurement of the phosphate-rich compounds of muscle energy metabolism-adenosine triphosphate (ATP), adenosine diphosphate (ADP), phosphocreatine (PCr), and pH-in the noninvasive investigation of this hypothesis.

Methods.—Bioenergetics in the calf muscle were studied in 12 men with moderate claudication and 14 normal control subjects by means of phosphorus MRS (^{31}P MRS) evaluation and standard treadmill testing. Phosphocreatine and ADP recovery time constants (t.c.) and intracellular pH and ATP production via anaerobic glycolysis were determined during 3 exercise sessions. The results were then averaged and compared to known values obtained from a control population.

Results.—The end exercise intracellular pH and ATP glycolysis during the ^{31}P MRS in patients with PAOD did not differ from those values in control subjects, which demonstrated that the oxygen supply was not significantly reduced by the protocol exercise. The phosphocreatine and ADP recovery t.c. were significantly slower in the patients with PAOD compared with control subjects; however, no correlation was found between these measures of mitochondrial function and any treadmill parameter (Fig 1).

Conclusions.—^{31}P MRS demonstrated the first direct evidence of defective energy metabolism in the mitochondria of claudicating calf muscle cells. In patients with mild to moderate claudication, the defect appeared

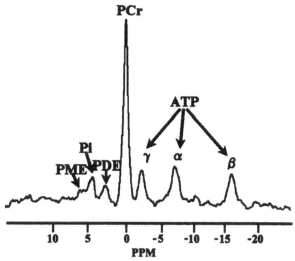

FIGURE 1.—³¹P spectrum collected from the calf muscle of a patient with moderate claudication. (Courtesy of Pipinos II, Shepard AD, Anagnostopoulos PV, et al: Phosphorus 31 nuclear magnetic resonance spectroscopy suggests a mitochondrial defect in claudicating skeletal muscle. *J Vasc Surg* 31:944-952, 2000.)

to be independent of both arterial flow and the severity of occlusive disease. These data, when viewed in light of the documented ultrastructural and DNA abnormalities in the mitochondria of claudicating skeletal muscle cells, are supportive of a secondary cause of muscle dysfunction in intermittent claudication.

▶ Many of us have suspected for years that claudication is undoubtedly not as simple as deprivation of oxygenated blood from exercising muscle. There must be more to it than that to explain the wide discrepancy in symptoms experienced by patients with similar degrees of arterial blockage. Morphologic alterations in muscle mitochondria have been noted for decades. These investigators present convincing evidence using a ³¹P MRS that there is a metabolic defect in the mitochondria of most claudicants. This defect appears to occur in most, but not all claudicants, and to be relieved with time after revascularization. Thus, available evidence suggests that ischemia induces chronic changes in mitochondrial morphology and function, and these ischemia-induced mitochondrial changes are the proximate cause of symptoms in patients who claudicate. This is interesting new information.

Platelet

Increased Platelet Aggregability During Exercise in Patients With Previous Myocardial Infarction: Lack of Inhibition by Aspirin

Hurlen M, Seljeflot I, Arnesen H (Ullevaal Univ, Oslo, Norway)
Thromb Res 99:487-494, 2000   1–53

Objective.—Platelet activation, blood coagulation, and fibrinogen increase after exercise. Platelet inhibitors are prescribed for patients with both stable and unstable coronary artery disease, but platelets can be activated by other pathways by agonists such as thrombin, epinephrine, and norepinephrine. The effects of a standardized exercise test on platelet aggregability, blood coagulation, and fibrinolysis were examined in patients in a stable phase after acute myocardial infarction (AMI).

Methods.—Three months after AMI, 40 patients (32 men), average age 60 years, were randomly assigned to receive daily 160 mg aspirin or warfarin (international normalized ratio, 2.0-2.5). Platelet function tests were performed on venous blood drawn before and after patients performed a fasting standard ergometer bicycle test. Hematocrit, platelet count, mean platelet volume (MPV), platelet aggregate ratio (PAR), plasma epinephrine, beta thromboglobulin (BTG), and plasma norepinephrine were measured. Hemostatic variables before and after exercise were compared statistically.

Results.—Hematocrit and platelet count increased significantly, MPV was unchanged, and BTG and PAR decreased significantly. Fibrinogen and plasma D-dimer decreased slightly. Serum D-dimer, tissue plasminogen activator, epinephrine, and norepinephrine increased significantly. Baseline PAR was significantly lower in the warfarin group than in the aspirin group (0.89 vs 1.00). Changes during exercise were similar for both groups, implying that aspirin did not completely prevent changes in platelet function. Both the warfarin and aspirin groups showed significantly reduced exercise PAR (0.75 vs 0.80) and BTG (22 vs 18 IU/mL) levels. Catecholamine levels increased similarly in both groups.

Conclusion.—Aspirin appears to have limited antithrombic activity during exercise in AMI patients. Its effect may be limited in all situations involving increased levels of catecholamines.

▶ This is worrisome information. Exercise induces an activation of platelets, probably related to catecholamines, which is not affected by aspirin. We have all heard increasingly the horror stories of apparently healthy people who dropped dead jogging. I suspect in a number of these cases the adverse event was related to thrombosis induced by catecholamine platelet activation unrelated to the presence of aspirin. (See also Abstract 1–54.)

A New Role for P-Selectin in Shear-Induced Platelet Aggregation

Merten M, Chow T, Hellums JD, et al (Univ of Texas Houston Med School; Rice Univ, Houston)
Circulation 102:2045-2050, 2000

Background.—The 140 kDa glycoprotein P-selectin is expressed on the surface of activated platelets. It is known to mediate rolling of platelets on endothelial cells. However, it is unknown whether P-selectin contributes to shear-induced platelet aggregation. An in vitro study was performed to examine the role of P-selectin in platelet aggregation in response to high and low shear stress.

Methods.—To simulate the in vivo conditions associated with arterial stenosis, platelets were exposed to pulsatile shear stress at 37°C. In the model, platelets were exposed to a single, 30-s pulse or to three 10-s pulses of high shear stress, 150 to 200 dynes/cm², followed by 4.5 min or 90 s of low shear stress, 10 dynes/cm². The same model was used to evaluate the effects of monoclonal anti-P-selectin antibodies on shear-induced platelet aggregation.

Results.—Pulsatile shear stress resulted in significantly greater platelet aggregation than low or high shear stress alone (Fig 3). Shear-induced platelet aggregation was reduced about 70% in response to anti-P-selectin antibodies. The effect of anti-P-selectin antibodies was especially strong for aggregation induced by the combination of high and low shear stress and was additive to the inhibitory effect of abciximab, the antiglycoprotein IIb/IIIa antibody. However, abciximab also inhibited shear-induced platelet aggregation at a temperature of 22°C, whereas anti-P-selectin had

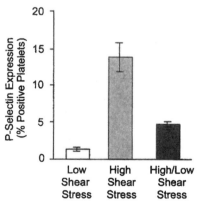

FIGURE 3.—P-selectin expression on platelets exposed to high, low, and combined shear stresses. Platelets were exposed to low shear stress (*open bar*), high shear stress (*shaded bar*), or combination of high shear stress and low shear stress (*solid bar*) in rotational viscometer at 37°C. Low shear stress or high shear stress alone increased P-selectin expression on platelets by 0.4% ± 0.2% or 12.8% ± 2.0%, respectively. When platelets were exposed to combination of high and low shear stress, P-selectin expression was increased by 3.8% ± 0.4%, significantly more than with low shear stress alone (n = 3, P < .001). (Courtesy of Merten M, Chow T, Hellums JD, et al: A new role for P-selectin in shear-induced platelet aggregation. *Circulation* 102:2045-2050, 2000.)

this effect only at 37°C. Platelets expressed shear-induced P-selectin only at the warmer temperature.

Conclusions.—This in vitro model suggests that pulsatile shear stress—similar to that present in arterial stenosis—leads to significantly greater platelet aggregation at 37°C than does monophasic shear stress. P-selectin may have a unique role in platelet aggregation separate from that of glycoprotein IIb/IIIa. P-selectin may be especially important in the development of thrombosis associated with atherosclerotic lesions.

▶ To state merely that platelet aggregation is a complex phenomenon grossly understates the issue. A complex series of events may induce activation of GBIIb/IIIa. This activated complex then appears to bind von Willebrand factor, which may act as a bridge between these receptors on adjacent platelets. Under low shear stress conditions, fibrinogen mediates the bridging of these complexes. These authors show here that in conditions of alternating high shear stress, followed by low shear stress, P-selectin has a role in platelet aggregation distinct from GBIIb/IIIa and may be of considerable importance in the initiation of thrombosis. These investigators speculate that P-selectin has an additive role in shear stress induced platelet aggregation with GBIIb/IIIa and that specific P-selectin antagonists may result in significant patient benefit under selected circumstances. I suspect they are correct.

Double-blind Study of the Safety of Clopidogrel With and Without a Loading Dose in Combination With Aspirin Compared With Ticlopidine in Combination With Aspirin After Coronary Stenting: The Clopidogrel Aspirin Stent International Cooperative Study (CLASSICS)
Bertrand ME, for the CLASSICS Investigators (Hôpital Cardiologique, Lille, France; et al)
Circulation 102:624-629, 2000   1–55

Introduction.—The combination of ticlopidine plus aspirin is associated with fewer hemorrhagic or peripheral complications compared with the conventional regimen of oral anticoagulant plus aspirin for patients undergoing coronary stenting. A full antiplatelet effect takes a few days because of the delayed onset of action of ticlopidine. Clopidogrel (Plavix/Iscover) is a new platelet adenosine diphosphate receptor antagonist that has a more potent antiaggregant effect than ticlopidine; it has a faster onset of action and does not cause the adverse events that limit the use of ticlopidine. The safety of clopidogrel (with or without a loading dose) plus aspirin was compared with that of ticlopidine plus aspirin for 1020 patients who had undergone successful coronary stenting.

Methods.—Patients in this multicenter, controlled, double-blind, parallel-group trial were randomly assigned to a 28-day treatment with either of the following regimens: (1) a 300 mg clopidogrel loading dose and 325 mg/d aspirin on day 1, followed by 75 mg/d clopidogrel and 325 mg/d aspirin; (2) 75 mg/d clopidogrel and 325 mg/d aspirin; or (3) 250 mg ticlopidine BID and 325 mg/d aspirin. The primary end points were the occurrence of major peripheral or bleeding complications, neutropenia, thrombocytopenia, or the early discontinuation of the study drug as the result of a noncardiac adverse event during the treatment phase.

Results.—Significant primary end point events occurred in 31 (9.1%) of patients in the ticlopidine group and 31 (4.6%) of patients in the combined clopidogrel group. The overall rates of major adverse cardiac events (cardiac death, myocardial infarction, target lesion revascularization) were low and similar among treatment groups (0.9%, 1.5%, and 1.2%, respectively, for the ticlopidine, clopidogrel, and the clopidogrel loading dose groups).

Conclusion.—The safety and tolerability of clopidogrel plus aspirin significantly exceeds that of ticlopidine plus aspirin. The 300-mg loading dose was well tolerated and did not result in higher risk of bleeding. Clopidogrel and ticlopidine had comparable efficacy in reducing cardiac events after successful stent placement.

▶ Several randomized trials have consistently shown that combination therapy with aspirin-ticlopidine is superior to heparin and warfarin in preventing subacute stent occlusion. Certainly, the dual antiplatelet approach has been more effective than the use of aspirin alone. Clopidogrel is a new platelet ADP receptor and appears to be more potent than ticlopidine and have a better safety profile. These investigators have concluded from this study of over 1000 patients undergoing coronary stent placement the safety and tolerability of clopidogrel plus aspirin is superior to that of ticlopidine plus aspirin. A real question in vascular surgery is going to become the use of combined antiplatelet agents. In a large majority of cases, we use simply aspirin or, occasionally, aspirin in combination with warfarin. The concept of using 2 antiplatelet drugs together is only beginning to emerge. Because clopidogrel and aspirin have distinctly different mechanisms of action, it does appear reasonable in certain extreme cases to combine them at the present time. If we ever develop a safe IIb/IIIa receptor blocker that can be given orally, perhaps that will become the single agent of choice.[1]

Reference

1. 2001 YEAR BOOK OF VASCULAR SURGERY, p 27.

Radiation

Inhibition of Restenosis With β-Emitting Radiotherapy: Report of the Proliferation Reduction With Vascular Energy Trial (PREVENT)

Raizner AE, Oesterle SN, Waksman R, et al (Baylor College of Medicine, Houston; Stanford Univ, Calif; Washington Hosp Ctr, Washington DC; et al)
Circulation 102:951-958, 2000   1–56

Background.—Animal studies demonstrated the possibility of reducing restenosis by intracoronary γ- and β-radiation. Clinical trials have yet to assess the effects of β-emitting radiation sources across a wide range of patients, including those with stents. A randomized controlled trial of intracoronary β-radiation therapy for patients undergoing various percutaneous coronary interventions was reported.

Methods.—The Proliferation Reduction With Vascular Energy Trial included 105 patients undergoing successful percutaneous transluminal coronary angioplasty. The lesions were de novo in 70% of cases and restenotic in 30%; treatment consisted of stenting in 61% of cases and balloon angioplasty in 39%. Intracoronary radiotherapy was performed with a β-emitting ^{32}P source wire. The source was implanted by means of an automated delivery unit and a source-centering mechanism (Fig 1). Patients were randomly assigned to receive no radiation (control) or a radiation dose of 16, 20, or 24 Gy to a depth of 1 mm within the arterial wall. Assessment included quantitative coronary angiography of the radiation target site and adjacent segments (Fig 3).

Results.—According to 6-month angiograms, the target site late loss index was 11% in patients receiving radiotherapy, compared with 55% in controls (Fig 4). This advantage was present in both patients with stents and those with balloon treatment, with similar benefit across the 3 radiation dose groups. Only 8% of radiation-treated patients had restenosis of 50% or greater at the target site, compared with 39% of controls. The restenosis rates at the target site plus adjacent segments were 22% and

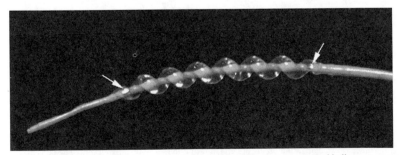

FIGURE 1.—The rapid-exchange centering balloon catheter incorporates a spiral balloon to center the source. Radio-opaque markers identify the radiation treatment zone (*arrows*). A closed lumen within the shaft serves as the conduit for the source wire, which is delivered by the source-delivery unit. (Courtesy of Raizner AE, Oesterle SN, Waksman R, et al: Inhibition of restenosis with β-emitting radiotherapy: Report of the Proliferation Reduction with Vascular Energy Trial (PREVENT). *Circulation* 102:951-958, 2000.)

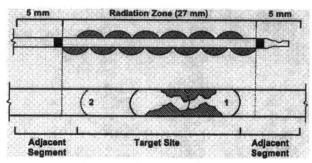

FIGURE 3.—Schematic diagram of defined segments on quantitative coronary angiography. Shown is an example of a balloon which was inflated in 2 different positions (numbers *1* and *2*) in the course of the procedure. The "target site" spans the length of these documented inflations. (Courtesy of Raizner AE, Oesterle SN, Waksman R, et al: Inhibition of restenosis with β-emitting radiotherapy: Report of the Proliferation Reduction with Vascular Energy Trial (PREVENT). *Circulation* 102:951-958, 2000.)

50%, respectively. Revascularization of the target site was required in 6% of the radiotherapy group versus 24% of the control group. However, patients receiving radiotherapy remained at risk for stenosis adjacent to the target site and for late thrombosis.

Conclusion.—This technique of intracoronary β-radiotherapy using a centered ^{32}P source effectively reduces the rate of restenosis after percuta-

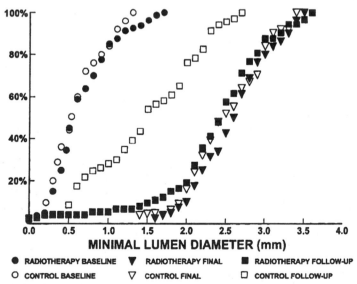

FIGURE 4.—The cumulative distribution curves of the minimal lumen diameter (MLD) before and after the index revascularization procedure and at 6-month follow-up angiography. The percentage on the vertical axis indicates the fraction of patients seen with an MLD equal to or smaller than a given value on the horizontal axis. The curves are similar for the radiofrequency and control groups before and after the procedure. However, at 6 months, the control patients had regressed toward preprocedure MLD values, whereas the radiotherapy patients remained close to the post procedure MLD curve. (Courtesy of Raizner AE, Oesterle SN, Waksman R, et al: Inhibition of restenosis with β-emitting radiotherapy: Report of the Proliferation Reduction with Vascular Energy Trial (PREVENT). *Circulation* 102:951-958, 2000.)

neous interventions. It is effective in patients who have undergone stent placement or balloon angioplasty. To achieve maximal benefit from intracoronary β-radiotherapy, new approaches are needed to reduce edge narrowing and late thrombotic events.

▶ Few topics in cardiology have attracted more attention in recent years than the use of radiation at sites of coronary angioplasty and stent insertion to minimize restenosis. The results reported in this article are rather typical. This β-emitting source achieved an admirable decrease in restenosis directly within the radiated site, but the findings were complicated by high evidence of restenosis immediately adjacent to the irradiated site, and by the lack of demonstration of a statistical decrease in major adverse clinical events in the radiated patients. In addition, I do not believe radiation therapy has been used long enough for us to fully appreciate potentially adverse events occurring at the site of radiation. I keep having the notion that using radiation to prevent restenosis is like using a large-gauge shotgun to kill a sparrow. While you may render the sparrow extremely dead, you may generate considerable collateral damage to the neighborhood. I strongly suspect we have not yet appreciated the magnitude of collateral damage associated with this nonspecific therapy.

Residual Plaque Burden, Delivered Dose, and Tissue Composition Predict 6-Month Outcome After Balloon Angioplasty and β-Radiation Therapy
Sabaté M, Marijnissen JPA, Carlier SG, et al (Thoraxcenter, Heartcenter, Rotterdam, The Netherlands; Daniel den Hoed Cancer Ctr, Rotterdam, The Netherlands)
Circulation 101:2472-2477, 2000   1–57

Background.—Endovascular radiation therapy is a promising new technique that is designed for the prevention of restenosis after percutaneous coronary intervention. The effectiveness of this technique has been proved in the treatment of in-stent restenosis, but the value of intracoronary irradiation in de novo coronary lesions has yet to be established. Radiation can be delivered to the coronary artery by catheter-based systems that use either γ-emitters or β-emitters. Long-term results may be influenced by absolute dose and by the homogeneity in dose distribution. The dose fall-off from β-emitters is more rapid than the fall-off from γ-emitters because of the short range of electrons. This difference in fall-off may result in a less homogeneous dose distribution during treatment of coronary segments with varying degrees of curvature, tapering, remodeling, and plaque extent. This inhomogeneity of dose distribution and anatomic aspects of the atherosclerotic plaque may affect the outcome of irradiated lesions after balloon angioplasty (BA). The influence of delivered dose and morphologic characteristics of coronary stenoses treated with β-radiation after BA was evaluated.

Methods.—Eighteen consecutive patients were treated according to the Beta Energy Restenosis Trial 1.5. The angioplasty site was irradiated with a β-emitting $^{90}SR/^{90}Y$ source. The irradiated areas were identified and volumetric assessment was performed by 3-dimensional intracoronary US imaging after treatment and again at 6 months. Tissue type, presence of dissection, and vessel volumes were assessed every 2 mm within the irradiated area. The minimal dose absorbed by 90% of the adventitial volume ($D_{v90}Adv$) was calculated in each 2-mm segment.

Results.—A total of 206 coronary subsegments were studied, and 55 were defined as soft, 129 as hard, and 22 as normal/intimal thickening segments. The increase in plaque volume was less in hard segments than in soft and normal/intimal thickening segments. $D_{v90}Adv$ was correlated with plaque volume at follow-up after a polynomial equation with linear and nonlinear components. Multivariate regression analysis identified plaque volume after treatment, $D_{v90}Adv$, and type of plaque as independent predictors of plaque volume at follow-up.

Conclusions.—Residual plaque burden, delivered dose, and tissue composition all have a significant effect on outcome at 6-month follow-up after β-radiation therapy and BA.

▶ Not surprisingly, these investigators found, using complex 3-dimensional methodology, that residual plaque burden, delivered radiation dose, and tissue composition all have important roles to play in the volumetric outcome 6 months after β-irradiation therapy and balloon angioplasty to first-time treated coronary lesions. Who can argue with this? I suspect before this is all over the type of radiation, the dose of radiation, the length over which the radiation is administered, and the type of lesion being treated, among other variables, will all assume increasing importance. In my opinion, we are now at the point of beginning to stick our toe in the water. We are going to have to learn much more about this potentially dangerous therapy before its use can be widely recommended.

Intracoronary γ-Radiation Therapy After Angioplasty Inhibits Recurrence in Patients With In-Stent Restenosis
Waksman R, for the Washington Radiation for In-Stent Restenosis Trial (WRIST) Investigators (Washington Hosp Ctr, Washington, DC; Erasmus Univ, Rotterdam, The Netherlands; Stanford Univ, Calif)
Circulation 101:2165-2171, 2000   1–58

Introduction.—In-stent restenosis after successful intracoronary stent implantation is an important clinical problem. It is primarily the result of neointimal tissue proliferation distributed either focally or diffusely over the entire length of the stent. Ionizing radiation has been shown to reduce neointimal formation within stents in animal models and in initial clinical trials. The effects of intracoronary γ-radiation versus placebo on clinical

TABLE 4.—Intravascular Ultrasound Results at 6 Months

| | WHC Core Lab | | Stanford Core Lab | | |
| | ^{192}Ir | Placebo | ^{192}Ir | Placebo | |
Variable	(n=54)	(n=57)	(n=37)	(n=38)	P
Change in mean stent CSA, mm^2	0.19±0.59	0.07±0.57	NA	NA	0.30
Change in mean luminal area, mm^2	0.61±1.64	1.97±1.58	0.18±0.91	1.87±1.75	0.0004
Change in mean minimal luminal CSA, mm^2	0.38±1.94	1.91±1.58	0.13±0.75	2.31±1.54	<0.0001
Change in volume of tissue growth, mm^3	3.13±38.43	54.98±60.13	2.16±19.17	50.0±69.3	<0.0001
Decrease in mean luminal volume, mm^3	7.87±42.08	56.37±65.19	NA	NA	<0.0001

Note: Values are mean ± SD. Values of *P* were calculated to the differences between placebo and ^{192}Ir for the Washington Hospital Center (WHC) core lab. CSA indicates cross-sectional areas. There were no statistically significant differences between the laboratories.

(Courtesy of Waksman R, for the Washington Radiation for In-Stent Restenosis Trial (WRIST) Investigators. *Circulation* 101:2165-2171, 2000.)

and angiographic outcomes were investigated in patients with in-stent restenosis.

Methods.—The study included 130 patients with in-stent restenosis who underwent successful coronary intervention and were randomly assigned to treatment with either intracoronary γ-radiation with ^{192}Ir (15 Gy) or placebo. Four independent core laboratories blinded to treatment protocols examined the angiographic and intravascular US end points of restenosis.

Results.—At 6-month follow-up, patients who received radiation therapy required significantly less target lesion revascularization and target vessel revascularization (9 [13.8%] and 17 [26.2%], respectively), compared with patients who received placebo (41 [63.1%] and 44 [67.7%], respectively). An increase in luminal dimensions and a regression in the neointimal tissue was observed at 6 months in 25 (53.2%) irradiated lesions (Table 4). The binary angiographic restenosis was significantly lower in patients who received irradiation versus those who received placebo (19% vs 58%). Freedom from major cardiac events was also significantly lower in irradiated patients versus those who received placebo (29.2% vs 67.7%).

Conclusion.—Intracoronary γ-radiation used as adjunctive therapy in patients with in-stent restenosis significantly diminishes both angiographic and clinical restenosis.

▶ This study convinces me that in-stent restenosis patients have much less restenosis at 6 months than do placebo treated patients. Remarkably, placebo patients had a 65% incidence of major coronary events compared with 30% in the radiation group, hardly the stuff dreams are made of. As noted in the preceding commentary, I am still having trouble putting this treatment in perspective. It is noteworthy that these investigators use γ-radiation as opposed to the β-radiation used by others.

Intracoronary β-Radiation Therapy Inhibits Recurrence of In-Stent Restenosis

Waksman R, Bhargava B, White L, et al (Washington Hosp Ctr, Washington DC)

Circulation 101:1895-1898, 2000   1–59

Background.—With regard to in-stent restenosis (ISR), the use of intracoronary γ-ionizing radiation (Ir-192) reduces angiographic late loss, binary restenosis, and the need to perform target lesion revascularization and target vessel revascularization. The safety and effectiveness of the β-emitter 90-yttrium were evaluated for prevention of recurrent ISR by a comparison of results with those seen in the placebo group in the Washington Radiation for In-Stent Restenosis Trial (WRIST).

Methods.—Percutaneous transluminal coronary angioplasty, laser angioplasty, rotational atherectomy, and/or stent implantation procedures were performed in 50 consecutive patients with ISR in native coronary vessels. After these procedures, a segmented balloon catheter was positioned and loaded with a 90-yttrium, 0.014-inch source wire (length, 29 mm) that delivered a dose of 20.6 Gy at a distance of 1.0 mm from the balloon's surface. Seventeen patients had lesions exceeding 25 mm in length that required manual stepping of the radiation catheter. The primary end point was the occurrence of major adverse clinical events (MACE) such as death or myocardial infarction or repeat target lesion revascularization at 6 months.

Results.—Delivery of the radiation was successful in all patients; the mean dwell time was 3.0 minutes. Ischemia forced fractionation of the dose in 11 patients. At 6 months, MACE had occurred in 17 patients. ISR was seen in 9 patients, and 14 had in-lesion restenosis. Both the MACE and angiographic restenosis findings were significantly less in the treated group than in those not treated in the WRIST study. The binary angiographic restenosis rate was 22%, the target lesion revascularization rate was 26%, and the target vessel revascularization rate was 34%.

Conclusions.—Patients with ISR may be treated successfully with intracoronary 90-yttrium β-radiation.

▶ Using a similar ISR model, but this time with β-radiation instead of γ-radiation, the same investigators described in the preceding abstract achieved equally good results. These investigators simply appear prone to get good results with intracoronary radiation no matter what the circumstances or what the radiation source. God love them.

Safety of Intracoronary γ-Radiation on Uninjured Reference Segments During the First 6 Months After Treatment of In-Stent Restenosis: A Serial Intravascular Ultrasound Study

Ahmed JM, Mintz GS, Waksman R, et al (Washington Hosp Ctr, Washington DC)
Circulation 101:2227-2230, 2000   1–60

Background.—In randomized placebo-controlled clinical trials, it has been shown that recurrent in-stent restenosis after primary catheter-based intervention can be reduced by adjunct brachytherapy. However, there are concerns about adverse effects that may result from brachytherapy, including late thrombosis, edge effects, formation of aneurysm, and premature atherosclerosis. The necessity for coverage of an entire treated area so that "geographical miss" and edge areas can be avoided and the limited selection of ^{192}Ir source lengths has led to the use of longer radioactive seed trains. The use of the longer seed trains has, in turn, resulted in exposure of angiographically normal reference segments to γ-irradiation. The effects of endovascular irradiation on uninjured reference segments during primary catheter-based treatment of restenosis were investigated.

Methods.—Patients who participated in the Washington Radiation for In-Stent restenosis Trial were treated by a conventional, catheter-based technique, then randomly assigned to receive either γ-irradiation (^{192}Ir) or a placebo (dummy seeds). Patients in whom the active (19 patients) or dummy seeds (19 patients) extended more than 10 mm proximal and distal to the in-stent restenosis were identified.

Results.—Serial external elastic membrane (EEM), lumen, and plaque and media (EEM—lumen) areas were measured by intravascular US every 1 mm over reference segments that were 5 mm long and 6 to 10 mm proximal and distal to the in-stent restenosis lesion. A similar increase was observed in the plaque and media area in the proximal and distal reference segments, not only in the ^{192}Ir patients but also in the placebo patients. In the ^{192}Ir patients, however, there was an increase in both the proximal and distal EEM areas, resulting in no changes in lumen area. In placebo patients, a decrease in the proximal reference EEM area, with no change in the distal reference EEM area, was observed and resulted in a decrease in lumen area.

Conclusion.—No evidence was found of an adverse effect of γ-irradiation on angiographically normal, uninjured reference segments in the first 6 months after treatment of in-stent restenosis.

▶ Dr Waksman reappears. In this variant of their preceding studies, the authors describe external elastic membrane areas by using intravascular US performed after radiation with γ-radiation. Predictably, they claim superiority for the radiation treatment group.

Endovascular Irradiation From β-Particle–Emitting Gold Stents Results in Increased Neointima Formation in a Porcine Restenosis Model

Schulz C, Niederer C, Andres C, et al (Technische Universität München; GSF-Forschungszentrum für Umwelt und Gesundheit, Neuherberg, Germany)

Circulation 101:1970-1975, 2000

1–61

Introduction.—Recent studies have demonstrated that ionizing radiation diminishes neointimal formation after balloon angioplasty and stent implantation in both experimental models of restenosis and first clinical trials. The dose distribution of a new β-particle-emitting radioactive gold stent and its dose-dependent vascular response in a coronary overstretch pig model were assessed.

Methods.—The study included 16 Gottingen Minipigs who underwent placement of 11 nonradioactive and 36 β-particle-emitting stents in the left anterior descending, left circumflex, or right coronary artery. The radio-

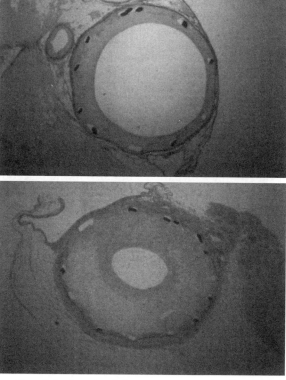

FIGURE 4.—van Gieson's elastica stains of pig coronary artery sections from control (**Top**) and 55-µCi [198]Au stent (**Bottom**) 12 weeks after implantation. Magnification × 25. (Courtesy of Schultz C, Niederer C, Andres C, et al: Endovascular irradiation from β-particle–emitting gold stents results in increased neointima formation in a porcine restenosis model. *Circulation* 101:1970-1975, 2000.)

active stents were implanted at mean 10.4, 14.9, 22.8, 35.8, and 55.4 µCi of ^{198}Au. At 3 months after implantation, the percent area of stenosis, neointimal thickness, neointimal area, and vessel injury were determined by quantitative histomorphometry.

Results.—For the various radioactivity levels indicated above, the mean lifetime radiation doses at 1-mm depth were 3.3, 4.7, 7.2, 11.4, and 17.6 Gy, respectively. No significant dose-response relationship was seen in the radioactive stents with respect to the percent area of stenosis, the mean neointimal thickness, or the mean neointimal area. Significantly less neointimal formation and less luminal narrowing was observed in the control stents compared with the β-particle-emitting stents (Fig 4). Multilinear regression analysis demonstrated that only the radioactivity level made a significant independent contribution to the degree of percent area stenosis.

Conclusion.—Neointimal formation in pigs is significantly increased by β-particle-emitting stents with ^{198}Au as the radioisotope. Doses of 3 to 18 Gy of low-dose-rate β-particle irradiation via endovascular stents caused pronounced luminal narrowing in the animal model at 3 months.

▶ Having achieved reasonable phase I results in humans, the radiation protocol has now been taken to the laboratory. Mini pigs received placement of nonradioactive or β-particle-emitting coronary stents and observations were carried out over time. Significantly lower neointimal formation and less luminal narrowing was seen in the control group than in the β-particle-emitting group. This is certainly information contrary to the mainstream and suggests that perhaps all is not well. Despite the multiple apologias pointing out the difference between animals and humans, we are left with disturbing information. I subscribe to the authors' suggestion that there is doubtless complex interaction between radiation dose, dose rate, and vessel wall cellular elements. I suspect we know a bit less about this than we may imagine.

Gene Therapy Enhances the Antiproliferative Effect of Radiation in Intimal Hyperplasia

Fortunato JE, Mauceri HJ, Kocharyan H, et al (Univ of Chicago)
J Surg Res 89:155-162, 2000   1–62

Background.—Intimal hyperplasia after vessel injury is associated with a transformation of vascular smooth muscle cells (VSMCs) from a quiescent state to a proliferative state. Ionizing radiation (IR) can attenuate the hyperplastic response of VSMCs but causes dose-related side effects such as medial and advential hemorrhage. Recent reports suggest that IR combined with radiosensitizing gene therapy can improve local tumor control in patients with cancer. A rabbit model was used to investigate whether IR in combination with radiosensitizing gene therapy can improve the inhibition of VSMCs and reduce intimal hyperplasia after arterial injury.

TABLE 1.—Comparison of Intimal-to-Medial Area and Thickness Ratios for
4 Sets of Animals

Histomorphometric Variable	Control	CD/5-FC	5 Gy IR	5 Gy IR + CD/5-FC
I/M area	0.37 ± 0.15	0.25 ± 0.08	0.19 ± 0.09*	0.18 ± 0.06*
I/M maximum thickness	0.61 ± 0.17	0.56 ± 0.12	0.47 ± 0.13†	0.41 ± 0.11†

Note: Results are expressed as mean ± standard deviation.
*P = .005.
†P = .007 compared with nonirradiated animals.
Abbreviations: CD/5-FC, Rabbits transfected with an adenoviral vector incorporated into the cytosine diaminase gene and subsequently injected with 5-fluorocytosteine; *5 GY IR*, animals exposed to ionizing radiation; *I/M*, intimal-to-medial.
(Courtesy of Fortunato JE, Mauceri HJ, Kocharyan H, et al: Gene therapy enhances the antiproliferative effect of radiation in intimal hyperplasia. *J Surg Res* 89:155-162, 2000.)

Methods.—The animals were 28 New Zealand White rabbits in which the entire length of the right common carotid artery was injured. Three of the 4 terminal internal and external branches were ligated to reduce flow and thus induce intimal hyperplasia. Seven of the animals were left untreated (controls). Another 7 animals were exposed to 5 Gy of IR at 24 hours. The remaining 14 animals were injected with an adenoviral vector incorporating the cytosine deaminase (CD) gene, then injected with 5-fluorocytosine (5-FC). CD converts 5-FC into 5-fluorouracil, a cytotoxic agent that disrupts DNA synthesis and causes cell death. Half of these animals received no other treatment (CD/5-FC group), whereas the other 7 were exposed to 5 Gy of IR at 24 hours (CD/5-FC + 5 Gy IR group). On day 14, arteries were harvested and intimal-medial (I/M) area and thickness ratios were determined. Immunohistochemical analysis was used to determine VSMC proliferative and apoptotic indexes.

Results.—Radiosensitizing gene therapy by itself did not have any effect on I/M area or maximal thickness compared with controls. However, compared with controls, IR with or without gene therapy caused a 50% reduction in I/M area and significantly attenuated I/M thickness (Table 1). In the 2 groups exposed to IR, I/M area and maximum thickness did not differ significantly in those who did or did not receive gene therapy. However, combining radiosensitizing gene therapy with IR caused a significant 70% reduction of the total number of proliferating VSMCs. There were 4.17 log-transformed cells/mm² in the animals exposed to IR only, compared with 2.97 log-transformed cells/mm² in the animals exposed to gene therapy and IR. VSMC apoptosis did not differ significantly among the 4 groups.

Conclusion.—Ionizing radiation, alone or in combination with radiosensitizing gene therapy, was effective in attenuating the intimal hyperplasia induced in these rabbits. The combination of IR with radiosensitizing gene therapy had a greater effect on the inhibition of VSMCs than IR alone, possibly because of selective killing of radioresistant S-phase VSMCs. Thus, IR plus radiosensitizing gene therapy may be a new strategy for controlling intimal hyperplasia after vessel wall injury.

► No effect was observed on intimal/medial area or thickness and the reduction of smooth muscle cell proliferation was modest at best; however, this is a rational approach that bears further evaluation. The potential to reduce dosage levels of radiation should certainly be welcome by the interventionalist and the use of a radiosensitizing agent might well reduce the high rates of "edge restenosis" that appear to be a limitation of intravascular radiation.

E. L. Chaikof, MD

Late Arterial Responses (6 and 12 Months) After ³²P β-Emitting Stent Placement: Sustained Intimal Suppression With Incomplete Healing
Farb A, Shroff S, John M, et al (Armed Forces Inst of Pathology, Washington, DC; Isostent Corp, Belmont, Calif)
Circulation 103:1912-1919, 2001   1–63

Background.—Previous studies of stent-based brachytherapy in rabbits have revealed decreases in neointimal growth at 3 months' follow-up. At the same time, delays in intimal healing suggest possible delay, rather than prevention, of intimal inhibition. The 6- and 12-month follow-up observations of β-emitting stents in the rabbit iliac artery were presented.

Methods.—Three-millimeter stents were placed in the normal iliac arteries of rabbits. The rabbits received either 6, 24, or 48 μCi β-emitting stents or nonradioactive control stents. The animals were killed for histologic evaluation after 6 or 12 months.

Results.—Compared with those of control stents, arteries with 24- and 48-μCi stents showed greater than 50% reduction in intimal growth and percentage of luminal stenosis. These higher-radioactivity stents were also associated with delayed intimal healing. Findings included persistent fibrin thrombus with nonconfluent matrix areas and incomplete endothelialization and increased intimal cellular proliferation. Twelve-month examination showed stent-edge restenosis—with associated intimal thickening and negative arterial remodeling—in the 24- and 48-μCi groups.

Discussion.—As in 3-month studies, β-emitting stents in rabbits continue to inhibit intimal growth at 6 to 12 months' follow-up. Long-term stent placement is also associated with delayed arterial healing, incomplete endothelialization, and edge restenosis.

► This report involves relatively long-term follow-up of β-emitting stent placement in the normal iliac arteries of rabbits and the comparison of their performance with that of control nonradioactive stents. The vessels were examined at 6 months and 1 year after placement, which are chronic times for animal models but not especially generous outcome measures for humans. There was observed an inhibition of intimal thickening in the "in stent" region, but that was associated with a prolonged inhibition of reendothelialization with fibrin-coated luminal surface and an increased inflammatory response in the arterial wall. The radiation-emitting stents were also found to induce increased negative remodeling at the edges of the stent and also increased intimal thickening at those sites.

The net effect of adding β-emission to stents is not clear. It is certainly desirable to achieve inhibition of intimal thickening after stenting; however, the other effects of β-emission, as mentioned above, may result in a net deleterious result. This article contains a good discussion of the concepts and competing goals that need to be considered, which is important as the future role of this technique in the treatment of human vascular disease is unclear.

M. A. Golden, MD

The 90-Day Coronary Vascular Response to 90Y-β Particle-Emitting Stents in the Canine Model
Taylor AJ, Gorman PD, Hudak C, et al (Walter Reed Army Med Ctr, Washington, DC; Isostent Inc, Belont, Calif; Armed Forces Inst of Pathology, Washington, DC)
Int J Radiat Oncol Biol Phys 46:1019-1024, 2000   1–64

Background.—Vascular brachytherapy is being studied for use in the prevention of restenosis. Preclinical trials using continuous, low-dose-rate ^{32}P β-emitting stents have produced disappointing results. A more promising brachytherapy device might be the ^{90}Y β-emitting stent, which offers a shorter half-life with a higher dose rate. The dose-response characteristics of a ^{90}Y β-emitting stent in a dog model, including the device's effects on neointimal formation, were assessed.

Methods.—A total of 77 ^{90}Y β-emitting coronary stents were placed in 26 normal dogs. The Fischell BX stainless steel stents had a length of 15 mm. Radioactivity ranged from 4.5 to 32 µCi, with nonradioactive stents used as control units. Histologic responses to stent placement were assessed after 3 months.

Results.—No significant differences were observed in luminal stenosis and neointimal area associated with control stents and low-activity ^{90}Y stents (4.5 and 8 µCi). The highest-activity stents (16 and 32 µCi) produced significant adverse effects. The 16 µCi stents were associated with total occlusion in 28% of placements and a 40% increase in neointimal area compared with the same variables with nonactive stents. Only the 16 and 32 µCi stents were associated with incomplete healing and a trend toward reduced neointimal cell density.

Conclusions.—These experiments suggest that ^{90}Y β-emitting coronary stents have an adverse impact on neointimal formation. High-activity-level stents are associated with a high rate of occlusion. Healing remains incomplete 90 days after stent placement, suggesting prolonged recovery from radiation injury. Despite their unique characteristics, ^{90}Y β-emitting stents are not a promising alternative vascular brachytherapy device.

▶ In contrast to the prior protocol, these investigators used ^{90}Y-β-emitting stents instead of P-β-emitting stents. These were implanted in the coronary arteries of dogs. Stent dosage in the range of 16 and 32 μCi were associated with total occlusions, incomplete neointimal healing, and a trend toward reduced neointimal cell density. These investigators conclude that these β-emitting stents have an adverse effect on neointimal formation at high activity levels. Once again, a drop of rain falls.

Prevention of Intimal Hyperplasia by Single-Dose Pre-insertion External Radiation in Canine-Vein Interposition Grafts
Ulus AT, Tütün U, Zorlu F, et al (Türkiye Yüksek Ihtisas Hosp, Ankara, Turkey; Hacettepe Univ, Ankara, Turkey; Gülhane Askeri Tip Akademisi, Ankara, Turkey; et al)
Eur J Vasc Endovasc Surg 19:456-460, 2000   1–65

Introduction.—Intimal hyperplasia can cause stenosis at the site of vascular or endovascular interventions and can compromise the vessel lumen by ultimate failure of the reconstruction. External beam or intravascular radiation therapy after vascular reconstructions has been shown to decrease intimal hyperplasia in numerous experimental and clinical trials. The efficacy of single-dose preinsertion gamma radiation of vein grafts for the prevention of intimal hyperplasia was studied in a canine model.

Methods.—Twelve mongrel dogs were randomized to either radiotherapy or no radiotherapy after insertion of femoral artery interposition grafts with internal jugular veins. Animals in the radiotherapy group received a single dose of cobalt-60 radiation at 14 Gy. The control group received no radiation. At 6 weeks after graft insertion, the vein grafts were fixed by pressure-perfusion, then harvested for histomorphometric analysis. Quantitative data on anastomotic stenosis were determined using Gilman parameters after cross-sectional image analysis.

Results.—Neointima formation was significantly reduced in vein grafts treated with radiation. The mean Gilman parameter was 1.09 for the control group and 0.65 for the radiotherapy group. All vein grafts in the radiotherapy group had a reduced amount of intimal and cellular infiltration.

Conclusion.—The amount of intimal hyperplasia in vein grafts was diminished using single-dose external preinsertion gamma radiation in a canine model.

▶ External radiation applied to veins being placed in an arterial graft in mongrel dogs was calculated to mimic the dose used in the coronary studies performed in humans. After 6 weeks, greatly decreased neointimal formation was noted in the radiated grafts compared with the control grafts. These authors enthusiastically conclude that this treatment reduces the rate of intimal hyperplasia, and I suspect they are correct. Unfortunately, their animal model did not permit detection of any potential adverse effects.

Stroke

Reduction of Stroke Events With Pravastatin: The Prospective Pravastatin Pooling (PPP) Project

Byington RP, for the PPP Investigators (Wake Forest Univ, Winston-Salem, NC; Univ of Texas, Houston; St Francis Hosp, Roslyn, NY; et al)
Circulation 103:387-392, 2001   1–66

Background.—Lipid-lowering therapy has been found to reduce the risk of coronary heart disease, but its effect on the risk of having a stroke has not been evaluated. The Prospective Pravastatin Pooling Project analyzed stroke data from 3 trials evaluating pravastatin (1 focused on primary prevention and 2 on secondary prevention) that have recently concluded.

Methods.—The 3 trials were large, placebo controlled, and randomized and included 19,768 patients over 102,559 person-years of follow-up. Each focused on the effectiveness of 40 mg/d of pravastatin. The objectives of this study were to gauge the effect of pravastatin on the total stroke rate for the 3 trials combined and for the combination of the 2 secondary trials, Cholesterol And Recurrent Events (CARE) and Long-term Intervention with Pravastatin in Ischemic Disease (LIPID).

Results.—During the approximately 5 years evaluated, 598 participants had fatal or nonfatal strokes; more than half of them were from the LIPID study, although LIPID and CARE shared similar placebo group event rates. The fewest strokes and the lowest rate of strokes were found in the West Of Scotland Coronary Prevention Study (WOSCOPS). For each trial, the risk of a stroke was reduced, although the CI for the hazard ratio from WOSCOPS was large. In the CARE trial, risk reduction ranged from 4% to 52% (average, 32%), and in the LIPID trial, the reduction ranged from 0% to 33% (average, 18%). The combined risk reduction of all 3 trials was 20% (range, 7%-32%). For 1 stroke to be averted, according to the CARE/LIPID database, 588 patients would have to be treated annually; according to WOSCOPS data, for 1 stroke to be averted would require treatment of 3333 patients per year. The cumulative fatal/nonfatal stroke curves (Fig 1) reveal that event rates in the WOSCOPS primary prevention trial were consistently lower than those in the secondary trials. Stroke rates were generally consistent in the secondary trials in terms of the long-term absolute risk of a stroke and the benefit derived from the use of pravastatin. Pravastatin produced obvious and consistent reductions in stroke rates in all subgroups, and no interaction was apparent between any specific baseline characteristic and any treatment group assignment.

Conclusions.—Among these patients with documented coronary disease, the risk of a stroke was reduced by using pravastatin, regardless of the lipid value. Nonfatal nonhemorrhagic stroke reduction was the principal factor.

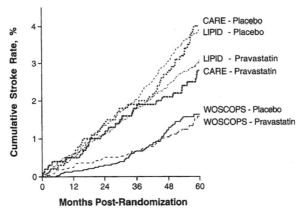

FIGURE 1.—Occurrence of any stroke (fatal or nonfatal) by clinical trial and treatment assignment. *Abbreviations: CARE,* Cholesterol And Recurrent Events trial; *LIPID,* Long-term Intervention with Pravastatin in Ischemic Disease trial; *WOSCOPS,* West Of Scotland Coronary Prevention Study. (Courtesy of Byington RP, for the PPP Investigators: Reduction of stroke events with pravastatin: The Prospective Pravastatin Pooling (PPP) Project. *Circulation* 103(3):387-392, 2001.)

▶ A series of observations have combined to make this a particularly interesting study. Without question, stroke continues to be a massive problem in the Western world, being the second leading cause of death in the Americas and killing over 160,000 persons per year. About 600,000 persons have a stroke annually in the United States. Stroke is obviously a leading cause of disability and increased health care costs. In recent years, a number of studies have indicated that the statin therapy associated with lipid lowering has markedly reduced the risk of coronary heart disease. The investigators reporting here did a pooled analysis of 3 recently completed event trials by using the specific drug pravastatin. These trials indicated that the use of pravastatin was associated with a 22% reduction in total strokes and a 25% reduction in nonfatal strokes. This led the authors to conclude that pravastatin reduces the risk of stroke over a wide range of lipid values among patients with documented coronary disease. The benefit is seen primarily as a reduction in nonfatal, nonhemorrhagic strokes. Here we have another indication for the increasing use of statins in clinical practice.

Effects of Tissue Plasminogen Activator for Acute Ischemic Stroke at One Year

Kwiatkowski TG, for the National Institute of Neurological Disorders and Stroke Recombinant Tissue Plasminogen Activator Stroke Study Group (Long Island Jewish Med Ctr, New Hyde Park, NY; et al)
N Engl J Med 340:1781-1787, 1999   1–67

Introduction.—The 2-part National Institute of Neurological Disorders and Stroke (NINDS) Recombinant Tissue Plasminogen Activator Stroke investigation of 1995 determined that patients treated with tissue plasmi-

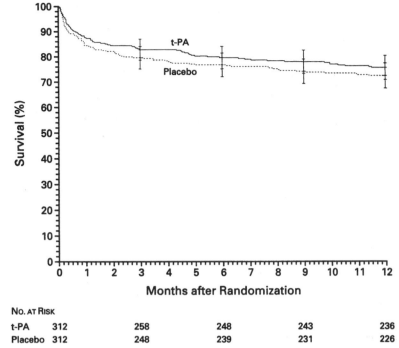

NO. AT RISK

t-PA 312	258	248	243	236
Placebo 312	248	239	231	226

FIGURE 2.—Kaplan-Meier estimate of survival after stroke in the tissue plasminogen activator (*t-PA*) and placebo groups. *I-bars* represent the standard errors of the point estimates of survival at 3, 6, 9, and 12 months. (Reprinted by permission of *The New England Journal of Medicine* from Kwiatkowski TG, for the National Institute of Neurological Disorders and Stroke Recombinant Tissue Plasminogen Activator Stroke Study Group: Effects of tissue plasminogen activator for acute ischemic stroke at one year. *N Engl J Med* 340:1781-1787, 1999. Copyright 1999, Massachusetts Medical Society. All rights reserved.)

nogen activator (t-PA) within 3 hours after symptom onset of an acute ischemic stroke were about 30% more likely to have minimal or no disability at 3 months after the stroke when compared with patients who received placebo. The mortality rate at 3 months was similar for both groups. It was not known whether the benefit seen at 3 months could be sustained over a longer follow-up. Six- and 12-month outcomes were examined.

Methods.—The 624 patients with stroke who were evaluated during the NINDS trial had been randomly assigned to receive either t-PA or placebo. Outcome data were collected during the 12-month period after the stroke. The primary outcome measure was a favorable outcome, which was defined as minimal or no disability. The Barthel Index, modified Rankin Scale, and the Glasgow Outcome Scale were used. The treatment effect was determined using a global statistic.

Results.—The t-PA group was favored over the placebo group by the global statistic, as determined by an intention-to-treat analysis for the combined results of the 2 parts of the trial at 6 and 12 months. Patients treated with t-PA were at least 30% more likely to experience minimal or no disability at 12 months, compared with patients treated with placebo. There were no significant between-group differences in mortality at 12 months (Fig 2). There was no association between the type of stroke at baseline and treatment in terms of long-term response. The rate of recurrent strokes at 12 months was similar in the 2 groups.

Conclusion.—During the 12-month follow-up, patients with acute ischemic strokes treated with t-PA within 3 hours after symptom onset were more likely to experience minimal or no disability compared with patients who received placebo. This suggests that patients treated with t-PA have a sustained benefit.

▶ This is a follow-up report on the NINDS Recombinant Tissue Plasminogen Activator Stroke Study. Six hundred twenty-four patients with new stroke were assigned to t-PA or placebo within 3 hours of stroke onset and monitored for 12 months. At both 6 and 12 months with intention to treat analysis, the odds ratio for a favorable outcome was 1.7 at both time intervals compared with placebo. The patients treated with t-PA were at least 30% more likely to have minimal or no disability at 12 months than were the placebo treated patients. I believe this substantially confirms the favorable effect of t-PA when it can be started within 3 hours of the onset of symptoms of an acute ischemic stroke. Interestingly, there was no difference in overall mortality between those receiving t-PA and those receiving placebo. Now, of course, the problem continues to be our ability to get patients entered into t-PA treatment within the 3-hour window of opportunity. In most settings, this has proven extremely difficult.

Retrograde Venous Perfusion With Hypothermic Saline and Adenosine for Protection of the Ischemic Spinal Cord
Parrino PE, Kron IL, Ross SD, et al (Univ of Virginia, Charlottesville)
J Vasc Surg 32:171-178, 2000   1–68

Background.—A spinal cord injury leading to paraplegia is a common complication of surgery on the thoracic artery. Numerous pharmacologic and mechanical protective strategies have been tried, but none is widely accepted. The capability of retrograde venous perfusion-cooling of the spinal cord with use of hypothermic saline and adenosine to protect against thoracic artery occlusion in swine was evaluated.

Methods.—Left thoracotomy was performed in anesthetized and intubated adult domestic swine. After division of the accessory hemiazygous vein, a catheter was placed distally and the aorta was clamped at the left subclavian artery. Seven animals, comprising the experimental group, underwent infusion of a 4°C saline/adenosine solution into the accessory hemiazygous vein. In the 7 animals in the control group, no venous catheter was placed. The aortic clamp and venous catheter were removed after 30 minutes, at which time the chest was closed. At 24 hours postoperatively, hindlimb activity was graded in a blind fashion on the Tarlov

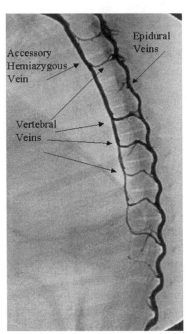

FIGURE 2.—Lateral view of chest. Contrast is present in the accessory hemiazygous vein, vertebral veins, and epidural veins. (Courtesy of Parrino PE, Kron IL, Ross SD, et al: Retrograde venous perfusion with hypothermic saline and adenosine for protection of the ischemic spinal cord. *J Vasc Surg* 32:171-178, 2000.)

scale (from 0 = complete paralysis to 5 = normal gait). Rectal temperatures and blood pressures were measured as well. In addition, 2 more groups were studied to evaluate the effects of retrograde venous perfusion on spinal cord temperature.

Results.—At the 24-hour evaluation, the mean Tarlov score was 1.7 in the control group versus 4.9 in the intervention group; mean decreases in spinal cord temperature were 4.05°C versus 0.58°C, respectively. Rectal temperatures were similar between groups. None of the animals developed arrhythmias or episodes of hypotension. Additional angiographic studies were performed to document retrograde venous perfusion of the spinal cord (Figs 2 and 3).

Conclusions.—This animal model suggests that retrograde venous perfusion-cooling of the spinal cord, with use of hypothermic saline and adenosine, as a new approach to preventing spinal cord ischemia during clamping of the thoracic aorta is effective. The retrograde perfusion technique has several potential advantages: it does not require access to the paraspinal spaces, induce systemic hypothermia, or require perfusion via diseased vessels.

▶ The search continues for a technique that will provide spinal cord protection during occlusion of the thoracic aorta, as in thoracoabdominal aneurysm

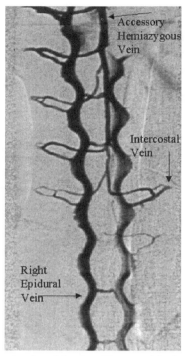

FIGURE 3.—Anterior-posterior view of the chest. (Courtesy of Parrino PE, Kron IL, Ross SD, et al: Retrograde venous perfusion with hypothermic saline and adenosine for protection of the ischemic spinal cord. *J Vasc Surg* 32:171-178, 2000.)

repair. The technique of retrograde venous perfusion has received some support in human studies of acute hypothermic arrest during complicated arch repairs. These investigators, using an animal model, have perfused the hemiazygous vein in the chest, with a cold solution of normal saline and adenosine at the rate of 16.65 mL/min during 30 minutes of thoracic aortic occlusion. The perfused animals had a markedly improved hind leg neurologic function compared with the placebo animals. I, of course, have no idea if this technique will be applicable in patients, although the authors believe it will be. It is interesting to make a list of the techniques recommended to minimize spinal cord injury during thoracoabdominal surgery. We have settled on spinal cord drainage and the use of narcan. We also put in a temporary right ax-fem bypass before performance of thoracotomy. We have no experience with hypothermic spinal canal perfusion, nor with retrograde venous perfusion as advocated in this article. Without question, the sporadic occurrence of spinal cord injury during thoracoabdominal surgery remains a devastating problem. I am glad the number of patients we see with thoracoabdominal aneurysms is small.

Vascular Biology

Accelerated Replicative Senescence of Medial Smooth Muscle Cells Derived From Abdominal Aortic Aneurysms Compared to the Adjacent Inferior Mesenteric Artery

Liao S, Curci JA, Kelley BJ, et al (Washington Univ, St Louis)
J Surg Res 92:85-95, 2000   1–69

Introduction.—Abdominal aortic aneurysms (AAAs) are correlated with aging and atherosclerosis. Current data indicate that the degradation of medial elastin has an important role in aneurysmal dilatation and that collagen degradation is ultimately responsible for aneurysm rupture. The degenerative process in AAAs is partly characterized by depletion of medial smooth muscle cells (SMCs), suggesting that generalized aging and SMC senescence represent potential mechanisms contributing to aneurysmal degeneration. It is not known whether SMCs from AAA tissue demonstrate a difference in proliferative capacity compared with SMCs from nonaneurysmal vessels or to what extent these differences may be caused by aging alone or other patient-specific factors. These issues were investigated by a comparison of aneurysmal wall tissue with nondiseased arterial tissue.

Methods.—Aneurysmal wall tissues were collected from 15 patients undergoing AAA repair. A segment of the adjacent (nonaneurysmal) inferior mesenteric artery (IMA) of each patient was used as a control. Paired AAA- and IMA-derived SMC strains were collected by explant techniques; their proliferative capacities were compared during serial passage in culture.

Results.—Sustainable SMC cultures were produced from all IMA explants and from 9 of the 15 AAAs ($P < .05$). The interval needed to achieve primary explant growth was significantly longer for AAAs than IMAs (16.4 vs 6.4 days). The interval was not related to patient age, gender, or aneurysm size. The AAA-derived SMCs seemed larger and rounder, compared with the corresponding IMA-derived culture; their maximal proliferation was significantly decreased by 44.2% in 5 pairs. Serum-stimulated [^{3}H]thymidine uptake in AAA-derived SMCs was also significantly diminished by 54.9% in 5 pairs. Flow cytometry showed no differences in SMC viability, apoptosis, or necrosis. The IMA-derived SMCs continued to proliferate beyond passage 20 during serial subculture; all AAA-derived SMCs developed replicative senescence by passage 12.

Conclusion.—Along with having a distinct morphologic appearance in culture and a limited in-vitro lifespan, AAA-derived SMCs demonstrate a reduced proliferative capacity, compared with SMCs from the adjacent IMA. These differences reveal an intrinsic alteration in SMC growth capacity independent of age alone. Tissue-specific processes leading to accelerated replicative senescence might be responsible for increasing the selective medial SMC depletion seen in AAAs.

▶ SMCs from an aneurysm demonstrate a diminished proliferative capacity compared with smooth muscle cells taken from the adjacent Inferior mesenteric artery in this interesting study. Hypotheses abound as to why aneurysm cells may have a diminished proliferative capacity in subsequent tissue culture. It is interesting to note that cells from the aorta which became aneurysmal and cells from the inferior mesenteric artery certainly had a similar embryologic origin. These cell populations clearly experienced different circumstances from that point on. The authors of this article speculate basically that the aneurysm cells have "used up" their replicative potential, whereas the IMA cells have not. Perhaps. For now, I am willing to accept without further explanation their observation that SMCs taken directly from an infrarenal AAA have diminished proliferative potential.

Localization of Matrix Metalloproteinase 2 Within the Aneurysmal and Normal Aortic Wall

Crowther M, Goodall S, Jones JL, et al (Leicester Royal Infirmary, England)
Br J Surg 87:1391-1400, 2000   1–70

Background.—Recent studies suggest that matrix metalloproteinase (MMP)-2 plays a key role in the development of abdominal aortic aneurysms (AAA). Smooth muscle cells from AAAs produce more MMP than control cells. The cell membrane-bound enzyme membrane type 1 MMP (MT1-MMP) is the major activator of the MMP-2 proenzyme in vivo. Arterial tissues from patients with AAAs were studied to examine production of the MMP-2–MT1-MMP–tissue inhibitor of metalloproteinase (TIMP)-2 system.

Methods.—Immunohistochemistry, in situ hybridization, and in situ zymography were performed to analyze production and expression of MMP-2, TIMP-2, and MT1-MMP proteins in samples of arterial tissue from 4 patients with AAAs. Samples from 4 normal controls were studied for comparison.

Results.—Both aneurysm and control tissues expressed all components of the MMP-2–TIMP-2–MT1-MMP system. Enzyme expression was found mainly in the medial tissues, co-localized with medial smooth muscle cells. Also, in normal and aneurysmal tissues, gelatinolytic activity was localized to elastin fibers.

Conclusions.—The study demonstrates MT1-MMP within the media of the arterial wall in both normal and aneurysmal tissues. This finding may explain the activation of MMP-2 in AAAs. The results strengthen the hypothesis that the MMP-2–TIMP-2–MT1-MMP enzyme system plays a key pathogenic role in AAA.

▶ These investigators suggest that MMP-2 may have a central role in aneurysm production. MMP-2 is activated in the complex fashion by a cell membrane-bound enzyme named MT1-MMP. In studying human aneurysmal tissue, they found both the MMP-2 and its activator present in the aneurysmal wall. Perhaps MMP-2 is going to prove to be an important substance in the production of aortic aneurysms.

Endothelial Cell Response to Different Mechanical Forces

Azuma N, Duzgun SA, Ikeda M, et al (Yale Univ, New Haven, Conn)
J Vasc Surg 32:789-794, 2000   1–71

Introduction.—The mechanism by which vascular cells sense and respond to external force has not been clearly defined. Endothelial cells (ECs) are exposed to the physical forces caused by blood flow. Systemic and local abnormalities of mechanical forces have been implicated in several pathologic events (including atherosclerosis and intimal hyperplasia) and may even be involved in the arterialization and development of anastomotic intimal hyperplasia of vein grafts. The EC signaling pathway in response to cyclic strain and shear stress was examined in cultured bovine aortic ECs.

Methods.—The ECs were seeded on flexible collagen I-coated silicone membranes to analyze the effect of cycle strain. The membranes were deformed with a 150 mm Hg vacuum at 60 cycles/min for up to 120 min. To compare the effect of shear stress, ECs from the same batch as used in the strain experiments were seeded on collagen I-coated silicone sheets. The ECs then underwent 10 dyne/cm^2 shear with a parallel flow chamber for up to 120 min. Activation of the mitogen-activated protein kinases was examined by ascertaining phosphorylation of extracellular signal-regulated kinase (ERK), c-jun N-terminal kinase (JNK), and p38 with immunoblotting.

Results.—Cyclic strain and shear stress activated ERK, JNK, and p38. Both these factors activated JNK with a similar temporal pattern and magnitude and a peak at 30 min. Shear stress caused a more robust and rapid activation of ERK and p38 compared with cyclic strain.

Conclusion.—Different mechanical forces caused differential activation of mitogenic-activated protein kinases. It is possible that there are different mechanoreceptors in ECs to detect the different forces or alternative coupling pathways from a single receptor.

▶ This very artificial study, with the use of the standard New Haven model, grew ECs on silicone membranes, and these cells were then subjected to a variety of cyclic strains, as well as of varying shear forces. The investigators specifically assessed the ability of these forces to induce phosphorylation of extracellular signaling of related kinases. The fact that different mechanical forces appeared to induce differential activation of mitogen-activated protein kinases is about what one would expect. The authors suggest, and I suspect quite accurately, that there are probably a variety of mechanoreceptors in endothelial cells detecting different forces, which result in differential activation of signaling mechanisms. It is an article of faith that a blood vessel is an organ and that ECs are remarkably complex. We are just beginning to scratch the surface in our understanding of mechanoreceptors. While we are beginning to learn some of the things mechanoreceptors seem to do, we have yet to fully characterize the mechanoreceptors themselves. I suspect this will occupy another generation of vascular wall investigators.

The Plasma Level of Matrix Metalloproteinase 9 May Predict the Natural History of Small Abdominal Aortic Aneurysms: A Preliminary Study
Lindholt JS, Vammen S, Fasting H, et al (Aarhus Univ, Denmark)
Eur J Vasc Endovasc Surg 20:281-285, 2000   1–72

Objective.—The decision to operate on abdominal aortic aneurysms (AAA) is based on size, but AAA less than 5 cm in diameter have an annual 0.5% rupture rate. Because increased elastase and matrix metalloproteinases MMP2 and MMP9 have been found in AAA, systemic measurements of these proteinases and their inhibitors may predict the natural history of aneurysms and improve patient selection for surgery or conservative management.

Methods.—Of 4404 men, aged 65 to 73 years, invited in 1994 to participate in a random screening, 3344 (76%) attended and 141 (4.2%) had AAAs. Serum and plasma samples in a random group of 36 men were analyzed for S-α_1-antitrypsin; S- and P-matrix metalloproteinase 2 (MMP2) and P-MMP9; S and P-tissue-inhibitor-metalloproteinases 1 and 2 (TIMP1 and 2); S-elastin-peptides; and S-procollagen III-N-terminal propeptide (PIINP) concentrations with enzyme-linked immunosorbent assay. Aneurysm size and average annual expansion rates were compared for concentrations above and below the median assay concentrations.

Results.—Plasma and serum levels of elastase complexes, MMP2 levels, and total MMP/total TIMP were not associated with AAA size or expansion, and PIINP-propeptide concentrations were not associated with expansion, but α_1-antitrypsin levels were significantly related to AAA expansion, P-MMP2 levels were significantly associated with both size and expansion, and systemic S-elastin peptide concentrations were predictive of expansion.

Conclusion.—P-MMP9, S-elastin peptides and P-α_1-antitrypsin were significantly related to initial aneurysm size and to annual expansion.

▶ Interestingly, in this study the major inhibitor of elastase complexes, namely, α_1-antitrypsin, was significantly associated with the expansion of small aneurysms, as was the plasma level of MMP-9. This study was simplistic and was a shotgun approach analyzing a variety of things in patients with small aneurysms to see which might fall out in a positive fashion. I consider this at best a hypothesis-seeking exercise. Nonetheless, the fact that α_1-antitrypsin and MMP-9 did appear related to aneurysm expansion is in itself an important observation and suggests the basis for a number of future studies.

Plasma MMP-9—A Marker of Carotid Plaque Instability

Loftus IM, Naylor AR, Bell PRF, et al (Leicester Univ, England)
Eur J Vasc Endovasc Surg 21:17-21, 2001   1–73

Background.—The atherosclerotic process can be broken down into phases, and each phase may be mediated by enzymes called matrix metalloproteinases (MMPs), which are the principal physiologic controls for the extracellular matrix. These MMPs are activated by limited proteolysis and may be associated with specific disease states in which tissue degradation is a key feature. MMP-2 is associated with vascular smooth muscle cells and is found in increased quantities in plaque. Plaques susceptible to rapidly occurring disruption show induction and activation of MMP-9 in smooth muscle cells and inflammatory macrophages. MMP-9 levels are 4 times higher in the most unstable plaques. The association of higher levels of MMPs in the peripheral blood of individuals with various disorders (eg, cancer, arthritis, and acute coronary syndromes) has led to speculation that MMPs may be a marker for patients at risk of rapidly occurring plaque disruption. Plasma levels of the major MMPs and of the tissue inhibitors of MMP (TIMPs) in patients who were undergoing carotid endarterectomy were evaluated for any characteristics that would distinguish individuals with spontaneous particulate embolization, the most sensitive indicator of plaque instability.

Methods.—Seventy consecutive patients undergoing carotid endarterectomy were evaluated with use of a sandwich enzyme immunoassay to ascertain plasma levels of MMP-1, MMP-2, MMP-3, MMP-9, TIMP-1, and TIMP-2. Transcranial Doppler (TCD) was used to monitor the patients preoperatively and during the dissection phase of the operation for

TABLE 2.—The Concentrations (ng/mL, Median [iqr]) of the Major
MMP and TIMP Subtypes Excluding MMP-9

	Emboli Positive $n = 21$	Emboli Negative $n = 49$
MMP-1	4.6	5.4
	(4.4-6.4)	(3.3-6.4)
MMP-2	991	921
	(787-1088)	(719-1088)
MMP-3	10.0	10.2
	(7.3-14.4)	(7.3-14.1)
MMP-1/TIMP-1	2.9	2.2
complex	(1.7-4.1)	(0.4-4.7)
TIMP-1	249	254
	(182-362)	(182-351)
TIMP-2	499	532
	(469-583)	(475-584)

Note: There were no significant differences between the groups.
Abbreviations: MMP, Matrix metalloproteinases; *TIMP*, tissue inhibitor of MMP.
(Reprinted from Loftus IM, Naylor AR, Bell PRF, et al: Plasma MMP-9—a marker of carotid plaque instability. *Eur J Vasc Endovasc Surg* 21(1):17-21, copyright 2001 by permission of the publisher W B Saunders Company Limited London.)

the purpose of identifying any who had spontaneous particulate embolization.

Results.—Twenty-one patients had spontaneous particulate embolization, and their plasma levels of MMP-9 were significantly higher than those found in patients who did not have embolization. None of the other MMP or TIMP plasma concentrations correlated with this finding (Table 2).

Conclusions.—Increased plasma levels of MMP-9 were associated with significant carotid stenoses that led to spontaneous particulate embolization. None of the other MMPs or TIMPs were found to differ between those patients with and without embolization. Thus, MMP-9 may be a marker for identifying plaque instability or other serious situations that require urgent intervention.

▶ The authors have found an association between increased plasma MMP-9 levels and carotid embolic events as detected by transcranial continuous wave Doppler in patients with significant carotid arterial occlusive disease who are undergoing surgery. They conclude that plasma MMP-9 levels may be useful in stratifying patients for high risk of embolization. It is not clear whether the source of the MMP-9 is the carotid plaque, or the distal organ after embolization, or alternatively from another source that correlated well with the embolization noted by transcranial Doppler.

Having a marker of high risk for symptomatic embolic events would be very valuable for patient management. MMP-9 may be such a marker, although many patients with embolic events were not found to have elevated plasma MMP-9. Just as we use measurements of several blood lipid moieties to assess the lipid risk for development of cardiovascular disease, it may require a combination of markers—possibly including MMP-9—to more clearly define the risk of plaque rupture and induction of clinical events. Larger studies would also need to confirm this work before it would be useful clinically.

M. A. Golden, MD

Direct Proinflammatory Effect of C-Reactive Protein on Human Endothelial Cells
Pasceri V, Willerson JT, Yeh ETH (Univ of Texas, Houston; Univ of Texas Health Sciences Ctr, Houston; Texas Heart Inst, Houston)
Circulation 102:2165-2168, 2000   1–74

Objective.—Acute-phase reactant C-reactive protein (CRP) is a risk factor for atherosclerosis and coronary heart disease. The effects of CRP on vascular cells have not been tested. The effects of CRP on the expression of adhesion molecules by human endothelial cells were tested in human umbilical vein endothelial cells (HUVECs) and human coronary artery endothelial cells.

Methods.—Endothelial cells were incubated with human CRP, and expression of vascular cell adhesion molecule (VCAM-1), intercellular adhesion molecule (ICAM-1), and E-selectin were detected by flow cytometry.

Results.—In unstimulated HUVECs, CRP (10 µg/mL) induced a 10-fold increase in expression of ICAM-1 and a significant expression of VCAM-1 at 24 hours and a significant expression of E-selectin at 6 hours. Unstimulated human coronary artery endothelial cells expressed significant levels of ICAM-1, no VCAM-1, and low levels of E-selectin that were increased only modestly by increases in CRP concentration up to 100 µg/mL. The proinflammatory effect of CRP was dependent on serum, whereas interleukin-1β induced adhesion molecule expression in the absence of serum.

Conclusion.—CRP induces adhesion molecule expression in the presence of serum at levels frequently found in high-risk patients.

▶ CRP is emerging as a marker of atherosclerosis not only of the coronary arteries but also of the peripheral arterial tree.[1] This study suggests not only that CRP can be elevated in response to an inflammatory state, but that CRP itself has a proinflammatory effect on human endothelial cells. So is CRP the chicken or the egg? Or maybe it is the chicken and the egg!

A. N. Sidawy, MD

Reference

1. Ridker PM, Stampfer MJ, Rifai N: Novel risk factors for systemic atherosclerosis: A comparison of C-reactive protein, fibrinogen, homocysteine, lipoprotein (a), and standard cholesterol screening as predictors of peripheral arterial disease. *JAMA* 285:2481-2485, 2001.

Increased Amount of Type III pN-Collagen in Human Abdominal Aortic Aneurysms: Evidence for Impaired Type III Collagen Fibrillogenesis
Bode MK, Soini Y, Melkko J, et al (Univ of Oulu, Finland)
J Vasc Surg 32:1201-1207, 2000   1–75

Objective.—Abdominal aortic aneurysms (AAAs) are characterized by destruction of aortic wall elastin and collagen that results in vessel dilatation and decreased distensibility that ultimately leads to rupture. The collagen content of the vessel wall is thus a measure of the net effects of synthesis and degradation. Antibodies against the aminoterminal propeptides of type I (PINP) and type III (PIIINP) procollagens were used to determine the distribution of these structural domains of collagens in the walls of AAAs, in aortoiliac occlusive disease, and in healthy aortas.

Methods.—Aminoterminal PINP and PIIINP procollagens and aminoterminal telopeptide of type III collagen (IIINTP) were determined in full-thickness longitudinal strips of the anterior wall of the infrarenal aorta from 19 consecutive patients (4 women), aged 59 to 79 years, with AAAs and in aneurysm specimens from 9 cadavers (3 women), aged 40 to 71 years. The amount of maturely cross-linked type III collagen fibrils was determined.

Results.—PINP, PIIINP, and IIINTP antigens were found in diseased aortas. Only IIINTP was found in healthy aortas. PINP was strongly localized in the intimal layer; PIIINP was found mostly in the medial layer. IIINTP was strongly positive in the adventitial and medial layers of the AAAs. Cross-linked type III collagen was most abundant in the medial layer of AAAs.

Conclusion.—Type III collagen synthesis appears to be enhanced in AAAs, particularly in the medial layer. PINP collagen was found in abundance in the intimal layer of AAAs, where atherosclerotic lesions develop.

▶ This report further supports the contention that collagen metabolism in the aortic wall is abnormal in aortic aneurysm disease. By immunohistochemistry, the authors noted increased amounts of type III procollagen and also cross-linked type III collagen in the aortic media in aortas of patients with AAA compared with healthy persons and with patients with aortoiliac occlusive disease. This increased amount of the procollagen and crosslinked form of type III collagen suggests that not only the quantity of collagen, but also the degree of organization and the integrity of collagen fibril formation may be critically important in preventing the formation of aneurysms. As this work demonstrates, aortic wall homeostasis is a complex process. It endeavors to balance the synthetic, degradative, and organizational processes in the wall to withstand the continuous and powerful attempt by physical forces and biologic processes to disrupt the vessel wall integrity.

M. A. Golden, MD

VEGF$_{121}$- and bFGF-Induced Increase in Collateral Blood Flow Requires Normal Nitric Oxide Production
Yang HT, Yan Z, Abraham JA, et al (Univ of Missouri-Columbia; Scios Inc, Sunnyvale, Calif)
Am J Physiol 280:H1097-H1104, 2001   1–76

Background.—Rat experiments have shown that the angiogenic proteins basic fibroblast growth factor (bFGF and FGF-2) and vascular endothelial growth factor 121 (VEGF$_{121}$) each enhance the collateral-dependent blood flow after bilateral femoral artery ligation. The effect of nitric oxide synthase inhibition on bFGF- or VEGF$_{121}$-induced blood flow expansion was investigated.

Methods.—After bilateral ligation of the femoral arteries in male Sprague-Dawley rats, the animals received tap water or tap water plus non-N^G-nitro-L-arginine methyl ester (L-NAME). Each group was subdivided into 3 groups: vehicle, bFGF, or VEGF$_{121}$. Growth factors were given by intra-arterial infusion with osmotic pumps on days 1 through 14. On day 16, maximal collateral blood flow was assessed.

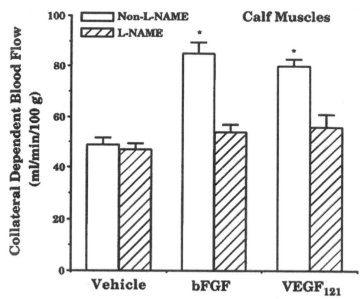

FIGURE 1.—Collateral-dependent blood flow to calf muscle (gastrocnemius-plantaris-soleus muscle group) during treadmill running. Data are expressed as means ±SE. *Asterisk* indicates significant difference from non-N^G-nitro-L-arginine methyl ester (L-NAME) vehicle group and L-NAME groups ($P < .001$). *Abbreviations:* VEGF, vascular endothelial growth factor; *bFGF*, basic fibroblast growth factor. (Courtesy of Yang HT, Yan Z, Abraham JA, et al: VEGF$_{121}$- and bFGF-induced increase in collateral blood flow requires normal nitric oxide production. *Am J Physiol* 280:H1097-H1104, 2001. Copyright, The American Physiological Society.)

Findings.—The administration of L-NAME for 18 days increased systemic blood pressure. In the absence of L-NAME, collateral-dependent blood flows to the calf muscles were higher in the VEGF$_{121}$ and bFGF subgroups than in the vehicle subgroup. For animals with nitric oxidase synthase inhibition by L-NAME, blood flows to the calf muscles were about the same among subgroups and did not differ from blood flow in the non–L-NAME vehicle subgroup (Fig 1).

Conclusion.—Normal nitric oxide production appears to be essential for the increased vascular remodeling induced by exogenous bFGF or VEGF$_{121}$ in a rat model of peripheral arterial insufficiency. A blunted endothelial nitric oxide production may temper vascular remodeling in response to these growth factors.

▶ Few substances in the field of vascular biology have attracted more interest in recent years than bFGF and VEGF, both potent angiogenic proteins that appear capable of inducing vascular remodeling to improve collateral blood flow. It is interesting to recollect that angiogenesis defines the sprouting of new capillaries from existing capillaries, while the enlargement of existing vessels is a process termed arteriogenesis. Using a rat model, these investigators found that the favorable blood flow–enhancing effect of either of these substances was eliminated by blocking nitric oxide production by the administration of L-NAME, a substance that totally blocks the synthesis of nitric oxide. Indeed, in this experiment, L-NAME inhibited the increased flow suggested by microsphere studies after VEGF and bFGF administration. I am forced to conclude that nitric oxide appears essential for whatever it is that results in the increased isotope counts in tissue after growth factor administration. Are these new blood vessels? I have no idea.

VEGF Gene Delivery to Myocardium: Deleterious Effects of Unregulated Expression
Lee RJ, Springer ML, Blanco-Bose WE, et al (Univ of California, San Francisco; Stanford Univ, Calif)
Circulation 102:898-901, 2000   1–77

Background.—Vascular endothelial growth factor (VEGF) potently stimulates angiogenesis and has been used via various modes to improve blood flow in patients with ischemic myocardium. Transient methods of delivery have been tested, but the effects of VEGF expressed continuously via myoblast-mediated delivery were investigated.

Methods.—Eleven immunodeficient mice were implanted subdiaphragmatically with primary murine myoblasts that expressed both the murine VEGF gene and the β-galactosidase (β-gal) gene from a retroviral promoter. A control group of 12 mice received the same number of myoblasts that expressed only the β-gal gene. Mice that survived 14 to 16 days were killed; their hearts were studied histologically.

Results.—Failure to thrive was noted in all 11 mice by the 13th day, and 5 died between 8 and 15 days after implantation. The control mice had no deaths or complications. The 6 surviving experimental mice and the 12 controls had successful implantation of the myoblasts, as noted by a positive β-gal reaction product. All experimental mice had vascular tumors that resembled hemangiomas in the myocardium receiving the VEGF myoblasts, and cells expressing β-gal were present. On immunohistochemical assessment, abundant endothelial nitric oxide synthase and CD31 were found in the lesion, which is consistent with endothelial cells being present.

Conclusions.—Both failure to thrive and the formation of vascular tumors derived from endothelial cells complicated the continuous expression of VEGF. Thus, VEGF expression must be closely monitored when used for therapeutic angiogenesis.

▶ New is not necessarily *improved* and more not always *better*. The effect of intracoronary administration of recombinant VEGF protein has been limited, and its short circulating half-life, reduced bioavailability, hypotensive effects, and the potential for undesirable angiogenic responses in non-target tissues has supported local drug delivery strategies with the use of a gene therapy approach. Thus, the transplantation of muscle cells expressing angiogenic proteins is an attractive method for the repair of ischemic muscle, but these authors clearly demonstrate that unregulated overexpression of VEGF leads to the formation of vascular tumors. Thankfully, current clinical trials continue to use transient modes of VEGF expression, based on expression from plasmid DNA or adenoviral vector. Whether therapeutic angiogenesis will have a role in clinical practice remains to be seen. However, I suspect that the road to determine appropriate routes, protein combinations, dosage levels, and clinical populations that will have greatest benefit from angiogenic therapy will be a long one. I wonder if the pharmaceutical industry has the stomach to persist.

E. L. Chaikof, MD

Direct Evidence for Cytokine Involvement in Neointimal Hyperplasia
Rectenwald JE, Moldawer LL, Huber TS, et al (Univ of Florida, Gainesville)
Circulation 102:1697-1702, 2000   1–78

Background.—The inflammatory cytokines tumor necrosis factor-α (TNF-α) and interleukin-1 (IL-1) act to stimulate expression of adhesion molecules, in addition to stimulating production of other proinflammatory cytokines. In vitro studies have shown that TNF-α and IL-1 also affect the migration and proliferation of vascular smooth muscle cells. The impact of endogenous TNF-α and IL-1 on low shear stress–induced neointimal hyperplasia (NIH) was examined in an in vivo study of mice.

Methods and Results.—A model of low shear stress in the patent, ligated common carotid artery in mice was used. This model has previously been demonstrated to lead to remodeling and NIH. The ligated arteries showed mRNA for both TNF-α and IL-1α, based on the results of reverse transcriptase–polymerase chain reaction assays. These cytokines were absent in normal arteries. In TNF−/− mice without functional TNF-α, neointimal area was reduced 14-fold, compared with wild-type control mice. Neointimal area was reduced 7-fold in p80 IL-1 type I receptor (IL-1RI) knockout mice. The common carotid arteries of TNF−/− mice showed no IL-1α mRNA, but the arteries of IL-1RI knockout mice did express TNF-α mRNA. The low shear stress–induced fibroproliferative response was increased in mice overexpressing membrane-bound TNF-α but not producing soluble TNF-α.

Conclusions.—This in vivo model supports the involvement of TNF-α and IL-1 in low shear stress–induced NIH. In addition, the results suggest that NIH can develop independent of soluble TNF-α. The results raise the possibility of treatments specifically directed against TNF-α and IL-1 to reduce NIH.

▶ I fully agree with the authors; they did provide a "direct" evidence to the involvement of TNF-α and IL-1α in the development of the intimal hypoplastic lesion in response to low sheer stress. Over the last few years there has been a plethora of information regarding control of the hyperplastic process in animal models. I am waiting for the day when control of this process is effectively achieved in humans.

A. N. Sidawy, MD

Integrin-Mediated Mechanotransduction Requires Its Dynamic Interaction With Specific Extracellular Matrix (ECM) Ligands
Jalali S, del Pozo MA, Chen K-D, et al (Univ of California, San Diego, La Jolla; Scripps Research Inst, La Jolla, Calif; Univ of California, Riverside)
Proc Natl Acad Sci U S A 98:1042-1046, 2001   1–79

Background.—The molecular mechanism by which integrins mediate mechanotransduction has not been established. The role of integrins in transducing fluid shear stress into intracellular signals in vascular endothelial cells was investigated.

Methods and Findings.—Experiments were performed on human umbilical vein epithelial cells. Shear stress activates integrins in endothelial cells plated on substrates containing the cognate extracellular matrix (ECM) ligands. Preventing new integrin-ECM ligand interactions by blocking the integrin-binding sites of ECM ligands or conjugating the integrins to immobilized antibodies eliminated the shear stress–induced mechanotransduction, as indicated by integrin-Shc association.

Conclusion.—Integrins play a crucial role in transmitting the mechanically initiated signals into the cell to trigger the intracellular signal transduction pathways for the modulation of gene expression and cellular functions. Integrins perform this role through their specific and dynamic connections with ECM ligands.

▶ In a simple but elegant study, these investigators demonstrate that endothelial cells require the dynamic formation of new integrin-ligand interactions to sense mechanical stimuli and initiate intracellular signals that control gene expression and cellular function. I have always wondered how this line of research might lead to new pharmacotherapeutics directed at reducing lesion formation. Mechanically sensitive control elements appear to be ill defined, nonspecific, or vary from gene to gene. Perhaps there is a small glimmer of hope that modulating the dynamics of integrin-ligand bindings might form a rational drug design strategy to limit the maladaptive effects of hemodynamic forces.

E. L. Chaikof, MD

IFN-γ Action in the Media of the Great Elastic Arteries, a Novel Immunoprivileged Site

Dal Canto AJ, Swanson PE, O'Guin AK, et al (Washington Univ, St Louis)
J Clin Invest 107:R15-R22, 2001   1–80

Introduction.—Infection of medial smooth muscle cells with γ-herpesvirus 68 (γHV68) produces severe chronic vasculitis that is confined to the great elastic vessels. A new animal model of chronic viral vasculitis restricted to the great elastic arteries has been created. This model of IFN-γ receptor-deficient mice infected with doses of γHV68 was used to assess the role of IFN-γ within the vasculature to help understand chronic inflammatory diseases of the great vessels.

Findings.—The persistence of disease in the greater elastic arteries was: a) caused by inefficient clearance of viral infection from the site, compared with other organs and other vascular sites; and b) related to failure of T cells and macrophages to enter the virus-infected elastic media. These results reveal the immunoprivilege of the media of the great elastic arteries. It was determined that IFN-γ acted on somatic cells during acute infection to hinder the establishment of medial infection and on hematopoietic cells to determine disease severity at the site. This immunoprivileged elastic media may offer a site for persistence of pathogens or self-antigens, thus predisposing the patient to chronic vascular disease, a process regulated by IFN-γ actions on both somatic and hematopoietic cells.

Conclusion.—The tropism of γHV68 for the media of the elastic arteries during chronic infection was caused by failure of the immune response to effectively clear the virus from the elastic media, despite effective clearance of other vascular sites and other organs. This may have significant implications for understanding immune responses contributing to controlling chronic inflammatory diseases of the great vessels.

▶ This remarkable article suggests that the body's immune system functions less efficiently in the elastic media of the great vessels than in small vessels or the adventitia of great vessels or visceral organs. This may be the explanation for the localization of chronic vasculitis to the media of the great elastic arteries. There appears to be a failure of T cells and macrophages to efficiently enter this area and, in fact, this leads these authors to conclude that the media of these arteries may be an immunoprivileged site. This certainly may have great significance for certain clinical syndromes, such as perhaps Kawasaki disease and giant-cell arteritis.

Left Ventricular Electromechanical Mapping to Assess Efficacy of phVEGH$_{165}$ Gene Transfer for Therapeutic Angiogenesis in Chronic Myocardial Ischemia

Vale PR, Losordo DW, Milliken CE, et al (St Elizabeth's Med Ctr, Boston; Tufts Univ, Boston)
Circulation 102:965-974, 2000   1–81

Introduction.—The NOGA system is a novel strategy of catheter-based electromechanical assessment of myocardial perfusion that uses electromagnetic field sensors to combine and integrate real-time information from percutaneous intracardiac electrograms acquired at several endocardial locations. Thirteen consecutive patients with chronic myocardial ischemia underwent NOGA electromechanical mapping (EMM) before and 60 days after gene transfer (GTx) of naked DNA encoding for the 165-amino acid isoform of vascular endothelial growth factor (phVEGF$_{165}$).

Methods.—Eight patients were male. The mean patient age was 60.1 years. All patients had chronic stable angina caused by angiographically documented coronary artery disease. All patients had failed conventional therapy with drugs, percutaneous transluminal coronary angioplasty, or coronary artery bypass grafting. Patients were treated with phVEGF$_{165}$, which was administered during surgery by direct myocardial injection during a minithoracotomy.

Results.—Foci of ischemic myocardium were observed on left ventricular EMM by preserved viability correlated with an impairment in linear local shortening. Myocardial viability, defined via unipolar and bipolar voltage recordings of 5 or more and 2 or more mV, respectively, was not significantly altered after GTx. Analysis of linear local shortening in areas of myocardial ischemia showed significant improvement after (vs before) phVEGF$_{165}$ GTx (15.26% vs 9.94%; P = .004). The area of ischemic myocardium was consequently decreased from 6.45 cm^2 before GTx to 0.95 cm^2 after GTx (P = .001).

These findings were in agreement with improved perfusion scores determined by single-photon emission CT-sestamibi myocardial perfusion scans recorded at rest (7.4 before GTx vs 4.5 after GTx; P = .009) and after pharmacologic stress (12.8 before GTx vs 8.5 after GTx; P = .047). Patients reported significant decreases in anginal episodes per week (48.1 vs 2.0; P < .0001) and in weekly consumption of nitroglycerin tablets (55 vs 1.9; P < .0001). The mean duration of exercise (Bruce protocol exercise tolerance testing) rose from 272 to 453 seconds (P = .001) up to 180 days after GTx.

Conclusion.—The EMM findings provide objective evidence that phVEGF$_{165}$ GTx enhances perfusion of ischemic myocardium. It is possible that GTx may successfully rescue foci of hibernating myocardium.

▶ By using a complex EMM system based on intracardiac electrograms acquired at multiple locations, these investigators, at least one of whom is a major owner of the pharmaceutical start-up company manufacturing the agent, purport to show that intracardiac injection of naked plasmid DNA encoding for VEGF produced objective improvement in myocardial performance at 60 days. In addition to experiencing clinical improvement in angina, the patients also were found to have increased exercise tolerance on the treadmill that persisted up to 180 days. Left ventricular ejection fraction did not significantly change.

Basic Fibroblast Growth Factor Increases Tissue Factor Expression in Circulating Monocytes and in Vascular Wall
Corseaux D, Meurice T, Six I, et al (Centre Hospitalier Régional Universitaire, Lille, France; Yale Univ, New Haven, Conn)
Circulation 101:2000-2006, 2000   1–82

Background.—Basic fibroblast growth factor (bFGF) can promote re-endothelialization with functional endothelium after balloon injury or induced atherosclerosis, but it may also activate tissue factor (TF), which may be instrumental in thrombogenesis and angiogenesis, with negative connotations. This study assessed whether giving bFGF induced TF expression by monocytes and vascular cells in rabbits.

Methods.—Sixteen New Zealand White rabbits ate standard rabbit food and were randomly assigned to receive 3-week treatment with either placebo or bFGF (2.5 µg twice weekly). Sixteen others were fed a cholesterol-increasing diet before random assignment to the same 2 groups. Immunohistochemical assay with a monoclonal anti-rabbit TF antibody

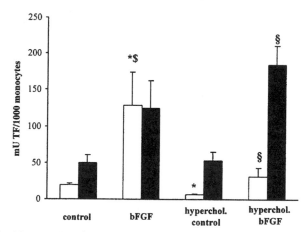

FIGURE 1.—Monocyte tissue factor (*TF*) expression in control basic fibroblast growth factor (*bFGF*), hypercholesterolemic control, and hypercholesterolemic bFGF rabbits. *Open bars* represent mononuclear cells cultured without endotoxin; *solid bars,* mononuclear cells cultured with endotoxin (5000 EU/mL). Results are expressed as milliunits of TF/1000 monocytes. *Asterisk* indicates *P* < .05 versus control group. *Section mark* indicates *P* < .005 versus hypercholesterolemic control group. *Dollar sign* indicates *P* < .05 versus hypercholesterolemic bFGF group. (Courtesy of Corseaux D, Meurice T, Six I, et al: Basic fibroblast growth factor increases tissue factor expression in circulating monocytes and in vascular wall. *Circulation* 101:2000-2006, 2000.)

was used to evaluate TF expression in mononuclear cells from arterial blood and aortic sections.

Results.—In both the normal and the hypercholesterolemic rabbits, bFGF administration increased monocyte TF expression (Fig 1). Further increase occurred when monocytes were stimulated by endotoxin in vitro. Hypercholesterolemic rabbits had lower TF expression than normal rabbits, but in the vascular wall, bFGF induced only a weak TF expression in the rabbits with high cholesterol levels but a strong response in normal rabbits.

Conclusion.—Circulating monocytes are incited to dramatically increase TF expression when bFGF is given. Normal rabbits also have a strong response in the vascular wall, but in rabbits with high cholesterol levels, the response is less vigorous.

▶ We are only beginning to understand the complex interrelation between many vascular wall substances. We are beginning to learn that there seems to be a light side and a dark side to almost everything. For example, bFGF, which may have the most desirable effect of inducing angiogenesis, may also activate less desirable substances. This publication convinces me that bFGF administration significantly upregulates tissue factor expression in both monocytes and in the vascular wall. TF is a potent activator of blood coagulation, and its abnormal presence could lead to thrombosis. In various complicated ways, TF also appears to interact in angiogenesis and vascular endothelial growth factor production. I suppose we must remember the old adage: Beware of what you ask for, you may get it. It is entirely possible that the angiogenesis factors will have far-ranging effects in addition to any basic effects they may or may not have on producing tiny new blood vessels.

The Response of Adult Human Saphenous Vein Endothelial Cells to Combined Pressurized Pulsatile Flow and Cyclic Strain, In Vitro

Tsukurov OI, Kwolek CJ, L'Italien GJ, et al (Massachusetts Gen Hosp, Boston; Harvard Med School, Boston)
Ann Vasc Surg 14:260-267, 2000   1–83

Background.—Several in vitro studies have examined the effects of isolated biomechanical forces on vascular wall cells. However, none of these studies have examined the response to simultaneous application of pressure, flow, and tensional deformation. Autogenous greater saphenous veins are the standard conduit for peripheral and coronary artery bypass grafting. The response of adult human saphenous vein endothelial cells (HVECs) to combined pressurized pulsatile flow and cyclic strain was examined.

Methods.—Adult HVECs were cultured in a compliant tubular device and subjected to simultaneous pressurized pulsatile flow and cyclic strain. These forces were designed to simulate the shear stress conditions present at the distal anastomosis of a saphenous vein graft, where intimal proliferation is common. The cell response was analyzed by Northern hybridization studies of mRNA for endothelin-1 (ET-1), endothelial cell nitric oxide synthase (ecNOS), tissue plasminogen activator (t-PA), and plasminogen activator inhibitor type 1 (PAI-1).

Results.—ET-1 mRNA was not significantly altered at 1 and 24 hours after hemodynamic forces were applied but did decrease by about 50% (compared with control tubes) by 48 hours. A similar pattern was noted for ecNOS mRNA, although 4 of 11 specimens exhibited a reduction of greater than 50% within 24 hours. Expression of t-PA mRNA was unchanged at 1 hour, was decreased by more than 60% at 24 hours, and was unexpressed after 48 hours. There was no significant change in PAI-1 mRNA.

Conclusions.—The combination of pressure, pulsatile flow, and cyclic strain has significant effects on HVEC vasoactive mediators and fibrinolytic agents. Steady-state t-PA mRNA levels are markedly reduced under hemodynamic conditions similar to those observed around vascular anastomoses, which is consistent with a prothrombotic state. Further study is needed, but these changes may contribute to the development of occlusion in saphenous vein grafts.

▶ I have trouble generating much enthusiasm for studies conducted with disassociated endothelial cells. In this case, the cells were grown in a silicone tube subjected to shear stress that was compatible with normal saphenous vein graft insertion. The finding of changes in the mRNA for various substances, while interesting, is difficult to relate directly to the intact saphenous vein. I have little confidence that the results obtained in this artificial environment have any particular relationship to what may occur in vivo, where endothelial cell activity is modulated by the full force of the vascular wall. Overall, this strikes me as a rather clumsy first effort in attempting to learn the cellular changes induced by saphenous vein grafting. I suppose it is better than nothing.

Induction of Angiogenesis by Cationic Lipid-Mediated VEGF$_{165}$ Gene Transfer in the Rabbit Ischemic Hindlimb Model

Gowdak LHW, Poliakova L, Li Z, et al (NIH, Baltimore, Md; Valentis Inc, Burlingame, Calif)
J Vasc Surg 32:343-352, 2000   1–84

Background.—Gene therapy is a promising new approach to treatment of a wide range of diseases, including arterial insufficiency. Previous studies have assessed the possibility of therapeutic angiogenesis, but the development of efficient gene transfer vectors has been a stumbling block. A new cationic lipid formulation with cDNA encoding for the 165-residue form of vascular endothelial growth factor (VEGF$_{165}$) was evaluated in a rabbit model.

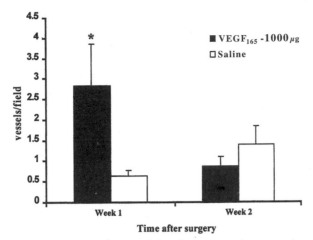

FIGURE 4.—Vascular density as a function of time after surgery and treatment. At week 1, a 3-fold increase in number of vessels was found in VEGF$_{165}$-treated animals relative to controls. At week 2, no differences were found among groups. *P < .005. (Courtesy of Gowdak LHW, Poliakova L, Li Z, et al: Induction of angiogenesis by cationic lipid-mediated VEGF$_{165}$ gene transfer in the rabbit ischemic hindlimb model. *J Vasc Surg* 32:343-352, 2000.)

Methods.—Hindlimb ischemia was induced in rabbits by removal of the right femoral artery. This was followed 2 days later by injection of VEGF$_{165}$ or saline solution into the ischemic thigh muscle. The response was assessed in terms of tissue perfusion and neovascularization of the ischemic limb.

Results.—Rabbits treated with 1000 µg of VEGF$_{165}$ showed a 1.5-fold increase in regional blood flow to the ischemic adductor and gastrocnemius muscles after 1 week. By 2 weeks, flow had increased by 2.5-fold. The VEGF$_{165}$-treated animals also showed a significantly greater blood pressure ratio at 2 and 3 weeks, compared with controls. Other evidence of early neovascularization in rabbits treated with VEGF$_{165}$ included increases in angiographically demonstrated collaterals and in number of capillaries, compared with controls (Fig 4).

Conclusions.—Initial evaluation of a gene therapy approach using plasmid-liposomes encoding for VEGF$_{165}$ suggests significant acceleration of angiogenesis and increased blood flow. This nonviral vector warrants further evaluation for therapeutic angiogenesis.

▶ The first thing we need to do is to satisfy ourselves that angiogenesis is real and that VEGF and bFGF can indeed induce the formation of new blood vessels. Once we satisfy ourselves that this is true, then we need to concern ourselves with the mechanics of how to transfer the genetic fragment into the ischemic tissue. In recent years, viral vectors appear to have fallen from favor, and the current preferred method seems to be the use of various cationic liposomes forming complexes with DNA, or else the injection of naked DNA itself. The study reported here used a complex plasmid liposome complex encoding for VEGF. The authors have concluded that this method of DNA injection is superior to previous ones tested. Perhaps it is, but I continue to have considerable reservations about the entire field of angiogenesis as now practiced. The field is ripe with apparent conflicts of interest as so many of the investigators seem to have ownership or other close relationships with a variety of manufacturers; in fact, I remain unconvinced that the wispy new vessels possibly induced by the angiogenesis factors are of any clinical significance whatsoever. Hard-nosed properly controlled studies are awfully hard to come by in this field.

2 Endovascular

AAA Endografts

Freedom From Endoleak After Endovascular Aneursym Repair Does Not Equal Treatment Success
Gilling-Smith GL, Martin J, Sudhindran S, et al (Royal Liverpool Univ, England)
Eur J Vasc Endovasc Surg 19:421-425, 2000   2–1

Background.—The presence of endoleak after endovascular repair of abdominal aortic aneurysm is generally taken as a sign of treatment failure. But is the absence of endoleak a sign of treatment success? These authors reviewed their records to correlate the presence or absence of endoleak with postoperative changes in the diameter of the aneurysm.

Methods.—The subjects were 55 patients (44 men and 11 women; median age, 71 years) who had undergone endovascular aneurysm repair and who had been followed up for 3 months or greater (median, 18 months). CT scans and angiograms during follow-up were reviewed to identify any endoleaks and to measure changes in the morphology of the aneurysm sac and the stent-graft. Aneurysms in which the maximum diameter (DMAX) increased by 2 mm or greater on 2 or more follow-up scans were defined as enlarging aneurysms, presumably the result of continued or recurrent pressurization of the aneurysm sac (ie, increased endotension).

Results.—Eight of the 55 patients died. Two deaths were related to aneurysm repair; 1 patient died as the result of fatal rupture of the aneurysm 4 months after repair, and 1 died of systemic sepsis from graft infection 12 months after repair. Also, 2 patients were lost to follow-up. Patients were examined according to whether DMAX stayed the same (group 1; 22 patients), shrank (group 2; 18 patients), or expanded (group 3; 15 patients). In group 1, 21 of the 22 patients with no change in DMAX had no endoleaks during follow-up (Table 1). The other patient sustained a secondary type II endoleak and was placed under observation. In group 2, 13 of the 18 patients with a shrinking aneurysm (median decrease, 7 mm) had no endoleaks. However, in 4 patients, secondary type I endoleak that required treatment developed, and 1 patient with a persistent primary type I endoleak died of a fatal aneurysm rupture 3 days before planned reoperation.

TABLE 1.—Relationship Between Change in Aneurysm Diameter and Presence or
Absence of Endoleak

Group 1 (*n* = 22)	No change	21	No endoleak on CT/angio	
		1	Secondary Type II endoleak	(not treated)
Group 2 (*n* = 18)	Aneurysm shrinking	13	No endoleak on CT/angio	
		4	Secondary Type I endoleak	(treated)
		1	Persistent primary Type endoleak	(fatal rupture)
Group 3 (*n* = 15)	Aneurysm expanding	10	No endoleak on CT/angio	
		4	sudden death (? Cause)	
		1	late conversion (sealed endoleak)	
		2	Type II endoleak on duplex scan	
		3	under observation	
		3	Secondary Type I endoleak	(treated)
		1	Secondary Type II endoleak	(treated)
		1	Persistent primary Type II endoleak	(lost to follow-up)

(Reprinted from the *European Journal of Vascular and Endovascular Surgery* courtesy of Gilling-Smith GL, Martin J, Sudhindran S, et al: Freedom from endoleak after endovascular aneurysm repair does not equal treatment success. *Eur J Vasc Surg* 19:421-425, 2000. Copyright 2000, by permission of the publisher, W B Saunders Company Limited London.)

In group 3, 10 of the 15 patients with an expanding aneurysm (median increase, 9 mm) had no endoleak on CT or angiography. However, an endoleak was noted during duplex scanning in 2 of these 10 patients, and 4 of these patients died suddenly from unknown cause (their DMAX ranged from 65-95 mm). Five patients in group 3 had endoleak; 4 were treated and 1 was lost to follow-up. Overall, 44 of the 55 patients (80%) had no endoleak. "Freedom from endoleak" correctly identified 34 patients (62%) with no increase in aneurysm size. However, "freedom from endoleak" also incorrectly identified 10 patients (18%) who had enlarging aneurysm, and who are thus presumed to be at greater risk of aneurysm rupture.

Conclusion.—The absence of an endoleak cannot be taken to indicate that a patient is free of endotension, as 10 of 44 patients with no endoleak (23%) had enlarging aneurysms. Aneurysm diameter and/or volume must be assessed regularly during follow-up to identify patients who are at increased risk of rupture.

▶ One may simplistically assume that after endograft placement for abdominal aortic aneurysms, generally an aneurysm decreasing in diameter would be one with no endoleak, and these patients should be relatively protected from rupture. An aneurysm remaining the same size may or may not have a leak but would be presumed at minimal rupture risk, while an aneurysm enlarging would be one which does have an endoleak and would have significantly increased rupture potential. A detailed analysis of a group of patients undergoing endovascular aneurysm repair was conducted. Unfortunately, freedom from demonstrable endoleak incorrectly implied freedom from endotension in 18% of patients. It is becoming more and more obvious that information on intrasac pressure is the information which we really require in following up these patients. Some method of routine monitoring of intrasac pressure after graft placement is going to be essential, even if this has to be done percutaneously. (See also Abstract 2–2.)

Aneurysm Sac Pressure Measurements After Endovascular Repair of Abdominal Aortic Aneuryms

Baum RA, Carpenter JP, Cope C, et al (Univ of Pennsylvania, Philadelphia)
J Vasc Surg 33:32-41, 2001   2–2

Background.—In endovascular grafting of abdominal aortic aneurysms (AAAs), unlike in the case of conventional open surgery, branch vessels in the sac are not ligated and may transmit pressure. The feasibility of various interventional methods for assessing pressure in the aneurysm sac was investigated for patients who had had endovascular AAA repair.

Methods.—Sac pressures for 21 patients who had had stent graft repair of AAA were measured. For 17 patients, 30-day CT scans showed endoleaks. For this group, access to the aneurysm sac was through direct translumbar sac puncture for 5 patients, a patent inferior mesenteric artery accessed via the superior mesenteric artery for 9, and direct cannulation around attachment sites in 3. For 4 patients, perioperative pressure measures were obtained through catheters alongside the endovascular graft at the time of deployment. Two catheters were left in place for 30 hours, during which time CT and conventional angiography were performed. Standard arterial-line pressure transduction methods were used to determine pressures, which were compared with systemic pressure for each patient.

Findings.—All patients had increased sac pressure. Sac pressure for patients with endoleaks was systemic for 15 patients and near systemic for 1 (Fig 2). All had pulsatile waveforms. Sac pressures were also increased for patients without CT or angiographic evidence of endoleak. For 2 of these patients, sac injection revealed a patent lumbar artery and an inferior mesenteric artery.

Conclusion.—Pressures from inside the aneurysm sac for patients with stent grafts can be measured by a variety of methods. Pressurized AAA sacs may persist, despite endovascular AAA repair.

▶ These investigators at the University of Pennsylvania performed sac pressure measurements in 21 patients up to 30 days post placement. Seventeen of these 21 patients had endoleaks demonstrable on CT scans. The critical information is that every patient had elevated sac pressure, including several patients who had no CT or angiographic evidence of endoleak. It is obvious that the objective of endograft placement is to prevent future rupture, and this can only be assured if the sac pressure is close to zero. It is important to note that these investigators demonstrated systemic sac pressure in both attachment and collateral leaks, regardless of their size or type. On balance, this is a very sobering study that has potentially profound implications.

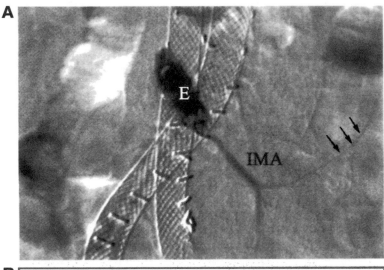

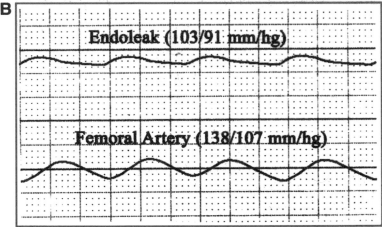

FIGURE 2.—Systemic pressure in inferior mesenteric artery (IMA) endoleak. **A,** A transarterial catheter (*arrow*) is placed through the IMA and into an endoleak (E) through the superior mesenteric artery. **B,** Systemic pressure is measured from within IMA endoleak. (Courtesy of Baum RA, Carpenter JP, Cope C, et al: Aneurysm sac pressure measurements after endovascular repair of abdominal aortic aneurysms. *J Vasc Surg* 33:32-41, 2001.)

Anatomical Risk Factors for Proximal Perigraft Endoleak and Graft Migration Following Endovascular Repair of Abdominal Aortic Aneurysms

Albertini J-N, Kalliafas S, Travis S, et al (Queen's Med Centre, Nottingham, England)

Eur J Vasc Endovasc Surg 19:308-312, 2000   2–3

Introduction.—Proximal perigraft endoleak (PPE) and graft migration are correlated with significant morbidity and mortality rates. Objective data establishing the correlation between neck anatomy and these complications are sparse. The anatomy of the neck was evaluated to determine which variables were significantly related to PPE and graft migration.

Methods.—An in-house custom-made stent graft (Gianturco stents plus Dacron) was used for endovascular repair of infrarenal abdominal aortic aneurysms (AAA) in 184 patients. Of these, 31 had PPE, and 15 had graft migration. Neck diameter was measured at the level of renal arteries and at the lower limit of the neck. Aortic necks were classified by shape (Fig 1). Neck angulation was determined by spiral CT, MRI reconstructions, or angiograms. Thrombus or atheroma lining and the presence of calcifications were noted.

Results.—The mean neck angulation was significantly greater in patients with PPE (50°) or graft migration (54°) compared with those who did not experience these complications (37°). Neck migration occurred

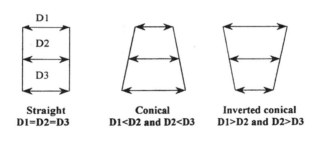

Straight
D1=D2=D3

Conical
D1<D2 and D2<D3

Inverted conical
D1>D2 and D2>D3

Hourglass
D1>D2 and D3>D2

Barrel
D1<D2 and D3<D2

FIGURE 1.—Classification of proximal aortic necks according to shape: *D1*, diameter at the level of the renal arteries. *D3*, diameter at the distal end of the neck. *D2*, intermediate diameter (maximum neck diameter for the "barrel" type and minimum for the "hourglass" type). (Reprinted from Albertini J-N, Kalliafas S, Travis S, et al: Anatomical risk factors for proximal perigraft endoleak and graft migration following endovascular repair of abdominal aortic aneurysms. *Eur J Vasc Endovasc Surg* 19:308-312, 2000. Copyright 2000, by permission of the publisher WB Saunders Company Limited London.)

TABLE 2.—Anatomical Characteristic of the Proximal Aneurysm Neck in
163 Patients

Max. diameter (mm)	26 ± 4
Length (mm)	30 ± 13
Max. angle (degrees)	41 ± 19
Thrombus or atheroma lining	72
Calcifications	16
Shape:	
Straight	109
Conical	33
Inverted conical	7
Barrel	8
Hourglass	6

Note: For quantitative variables, results are mean ± SD. For categorical variables the number of patients is indicated.
(Reprinted from Albertini J-N, Kalliafas S, Travis S, et al: Anatomical risk factors for proximal perigraft endoleak and graft migration following endovascular repair of abdominal aortic aneurysms. *Eur J Vasc Endovasc Surg* 19:308-312, 2000. Copyright 2000, by permission of the publisher W B Saunders Company Limited London.)

significantly more frequently in patients with PPE. The incidence of PPE or graft migration was not significantly higher for patients with a conical-shaped aortic neck, thrombus, or atheroma lining and calcifications (Table 2).

Conclusion.—Neck angulation was the risk factor most significantly associated with PPE and graft migration.

▶ This is an excellent retrospective analysis of anatomical factors that may influence the development of PPE in the setting of endograft treatment of AAAs with an in-house custom-made device. That neck angulation was found to be associated with a higher incidence of PPE is not surprising. It has been my impression that neck angulation has been an important factor, but it is also important to consider the other factors such as diameter and length. The authors also noted an association of larger neck diameters with PPE. It stands to reason that as the neck becomes more dilated, more angulated, and shorter, these and possibly other factors will combine to sabotage the integrity of the proximal fixation and seal, yielding PPE or device migration or both.

The authors' data apply to their particular device and would need to be examined together with different devices to determine which factors might be most important. It is our experience that different device designs have different tolerances for the various anatomical characteristics, and we have used this to aid in selecting the specific device type for each individual patient. Studies such as this will allow us to more accurately predict outcomes and therefore hopefully avoid problems such as PPE or device migration.

M. A. Golden, MD

Suitability for Endovascular Aneurysm Repair in an Unselected Population

Woodburn KR, Chant H, Davies JN, et al (Royal Cornwall Hosp, Truro, England)
Br J Surg 88:77-81, 2001   2–4

Introduction.—Tertiary referral centers indicate that up to 60% of patients with abdominal aortic aneurysms (AAAs) may be suitable for endovascular repair (EVAR). These patients may not represent the AAA population seen in most vascular practices. The percentage of AAAs presenting to a countywide vascular service who were suitable for EVAR was examined, along with the outcome of subsequent AAA repair in relation to aneurysm morphology.

Methods.—All patients undergoing AAA repair from January 1998 to December 1999 underwent spiral CT angiography to ascertain aneurysm morphology and suitability for EVAR. A prospective vascular database was used to record subsequent outcome.

Results.—Of 115 patients evaluated, 63 (55%) had at least 1 absolute contraindication to EVAR (Table 1). An additional 13 (11%) had at least 1 relative contraindication. There was no contraindication to EVAR in 39 patients (34%). Of the 52 patients with no absolute contraindication, 10 underwent successful EVAR, 5 did not meet recognized criteria for surgery, 1 was awaiting EVAR, 4 remained under observation, 1 was awaiting open repair, and 31 underwent open repair with no mortality.

Conclusion.—Only 30% of unselected patients with AAA evaluated in a vascular service are entirely suitable for EVAR. The increased use of EVAR may result from surgeons offering surgery to a group of patients with AAA who would previously have been treated conservatively.

▶ The percentage of patients who would be suitable for EVAR of an AAA remains an unanswered question. Referral centers that specialize in this type of aneurysm repair report very high percentages of suitable patients. This study reports the experience of a county-wide vascular service that was not a referral center. The authors report that 30% of unselected patients

TABLE 1.—Absolute Contraindication

Absolute Contraindication	Number of AAAs With Contraindication on CT
Proximal neck <15 mm	40*
Infrarenal aortic diameter >28 mm	10
Thoracoabdominal aortic aneurysm (suprarenal aortic diameter >30 mm)	7
External iliac diameter <9 mm or >16 mm	3
Bilateral internal and external iliac aneurysms	1
Prosthetic graft material in both groins	1
Evidence of retroperitoneal leak on CT	1

*In 12 abdominal aortic aneurysms (AAAs), the infrarenal aortic diameter was also greater than 28 mm.
(Courtesy of Woodburn KR, Chant H, Davies JN, et al: Suitability for endovascular aneurysm repair in an unselected population. *Br J Surg* 88:77-81, 2001. Blackwell Science Ltd.)

with AAAs were suitable for EVAR, which appears to be far lower than the reported experience from referral centers. Their mortality rate for elective open AAA repair was a very respectable 6%, and very interestingly the authors point out that in the patients deemed appropriate for EVAR who underwent traditional open repair, there were no mortalities.

This report raises some very interesting considerations. Could it be that the large percentage of EVARs in some centers are done for patients who have relative contraindications to this type of repair? Could it be that some of the patients undergoing EVAR would not have been considered for conventional open repair because they did not have the usual, accepted indications for aneurysm surgery? Could it be that the low morbidity and mortality reported in some centers from EVAR results from the fact that many of these patients are highly selected and would have also done well with conventional open repair? We need to be sure that EVAR with devices that are probably going to be modified and become safer should be reserved for patients who truly represent a prohibitive risk from conventional open aneurysm surgery.

J. O. Menzoian, MD

Endovascular Repair of Abdominal Aortic Aneurysms: Eligibility Rate and Impact on the Rate of Open Repair
Wolf YG, Fogarty TJ, Olcott C IV, et al (Stanford Univ, Calif)
J Vasc Surg 32:519-523, 2000   2–5

Objective.—There are widely varying estimates of the number of patients with abdominal aortic aneurysms (AAAs) that are eligible for endovascular repair. The number and type of open abdominal aneurysm repairs before and after the inception of Stanford's endovascular program were analyzed in a retrospective study.

Methods.—The endovascular repair program began in November 1996. Records of all 324 patients considered for endovascular repair between November 1, 1996, and October 31, 1999, were reviewed by a panel of vascular surgeons and radiologists. Open AAA repairs were categorized as simple, complex (juxtarenal, suprarenal, thoracoabdominal, and infected), or ruptured aneurysms.

TABLE 1.—Eligibility for Endovascular Repair*

Period	Candidates	Noncandidates	Incomplete Evaluation	Total
First 18 mo	66 (45%)	78 (53%)	4 (3%)	148
Second 18 mo	110 (63%)	60 (34%)	6 (3%)	176
Entire period	176 (54%)	138 (43%)	10 (3%)	324

*The rate of eligibility was significantly higher in the second period ($P < .001$).
(Courtesy of Wolf YG, Fogarty TJ, Olcott C IV, et al: Endovascular repair of abdominal aortic aneurysms: Eligibility rate and impact on the rate of open repair. *J Vasc Surg* 32:519-523, 2000.)

TABLE 4.—Open Abdominal Aneurysm Repair

Period	Simple	Complex	Rupture	Total
Pre-EV program	213 (80%)	43 (16%)	9 (3%)	265
Post-EV program	216 (78%)	43 (16%)	18 (6%)	277
Overall	429 (79%)	86 (16%)	27 (5%)	542

Abbreviation: EV, Endovascular.
(Courtesy of Wolf YG, Fogarty TJ, Olcott C IV, et al: Endovascular repair of abdominal aortic aneurysms: Eligibility rate and impact on the rate of open repair. *J Vasc Surg* 32:519-523, 2000.)

Results.—One hundred seventy-six (54%) patients were eligible for endovascular repair (Table 1). The main reason for disqualification was a short aortic neck. Eligible patients were significantly younger (74.4 vs 78.3 years) and had aneurysms with a smaller diameter (57.6 vs 60.8 mm). Among the candidates, 78% had endovascular repair, 6% had open repair, and 11% had no treatment. Among noncandidates, 54% had open repair and 19% had no treatment. During a 6-year period, 542 open AAA repairs were performed: 429 simple, 86 complex, and 27 ruptured. The data before and after initiation of the endovascular program were not significantly different (Table 4).

Conclusion.—The percentage of individuals eligible for endovascular AAA repair (54%) is higher than previously reported. The proportion of patients requiring open repair has not changed.

▶ Over a 3-year period, this aggressive endovascular center found that 54% of 324 patients with AAAs were candidates for endovascular repair. Since these were generally referral patients, we have to assume that a significant amount of preselection had occurred prior to referral. I stand by my suspicion that no more than 40% of patients with AAAs, overall, are going to be eligible for endovascular repair with the use of current standards. Should the standards change because of surgical experience or device improvement, this 40% number may, of course, also change.

Mid-term Results of Endovascular Versus Open Repair for Abdominal Aortic Aneurysm in Patients Anatomically Suitable for Endovascular Repair

Becquemin J-P, Bourriez A, D'Audiffret A, et al (Univ Paris Val de Marne)
Eur J Vasc Endovasc Surg 19:656-661, 2000   2–6

Background.—Few data are available on the midterm results of endovascular repair of abdominal aortic aneurysms (AAAs). The midterm results of endovascular repair of AAAs were compared with those of open AAA repair.

Methods.—The study included 180 of a series of 438 patients with AAA who were candidates for endovascular repair, as identified by CT and angiographic criteria. Repair was done by various endovascular graft techniques in 73 patients and by the open repair technique in 107. The postoperative follow-up included a biannual clinical examination, duplex scanning, and, for patients in the endovascular repair group, CT scanning.

Results.—At baseline, the 2 groups were similar in age, sex, preoperative risk factors, and aneurysm diameter. Operative time was also similar, 149 minutes in the endovascular group (EV) and 133 minutes in the open repair (OR) group. However, operative blood loss was 96 mL with endovascular repair versus 985 mL with open repair. Length of hospital stay was 7 versus 13 days, respectively. The 1-month mortality rate was approximately 3% in both groups, but cardiac and pulmonary complications were more frequent in the open repair group (7% vs 20%).

Cumulative 1-year survival was 82% in the EV group versus 96% in the OR group. No deaths resulted from AAA rupture, but 3 patients required conversion to open surgery. Subsequent intervention, major or minor, was needed in 22% of the EV group versus 7.5% of the OR group. The 1-year cumulative freedom from any reintervention was 79% for the EV group versus 93% for the OR group. The rate of early endoleaks in the EV group was 23%, with a 10% rate of persistent endoleaks at the end of follow-up. The rate of primary success—that is, no endoleak and no reintervention— was 74% in the EV group versus 94% in the OR group.

Conclusions.—For patients undergoing AAA repair, endovascular techniques offer several immediate advantages, including reduced blood loss, fewer pulmonary and cardiac complications, and a shorter hospital stay time. However, at midterm follow-up, patients undergoing endovascular repair require more repeat interventions to manage endoleaks or to maintain graft patency.

▶ Exercises such as this are valuable but are invariably dismissed by enthusiasts as covering a period of start-up learning curve activity and a period during which time devices were improving. Thus, we have the eternal moving target. This remarkably objective evaluation—amazingly enough from France—appears to be filled with EV enthusiasts and concludes reasonably that for the present, OR of AAAs presents an overall more attractive option during follow-up than does EV repair.

Since EV repair does, of course, present the long-term problem of endoleak and aneurysm rupture, it seems clear to me that we should not adopt this technique unless there are palpable benefits. Clearly, mortality is equal between OR and EV repair, cost is probably higher for EV repair, and freedom from adverse events during follow-up is distinctly superior for OR repair. Thus, the only advantage one can cite in favor of EV repair from the patient's standpoint is ease of procedural recovery. Just how important is this? In my opinion, it is not sufficiently important to warrant the use of an inferior technique. I wonder if anyone has a different opinion?

Comparison of First- and Second-Generation Prostheses for Endoluminal Repair of Abdominal Aortic Aneurysms: A 6-Year Study With Life Table Analysis

May J, White GH, Waugh R, et al (Univ of Sydney, Australia)

J Vasc Surg 32:124-129, 2000   2–7

Background.—With the introduction of new and improved techniques for endoluminal treatment of abdominal aortic aneurysms (AAAs), problems in the reporting of outcomes have developed. Many excellent reports unfortunately have a relatively short period of follow-up. The longest period of follow-up is desirable, but it requires the inclusion of patients who were treated with older prostheses that are no longer in use. Thus, the overall outcome may not be reflective of results that are possible with recently developed prostheses. The outcomes of endoluminal repair of AAAs with 2 generations of prostheses were compared.

Methods.—From May 1992 to December 1998, 266 patients underwent elective endoluminal repair of an AAA. Group I was composed of 118 patients who received first-generation prostheses, and group II was composed of 148 patients who received second-generation prostheses. The 2 groups were similar in demographic characteristics and in the size of AAA. There was a higher proportion of patients with comorbidities in group I than in group II, but the difference was not significant. The first-generation prostheses had large delivery systems (24F internal diameter) and 1-piece construction and lacked metallic support throughout their length. In contrast, the second-generation devices had smaller delivery systems (921F or smaller internal diameter), modular construction, and a metallic frame throughout the length of the prosthesis. The primary end point criteria were survival and successful endoluminal repair, and success was defined as exclusion of the aneurysm sac from the circulation and stability or reduction in AAA maximum transverse diameter. Persistent endoleaks

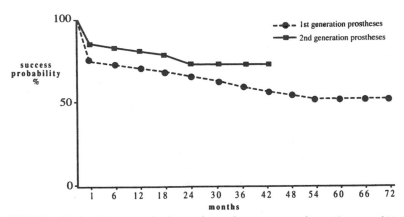

FIGURE 2.—Kaplan-Meier curves for first- and second-generation prostheses. (Courtesy of May J, White GH, Waugh R, et al: Comparison of first- and second-generation prostheses for endoluminal repair of abdominal aortic aneurysms: A 6-year study with life table analysis. *J Vasc Surg* 32:124-129, 2000.)

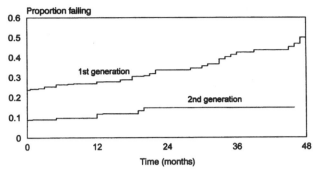

FIGURE 3.—Cumulative incidence of primary graft failure. (Courtesy of May J, White GH, Waugh R, et al: Comparison of first- and second-generation protheses for endoluminal repair of abdominal aortic aneurysms: A 6-year study with life table analysis. *J Vasc Surg* 32:124-129, 2000.)

were considered as failures. The minimum period of follow-up was 5 months, and analysis was performed with the life-table method.

Results.—There was no significant difference in perioperative mortality rate between the 2 groups (group I, 4.2%; group II, 2.7%). However, the difference in survival curves for the 2 generations was statistically significant (Fig 2). A significant difference was also seen between the 2 generations of patients in their conditional probability of graft failure when the competing risk of all-cause mortality was taken into consideration (Fig 3). Second-generation patients had a lower risk for graft failure than first-generation patients. Probablility of failure was expressed as a proportion of graft failure at 2 years and was 0.15 for second-generation patients compared with 0.33 for first-generation patients.

Conclusions.—Endoluminal repair of AAAs is a safe procedure regardless of whether first- or second-generation prostheses are used. However, these data indicated that the survival and probability of graft survival were significantly higher for second-generation prostheses than for first-generation prostheses, which is a result of a combination of improved technology and increasing clinical experience. For a more accurate evaluation of the role of the endoluminal technique in AAA repair, studies should focus on patients in whom second-generation devices were used, rather than on longer term results in patients in whom first- and second-generation prostheses were used.

▶ The significant experience of the Sydney group continues to provide the vascular community with important lessons regarding the endovascular management of AAAs. With that said, in attempting to assess the impact of changes in endograft technology, this report is of limited value. As anticipated, conversion rates are higher during the early phase of the clinical experience and with devices that are dependent on larger delivery systems. However, beyond the initial implant period, failure rates appear to be similar during the first 24 months of observation.

So what do we learn about "first" versus "second" generation systems? Not much that is particularly insightful. The desire to arbitrarily lump devices into "generations" is unfortunate. In the process, we risk the loss of important insight gained from careful analysis of individual early and late failure modes that are uniquely associated with a given endograft design. It is of interest that of the new and presumably improved *second-generation* devices presented in this review, the Stentor/Vanguard endograft has been pulled from the market and the AneuRx endograft has since been redesigned.

E. L. Chaikof, MD

Incidence and Risk Factors of Late Rupture, Conversion, and Death After Endovascular Repair of Infrarenal Aortic Aneurysms: The EURO-STAR Experience
Harris PL, for the EUROSTAR Collaborators (Royal Liverpool Univ, England; et al)
J Vasc Surg 32:739-749, 2000   2–8

Objective.—The feasibility and short-term benefits of endovascular repair of abdominal aortic aneurysms have been established. An assessment of the 4-year results of the European Collaborators on Stent/Graft Techniques for Aortic Aneurysm Repair (EUROSTAR) organization was presented, and the risk factors for rupture, late conversion, and death were identified.

Methods.—Operative risk profiles, according to the American Society of Anesthesiologists (ASA), were determined for 2464 patients (197 women), aged 37 to 93 years. Bifurcated endovascular stent-grafts were employed in 2261 (92%) patients. Patients were assessed clinically and with contrast-enhanced CT scans at 1, 3, 6, 12, and 18 months and yearly thereafter. Expected overall survival rates at 1 and 2 years were 77.2% and 73.7%, respectively. Results of treatment at 30 days, death from all causes and sudden death from unknown causes at more than 30 days, rupture and outcome, risk factors for late rupture, conversion to open repair, and risk factors for later conversion to open repair were recorded. Risk ratios were calculated to correlate procedural complications and potential risk factors such as stent-graft kinking, migration, stenosis, thrombosis, and endoleak. Survival analysis was calculated by the Kaplan-Meier method.

Results.—Deployment was successful in 97.6% of patients. Thirty-four patients initially required conversion to open repair. There were 79 (3.2%) deaths in the first month, with 11.4% of deaths occurring in ASA class 4 patients. There were 419 endoleaks in 2404 patients with successful deployment; there were 140 (8.3%) endoleaks in 1688 patients at 1 month. Between 1 and 48 months of follow-up, there were 136 deaths. There was 1 rupture within 30 days and 13 after 30 days. Most ruptures occurred 18 months after surgery. The early rupture patient died. Twelve rupture patients had emergency open surgery, and 5 (41.6%) died. The 2 nonoperated rupture patients also died, for an overall death rate of 64.5%. Significant risk factors for late rupture were proximal type I endoleak, midgraft (type III) endoleak, stent-graft migration, and kinked endograft. There were a total of 41 conversions to open repair. Conversions peaked at 18 months. The average annual risk of conversion was 2.1%; 10 (24.4%) conversion patients died within 30 days of surgery. Significant risk factors for late conversion were proximal type I endoleak, midgraft (type III) endoleak, stent-graft migration, kinked endograft, type II endoleak, and distal type I endoleak.

Conclusion.—Endovascular repair of infrarenal aortic aneurysms results in a combined cumulative risk of a potential fatal adverse event of 3% per year.

▶ This report outlines an extensive evaluation of a large experience with the endovascular repair of abdominal aortic aneurysms. The large number of patients in this study (2464), with a mean duration of follow-up of 12.19 months, makes this a valuable report. One problem of an analysis such as is done in this report is that there were many devices placed at many centers by many different surgeons. As a simplification of all of the data in this article, "hard" end points of rupture, late conversion, and death were at a rate of 3% per year. Deployment of the endoluminal device was possible in 97.6% of the attempts. The 30-day death rate was 3.2%.

This report clearly points out to me that this is a changing and rapidly evolving field. The devices are varied; they have been modified and continue to be modified, and the indications at various centers are very variable. The results are good but the morbidity and mortality rates are real. Continued lifelong surveillance is a fact of life. To quote the authors of this article, "Until the long-term efficacy of this approach has been established through further analysis of reliable hard end points, caution should be exercised with respect to its application in routine clinical practice."

J. O. Menzoian, MD

Need for Secondary Interventions After Endovascular Repair of Abdominal Aortic Aneurysms: Intermediate-term Follow-up Results of a European Collaborative Registry (EUROSTAR)
Buth J, for the EUROSTAR Collaborators (Catharina Hosp, Eindhoven, The Netherlands; et al)
Br J Surg 87:1666-1673, 2000   2–9

Objective.—The need for secondary interventions after endovascular aneurysm repair can increase the annual rupture rate and place an additional burden on patients and the health care system. Late interventions in patients included in the multicenter collaborative European registry (EUROSTAR) were analyzed and correlated with clinical and imaging findings at follow-up.

TABLE 1.—Baseline Characteristics in 1023 Patients With Follow-up of
More than 12 Months After Endovascular Aneurysm Repair

	No. of Patients
Male sex	925 (90)
ASA physical status classification	
I	88 (9)
II	400 (39)
III	437 (43)
IV	61 (6)
Not defined	37 (4)
Device type	
Vanguard	521 (51)
Stentor	243 (24)
AneuRx	125 (12)
Talent	78 (8)
Ancure	28 (3)
Zenith	10 (1)
Other	18 (2)

Values in parentheses are percentages.
Abbreviation: ASA, American Society of Anesthesiologists. Device manufacturers are as follows:
Vanguard, Boston Scientific, Natick, MA, USA; Stentor, Mintec, Freeport, Bahamas; AneuRx,
Medtronic, Santa Rosa, CA, USA; Talent, World Medical, Sunrise, FL, USA; Ancure, Guidant, Menlo
Park, CA, USA; Zenith, Cook, Karlslunde, Denmark.
(Courtesy of Buth J, for the EUROSTAR Collaborators: Need for secondary interventions after
endovascular repair of abdominal aortic aneurysms: Intermediate-term follow-up results of a European
collaborative registry (EUROSTAR). *Br J Surg* 87:1666-1673, 2000, Blackwell Science Ltd.)

Methods.—Among 1023 patients whose status was followed for at least
12 months in the period from January 1994 to November 1999, 186
patients (18%), aged 42 to 90, (90% male) had secondary interventions
(Table 1). Differences in clinical and imaging findings between subgroups
with and without specific secondary interventions were compared, and
relative risks were assessed.

Results.—The average follow-up was 12 months, and interventions
occurred at an average of 14 months. The average number of initial
procedures per center was 18, and the average percentage of secondary
procedures was 15. Intervention rates were similar regardless of duration
of follow-up, devices used, graft configuration, or graft type. Interventions
used a transabdominal approach (12%), extra-abdominal bypass (11%),
or transfemoral procedure (76%). Rates of freedom from intervention at
1, 3, and 4 years were 89%, 67%, and 62%, respectively. The major
reasons for secondary interventions were proximal endoleak (relative risk
[RR], 12.6), midgraft endoleak (RR, 4.5), migration (RR, 8.9), and aneurysm rupture (RR, 22.6). All 21 extra-anatomic interventions (femorofemoral bypass) were performed for thrombosis or stenosis of a limb of the
graft (RR, 5.6). The relative risks of transfemoral secondary interventions
ranged from 2.5 to 6.9 (Table 2).

Conclusion.—The rate of secondary intervention in the EUROSTAR
study is a constant 10% per year. Patients undergoing endovascular aneurysm repair require lifelong surveillance.

TABLE 2.—Secondary Interventions and Findings at Follow-up Surveillance

Secondary Interventions	Surveillance Variables Correlated
Transabdominal secondary intervention	Endoleak proximal
With conversion to open procedure	Endoleak midgraft
With preservation of endograft function	Endoleak distal
Extra-anatomic secondary intervention	Reinjection from side branch
Transfemoral secondary intervention	Kinking of endograft
	Stenosis/thrombosis of device (limb)
	Migration of device

(Courtesy of Buth J, for the EUROSTAR Collaborators: Need for secondary interventions after endovascular repair of abdominal aortic aneurysms: Intermediate-term follow-up results of a European collaborative registry (EUROSTAR). *Br J Surg* 87:1666-1673, 2000, Blackwell Science Ltd.)

▶ Interestingly, this article was published almost simultaneously with the preceding one (see Abstract 2–8). This study was limited to slightly over 1000 patients who had passed the first postoperative year. Remarkably, at 24 and 36 months, the freedom from all secondary reinterventions was about 70% and 65% respectively. These investigators conclude that the requirement for reintervention seems to be holding steady at about 10% per year through the short- and intermediate-term follow-ups. I continue to ask the question, "O Lord, how much is enough?"

Failure of Endovascular Abdominal Aortic Aneurysm Graft Limbs

Carpenter JP, Neschis DG, Fairman RM, et al (Univ of Pennsylvania, Philadelphia)

J Vasc Surg 33:296-303, 2001   2–10

Background.—Many types of graft designs are used for endovascular repair of abdominal aortic aneurysm (AAA), including fully supported graft limbs (with a stented endoskeleton or exoskeleton) and unsupported graft limbs. However, these and other authors have noted that these grafts are subject to endograft limb failure. An experience with patients undergoing endovascular AAA repair and femorofemoral bypass grafting was reviewed to determine whether certain design features of the graft are associated with better patency of endograft limbs.

Methods.—Medical records were reviewed to identify all patients undergoing endovascular AAA repair between April 1998 and March 2000 and all patients undergoing femorofemoral bypass grafting for arterial occlusive disease or in conjunction with an aortomonoiliac (AI) endograft for aneurysm between September 1994 and July 1999. Graft designs were examined according to graft patency.

Results.—During the 2-year interval examined, 173 patients underwent endovascular AAA repair. Bifurcated grafts were used for 137 patients (total of 301 aortic graft limbs), and AI grafts were used in association with femorofemoral bypass in 36 patients. Additionally, during the approximately 5-year interval examined, 39 patients underwent femorofemoral bypass grafting for occlusive disease. Primary patency rates for all

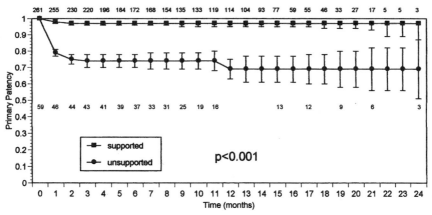

FIGURE 5.—Comparison of patency of endograft limbs: supported versus unsupported designs. Primary patency of supported graft limbs at 18 months was 97% and of unsupported limbs, 69% (P < .001). Assisted primary patency rate (not shown) for supported limbs was 99% and for unsupported, 91% (P = .01). Secondary patency was achieved in all cases. (Courtesy of Carpenter JP, Neschis DG, Fairman RM, et al: Failure of endovascular abdominal aortic aneurysm graft limbs. *J Vasc Surg* 33: 296-303, 2001.)

endografts performed for AAA repair ranged from 69% to 100% at 24 months (92% overall).

During a mean follow-up of 9.7 months, 24 endograft limbs failed. Of these failures, 17 with stenosis or kinks noted at graft placement required primary stenting to achieve patency, for an assisted primary patency rate of 97% at 18 months. The other 7 limbs thrombosed later and required thrombolysis or surgical thrombectomy followed by stenting. None of these cases was associated with long-term ischemic sequelae. All failed grafts achieved secondary patency. Among the different types of endograft limbs, primary patency rates at 18 months did not differ significantly between AI and bifurcated graft limbs (97% and 90%, respectively). Similarly, patency rates for fully supported graft limbs did not differ significantly according to manufacturer. However, compared with unsupported endograft limbs, fully supported endograft limbs at 18 months had significantly better primary patency rates (99% vs 69%) and assisted primary patency rates (99% vs 91%) (Fig 5).

Conclusion.—During endovascular AAA repair and femorofemoral by-pass grafting, the patency of AI graft limbs and bifurcated graft limbs is similar (97% and 90%, respectively, at 18 months). However, fully supported AAA endograft designs have significantly better endograft limb patency than unsupported endograft limbs. Furthermore, all 7 limbs that thrombosed after grafting had a kink or stenotic lesion noted at revision, and stenting was required in 17 limbs at the time of initial grafting because of kinks or stenoses. Thus, routine prophylactic stenting of all unsupported endograft limbs used during endovascular AAA repair and femo-rofemoral bypass grafting may be prudent.

▶ It looks as if these authors favor fully supported endografts over unsupported endografts and find that the AI with a femorofemoral artery seems to work well. I certainly cannot argue with their conclusions. The fully supported endograft is emerging as the graft of preference over the unsupported endograft. Whether a bifurcation graft or an AI is placed appears to have little influence on intermediate-term patency. Dr May from the University of Sydney asks some penetrating questions in the Discussion section of this article, which I commend to all of you who may be interested. There is a real problem with including the limb failures occurring and being corrected during insertion in the group of late limb failures that appeared perfect after initial deployment.

Comparison of Cognitive Function and Quality of Life After Endovascular or Conventional Aortic Aneurysm Repair

Lloyd AJ, Boyle J, Bell PRF, et al (Oxford Brookes Univ, England; Leicester Univ, England)

Br J Surg 87:443-447, 2000   2–11

Background.—Endovascular aortic aneurysm repair has some advantages over open repair, but its long-term effects on the patient's cognitive function and quality of life (QOL) have not been evaluated. Outcomes for patients undergoing conventional repair and those obtained with endovascular aortic aneurysm repair were compared.

Methods.—Eighty-two patients were studied; 34 had endovascular procedures and 48 had conventional procedures. Assessments of cognitive function and QOL were performed before operation and 6 months after-

TABLE 3.—Scores From the Cognitive Function Battery for Endovascular and Conventional Surgical Groups Before and 6 Months After Operation

| | Endovascular Group | | Conventional Group | |
	Preoperative	Postoperative	Preoperative	Postoperative
MMSE	28 (27-29)	28 (27-29)	27 (26-28)	27 (26-28)
Visual search				
Task 1	20·5 (16·6-24·4)	19·0 (15·8-22·2)	24·5 (21·3-27·7)	20·5 (17·0-24·0)
Task 2	41·5 (34·8-48·2)	36·0 (29·7-42·3)	43·5 (38·0-49·0)	37·5 (31·9-43·1)
Visual attention				
Task 1	8 (7-9)	9 (8-10)	6 (5-7)	7 (6-8)
Task 2	4·6 (3·7-5·5)	4·5 (3·9-5·1)	5·3 (4·7-5·9)	4·7 (4·3-5·1)
Immediate recall	4·5 (3·4-5·6)	7·0 (6·0-8·0)	5·0 (3·9-6·1)	5·5 (4·3-6·7)
Delayed recall	2·5 (1·6-3·4)	5·0 (4·1-5·9)	3·5 (2·3-4·7)	4·3 (3·2-5·4)
Naming	38 (37-39)	38 (37-39)	38 (37-39)	38 (37-39)

Note: Values are median (95% confidence interval). There were no significant differences between the groups.
Abbreviation: MMSE, Mini Mental State Examination.
(Courtesy of Lloyd AJ, Boyd J, Bell PRF, et al: Comparison of cognitive function and quality of life after endovascular or conventional aortic aneurysm repair. *Br J Surg* 87:443-447, 2000. Blackwell Science Ltd.)

ward. Various psychometric tests quantified cognitive function; the Medical Outcomes Short Form 36 questionnaire assessed QOL.

Results.—Only 78% of the patients had data available 6 months postoperatively. Compared with preoperative assessments, the visual search test showed significant declines for the patients as a group, as did the physical function and vitality domains of the Medical Outcomes Short Form 36 questionnaire. The procedure done appeared to have no significance for either cognitive function or QOL (Table 3).

Conclusion.—No differences were noted between the endovascular group and the conventional group with regard to cognitive function or QOL. Thus, while there was a negative impact on the patients' cognitive function and QOL, it could not be ascribed to either specific procedure.

▶ Without question, we are all going to be forced to become more aware of attempts to assess QOL after treatment of our vascular surgery patients. Using standard methodology, these experienced investigators at Oxford Brookes and Leicester universities concluded that both endovascular and open aneurysm repair result in a similar negative impact on health-related QOL and cognitive function assessment. I am not extremely surprised by this. Patients undergoing aneurysm repair are generally elderly and fragile and are frequently in a period of rapid decline in social functioning, exclusive of the need for any aneurysm surgery. It would certainly have been nice to have had a control group who had no aneurysm procedure at all who were age matched to make sure that the observed declines were not nonspecifically related to age rather than aneurysm.

Aneurysm Rupture After Endovascular Repair Using the AneuRx Stent Graft
Zarins CK, White RA, Fogarty TJ (Stanford Univ, Calif; Univ of California Los Angeles)
J Vasc Surg 31:960-970, 2000   2–12

Introduction.—Transluminal endovascular aneurysm repair significantly diminishes patient morbidity and offers rapid patient recovery and comparable mortality to the direct repair with the prosthetic graft. The long-term effectiveness of preventing aneurysm rupture has yet to be determined. The cause and frequency of aneurysm rupture after endovascular aneurysm repair was investigated.

Methods.—All patients with aneurysm rupture enrolled for endovascular aortic aneurysm repair in phases I, II, and III of the US AneuRx Multicenter Clinical Trial from June 1996 through October 1999 were evaluated.

Results.—The AneuRx stent graft was successfully implanted in 1046 patients (98%); the repair was not successful in 21 patients (2%). Thirteen (1%) patients were converted to an open aneurysm repair. Two patients (0.2%) experienced aneurysm rupture caused by procedure-related instru-

TABLE 2.—Aneurysm Rupture After Endovascular Repair

Patient	Time Since Implant	Endoleak	Aneurysm Diameter	Presentation At Rupture	Probable Cause	Comment	Outcome After Surgical Repair
1	23 mo	No	No change	Stable, back pain	Proximal extender cuff	Short angulated neck	Alive—10 mo
2	14 mo	No	No change	Unstable, shock	Proximal fixation	Short angulated neck	Died—2 mo, pneumonia
3	15 mo	Yes	Increase 7 mm	Stable, back pain	Distal fixation	Pt refused treatment	Alive—5 mo
4	23 mo	No	Decrease 31 mm	Unstable, back pain	Iliac junction gate	Shrinkage and angulation	Died—9 d
5	24 mo	Yes	Increase 6 mm	Unstable, shock	Distal fixation	Pt refused treatment	Died—3 d
6	3 wk	No	No data	Unstable, shock	Proximal fixation	Inadequate neck	Died—in OR
7	9 mo	No	No change	Stable, automobile crash	Proximal fixation	Angulated neck	Alive—8 mo

Abbreviations: OR, Operating room; *Pt*, patient.
(Courtesy of Zarins CK, White RA, Fogarty TJ: Aneurysm rupture after endovascular repair using the AneuRx stent graft. *J Vasc Surg* 31:960-970, 2000.)

mentation and required open surgical conversion. Seven patients (0.7%) experienced aneurysm rupture at 3 weeks to 24 months (mean, 16 months) after undergoing successful endovascular repair. Four patients survived the open procedure and 3 died within 30 days (Table 2). The overall rupture-related mortality rate was 0.5%, which included late deaths after rupture. There were 2 patients who had endoleak and aneurysm enlargement before rupture and 5 who had no endoleak and no aneurysm enlargement. After aneurysm rupture, all 7 patients had indication of poor fixation of the stent graft at the proximal, distal, or iliac junction fixation sites. The 2 patients with endoleak refused recommended open surgical or endovascular repair. The probability of no aneurysm rupture for all patients who underwent endovascular repair was .996 and .974 at 1 and 2 years by life table analysis with the longest follow-up of 41 months.

Conclusion.—The early risk of rupture after endovascular aneurysm repair was low. The possibility of rupture endures even in patients with endoleak who have undergone the procedure. Patients with evidence indicative of insecure stent graft fixation should undergo further endovascular treatment or open surgical repair.

▶ Remarkably, this article, published in May of 2000, was able to ferret out 2 patients undergoing aneurysm rupture with the AneuRx graft during implantation and 7 additional patients who experienced rupture at a later time after AneuRx placement. This information has been substantially supplanted by a letter from the US FDA dated April 27, 2001 and stating that the FDA has received reports of 25 aneurysm ruptures in patients with the AneuRx graft. The haunting question remains: How many ruptures are enough to keep one from using this graft? If EUROSTAR is correct in stating that we are experiencing about a 1% rupture rate per year and considering that these endografts are substantially being placed in patients who have smaller aneurysms, I wonder whether the endografts have favorably affected the rupture rate at all. It is quite likely that the rupture rate would have been about 1% per year had no treatment been undertaken. As I have said in the past, is it possible that we are kidding ourselves concerning the efficacy of endografts for abdominal aortic aneurysms?

Maximal Aneurysm Diameter Follow-up Is Inadequate After Endovascular Abdominal Aortic Aneurysm Repair

Wever JJ, Blankensteijn JD, Mali WPTM, et al (Univ Med Ctr, Utrecht, The Netherlands)
Eur J Vasc Endovasc Surg 20:177-182, 2000   2–13

Background.—Patients undergoing endovascular abdominal aortic aneurysm repair (EAR) are typically followed up with serial diameter measures. However, a change in size after EAR is caused by changes in the excluded aneurysm sac volume. The agreement between measures of diameter and volume after EAR was investigated.

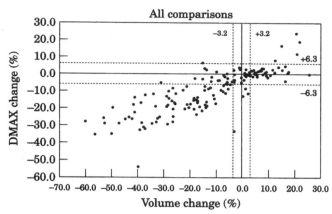

FIGURE 4.—Volume changes plotted against DMAX changes for all comparisons. The intraobserver limits are added to the graph. *Abbreviation: DMAX*, Maximal aneurysm diameter. (Reprinted from Wever JJ, Blankensteijn JD, Mali WPTM, et al: Maximal aneurysm diameter follow-up is inadequate after endovascular abdominal aortic aneurysm repair. *Eur J Vasc Endovasc Surg* 20:177-182, copyright 2000 by permission of the publisher W B Saunders Company Limited London.)

Methods.—Of 53 consecutive patients scheduled for EAR, 35 had follow-up data available for at least 6 months. CT angiography (CTA) was performed at discharge, at 6 months, and every year thereafter. The maximal aneurysm diameter (DMAX) was measured along the central lumen line, and the total aneurysm volume was determined by manual segmentation. All individual patients' measurements were compared with each other, which resulted in 149 comparisons.

Findings.—Volume measures and DMAX were discordant in 37% of the comparisons (Figs 4 and 5). When DMAX was used, aneurysm size

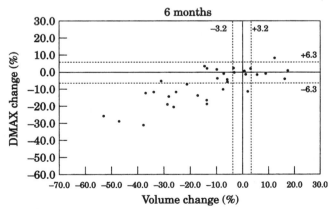

FIGURE 5.—Volume changes plotted against DMAX changes for the individual patients at 6 months of follow-up. *Abbreviation: DMAX*, Maximal aneurysm diameter. (Reprinted from Wever JJ, Blankensteijn JD, Mali WPTM, et al: Maximal aneurysm diameter follow-up is inadequate after endovascular abdominal aortic aneurysm repair. *Eur J Vasc Endovasc Surg* 20:177-182, copyright 2000 by permission of the publisher W B Saunders Company Limited London.)

decreases were missed in 14% of the cases and increases were missed in 19%.

Conclusions.—Assessing volume is more accurate than using DMAX in following up the evolution of the aneurysm sac. Follow-up with DMAX alone after EAR is not sufficient.

▶ I have always thought that the simple measurement of diameter is a rather crude method of characterizing the size of an infrarenal abdominal aortic aneurysm. With modern computer technology, it is possible to calculate total aneurysm volume using the CT scan. These investigators found that aneurysm volume calculations disagreed with simple DMAX measurements in about 37% of patients; in one half the DMAX was too large and in one half it was too small. These investigators and others feel we should be using total aneurysm volume as a superior means of calculating the residual sac compared with DMAX. I suspect they are correct.

Feasiblity of Using Dynamic Contrast-Enhanced Magnetic Resonance Angiography as the Sole Imaging Modality Prior to Endovascular Repair of Abdominal Aortic Aneurysms

Ludman CN, Yusuf SW, Whitaker SC, et al (Univ Hosp, Nottingham, England)
Eur J Vasc Endovasc Surg 19:524-530, 2000   2–14

Background.—Preoperative imaging is critical when evaluating candidates for the endovascular repair of abdominal aortic aneurysms. The most commonly used imaging method is helical CT angiography (CTA). CTA requires large volumes of hyperosmolar iodinated contrast material, which increases the risk of cardiovascular or renal failure. MR angiography (MRA) with dynamic contrast enhancement (DCE) does not have this disadvantage. Whether DCE MRA can be used as the sole preoperative imaging modality for patients being evaluated for endovascular repair of abdominal aortic aneurysms was investigated.

Methods.—The subjects were 14 men and 2 women (mean age, 73.1 years) with abdominal aortic aneurysm who were undergoing helical CTA to evaluate their suitability for endovascular management. Patients also underwent DCE MRA or MRI, and images were assessed to measure the length, diameter, and shape of the infrarenal neck; the internal and external diameters of the aneurysm; the distance from the inferior renal artery to the iliac bifurcation; and the lengths and diameters of the common and external iliac arteries (Fig 1). Patients in whom the infrarenal neck diameter was < 3.0 cm, there was at least 1.5 cm between the renal arteries and the proximal extent of the aneurysm, and there were no significant mural thrombi within the aneurysm neck that were considered suitable for endovascular treatment. Patient suitability was determined independently from helical CTA and DCE MRA/MRI images, then management decisions based on the 2 methods were compared.

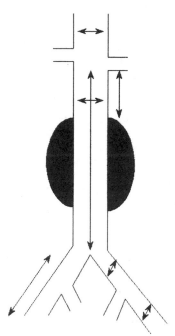

FIGURE 1.—Diagrammatic representation of the aortoiliac vasculature to illustrate the measurements necessary prior to planning an endovascular repair. (Reprinted from the *European Journal of Vascular and Endovascular Surgery* courtesy of Ludman CN, Yusuf SW, Whitaker SC, et al: Feasibility of using dynamic contrast-enhanced magnetic resonance angiography as the sole imaging modality prior to endovascular repair of abdominal aortic aneurysms. *Eur J Vasc Endovasc Surg* 19: 524-530, 2000. Copyright 2000, by permission of the publisher, W B Saunders Company Limited London.)

Results.—High-quality helical CTA and DCE MRA/MRI images were obtained in all 16 patients (Fig 2). In each case, management decisions based on helical CTA concurred with those based on DCE MRA/MRI. This included 6 patients who were considered candidates for endovascular repair, 1 patient with borderline measurements whose additional features justified an endovascular approach, and 9 patients who were deemed unsuitable because of neck morphology or a mural thrombus.

Conclusion.—In each of these 16 patients, decisions regarding the patient's suitability for an endovascular approach to abdominal aortic aneurysm repair were identical based on helical CTA and DCE MRA/MRI. Both techniques have their advantages and disadvantages, but the most significant advantage of DCE MRA/MRI is that it does not require the use of hyperosmolar iodinated contrast material and ionizing radiation. Thus, DCE MRA/MRI appears to be feasible as a sole preoperative imaging modality for patients being evaluated for endovascular repair of abdominal aortic aneurysm.

▶ I suppose in the right hands DCE MRA is about as good as contrast CTA in imaging for endovascular aneurysm graft insertion. I have been impressed that the clinical utility of MRA seems to be determined almost exclusively by

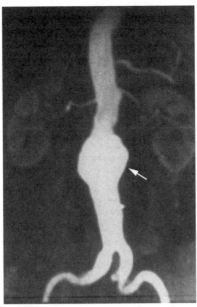

FIGURE 2.—Breath-held MR angiographic images acquired during dynamic administration of IV gadolinium-DTPA contrast. The vascular lumen of a small abdominal aortic aneurysm (*arrow*) and the aortoiliac and renal vasculature are clearly delineated. (Reprinted from the *European Journal of Vascular and Endovascular Surgery* courtesy of Ludman CN, Yusuf SW, Whitaker SC, et al: Feasibility of using dynamic contrast-enhanced magnetic resonance angiography as the sole imaging modality prior to endovascular repair of abdominal aortic aneurysms. *Eur J Vasc Endovasc Surg* 19: 524-530, 2000. Copyright 2000, by permission of the publisher, W B Saunders Company Limited, London.)

the expertise and the degree of interest of your local radiologist who operates the machine. No one at our institution has had much interest in it so, consequently, it has not been of much use to us to date. However, with the proper degree of interest, I suspect the images obtained are every bit as helpful as the CT angiogram, to which it is being compared.

Percutaneous Endovascular Repair of Infrarenal Abdominal Aortic Aneurysms: A Feasibility Study

Traul DK, Clair DG, Gray B, et al (Cleveland Clinic Found, Ohio)
J Vasc Surg 32:770-776, 2000   2–15

Objective.—The usual endovascular repair of abdominal aortic aneurysms involves a single or bilateral groin incision. The initial experience with a totally percutaneous approach to endovascular repair of abdominal aortic aneurysms was described.

Methods.—Percutaneous placement of the AneuRx endovascular graft (Medtronic, Sunnyvale, Calif), using a modification of the insertion technique for the Prostar device (Perclose, Redwood City, Calif), was attempted in 17 patients (1 woman), aged 62 to 93 years. Preoperative and postoperative records—including anatomical variables and operative events, operation times, and length of hospital stays—were reviewed and compared with those of patients having bilateral open femoral access.

> *Technique.*—Retrograde percutaneous arterial access was achieved with an 18-gauge needle, a 0.035-in guidewire, and an 8F sheath, which was exchanged for a 10F Prostar device that was deployed during insertion of the contralateral limb. The guidewire was reinserted in patients undergoing percutaneous insertion of the main body of the device and used to guide the advance of the 21F device. The device was deployed and rotated 45°. Patients were given systemic heparinization. In 5 patients, a second guidewire was reinserted, and a 22F sheath was placed. Hemostasis at the hub was achieved by insertion of an 8F sheath.

Results.—The procedure was successful in 14 patients, with successful deployment through the 22F sheath in 9 (75%) of 12 attempts and successful deployment through the 16F sheath in 11 (64.7%) of 17 attempts. Six attempts (46.2%) were successful in 13 patients having bilateral procedures. Operative times averaged 167 minutes for patients having bilateral open femoral access, 138 minutes for 17 attempts at percutaneous access, and 90 minutes for bilateral percutaneous success. Percutaneous vascular closure failure resulted from bleeding in 48 patients, vessel dissection in 15, device malfunction in 7, and inflow in 16. Patients were converted to the open procedure for bleeding in 6 procedures, iliofemoral dissection in 2, device failure in 1, and compromised distal flow in 1. Percutaneous deployment was problematic in small vessels (less than 7 mm in diameter), heavily calcified or diseased arteries, and tortuous arteries.

Conclusion.—Percutaneous endovascular repair of infrarenal abdominal aortic aneurysms was successful in 46.2% of attempts.

▶ The manually facile group at Cleveland Clinic has been able to achieve percutaneous endograft placement of the AneuRx graft in about 75% of patients. It is, however, sobering to note that the reasons for failure include inadequate percutaneous hemostasis, iliofemoral dissection, device failure, and compromised distal flow—not insignificant considerations. Perhaps one day there will be a much smaller device for insertion, but if so I wonder what we will use for graft fabric and for an attachment device. Clearly, the present generation of material will not be acceptable. Perhaps in the future we will have a cobweb like graft material that will fold down into almost invisibility and an attachment device made from an as yet unimagined alloy with infinite strength at minimal size. On balance, this whole thing sounds like someone getting ready to sell you a bridge in Brooklyn.

Duplex Ultrasound Scanning Versus Computed Tomographic Angiography for Postoperative Evaluation of Endovascular Abdominal Aortic Aneurysm Repair

Wolf YG, Johnson BL, Hill BB, et al (Stanford Univ, Calif)
J Vasc Surg 32:1142-1148, 2000   2–16

Background.—The long-term efficacy of endovascular aneurysm repair for preventing rupture has not been established. Because persistent flow in the aneurysm sac carries a risk of rupture, patients must be followed up with imaging after endovascular repair of abdominal aortic aneurysm (AAA). Duplex US scanning and CT angiography in the postoperative imaging and surveillance of patients after AAA endovascular repair were compared.

Methods.—One hundred consecutive patients with AAA underwent endovascular aneurysm repair. Both CT angiography and duplex US were performed at regular intervals after the procedure.

Findings.—Two hundred sixty-eight CT scans and 214 duplex scans were obtained 1 to 30 months after repair. All CT scans were technically adequate, as were 93% of the duplex scans. Scan pairs were obtained within 7 days of each other in 166 instances in 76 patients. The 2 methods correlated closely in maximal transverse aneurysm sac diameter (Fig 1). Measures were within 5 mm of each other in 92% of the scans. The 2 modalities were also correlated closely in diagnosing endoleaks (Table). Compared with CT, duplex scanning had an 81% sensitivity, 95% speci-

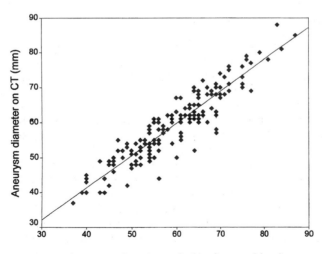

Aneurysm diameter on duplex ultrasound (mm)

FIGURE 1.—Maximal transverse diameter of aneurysm after endovascular exclusion of abdominal aortic aneurysm. Measurement by CT and duplex scan correlated closely (r, -0.93; $P < .001$), and on paired t test, no significant difference was found. In 92% of the scans, diameter measurements differed by less than 5 mm. (Courtesy of Wolf YG, Johnson BL, Hill BB, et al: Duplex ultrasound scanning versus computed tomographic angiography for postoperative evaluation of endovascular abdominal aortic aneurysm repair. *J Vasc Surg* 32:1142-1148, 2000.)

TABLE.—Identification of Endoleak on CT Angiography Versus Duplex US Scan in 166 Scan Pairs

	CT Angiography	
	No Endoleak	Endoleak
Duplex		
No endoleak	98	11
Endoleak	3	51
Indeterminate	2	1

Note: The tests had excellent correlation (χ^2 109; $P < .001$). Endoleaks missed on duplex scan were small, located posteriorly, and associated with lumbar arteries.

(Courtesy of Wolf YG, Johnson BL, Hill BB, et al: Duplex ultrasound scanning versus computed tomographic angiography for postoperative evaluation of endovascular abdominal aortic aneurysm repair. *J Vasc Surg* 32:1142-1148, 2000.)

ficity, and positive and negative predictive values of 94% and 90%, respectively. Findings were discordant in 8% of examinations. In all 8 patients with an endoleak considered severe enough to warrant arteriography, the endoleak was visualized on both studies. Graft patency was demonstrated in all patients by both modalities, with no discrepancy.

Conclusion.—High-quality duplex US scanning is comparable to CT angiography in assessing aneurysm size, endoleak, and graft patency after endovascular exclusion of AAA. This modality may be used for surveillance and routine follow-up.

▶ This is a very timely study in light of recent recommendations that patients undergoing endovascular repair of an AAA have frequent, if not lifelong, graft surveillance. This report compared detection of changes in aneurysm size, presence of endoleak, and graft patency by 2 modalities: CT angiography and duplex US scanning. The ideal and safe method for following up patients is a consideration, especially since CT angiography involves radiation exposure and possible contrast-related nephrotoxicity. However, some recent studies suggest that duplex US may not be accurate enough for surveillance of these grafts.

These authors demonstrate an excellent correlation between the 2 methods of evaluation from the point of view of aneurysm size, endoleak, and graft patency. There was a lack of concordance in 8% of the examinations for the diagnosis of endoleak but the authors point out that any significant endoleak was diagnosed by both techniques. All cases of endoleak that were thought to involve the attachment sites and to warrant arteriography and reintervention were detected by both methods. The only potential problem, as is well known, is that duplex US scanning is highly operator-dependent whereas CT angiography is not. If a service is going to adopt a policy of using duplex US scanning, it is essential that it offer high-quality reproducible scans.

J. O. Menzoian, MD

Lower Extremity Paraparesis or Paraplegia Subsequent to Endovascular Management of Abdominal Aortic Aneurysms

Rockman CB, Riles TS, Landis R (New York Univ)
J Vasc Surg 33:178-180, 2001   2–17

Background.—Paraplegia and paraparesis are rare but devastating complications of surgical repair of abdominal aortic aneurysms (AAAs). Two cases of paraparesis/paraplegia associated with endovascular AAA repair were reported.

Patients.—Both patients were elderly (aged 84 and 82 years) with 5-cm AAAs. Both patients had a history of previous neurologic conditions, although they had only mild deficits preoperatively. In the first patient, severe paraparesis and bladder dysfunction developed after apparently successful endovascular repair; it was attributed to spinal cord ischemic caused by atheroembolization. Endovascular repair was attempted in the second case but was converted to standard open repair because of technical problems. Postoperatively, the patient had severe paresis of the left lower extremity. Again, the neurologic diagnosis was spinal cord ischemia caused by atheroembolization.

Discussion.—These cases suggest that atheroembolization to the spinal cord may be more frequent with endovascular repair of AAAs than with open surgical management. The complication may result from manipulation of endovascular devices in severely atherosclerotic vessels. No patient or surgically related factors predictive of these events have yet been identified.

▶ The intraluminal placement and manipulation of guide wires, catheters, and endovascular device deployment systems is associated with a risk of embolization of debris. This observation has been previously reported. It is entirely logical that these devices might also involve the spinal cord, a devastating event with poor prospects for recovery. These devices are also not well understood with open surgery, where results also are unpredictable and tragic. It has been my experience, and that of others, that the risk of spinal ischemia is less with endovascular repair of thoracic aortic lesions than with open surgical repair. The incidence is sufficiently low in the abdominal aorta to make such a comparison difficult. There is less risk of hypotension, hypoperfusion, and blood loss with endovascular aortic aneurysm repair compared with open repair; however, it is likely that the risk of embolization is greater with endovascular procedures.

M. A. Golden, MD

Aortic Aneurysmal Disease: Assessment of Stent-Graft Treatment—CT Versus Conventional Angiography

Armerding MD, Rubin GD, Beaulieu CF, et al (Stanford Univ, Calif)
Radiology 215:138-146, 2000   2–18

Introduction.—CT angiography is being used with increasing frequency as an alternative to the more invasive conventional angiography. Conventional angiography has higher spatial resolution in comparison to CT angiography, but the volumetric acquisition of CT angiography eradicates

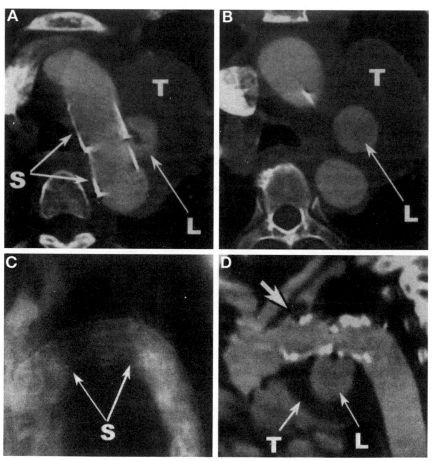

FIGURE 1.—**A, B,** Serial transverse CT scans demonstrate a large aortic arch aneurysm that is partially thrombosed following deployment of a stent-graft. All three CT angiography readers identified a large perigraft leak. **C,** Anterior 60° left oblique screen-film angiogram was read as positive for perigraft leakage by none of the three conventional angiography readers. **D,** Oblique curved planar reformation image shows leakage from a perspective similar to that in the conventional angiogram in **C** and also demonstrates the stent-graft occluding the origin of the left subclavian artery, where a thrombus (*thick arrow*) has formed. *Abbreviations:* L, Perigraft leak; *S* stent-graft; *T*, thrombosis. (Courtesy of Armerding MD, Rubin GD, Beaulieu CF, et al: Aortic aneurysmal disease: Assessment of stent-graft treatment—CT versus conventional angiography. *Radiology* 215:138-146, 2000. Radiological Society of North America.)

the limitations of conventional angiographic projections, which have poor discrimination of overlapping structures, limited contrast resolution, and parallax. The efficacy of CT angiography was compared with that of conventional angiography in ascertaining the success of endoluminal stent-graft treatment of aortic aneurysms.

Methods.—The study included 40 patients who underwent both conventional angiography and CT angiography after treatment of aneurysms with endoluminal stent-grafts. Six additional sets of these examinations were performed in 5 patients who underwent placement of additional stent-grafts or coil embolization to treat perigraft leakage. Three CT radiologists blinded to patient clinical data and outcome independently interpreted the CT angiograms; 3 angiographers not involved in the stent-graft deployment interpreted the conventional angiograms. Images were evaluated for the presence of postdeployment complications. A reference standard was created by experienced radiologists using all available images and clinical data. Sensitivities, specificities, and k values were determined.

Results.—The most commonly observed complication was perigraft leakage (Fig 1). Twenty perigraft leaks were seen in 46 examinations. Sensitivities and specificities for identifying perigraft leakage were 63% and 77%, respectively, for conventional angiography; for CT angiography, these rates were 92% and 90%, respectively. The k values were 0.41 and 0.81 for conventional angiography and CT angiography, respectively.

Conclusion.—CT angiography is the preferred technique for determining the presence of perigraft leakage after treatment of aortoiliac aneurysms with stent-grafts.

▶ In a further effort to comparatively evaluate various imaging modalities in patients after endovascular graft deployment, these extremely experienced investigators found that CT angiography was superior to conventional angiography, at least in detecting endoleaks, which was by far the most frequently observed complication. While I believe this conclusion is exactly correct, it does seem as if these investigators have worked rather hard to set up a straw man to knock down. I am not sure anyone thought that conventional angiography was superior to CT angiography in postoperative evaluation. I am glad that they seem to have come to the same conclusion reached by almost everyone else.

Special Iliac Artery Considerations During Aneurysm Endografting
Henretta JP, Karch LA, Hodgson KJ, et al (Southern Illinois Univ, Springfield)
Am J Surg 178:212-218, 1999   2–19

Background.—Endoluminal repair of infrarenal abdominal aortic aneurysms has been demonstrated to be effective and possibly advantageous in comparison with standard open surgical repair in terms of associated morbidity, hospital stay, and time to return to baseline health status.

However, there have been few data regarding the technical aspects of endoluminal repair in the literature thus far. Delivery of the graft through diseased or tortuous iliac arteries is challenging, as is the treatment of associated iliac aneurysmal disease. The types of iliac issues requiring special attention during endoluminal aortic aneurysm repair and specific techniques to address these challenging situations are presented.

Methods.—Records of all patients who underwent endoluminal repair of abdominal aortic aneurysms at a single institution were prospectively reviewed. Over 19 months, endoluminal repair of abdominal aortic aneurysms and/or iliac artery aneurysms was performed in 74 patients. All repairs were performed using a bifurcated, self-expanding modular device that was fully supported with an exoskeleton of nitinol "Z" stents. Iliac anatomy that required special consideration during endografting was reviewed.

Results.—Iliac anatomy that required special consideration was present in 35 of 74 patients (47%). Aneurysmal involvement of a common iliac artery was present in 13 of 74 patients (18%), and 11 of these patients required endograft extension into the external iliac artery (EIA) and hypogastric coil embolization because of the proximity of the aneurysm to the hypogastric origin. Aortic cuffs were used in 11 patients with ectatic, nonaneurysmal iliac arteries to achieve a distal seal in these oversized vessels. In 27 of 74 patients (36%), iliac artery tortuosity or stenosis were compelling factors, and, in 2 of these patients, the use of brachial guidewire tension was required to allow tracking of the delivery device. Crossed placement of the iliac limbs was required in 5 patients with severely splayed aortic bifurcations to prevent kinking of the endograft. Preprocedural dilatation and stenting were required in 3 patients, and postprocedural surgical EIA reconstruction was needed in 5 patients with occlusive atherosclerotic disease. In 3 patients who underwent successful endograft placement, subsequent endovascular repair of traumatized EIAs was required.

Conclusions.—The anatomy of the iliac artery has a significant role in the endoluminal treatment of infrarenal abdominal aortic aneurysms, which complicates the procedure in up to 47% of patients with otherwise suitable anatomy. Both surgical and endovascular supplemental procedures may be required for the facilitation of endograft placement. Proper planning and a unique understanding of the complicating factors in iliac artery anatomy are required if optimal therapy is to be delivered.

▶ Who could dispute the suggestion that careful preoperative evaluation of the iliac system is important to the delivery of optimal endografts? Almost 50% of the iliac arteries in patients receiving aortic endografts required special attention because of a combination of dilatation, tortuosity, and widening of the bifurcation. Clearly, successful endograft placement does not end with the aortic anchor. We have to also be fully cognizant of the details of iliac artery deployment. While the authors do appear to state the obvious, it is perhaps helpful to be periodically reminded of the importance of careful consideration of iliac anatomy in endograft deployment.

Carotid

Immediate and Late Clinical Outcomes of Carotid Artery Stenting in Patients With Symptomatic and Asymptomatic Carotid Artery Stenosis: A 5-Year Prospective Analysis

Roubin GS, New G, Iyer SS, et al (Lennox Hill Heart and Vascular Inst, New York; Univ of Alabama, Birmingham; Cleveland Clinic, Ohio; et al)
Circulation 103:532-537, 2001   2–20

Background.—For patients with carotid stenosis, carotid stenting (CS) offers a less-invasive alternative to carotid endarterectomy. Previous studies indicate little difference in the risk of periprocedural complications. A 5-year prospective study assessed the long-term outcomes of CS for patients with carotid stenosis.

Methods.—The experience included 528 consecutive patients undergoing CS; a total of 604 hemispheres/arteries were treated. The patients were 356 men and 172 women with a mean age of 69 years.

Results.—The 30-day fatal stroke rate was 0.6%, while the rate of death from causes other than stroke was 1.0%. Major stroke occurred for 1.0% of patients and minor stroke for 4.8%. Thus, the 30-day composite stroke and death rate was 7.4%. The 30-day risk of minor stroke decreased significantly as experience was gained; it ranged from 7.1% in the first year to 3.1% in the fifth. Patients aged 80 years or older were most likely to die or experience a stroke within 30 days. Beyond 30 days, the rate of fatal and nonfatal stroke was 3.2%. The Kaplan-Meier rate of freedom from ipsilateral or fatal stroke 3 years after CS was 92%.

Conclusion.—This experience suggests an acceptable 30-day complication rate for patients undergoing CS. The late risk of fatal and nonfatal stroke is low. The results support the ongoing National Institutes of Health study comparing CS with carotid endarterectomy for patients with carotid artery disease.

▶ There are many things wrong with this series. In the first place, the mean follow-up is quite short. Although never stated, it is probably little more than 12 months. The patients were not seen after 30 days but were followed up by telephone interviews. Routine CT or MRI of the head were not obtained. Within the limits of these severe problems, the perioperative death rate at 30 days was 1.6%. The major stroke rate was 1%, the minor stroke rate was, 4.8%, with an overall stroke and death rate of 7.4%. However, I consider all data in this series to be soft after 30 days. The absence of detailed neurologic examination during follow-up, the absence of adequate follow-up, and the absence of head imaging all suggest to me that these data are being presented in the most favorable light possible. One must keep in mind that angioplasty in this setting is being held out as superior treatment to surgery, when surgery typically takes 1 to 2 days in the hospital and is accomplished with a stroke/death rate of under 1.5% and excellent long-term clinical results. I really do not see how carotid angioplasty could be considered superior.

Carotid Artery Stenting: Technical Considerations

Vitek JJ, Roubin GS, Al-Mubarek N, et al (Lenox Hill Hosp, New York)
AJNR Am J Neuroradiol 21:1736-1743, 2000   2–21

Objective.—Carotid artery stenting (CAS) was prospectively investigated as an alternative to carotid endarterectomy (CEA) for preventing stroke. Complication-free results were emphasized.

Methods.—Between September 1994 and September 1998, 412 CAS procedures were performed on 390 patients (70% male; 421 carotid arteries), aged 35 to 89 years, with the use of a 7F 90-cm guiding sheath for predilation and stent placement and deployment (Fig 1). Antiplatelet therapy was administered 2 to 4 days prior to surgery. Technical success was defined as a residual stenosis no greater than 20%. Patients were discharged the next morning. Outcome measures were an occurrence within 30 days of minor stroke, major stroke, death, or myocardial infarction.

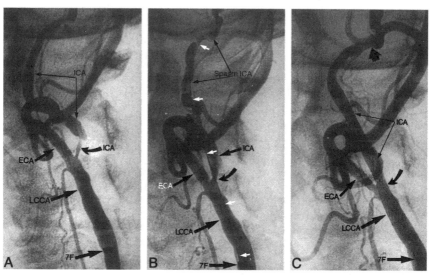

FIGURE 1.—Angiograms from the case of an 80-year-old man with bilateral internal carotid artery stenosis. **A,** Angiogram shows 80% stenoses in the left internal carotid artery *(ICA)* *(curved arrow)*. A 7F sheath *(7F)* was inserted into the left common carotid artery *(LCCA)*. Distal, independent stenosis on the internal carotid artery *(thick black arrow)* can be seen. *Abbreviation: ECA,* External carotid artery. **B,** Angiogram shows status after predilation *(curved arrow)* of the internal carotid artery with a 4-mm balloon over a 0.018-inch guidewire *(white arrows)*. Spasm on the distal internal carotid artery can be seen. **C,** Angiogram obtained after the carotid artery stenting control study. A 10 × 20 Wallstent was used, dilated with a 5 × 20 Symmetry balloon. Minimal residual spasm can be seen. Independent distal stenosis persists *(wide black arrow)*. (Courtesy of Vitek JJ, Roubin GS, Al-Mubarek N, et al: Carotid artery stenting: Technical considerations. *AJNR Am J Neuroradiol* 21:1736-1743, 2000. Copyright by American Society of Neuroradiology.)

TABLE.—Carotid Angioplasty With Stenting: Thirty-day Events

	Total	%
Asymptomatic hemispheres (vessels)	202	
Minor strokes	11	5.4%
Major strokes	2	1%
Neuro Death	0	
Non Neuro Death	2	1%
All strokes/death	15	7.4%
Symptomatic hemispheres (vessels)	249	
Minor strokes	14	5.6%
Major strokes	2	0.8%
Neuro Death	2	0.8%
Non Neuro Death	3	1.2%
All strokes/death	21	8.4%

(Courtesy of Vitek JJ, Roubin GS, Al-Mubarek N, et al: Carotid artery stenting: Technical considerations. *AJNR Am J Neuroradiol* 21:1736-1743, 2000. Copyright by American Society of Neuroradiology.)

Results.—Technical success was achieved in 98% of procedures. Stenosis was reduced on average from 74% to 5%. Self-expanding Wallstents were used in 72% of procedures. The combined stroke and death rate at 30 days was 7.9% (Table).

Conclusion.—CAS is a less invasive procedure than CEA and is an effective treatment for carotid stenosis.

▶ This article was published 3 months before the preceding article (Abstract 2–20) and reports on 390 patients, while the prior article reports on 528 patients. All internal data are the same. Data entry extended 1 additional year in the preceding article, indicating to me that these interventionists treated 138 patients during the last year. For regaling us with nearly identical data in nearly simultaneous publications, I am delighted to convey to these authors the coveted Camel Dung Award for duplicate publication. They obviously subscribe to the old Chicago motto: If you have salable data, publish early and often.

Endovascular Stenting for Carotid Artery Stenosis: Preliminary Experience Using the Shape-Memory–Alloy-Recoverable–Technology (SMART) Stent

Phatouros CC, Higashida RT, Malek AM, et al (Univ of California, San Francisco)

AJNR Am J Neuroradiol 21:732-738, 2000   2–22

Background.—Carotid artery stent-supported angioplasty shows promise as an alternative to carotid endarterectomy for patients with carotid artery occlusive disease. An initial experience with a new self-expanding stent—the shape–memory–alloy-recoverable–technology (SMART) stent (Cordis Endovascular, Miami Lakes, Fla)—in 5 patients with carotid occlusive disease was reported.

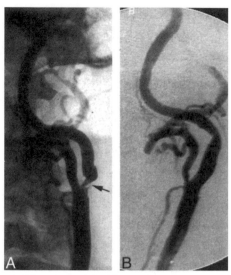

FIGURE 4.—Ipsilateral oblique views of the left carotid artery. A, Severe short-segment, circumferential, atherosclerotic stenosis of the internal carotid artery origin (*arrow*). B, Appearance after deployment of a SMART stent within the internal carotid artery. (Courtesy of Phatouros CC, Higashida RT, Malek AM, et al: Endovascular stenting for carotid artery stenosis: Preliminary experience using the shape-memory–alloy–recoverable–technology (SMART) stent. *AJNR Am J Neuroradiol* 21: 732-738, 2000. Copyright by American Society of Neuroradiology.)

Methods.—The basic procedure, in brief, is as follows: Three days preoperatively, patients began taking enteric-coated aspirin and clopidogrel. With the patient under conscious sedation, a groin sheath was inserted into the common femoral artery and clotting time was measured. Cerebral angiography was performed, then heparin was administered until the activated clotting time was 2 to 2.5 times the baseline value or 250 seconds or greater.

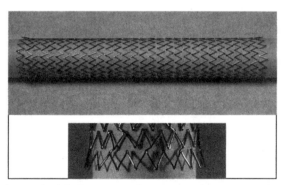

FIGURE 5.—Photograph of the SMART stent shows segmented geometry and flared margins. (Courtesy of Phatouros CC, Higashida RT, Malek AM, et al: Endovascular stenting for carotid artery stenosis: Preliminary experience using the shape-memory–alloy–recoverable technology (SMART) stent. *AJNR Am J Neuroradiol* 21: 732-738, 2000. Copyright by American Society of Neuroradiology.)

An 0.035-in, 300-cm exchange-length wire was placed in the ipsilateral external carotid artery, then a 9F guiding catheter was positioned in the common carotid artery over the wire. The stenosis was crossed with a 2.3F microcatheter and a 0.014-in. guidewire, which was exchanged with an 0.014-in., 300-cm exchange-length guidewire. Glycopyrrolate was administered before balloon inflation to prevent reflex bradycardia or asystole, then the balloons were predilated and the stent was advanced over the immobilized guidewire. Once the stent was deployed, balloon angioplasty was performed.

Patients continued receiving IV heparin overnight, then it was tapered. Once partial thromblastin times had returned to normal, the femoral sheaths were removed via an external compression device. Patients continued to take oral aspirin indefinitely and clopidogrel for 6 weeks. Patients were followed up at 6 months with carotid duplex US. This technique was used in 4 patients (2 men and 2 women aged 44-85 years) with carotid artery stenosis of 70% or greater. 1 patient required 2 SMART stents because the first one did not completely conform to the contour of the carotid bulb and caused partial luminal obstruction.

Results.—All procedures were successful, with less than 20% residual stenosis in all cases (Fig 4). There were no complications specifically related to the SMART stent, and none of the patients have died. During an average follow-up of 3 months, all patients remain free of symptoms, and none has experienced a transient ischemic attack or new stroke.

Conclusion.—The SMART stent was successful in the endovascular treatment of carotid occlusive disease in these 4 patients. This stent has numerous advantages over other self-expanding stents, such as the Wallstent (Schneider, Minneapolis, Minn). First, the SMART stent is made of Nitinol, which is a nickel-titanium metallic alloy that has shape memory: When exposed to body temperature, the stent assumes a predetermined shape that resists deformation and compression. Additionally, the SMART stent is generally easier to position accurately than other stents. It conforms better to the native vessel contour, in part because the SMART stent has a segmented geometrical design (Fig 5) that allows the individual stent hoops to behave somewhat independently of each other. Additional studies with more patients and longer follow-up are needed to validate these results, but these initial results indicate that the SMART stent appears to be an alternative to carotid endarterectomy for carotid occlusive disease.

▶ The authors describe a new self-expanding Nitinol stent for use in the carotid artery. Early results in a few patients appear quite positive. These authors suggest that this stent appears to be at least as good as the wall stent, which is frequently used for carotid disease treatment. I suppose they are correct.

Carotid Stenting for Radiation-Induced Stenoses: A Report of 7 Cases

Houdart E, Mounayer C, Chapot R, et al (Hôpital Lariboisière, Paris)
Stroke 32:118-121, 2001   2–23

Background.—External irradiation of the head and neck can lead to extracranial carotid stenoses. These lesions present with fibrosis of the arterial wall and normal tissue planes, posing a difficult challenge in management. An experience with carotid angioplasty stenting (CAS) in 7 patients with radiation-induced carotid stenoses was reported.

Methods.—The patients, treated over a 2-year period, underwent CAS for a total of 10 radiation-induced carotid stenoses of the common or internal carotid artery. Four patients had a history of previous radical neck dissection, while 3 had a permanent tracheostomy in place. All stenoses were 70% or greater; all but 1 of the patients had neurologic symptoms. Via a femoral approach, a self-expandable stent was placed, followed by carotid dilation.

Results.—All CAS procedures were successful (Figure). Residual stenoses were less than 20% in all cases, with no permanent complications. At a mean follow-up of 8 months, all patients were asymptomatic and had no Doppler evidence of restenosis.

Conclusion.—CAS offers a safe and effective treatment option for patients with radiation-induced carotid stenoses. The authors call for long-term follow-up studies of CAS in this high-risk group of patients.

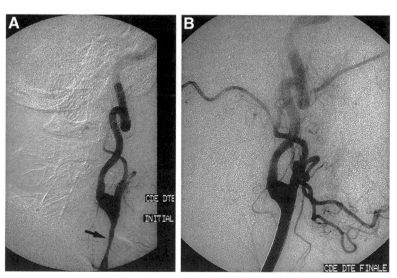

FIGURE.—**A,** Initial angiography of the right carotid artery shows a long tight stenosis of the common carotid artery (*arrow*), **B,** Angiography after carotid angioplasty stenting of the right common carotid artery. (Courtesy of Houdart E, Mounayer C, Chapot R, et al: Carotid stenting for radiation-induced stenoses: A report of 7 cases. *Stroke* 32:118-121, 2001. Reprinted with permission of *Stroke*. Copyright 2001, American Heart Association.)

▶ We have all been dismayed to receive increasing numbers of patients after radical neck cancer surgery and external irradiation who present with symptomatic carotid artery stenosis. In these patients, the carotid artery is often covered only by the skin. In most of these patients, the carotid disease is calcific and transmural. An endarterectomy is technically difficult to perform because of the frequent transmural nature of the calcification, and it is always challenging to get secure skin closure over the operative site. Finally, these operations have been notorious for early recurrences. For all these reasons, I am quite willing to consider angioplasty in symptomatic patients as described here. The results with 7 patients so treated and reported here appear excellent. I do believe the use of angioplasty in such a "hostile neck" environment is a sensible choice.

Carotid Stenting and "Extarterectomy" in the Management of Head and Neck Cancer Involving the Internal Carotid Artery: Technical Case Report

Nussbaum ES, Levine SC, Hamlar D, et al (Univ of Minnesota, Minneapolis)
Neurosurgery 47:981-984, 2000   2–24

Objective.—The treatment of patients with advanced head and neck cancer involving the internal carotid artery (ICA) is controversial. A novel technique for radical tumor removal that avoids the need to interrupt flow through the ICA is described.

> *Case Report.*—Man, 62, with extensive neck malignancy involving the ICA had pain, difficulty swallowing, and hoarseness. Preoperative chemotherapy shrank his malignant fibrous histocytoma by 50%. He had good collateral flow from the opposite hemisphere but reported vision loss in the ipsilateral eye during balloon test occlusion. The ICA was stented with an 8-mm-diameter 40-mm-long, self-expanding nitinol Smart stent to span the entire portion of the artery encased by the tumor. After 1 month, surgery was

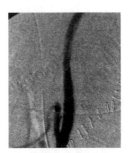

FIGURE 4.—Postoperative lateral left carotid arteriogram revealing normal filling of the ICA. The distal external carotid artery has been sacrificed as part of the tumor removal. (Courtesy of Nussbaum ES, Levine SC, Hamlar D, et al: Carotid stenting and "extarterectomy" in the management of head and neck cancer involving the internal carotid artery: Technical case report. *Neurosurgery* 47:981-984, 2000.)

performed using a transcondylar approach to expose the ICA at its cranial base and including an arteriotomy extending from the proximal ICA above the carotid bifurcation to below the cranial base. A neoendothelium that had formed below the stent prevented bleeding. The carotid wall was removed en bloc, and the artery was wrapped with a synthetic Hemashield patch. Postoperatively, the ICA demonstrated normal filling (Fig 4).

Conclusion.—Preoperative stenting and delayed tumor resection allow successful removal of an invasive head and neck malignancy involving the ICA without interrupting the flow in the ICA.

▶ This is indeed a novel use of a carotid stent. I congratulate the authors on their innovation. Even though this is only a single case report, it may point the way to a new means of therapy applicable to a modest number of patients with aggressive head and neck tumor. I commend it for your consideration.

In-Stent Restenosis After Carotid Angioplasty–Stenting: Incidence and Management
Chakhtoura EY, Hobson RW II, Goldstein J, et al (Univ of Medicine and Dentistry of New Jersey, Newark)
J Vasc Surg 33:220-226, 2001   2–25

Background.—Carotid angioplasty-stenting (CAS) seems to be a viable alternative to carotid endarterectomy (CEA) for select subgroups of patients with carotid occlusive disease. These subgroups include high-risk patients with significant comorbidities who have primary stenosis, patients with carotid restenosis after prior CEA, patients with anatomically inaccessible lesions above the second rib, and patients with radiation-induced stenosis. Nonetheless, the incidence of in-stent restenosis (ISR) after CAS and its optimal management are poorly defined. An experience with ISR after CAS is described.

Methods.—Between September 1996 and May 2000, 46 patients underwent 50 CAS procedures to treat asymptomatic (61%) and symptomatic (39%) carotid stenosis of 80% or more (Table 2). The 50 lesions included 40 post-CEA stenoses (80%), 9 primary lesions in patients with critical 2- or 3-vessel coronary artery disease (18%), and 1 stenosis caused by radiation in 1 patient (2%). After CAS, all patients were followed up at 3- to 6-month intervals via clinical examinations and duplex US. Patients with US evidence of ISR that was 80% or greater were evaluated by angiography to confirm the extent of stenosis.

Results.—None of the patients experienced a stroke during the first 30 postoperative days, but 1 patient (2%), a 72-year-old woman, died 10 days after discharge due to myocardial infarction. During a mean follow-up of 18 months, duplex US identified 4 cases (8%) of ISR that was

TABLE 2.—Baseline Clinical Characteristics of the Study Group (N = 46)

	n	%
Men	26	57
Women	20	43
Asymptomatic (> 80%)	28	61
Symptomatic	18	39
Hemispheric TIA	6	13
Amaurosis fugax	2	4
Global symptoms	10	22
Diabetes	15	33
Hypertension	39	85
Smoker	23	50
Hypercholesterolemia	23	50
Coronary artery disease	25	54

Abbreviation: TIA, Transient ischemic attack.
(Courtesy of Chakhtoura EY, Hobson RW II, Goldstein J, et al: In-stent restenosis after carotid angioplasty-stenting: Incidence and management. *J Vasc Surg* 33:220-226, 2001.)

80% or greater, all of which were confirmed by angiography. Three of these cases developed in patients after they had undergone CEA, whereas the fourth case occurred in the patient with radiation-induced stenosis. All ISRs were successfully treated with balloon angioplasty (3 cases) or angioplasty and restenting (1 case). During a mean follow-up of 10 months after revision, none of these patients have experienced recurrent ISR, and all remain asymptomatic.

Conclusions.—The efficacy and safety of CAS are confirmed for post-CEA restenosis, for primary stenoses in high-risk patients with comorbid conditions, and for radiation-induced stenosis. ISR developed in 4 patients (8% of procedures) and was effectively treated by angioplasty alone or in combination with restenting.

▶ This publication addresses what I am sure will become an increasingly important problem, namely, what to do with patients in whom ISR develops after CAS. In follow-up for a mean of 18 months of 50 patients undergoing CAS, recurrent ISR greater than 80% developed in 4 (8%). Each of these patients was treated successfully by repeat balloon angioplasty, with restenting in 1 patient. These patients have subsequently remained free of stenosis for a mean follow-up of 10 months. To date, no new recurrences have developed. Interestingly, all of the restenoses treated were asymptomatic. I wonder whether the treatment was essential? It seems that most interventionists have adopted the attitude that if an angioplasty fails, simply do it again, and do it over and over until there is no possibility of doing it anymore. We seem to be developing a new treatment paradigm.

Initial Evaluation of Carotid Angioplasty and Stenting With Three Different Cerebral Protection Devices

Parodi JC, La Mura R, Ferreira LM, et al (Instituto Cardiovascular Buenos Aires, Argentina; Palm Beach Surgical Group, West Palm Beach, Fla; Clínica "La Sagrada Familia," West Palm Beach, Fla)
J Vasc Surg 32:1127-1136, 2000   2–26

Background.—If carotid artery angioplasty and stenting (CAS) is to become a valid alternative to surgery for carotid occlusive disease, effective approaches for reducing the rate of procedure-related neuroembolism will be needed. Various approaches to cerebral protection have been proposed for this purpose, including filter devices placed in the internal carotid artery (ICA) (AngioGuard) (Fig 1A) and balloon occlusion of the ICA (PercuSurge) (Fig 2B). Recently, the Parodi Antiembolism System (PAES) was developed, which works by producing retrograde ICA flow and occlusion of the common and external carotid arteries (Fig 3A-C). These 3 approaches to cerebral protection were evaluated in patients undergoing CAS.

Methods.—The prospective study included 46 patients undergoing CAS for severe carotid stenosis, which was symptomatic in 39% of cases. In 25 patients, the procedure was performed using the PercuSurge, AngioGuard, or PAES for cerebral protection. All procedures used Wallstents with selective predilation. The main study outcomes were perioperative neurologic complications and deaths.

Results.—The overall rate of perioperative neurologic deficits was 4.34%. Two events occurred in patients who did not receive cerebral protection: a transient ischemic attack and a minor stroke, which yielded a rate of 9.53%. There were no events in the cerebral protection group,

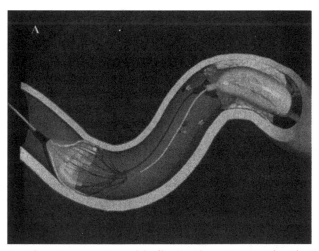

FIGURE 1A.—Schematic representation of the filter-type device (Angioguard) at the time of balloon predilation angioplasty. (Courtesy of Parodi JC, La Mura R, Ferreira LM, et al: Initial evaluation of carotid angioplasty and stenting with three different cerebral protection devices. *J Vasc Surg* 32:1127-1136, 2000.)

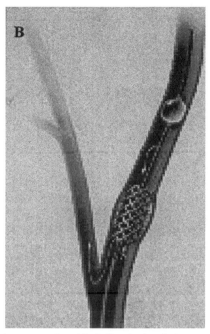

FIGURE 2B.—Schematic representation of the balloon in place during carotid angioplasty and stenting with blood flow redirected toward the external carotid artery. (Courtesy of Parodi JC, La Mura R, Ferreira LM, et al: Initial evaluation of carotid angioplasty and stenting with three different cerebral protection devices. *J Vasc Surg* 32:1127-1136, 2000.)

although the difference was nonsignificant. There were no deaths in either group. Intention-to-treat analysis showed that CAS was technically successful in 97.8% of cases. Cerebral protection devices were successfully placed in 100% of cases. With all 3 interventions, the cerebral protection device caught a significant number of particles of various sizes.

Conclusions.—This experience demonstrates a high technical success rate with 3 different systems for cerebral protection during CAS. All devices tested seem effective in preventing perioperative neurologic deficits. Further studies in larger numbers of patients will be needed.

▶ Several things are apparent. First, CAS seems to release an abundance of debris, which embolizes distally. And second, a number of innovative protection devices and methods have been developed to attempt to trap or in some other way prevent this debris released by angioplasty from entering the cerebral circulation. Three different cerebral protection devices are described in this article. On balance, this is a good review.

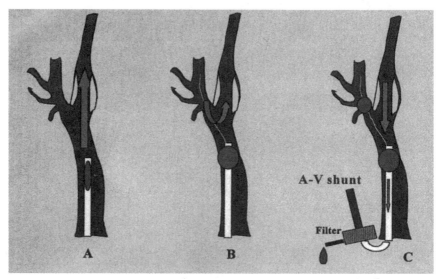

FIGURE 3.—Schematic sequence of the Parodi device. Placement of Parodi's guiding catheter in the CCA below the stenotic lesion (**A**). Inflation of the CCA balloon with forward ICA flow maintained based on retrograde ECA flow (**B**). Inflation of ECA balloon with inversion of ICA flow through Parodi's guiding catheter, which is then externally connected with a blood-filtered line to a femoral vein introducer (**C**). *Abbreviations:* CCA, Common carotid artery; *ICA*, internal carotid artery; *ECA*, external carotid artery; *A-V*, arteriovenous. (Courtesy of Parodi JC, La Mura R, Ferreira LM, et al: Initial evaluation of carotid angioplasty and stenting with three different cerebral protection devices. *J Vasc Surg* 32:1127-1136, 2000.)

Balloon-Protected Carotid Angioplasty

Albuquerque FC, Teitelbaum GP, Lavine SD, et al (St Joseph's Hosp and Med Ctr, Phoenix, Ariz; Univ of Southern California, Los Angeles)

Neurosurgery 46:918-923, 2000   2–27

Background.—Carotid angioplasty can be used in stroke prevention in selected patients, specifically those at highest risk for complications after carotid endarterectomy, the "gold standard" therapy. However, embolic complications can occur during carotid endarterectomy, so a technique was developed to protect the cerebral circulation.

Methods.—Seventeen procedures (1 bilateral) in 16 patients were studied. The patients had stenoses ranging from 70% to 95%. The distal internal carotid artery was occluded by a silicone balloon during the angioplasty phase, when most emboli are produced (Fig 1). The balloon remained inflated after angioplasty was completed, and debris was flushed into the external circulation. The balloon was deflated and an exchange guidewire passed through the angioplasty catheter to provide continuous guidewire access across the stenotic zone, easing stent placement.

Results.—Only 5 minutes or less was required to inflate the balloon. Sixteen (94%) of the procedures were successful. When a later angioplasty was performed without protection, the patient in whom the balloon could

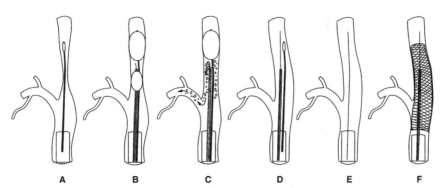

FIGURE 1.—Schematic representation of the balloon protection technique. A, The occlusion balloon catheter is advanced across the area of stenosis using digital roadmapping. B, Angioplasty is performed with the occlusion balloon inflated. C, The angioplasty catheter (with its balloon deflated) is advanced just proximal to the occlusion balloon. Angioplasty debris is then flushed into the external carotid circulation. D, With the occlusion balloon deflated, a guidewire is advanced through the angioplasty catheter into the distal internal carotid artery. E, The guidewire maintains access across the site of percutaneous transluminal angioplasty. F, The guidewire allows stent deployment across the site of stenosis. (Courtesy of Albuquerque FC, Teitelbaum GP, Lavine SD, et al: Balloon-protected carotid angioplasty. *Neurosurgery* 46:918-923, 2000.)

not be advanced across the stenotic area had a transient ischemic attack. No other complications occurred.

Conclusion.—Simultaneous stent placement is not possible with the technique described, but stent deployment is facilitated by placement of the continuous guidewire. The technique does protect the cerebral vessels, as evidenced by the high level of success without complications.

▶ One particular internal carotid artery occlusive balloon cerebral protective device is described in this experience with 17 patients. This has given generally satisfactory results in the authors' experience. A defect in this article, of course, is that the results are purely anecdotal. Performance of transcranial Doppler to monitor cerebral emboli would have been helpful. The ultimate evaluation of this or any other cerebral protection device is going to require both detailed neurologic examination and cerebral imaging, probably MRI, and all this probably combined with continuous transcranial Doppler examination. Simple anecdotal experience is not going to be adequate for the ultimate evaluation of any of these devices.

Atheroemboli to the Brain: Size Threshold for Causing Acute Neuronal Cell Death

Rapp JH, Pan XM, Sharp FR, et al (Univ of California, San Francisco; Albany Med College, NY; Univ of California, Davis)
J Vasc Surg 32:68-76, 2000   2–28

Objective.—Plaque fragments, released as a result of balloon angioplasty of carotid plaques, can have neurologic consequences. The number and size of plaque fragments released during ex vivo balloon angioplasty

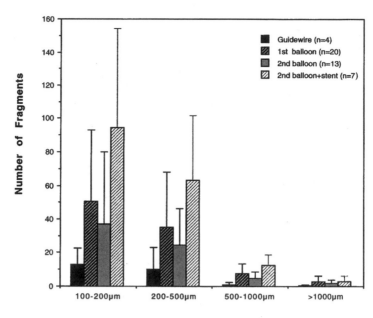

FIGURE 1.—The number and size of plaque fragments released with ex vivo angioplasty. Data are exposed as the mean plus or minus SD. (Courtesy of Rapp JH, Pan XM, Sharp FR, et al: Atheroemboli to the brain: Size threshold for causing acute neuronal cell death. *J Vasc Surg* 32:68-76, 2000.)

of human carotid plaques were determined, and the likelihood of neuronal injury was investigated in the rat model.

Methods.—Ex vivo angioplasty was performed on 20 carotid bifurcation endarterectomy specimens with more than 60% stenosis. Embolic fragments were collected, analyzed, and separated into 200- to 500-µm and smaller-than 200-µm fragments (Fig 1). Rats were injected in their carotid arteries with saline (group A), 100 fragments smaller than 200 µm (group B), or 100 fragments 200 to 500 µm (group C). Rats were killed at 1, 3, and 7 days. Brain sections were examined for neuronal damage by assaying for heat shock protein 72 (HSP72).

Results.—The number of fragments released varied from 11 to 323, depended on plaque architecture, and tended to increase with stent placement. Group A rats demonstrated no cerebral injury. Group B rats demonstrated no cerebral injury at days 1 and 3, but 2 of 3 group B rats showed evidence of injury at 7 days. In group C rats, cerebral damage was detected on day 1, in 1 of 3 rats on day 3, and in 2 of 3 rats on day 7.

Conclusion.—Carotid angioplasty can dislodge plaque fragments that can cause neuronal damage as long as 1 week after the procedure.

▶ The conclusions of this interesting study are clear: Angioplasty of carotid plaques releases lots of debris in the 1- to 500-µm size range and some particles considerably larger than this. And, following carotid injection in rats, some delayed neuronal damage is apparent after 7 days with particles under 200 μm, and a great deal of immediate neuronal damage is apparent with particles between 200 and 500 μm. I accept this as valid in the rat model, and I suspect that generally the same size relationships will hold true in patients.

There seems no doubt that the brain has a remarkable capacity to absorb emboli without producing near-term neurologic deficits. However, it strikes me as foolish to assume that these embolic events are entirely without consequence. Any time you annihilate significant populations of neurons, you should expect to pay some sort of a price, even if it is only a subtle decline in neurologic function, without gross stroke deficits.

Endovascular Management of Extracranial Carotid Artery Dissection Achieved Using Stent Angioplasty

Malek AM, Higashida RT, Phatouros CC, et al (Univ of California, San Francisco)

AJNR Am J Neuroradiol 21:1280-1292, 2000   2–29

Objective.—There is a subset of patients with a dissected cervical carotid artery who fail to heal spontaneously after systemic anticoagulation therapy. Focal or extensive stenosis can develop in these patients and lead to the formation of a pseudoaneurysm. Endovascular stents may be of benefit to these patients. The clinical and angiographic outcome of this type of therapy was retrospectively investigated.

Methods.—Between October 1997 and March 1999, 10 consecutive patients (5 men), aged 37 to 83 years, with carotid dissection, underwent percutaneous endovascular balloon angioplasty and intraluminal stent placement. The cause of the dissection was iatrogenic in 3, spontaneous in 5, and traumatic in 2. All patients had failed optimal medical therapy, were unable to undergo anticoagulation, or did not have other lower-risk options.

Results.—Seven patients had coexisting hypertension, and 7 had suffered a stroke. Seven dissections were located on the left side. Two patients had an intraprocedural vasospasm of the high cervical carotid artery, and 1 required angioplasty. One patient had a retroperitoneal hemorrhage requiring a blood transfusion and surgical repair. One patient required permanent sacrifice of the right internal carotid artery on day 3 after surgery for a left internal carotid dissection. This patient had a massive stroke of the right hemisphere 8 months later, but his deficits were mostly resolved at a follow-up of 24 months. No patient had worsening of symptoms during the postoperative period. At an average follow-up period of 16 months, there was no evidence of stent occlusion or stenosis. Modified Rankin scores had improved from 0.7 at baseline to 1.8, and Barthel indices had increased from 80.5 to 99.5.

Case Report.—Woman, 45, with hypertension, lupus, and migraine headaches, experienced acute dissection during diagnostic angiography. She was given heparin but hemiparesis developed. She was transferred to another institution and found to have a completely occluded previously dissected left internal carotid artery. She underwent recanalization and elimination of the inflow to the subintimal dissection. An 8-mm × 2 cm Wallstent was deployed at the proximal inflow zone. Blood flow resumed, her left hemiparesis improved, and she was symptom-free at last follow-up.

Conclusion.—Endovascular stent placement is safe and effective and leads to a good clinical outcome in a subset of patients with carotid dissection who fail medical management.

▶ Despite attempting to remain vigilant in both the clinic and the vascular laboratory, we see only a small number of extracranial carotid artery dissections per year. Almost all of these patients have typical narrowing of the artery at the time of diagnosis, but over a period of several months of warfarin, they recover a normal-appearing carotid artery. Clearly, however, in some patients, dissection can result in a severe stenosis. It seems clear that for the occasional selected patient, carotid stenting may restore a normal appearance to the carotid artery in patients with carotid dissection. I do believe the need for this procedure will be vanishingly small, but clearly we should be aware that the procedure is available for a subset of patients.

Femoropopliteal Brachytherapy

Endovascular Brachytherapy for Prophylaxis of Restenosis After Femoropopliteal Angioplasty: Results of a Prospective Randomized Study
Minar E, Pokrajac B, Maca T, et al (Univ of Vienna)
Circulation 102:2694-2699, 2000   2–30

Introduction.—Restenosis continues to significantly limit the clinical usefulness of percutaneous transluminal angioplasty (PTA). Endovascular brachytherapy (BT) has strong potential for controlling the pathologic proliferation of smooth-muscles cells that have been observed in animal models. The efficacy of endovascular BT for prophylaxis of restenosis after femoropopliteal PTA was examined in 113 patients with de novo or recurrent femoropopliteal lesions.

Methods.—The mean age of the 63 men and 50 women in the study was 71 years. Patients were randomly assigned to either PTA plus BT (PTA + BT group) or to PTA (PTA group) without stent implantation. The mean treated lengths were 16.7 cm and 14.8 cm for the PTA + BT and the PTA group, respectively. A dose of 12 Gy was applied from an ^{192}Ir source 3 mm from the source axis for patients in the PTA + BT group. During follow-up examinations, patients underwent measurement of the ankle-brachial index, color-flow duplex sonography, and angiography. The major end point was patency after 6 months.

Results.—The overall rates of restenosis at 6 months were 28.3% (15/53 patients) in the PTA + BT group and 53.7% (29/54) in the PTA group (*P*

< .05). Cumulative patency rates at 12 months were 63.6% and 35.3%, respectively, in the PTA + BT and the PTA group (P < .005).

Conclusion.—This is the first randomized trial to illustrate the efficacy of endovascular BT for prophylaxis of restenosis after femoropopliteal PTA. Before endovascular BT can be generally recommended for prophylaxis of restenosis after femoropopliteal PTA, these findings need to be verified by a double-blind, randomized, multi-institutional trial with the use of an adequate centering device.

▶ With the recent reported success of BT in the treatment of coronary lesions, it was only a matter of time before the same was tried in peripheral lesions. The randomized study reported here delivered intraluminal BT to femoropopliteal stenosis following angioplasty alone without stent placement. A significant improvement was noted in the 1-year follow-up in favor of the BT group. The authors modestly note that this is the first randomized study to demonstrate the efficacy of endovascular BT in the prevention of restenosis after femoropopliteal PTA. My prior comments on the efficacy of coronary BT not withstanding, this is impressive information. However, I do hasten to point out that the 12-month patency rates in both arms of the study are lousy compared with well-performed surgery. In examining individual trees, we should not lose track of the forest.

Intraarterial ^{192}Ir High-Dose-Rate Brachytherapy for Prophylaxis of Restenosis After Femoropopliteal Percutaneous Transluminal Angioplasty: The Prospective Randomized Vienna-2-Trial Radiotherapy Parameters and Risk Factors Analysis
Pokrajac B, Pötter R, Maca T, et al (Univ of Vienna)
Int J Radiat Oncol Biol Phys 48:923-931, 2000   2–31

Background.—Restenosis continues to be a major problem after femoropopliteal artery recanalization with percutaneous transluminal angioplasty (PTA). Previous studies suggest that external beam radiotherapy and endovascular brachytherapy (BT) are promising approaches to preventing restenosis. Intra-arterial BT using a high-dose-rate ^{192}Ir source was evaluated for use in the prevention of femoropopliteal artery restenosis after PTA.

Methods.—The randomized trial included 113 patients (63 men and 50 women; mean age, 71 years) who underwent successful PTA for claudication or critical limb ischemia with de novo stenosis or restenosis/occlusion after previous PTA. After PTA, the patients were randomly assigned to undergo BT or no further treatment. In the BT group, a radiation dose of 12 Gy was prescribed at a distance of 3 mm from the source axis, or 6.8 Gy at a 5 mm distance (Fig 2). The 2 groups were compared for the 6-month femoropopliteal patency rate, among other outcomes.

Results.—The 2 groups were well-stratified in terms of new stenosis versus restenosis, stenosis versus occlusion, claudication versus critical

FIGURE 2

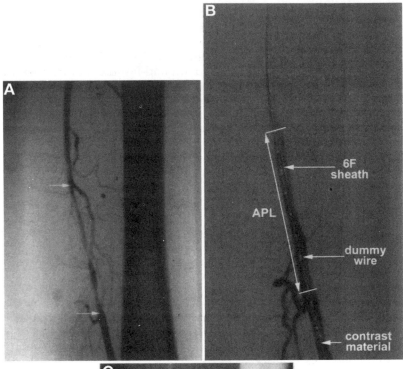

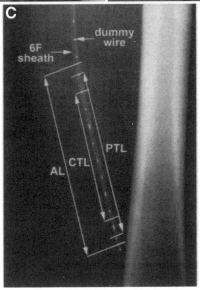

(Continued)

FIGURE 2 (cont.)

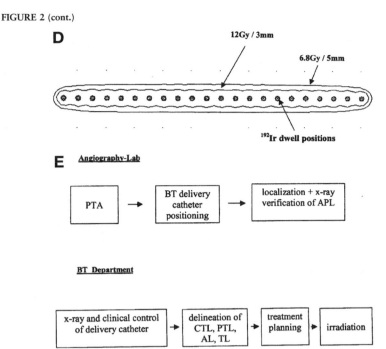

D

12Gy / 3mm

6.8Gy / 5mm

^{192}Ir dwell positions

E <u>Angiography-Lab</u>

| PTA | → | BT delivery catheter positioning | → | localization + x-ray verification of APL |

<u>BT Department</u>

| x-ray and clinical control of delivery catheter | → | delineation of CTL, PTL, AL, TL | → | treatment planning | → | irradiation |

FIGURE 2.—Procedure of PTA plus BT. Legend: measuring rod: A, B, C, 1:1.7 cm; measuring rod: D, 1:0.75 cm. *Abbreviations:* PTA, Percutaneous transluminal angioplasty; BT, brachytherapy; F, French (1F = 0.33 mm); CTL, clinical target length; PTL, planning target length; AL, active length; TL, treated length. A, Angiogram with femoropopliteal restenosis (7.5 cm) after former PTA (*between arrowheads*). B, PTA: x-ray documentation of the angioplasty site, 6F sheath, 5F radiation delivery catheter (not radio-opaque), and dummy wire (radio-opaque markers with 1-cm interval). C, BT: x-ray localization of the angioplasty site (ie, CTL and 6F sheath, 5F radiation delivery catheter with dummy wire). Definition of PTL and AL. D, Computer-assisted treatment planning for a dose of 12 Gy prescribed at 3 mm from the source axis and dwell time calculation of the stepping source to cover adequately the PTL. Dose to the adventitia (2 mm from intima) is 6.8 Gy. E, Flowchart of PTA and BT procedure. (Reprinted from Pokrajac B, Pötter R, Maca T, et al: Intraarterial ^{192}Ir high-dose-rate brachytherapy for prophylaxis of restenosis after femoropopliteal percutaneous transluminal angioplasty: The prospective randomized Vienna-2-Trial radiotherapy parameters and risk factors analysis. *Int J Radiat Oncol Biol Phys* 48:923-931, Copyright 2000, with permission from Elsevier Science.)

limb ischemia, and diabetes versus no diabetes. However, patients in the PTA group were more likely to have long stenoses. All patients tolerated the addition of BT to PTA, and no immediate, short-term, or long-term adverse effects occurred. By 6 months, restenosis had occurred in 54% of the PTA-only group versus 28% of the PTA plus BT group. Actuarial 6-month patency rates were 45% and 72% in the PTA only and PTA-plus-BT groups, respectively (Fig 4). The addition of BT significantly reduced the restenosis rate in various high-risk groups, including patients with restenosis after previous PTA, those with occlusion, and those with stenoses longer than 10 cm. No significant reduction was noted in patients with diabetes.

Conclusions.—This randomized trial demonstrates the safety and feasibility of adding BT with a ^{192}Ir source after femoropopliteal PTA. This

FIGURE 4

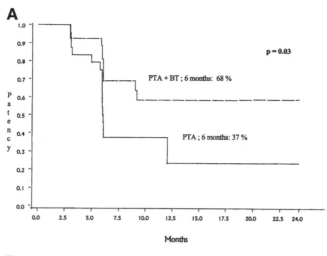

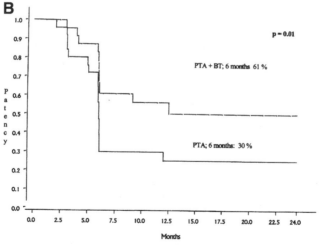

(Continued)

procedure carries no additional morbidity and significantly reduces the rate of restenosis, including that in certain groups of high-risk patients. Further benefits may be achievable through higher radiation doses and the use of a centering device for more consistent dosing.

▶ If you did not adequately understand this trial from Abstract 2–30, here is another version regarding the identical patients and published the same month in another journal. For harassing us with this egregious example of dual publication, I am delighted to present these authors the Camel Dung Award with eucalyptus cluster. The cluster has only been awarded once

FIGURE 4 (cont.)

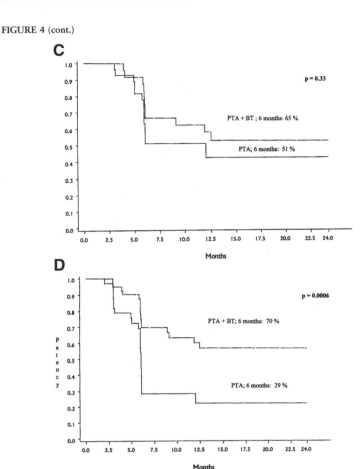

FIGURE 4.—Actuarial estimate of patency at 6 months in femoropopliteal arteries after PTA alone or PTA plus BT with ^{192}Ir source. *Abbreviations: PTA,* Percutaneous transluminal angioplasty; *BT,* brachytherapy. **A,** Restenosis after former PTA: 37% patency for PTA alone versus 68% patency for PTA + BT ($P = .03$); 45% increase of patency in PTA + BT arm. **B,** Occlusion: 30% patency for PTA versus 61% patency for PTA + BT ($P = .01$); 51% increase of patency in PTA + BT arm. **C,** Diabetes: 51% patency for PTA versus 65% patency for PTA + BT ($P = .33$); 21% increase of patency in PTA + BT arm. **D,** PTA length greater than 10 cm: 29% patency for PTA versus 70% patency for PTA + BT ($P = .0006$); 58% increase of patency in PTA + BT arm. (Reprinted from Pokrajac B, Pötter R, Maca T, et al: Intraarterial ^{192}Ir high-dose-rate brachytherapy for prophylaxis of restenosis after femoropopliteal percutaneous transluminal angioplasty: The prospective randomized Vienna-2-Trial radiotherapy parameters and risk factors analysis. *Int J Radiat Oncol Biol Phys* 48:923-931, Copyright 2000, with permission from Elsevier Science.)

before. However, the duplication in these 2 publications is so perfect that special recognition is in order. I hope they will accept this award in the spirit in which it is offered and never torture us again with such egregious duplicate publication.

Iliac Artery

Comparing Patency Rates Between External Iliac and Common Iliac Artery Stents

Lee ES, Steenson CC, Trimble KE, et al (Veterans Affairs Med Ctr, Minneapolis)

J Vasc Surg 31:889-894, 2000

2–32

Background.—Treatment of localized arterial stenoses involves placement of intraluminal stents in the common iliac artery (CIA) and the external iliac artery (EIA). Because the EIA has a smaller diameter and is more likely to have diffuse disease than is the CIA, EIA stents would be expected to have lower patency rates. Anatomical patency rates of EIA versus CIA stents in patients with occlusive disease were assessed.

Methods.—The 69 male patients studied had 98 stents placed for significant iliac artery occlusive disease and various degrees of chronic limb ischemia. The EIA patients' mean age was 69 years and that of the CIA patients was 66 years. Follow-up evaluation with duplex US was performed 1 day and 3 months after the procedure and then at 6-month intervals over a mean of 21.4 months. If velocities exceeded 300 cm/s, follow-up angiograms were performed. Those receiving EIA stents and those having CIA stents were compared with respect to patient risk factors, iliac artery runoff, concomitant outflow procedures, and anatomical patency rates.

Results.—No differences in the risk factor analyses were identified between the groups. More ischemic lower limbs were identified among the EIA group than the CIA group. The lengths of the lesions were similar between the 2 groups, with those of EIA patients being 4.6 cm and those of CIA patients being 5.3 cm. At 1 year, the primary patency rate for EIA was 93% and that for CIA was 88%; at 2 years, the rates were 91% and 78%, respectively; and at 3 years, the EIA rate was 90% and the CIA rate 78% (Fig 2). Cumulative patient survival rates were similar.

Conclusion.—The patency rates of EIA stents were comparable with those of CIA stents despite greater age and the presence of more ischemic limbs in the patients receiving EIA stents.

▶ There continues to be a debate as to whether angioplasty and stenting of the EIA has less favorable results than the same procedures performed in the CIA. The fact that the EIA is of a smaller diameter and often demonstrates more diffuse disease than the CIA has been the basis of why some reports have shown less favorable results. This study reports that the patency rates following angioplasty and stenting of the EIA and CIA are similar in both groups of patients. The authors report that there was no difference in the run-off score or the category of limb ischemia between the 2 groups.

One of the advantages of this study is the fact that the authors reported the anatomical patency rate as judged by follow-up angiograms and duplex

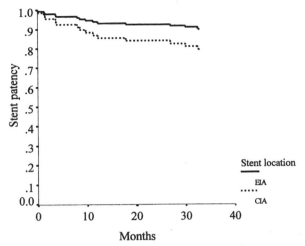

FIGURE 2.—Primary patency rates of iliac artery stents by anatomical location (*P* = .13). *Abbreviations: CIA,* Common iliac artery; *EIA,* external iliac artery. (Courtesy of Lee ES, Steenson CC, Trimble KE, et al: Comparing patency rates between external iliac and common iliac artery stents, *J Vasc Surg* 31:889-894, 2000.)

US studies. They do not report any hemodynamic comparison to assess patency rates because, as they point out, the multilevel nature of this disease could make hemodynamic assessment less accurate. Although this study has a relatively small number of patients (69), the authors report that the study has a 92% power of detecting a 10% difference in patency rates with a *P* value of less than .05. It appears that angioplasty and stenting of the EIA may have results at least as good as those of a similar procedure for the CIA.

J. O. Menzoian, MD

Iliac Occlusions: Stenting or Crossover Grafting? An Examination of Patency and Cost
Whatling PJ, Gibson M, Torrie EPH, et al (Royal Berkshire Hosp, Reading, England)
Eur J Vasc Endovasc Surg 20:36-40, 2000   2–33

Background.—There has been a trend in recent years away from aortofemoral bypass grafting and toward less invasive procedures for the treatment of aortoiliac disease. From 1988 to 1994, extra-anatomical bypass grafts were being used in preference to aortofemoral bypass. However, the number of crossover grafts declined from 1994 to 1996, with increasing use of percutaneous transluminal angioplasty with stents. Percutaneous transluminal angioplasty with stents is thought to be a less invasive and less expensive option compared with surgical reconstruction for the treatment of iliac artery occlusion. A prospective observational study was conducted of all patients undergoing an iliac stent or femoral crossover graft for iliac artery occlusion to assess the cost effectiveness of the 2 approaches.

Methods.—In a district general hospital, 51 patients underwent primary angioplasty with stenting. Another 87 patients underwent crossover grafting. All patients were assessed 2 months after the procedure and at intervals throughout the ensuing years.

Results.—In 13 patients, it was impossible to place the stent successfully. In another 10 patients, major complications occurred, primarily thromboembolic. Crossover grafting was performed in 15 patients after failure to insert a stent or stent occlusion. No major complications occurred after crossover grafting. The median hospital stay after successful crossover grafting was 4 days; for successful stenting, the median stay was 1 day. The mean stay was higher for each group (2.5 days for stenting, 5.8 days for crossover grafting) and is considered a more accurate parameter for cost estimation. The cost of iliac stenting was estimated at £1912, compared with £3072 for crossover grafting. For patients who suffered complications after stenting, the mean additional cost was £2481. Patency on an "intention-to-treat" basis was 52% after stent insertion, compared with 100% after bypass. The cost advantage of stenting is lost if any complication occurs after stenting. The initial cost benefit of iliac stenting is lost within 6 months for patients without complications, because these patients require additional intervention when the stent occludes.

Conclusion.—Crossover grafting was shown to be a durable low-risk procedure. It is suggested that stenting of occluded iliac arteries should only be performed on patients with limited life expectancy. Younger and fitter patients should be offered femorofemoral crossover grafting as an initial procedure until research advances to a point at which patients most likely to maintain long-term patency after stenting can be identified.

▶ When encountering a unilateral symptomatic occluded iliac artery, one obviously has a choice between angioplasty and stenting of the occluded iliac or crossover femorofemoral grafting. In the experience of these authors, crossover femorofemoral grafting proved to be a superior option. I really can find little to disagree with in their conclusions. While a femorofemoral graft is not the greatest graft in the world, it certainly does appear to be superior to dilatation of an occluded iliac artery segment. In our hands, we expect the femorofemoral graft to have about 60% patency at 3 to 5 years. As stated, this is not one of our better grafts. Nonetheless, I do believe it is superior to the patency anticipated following angioplasty of an occluded iliac segment.

Peripheral Arterial Obstruction: Prospective Study of Treatment With a Transluminally Placed Self-expanding Stent-Graft

Lammer J, for the International Trial Study Group (AKH Universitatskliniken, Vienna; et al)
Radiology 217:95-104, 2000   2–34

Objective.—Endovascular stents salvage acute failure of percutaneous transluminal angioplasty and increase its technical success rates to greater than 95%. Long-term patency depends, in several respects, on the stent used. The safety and efficacy of the HEMOBAHN Endoprosthesis (W. L. Gore and Associates, Flagstaff, Ariz), a flexible, expanding prosthesis, was tested in a prospective multicenter study.

Methods.—Between September 1996 and February 1998, the self-expanding HEMOBAHN Endoprosthesis was implanted in 141 limbs (61 iliac arteries and 80 femoral arteries) of 127 symptomatic patients (44 women), aged 37 to 89 years, in 17 centers in the United States and Europe

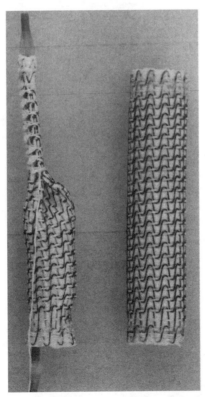

FIGURE 2.—Partially and completely deployed endoprostheses. As the deployment knob is pulled, the deployment line removes the knots over the device, and the prosthesis expands from the trailing toward the leading end of the catheter (catheter tip). (Courtesy of Lammer J, for the International Trial Study Group: Peripheral arterial obstruction: Prospective study of treatment with a transluminally placed self-expanding stent-graft. *Radiology* 217:95-104, 2000. Radiological Society of North America.)

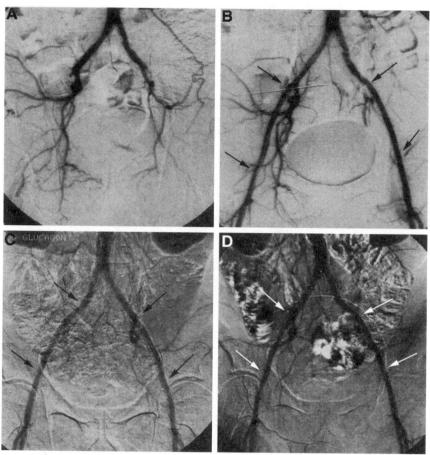

FIGURE 5.—**A,** Intra-arterial digital subtraction angiography (DSA) image shows bilateral occlusion of the external iliac arteries. **B,** Intra-arterial DSA image shows bilateral implantation of 8 × 100–mm endoprostheses (*arrows*). **C, D,** Follow-up IV DSA images obtained (C) 12 and (D) 24 months after implantation show the proximal and distal ends of the devices (*arrows*). (Courtesy of Lammer J, for the International Trial Study Group: Peripheral arterial obstruction: Prospective study of treatment with a transluminally placed self-expanding stent-graft. *Radiology* 217:95-104, 2000. Radiological Society of North America.)

(Fig 2). Clinical assessments, color duplex flow US, treadmill testing, and resting ankle-brachial index measurements were performed at baseline, and at 1, 3, 6, and 12 months. Functional results were assessed according to standard limb ischemia scores. Adverse events were recorded. Patency was recorded for at least 12 months.

Results.—All stent deployments were technically successful. One 8-mm device, which could not be advanced across a lesion, was removed and successfully replaced with a 7-mm device. There were 24 (17.0%) complications, 3 (2.1%) of them major. There were 4 (1 iliac and 3 femoral) primary reobstructions that recurred within 30 days. There were 22 (6 iliac and 16 femoral) primary reobstructions that recurred within 360 days (Fig

5). Cumulative primary patency rates at 6 months for iliac and femoral arteries were 98.4% and 89.7%, respectively. The corresponding rates at 12 months were 91.2% and 78.7%. The cumulative secondary patency rates at 6 months for iliac and femoral arteries were 98.4% and 96.1%, respectively. The corresponding rates at 12 months were 94.7% and 93.4%.

Conclusion.—The HEMOBAHN Endoprosthesis can safely be used to treat peripheral iliac and femoral arterial obstruction for as long as 12 months.

▶ The HEMOBAHN Endoprosthesis manufactured by W.L. Gore & Associates has been bouncing around the peripheral arterial circulation for several years. The results reported here by this experienced group of investigators are most impressive, including primary patency rates in femoral arteries of 90%, and 79% at 6 and 12 months, respectively, and iliac artery primary patency rates of 98% and 91% at 6 and 12 months, respectively. Presently, this particular device, consisting of an expanded polytetrafluoroethylene tube inside a nitinol sinusoidally shaped, helically wrapped stent, is not available for use in the United States. It is my tentative conclusion that this device may have some real applicability in selected patients. Generally, I am encouraged by these results.

The Durability of Endovascular Treatment of Multisegment Iliac Occlusive Disease

Powell RJ, Fillinger M, Bettmann M, et al (Dartmouth-Hitchcock Med Ctr, Lebanon, NH)

J Vasc Surg 31:1178-1184, 2000   2–35

Background.—Aortoiliac occlusive disease is most commonly treated with iliac artery angioplasty and selective stent placement. It has been demonstrated that the patency rates for iliac artery angioplasty are dependent on the indication, lesion severity, runoff, sex of the patient, and lesion location. In general, external iliac lesions have an inferior patency rate in comparison with common iliac lesions. Iliac angioplasty has a 4-year success rate of 44% to 65%, but with stent placement, the 5-year primary patency rate has been improved to from 53% to 77%. In 1 study, the secondary patency rate was improved to more than 80% at 32 months.

The use of endovascular techniques in the treatment of isolated iliac stenoses has become commonplace, but the use of these techniques in the treatment of patients with multisegment iliac disease has not been well-studied. The effectiveness of endovascular treatment of multisegment iliac occlusive disease was evaluated in patients with involvement of 2 or more common or external iliac arteries.

Methods.—All patients who underwent angioplasty or stenting of at least 2 separate iliac artery segments from July 1992 to December 1998

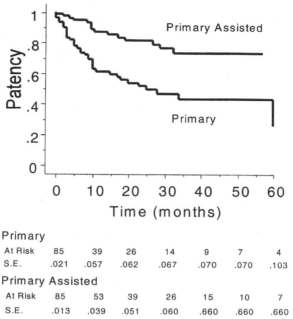

FIGURE 1.—Primary patency and assisted–primary patency of aortoiliac segments for all patients. *At risk* indicates the number of patients at risk at the end of each period. *Abbreviation: SE,* Standard error. (Courtesy of Powell RJ, Fillinger M, Bettmann M, et al: The durability of endovascular treatment of multisegment iliac occlusive disease. *J Vasc Surg* 31:1178-1184, 2000.)

were identified. In addition to demographic data, investigators gathered data regarding technical and hemodynamic success and aortoiliac primary and primary–assisted patency. These data were analyzed by Society for Vascular Surgery and International Society for Cardiovascular Surgery criteria. Outcome predictors were determined by multivariate life table analysis.

Results.—In the period under study, 87 patients underwent 207 iliac artery angioplasties and 115 iliac artery stents (Fig 1). These procedures were performed in 210 iliac segments for disabling claudication in 60% of patients, for rest pain in 17% of patients, and for tissue loss in 23% of patients. In 64% of patients, 2 iliac segments were treated; 3 segments were treated in 28% of patients and 4 segments were treated in 8% of patients. Initial hemodynamic success was achieved in 72% of patients; the complication rate was 11%. Eighty-eight percent of patients experienced clinical improvement.

Endovascular reintervention was required in 29% of patients, and surgical inflow procedures were required in 14%. the mean time from primary intervention to first reintervention was 10 ± 3 months. Primary patency rates at 6, 12, and 36 months after intervention were 95%, 87%, and 72%, respectively. The only factor that adversely affected both primary and assisted–primary patency was the presence of an external iliac artery stenosis. The aortoiliac primary patency rates in patients without the presence of an external iliac artery stenosis at 6, 12, and 36 months were 88%, 47%, and 18%, respectively. These rates compared with 68%, 47%, and 18%, respectively, in patients who had external iliac artery lesions.

Conclusion.—Patency rates for endovascular therapy for multisegment aortoiliac occlusive disease are acceptable, but reintervention is often needed. The presence of external iliac artery disease was found to be a significant predictor of poor outcome.

▶ These investigators appear to conclude that angioplasty of multiple stenoses in iliac arteries is less successful than angioplasty of a single stenosis. In fact, the patency rate and clinical benefits for the multisegment-dilated patients are only mediocre, with a 36-month primary patency rate of less than 70%. These investigators found that the presence of an external iliac stenosis appeared to adversely affect results.

Predicting Outcome of Angioplasty and Selective Stenting of Multisegment Iliac Artery Occlusive Disease
Powell RJ, Fillinger M, Walsh DB, et al (Dartmouth-Hitchcock Med Ctr, Lebanon, NH)
J Vasc Surg 32:564-569, 2000   2–36

Background.—To maintain long-term patency in patients who need angioplasty and stenting of multiple iliac arterial segments, it often requires reintervention. Morphological predictors of failure have not been established. Arteriographic predictors of angioplasty and selective stent failure were defined in the treatment of multisegment iliac occlusive disease.

Methods.—Seventy-five patients undergoing angioplasty and selective stent placement for multisegment iliac occlusive disease were included. All iliac segments were scored by means of a modified Society of Cardiovascular and Interventional Radiology classification for iliac angioplasty (Table 1). The total iliac score was determined by summing scores from each segment, and a separate external iliac score was determined by adding only the external iliac scores.

TABLE 1.—Modified SCVIR Guidelines for Grading Iliac Artery Lesions

Grade	Morphologic Description
0	No lesion
1	Symmetric lesion < 3 cm
2	Lesion 3-5 cm
3	Lesion > 5 cm
4	Occlusion

Abbreviation: SCVIR, Society of Cardiovascular and Interventional Radiology.
(Courtesy of Powell RJ, Fillinger M, Walsh DB, et al: Predicting outcome of angioplasty and selective stenting of multisegment iliac artery occlusive disease. *J Vasc Surg* 32:564-569, 2000.)

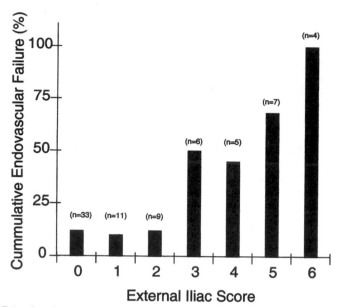

FIGURE 1.—Cumulative endovascular failure (%) based on preintervention external iliac score ($P = .01$; χ^2 test). n, Number of patients with score shown. (Courtesy of Powell RJ, Fillinger M, Walsh DB, et al: Predicting outcome of angioplasty and selective stenting of multisegment iliac artery occlusive disease. *J Vasc Surg* 32:564-569, 2000.)

Findings.—In three fourths of the patients, the recurrence was noted in the site of the previous endovascular intervention. New lesions, believed to be caused by progressive atherosclerosis, were noted in 15% of the patients. Lesions in new and previously treated iliac segments occurred in 10% of the patients. The only independent predictor of failed endovascular therapy, despite reintervention, was the external iliac score. Among patients with an external iliac score of 2 or less, the endovascular primary-assisted patency rates were 96% at 6 months, 92% at 12 months, and 89% at 24 months; among those with an external iliac score of 3 or more, the corresponding rates were 90%, 63%, and 45%. Patients with an external iliac score of 3 or more had a significantly lower incidence of hemodynamic and clinical improvement after intervention, as well as a 3-fold greater need for surgical inflow procedures, compared with patients with an external iliac score of 2 or less (Fig 1).

Conclusions.—Among patients treated for multisegment iliac occlusive disease, lesion formation occurs typically in the areas of the intervention. The degree of external iliac disease is useful for stratifying patients with multisegment iliac occlusive disease likely to respond to endovascular treatment with a lasting result.

▶ The same authors, using exactly the same patients described in Abstract 2–35, attempted to define arteriographic predictors of angioplasty and stent failure. Once again, they concluded primarily that external iliac disease was the finding leading to a poor result. I am surprised to detect our erudite colleagues from New Hampshire engaged in publication salami slicing so fine as to smack of duplicate publication. For this offense to the sensibility of discerning readers everywhere, I am pleased to present them with the Camel Dung Award for duplicate publication. As the material was not particularly boring, they are not awarded the Eucalyptus Leaf Cluster. Thus, they still have something to aspire toward.

Influence of Hormone Replacement Therapy on the Outcome of Iliac Angioplasty and Stenting
Timaran CH, Stevens SL, Grandas OH, et al (Univ of Tennessee, Knoxville)
J Vasc Surg 33:S85-S92, 2001   2–37

Background.—Among women with cardiovascular disease, hormone replacement therapy (HRT) is associated with an increased rate of thromboembolic events. However, there are few data on how HRT affects the outcomes of women with aortoiliac occlusive disease. A group of women undergoing iliac artery angioplasty and stenting were followed up to assess HRT and other risk factors.

Methods.—The 5-year follow-up study included 88 women who had undergone a total of 126 iliac angioplasties, including placement of 144 stents. The women averaged 63.2 years of age, with 43% receiving HRT.

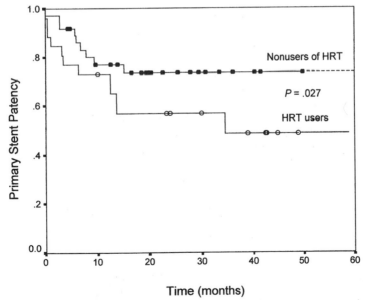

FIGURE 1.—Primary patency rates after iliac artery angioplasty and stenting were significantly lower in hormone replacement therapy (*HRT*) users compared with nonusers (Kaplan-Meier, log-rank test, P = .02). (Courtesy of Timaran CH, Stevens SL, Grandas OH, et al: Influence of hormone replacement therapy on the outcome of iliac angioplasty and stenting. *J Vasc Surg* 33:S85-S92, 2001.)

Claudication was the reason for iliac angioplasty in 65%; other indications included limb salvage in 32% and blue toe syndrome in 3%. Outcomes and potential risk factors were defined by the criteria of the Ad Hoc Committee on Reporting Standards of the Society for Vascular Surgery/International Society for Cardiovascular Surgery.

Results.—Ninety-five percent of procedures were technically successful. Twenty-two percent of patients underwent primary stent placement; other indications for postangioplasty stenting included residual stenosis or pressure gradient for 57%, iliac dissection for 8%, long segment occlusion for 8%, and eccentric lesions for 5%. Women taking HRT were more likely to be diabetic; otherwise, they were similar to non-HRT users in their risk factors. The primary patency rate was 76% at 1 year, decreasing to 67% at 3 years and 62% at 5 years (Fig 1). These rates were 75%, 57%, and 49%, respectively, for women using HRT; compared with 75%, 74%, and 74% for non-HRT users. The 5-year limb salvage rates were similar for HRT users and nonusers. HRT use was a significant risk factor for decreased primary patency (relative risk, 2.4). Stenting in the external iliac artery was also a significant risk factor (relative risk, 4.3).

Conclusion.—For women undergoing iliac angioplasty and stenting, HRT use is associated with a significant reduction in the primary patency rate. Women who use HRT are more likely to experience long-term failure, necessitating additional procedures for successful management. Stent placement in the external iliac artery is also a risk factor for reduced patency.

▶ The influence of posthormonal replacement therapy on the cardiovascular system of postmenopausal women remains controversial. For years, it was assumed that such therapy was beneficial and actually delayed the development of atherosclerosis. Recent randomized trials have questioned this assumption and have suggested that such therapy may actually be detrimental. Certainly, postmenopausal HRT has not had a favorable effect on the development of coronary disease. In the study reported here, women receiving HRT and undergoing iliac artery angioplasty did distinctly worse than those not receiving HRT. I do not believe this data to be sufficiently robust to justify discontinuing HRT in our patients. It is noteworthy that this was not a randomized trial.

Lower Extremity Arteries

Endoluminal Femoropopliteal Bypass for Intermittent Claudication
Tisi PV, Cowan AR, Morris GE (Southampton Gen Hosp, England)
Eur J Vasc Endovasc Surg 19:481-488, 2000   2–38

Background.—The options for patients whose intermittent claudication worsens despite conservative therapy are limited. Percutaneous transluminal angioplasty is associated with poor long-term graft patency, and conventional bypass surgery carries too many risks for the typical patient. Endoluminal bypass grafts have been successfully used to treat abdominal

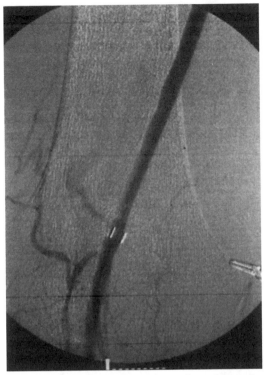

FIGURE 3.—Completion arteriogram following placement of an endoluminal graft. (Reprinted from the *European Journal of Vascular and Endovascular Surgery* courtesy of Tisi PV, Cowan AR, Morris GE: Endoluminal femoropopliteal bypass for intermittent claudication. *Eur J Vasc Endovasc Surg* 19: 481-488, 2000. Copyright 2000, by permission of the publisher, W B Saunders Company Limited London.)

aortic aneurysm. The use of endoluminal femoropopliteal bypass grafts to treat intermittent claudication was described.

Methods.—The subjects were 14 patients (11 men and 3 women; median age, 67 years) with disabling intermittent claudication of the calf and superficial femoral artery (SFA) occlusion. Endoluminal femoropopliteal bypass grafting was performed under the guidance of digital subtraction angiography. Briefly, the common femoral bifurcation is exposed and a small incision is made in the common femoral artery for the insertion of a 5F sheath. The diseased arterial segment is crossed into the healthy below-knee popliteal artery with the use of a guidewire. Angiography is used to determine the distal interface, then the SFA is mechanically dilated and endarterectomized in 5-cm increments up to the distal interface.

The distal end point is dilated and a specially designed instrument is used to place the polytetrafluoroethylene graft transluminally. The stent is inflated until it matches the diameter of the SFA, then the graft and the femoral artery are joined via a conventional end-to-end proximal anastomosis. Patency is confirmed by a completion arteriogram (Fig 3). Patients were followed up every 6 weeks for up to 6 months by duplex US and

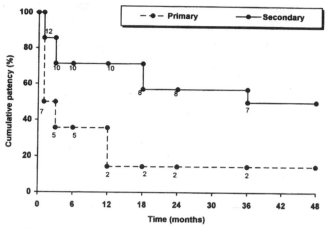

FIGURE 4.—Cumulative primary and secondary patency rates for endoluminal grafts. Number of grafts "at risk" for each time interval is shown. (Reprinted from the *European Journal of Vascular and Endovascular Surgery* courtesy of Tisi PV, Cowan AR, Morris GE: Endoluminal femoropopliteal bypass for intermittent claudication. *Eur J Vasc Endovasc Surg* 19: 481-488, 2000. Copyright 2000, by permission of the publisher, W B Saunders Company Limited London.)

arteriography. Radiologic interventions or surgery were used to maintain graft patency, and most patients (8) received postoperative warfarin.

Results.—Ten of the 14 cases (71%) were associated with perioperative complications, including difficulty crossing the lesion with a guidewire (6 patients), equipment failure (3 patients), and thromboembolism (3 patients). Conversion to open surgery was required for 2 procedural failures caused by graft thrombosis or vessel perforation. Cumulative primary and secondary patency rates at 1 year were 35.7% and 71.4%, respectively, and corresponding rates at 2 years were 14.3% and 57.1% (Fig 4). Of the remaining 12 cases, endovascular grafts remained patent in 7 patients at a mean follow-up of 50 months; however, these patients required 23 endovascular interventions to maintain graft patency. Five patients subsequently underwent reconstructive surgery for occlusion of a previously patent endovascular graft; graft infection in 2 of these patients required major amputation. To date, none of the patients has died.

Conclusion.—Endoluminal femoropopliteal bypass is a minimally invasive approach to treating disabling intermittent claudication. One- and 2-year patency rates are acceptable, although numerous interventions may be required to maintain graft patency. The learning curve associated with this procedure is significant, but increasing experience and improvements in technique and instrumentation may prove endoluminal femoropopliteal bypass to be a viable alternative to conventional surgery in these patients.

▶ The ideas described in this article have been hovering on the edge of endoluminal activity for years. Through a small groin incision, an essentially blind endarterectomy of the SFA is carried out, followed by placement of an endovascular prosthetic graft, in this case, polytetrafluoroethylene. The primary patency rate—the real test of a bypass procedure—was 35% at 1 year and 14% at 2 years. While the authors consider these results "acceptable," I think they are deceiving themselves. These results are awful and should be officially noted as such. Take notice, I hereby note that these results are awful.

Three-Year Outcome of Endovascular Treatment of Superficial Femoral Artery Occlusion

Gordon IL, Conroy RM, Arefi M, et al (Univ of California, Irvine; Veterans Affairs Med Ctr, Long Beach, Calif; Univ of California, Los Angeles)
Arch Surg 136:221-228, 2001   2–39

Background.—The use of percutaneous transluminal angioplasty (PTA) or PTA with stenting in the treatment of patients with stenosis and occlusion of the femoropopliteal segment of the arterial tree has increased in recent years. Previous studies have reported that many patients underwent stenting for management of suboptimal PTA results or after previous interventions had failed. While the long-term results of stenting of the superficial femoral artery (SFA) may be no better than PTA alone, it is possible that previous outcomes reflected an unfavorable bias, since the great majority of cases involved patients in whom stents were used after previous endovascular failures. This study was based on the hypothesis that patency after PTA and stenting of occlusions of the SFA is actually better than historical experience with PTA alone.

Methods.—In a consecutive case series conducted at a Veterans Affairs medical center, primary PTA with stenting was performed on 57 previously untreated men with 71 limbs having chronic atherosclerotic SFA occlusion with suprageniculate reconstitution and patent tibial runoff. Critical ischemia was present in 10% of patients, while the rest had only intermittent claudication. Guidewire recanalization was followed by PTA, deployment of a stent (Wallstent), and adjunctive thrombolysis as needed. Thrombolysis was required in 19 limbs (27%) for management of periprocedural thrombosis. The primary outcome measures were cumulative patency, limb salvage, and complications.

Results.—The average length of the occlusion was 14.4 ± 9.9 cm, and the length of the stented artery was 24.3 ± 11.1 cm. After stenting, the ankle brachial index increased from 0.59 ± 0.14 to 0.86 ± 0.16. One-year patency rates were primary (54.6% ± 6.3%), assisted primary (72.3% ± 5.6%), and secondary (81.6% ± 4.8%). Three-year patency rates were primary (29.9% ± 6.6%), assisted primary (59.0% ± 6.8%), and secondary (68.3% ± 6.5%). The 3-year secondary patency rate for limbs that required periprocedural thrombolysis was 35.7% ± 12.5%, compared with 70.6% ± 7.4% for limbs that did not. There were no significant differences between these groups in occlusion length and severity of ischemia. In limbs that underwent adjunctive PTA during angiography 6 to 12 months after initial stenting, the patency rate at 3 years was 63.0% ±

13.3%, compared with 100% patency in limbs that did not require PTA during that time.

Periprocedural mortality and morbidity were 2.8% and 15.5%, respectively. Amputation during follow-up was performed in 3 of 7 limbs with critical ischemia, compared with 2 of 64 limbs with functional ischemia. There was a mean of 1.8 endovascular interventions per limb.

Conclusion.—The patency rates with PTA and stenting were higher than with PTA alone in historical controls. However, subsequent patency appears to be significantly worse when periprocedural thrombolysis is required. The usefulness of the technique is limited by poor results after PTA and stenting of limbs with critical ischemia and the need for additional endovascular therapy.

▶ Reported here is the use of endovascular stenting for suprageniculate SFA occlusive disease. This was the primary treatment for these patients who had never undergone a previous intervention, either angioplasty or bypass surgery. Ninety percent of the patients were claudicants and 10% had critical ischemia. I believe this to be an honest appraisal of a technique that probably should play little role in the treatment of patients with symptomatic peripheral vascular disease. The results are especially poor in patients with critical limb ischemia.

The authors are to be commended for their conclusion that patients with intermittent claudication should not be managed by current endovascular methods. This study was carried out with an excellent design and the data reported are well evaluated, and even though the results are somewhat negative, this type of honest appraisal is critical in helping us clinicians decide the best treatment for patients with chronic lower-extremity ischemia. The relatively poor patency rates, the risk of the procedure, and the risk of the obligatory use of warfarin for 30 days clearly point out that at the current time, endovascular treatment of SFA occlusion cannot be recommended.

J. O. Menzoian, MD

Clinical Failure After Percutaneous Transluminal Angioplasty of the Superficial Femoral and Popliteal Arteries

Karch LA, Mattos MA, Henretta JP, et al (Southern Illinois Univ, Springfield)
J Vasc Surg 31:880-888, 2000   2–40

Background.—Percutaneous transluminal angioplasty (PTA) is used in the treatment of focal occlusive disease of the superficial femoral and popliteal arteries. However, there is no guarantee of clinical success, even if anatomical patency is achieved following PTA. The factors that produce clinical failure after PTA were evaluated.

Methods.—A retrospective review was performed of the medical records of all patients having PTA of the femoropopliteal arterial segment. Eighty-five patients with 112 lesions were identified. Criteria for inclusion were

TABLE 2.—Life-table Analysis of Clinical Success After Percutaneous Transluminal Angioplasty of the Femoropopliteal Arterial Segment

Interval (Mo)	No. at Risk at Start of Interval	No. of Failures	No. Withdrawn Successfully	Interval Failure Rate (%)	Interval Success Rate (%)	Cumulative Success (%)	SE (%)
0-1	112	2	2	1.8	98.2	98.2	1.2
1-6	108	20	17	20.1	79.9	78.5	3.5
6-12	71	8	11	12.2	87.8	68.9	4.6
12-24	52	9	18	20.9	79.1	54.5	5.1
24-36	25	2	7	9.3	90.7	49.4	7.0
36-48	16	2	9	17.4	82.6	40.8	7.8
48-60	5	0	3	0	100.0	40.8	14.0
> 60	2	2	0	100.0	0	0	0

(Courtesy of Karch LA, Mattos MA, Henretta JP, et al: Clinical failure after percutaneous transluminal angioplasty of the superficial femoral and popliteal arteries, *J Vasc Surg* 31:880-888, 2000.)

complete records and at least 1 postprocedure assessment in the same 30-day period. The standards set by the Society for Vascular Surgery/ International Society for Cardiovascular Surgery Ad Hoc Subcommittee on Reporting Standards for Endovascular Procedures were used to define success. A life-table analysis (intent-to-treat basis) was applied to determine anatomical cumulative patency and clinical success rate.

Results.—Average stenosis was 80% and length of lesion was 2.3 cm. Six lesions had technical failure; 45 had clinical failure, 27 of which were associated with anatomical failure. At 1 year, the cumulative clinical success rate was 69%; at 2 years, it was 54%; at 3 years, it was 49%; and at 4 years, it was 40% (Table 2). Anatomical patency rates at 1 year were 74%; at 2 years, 62%; at 3 years, 57%; and at 4 years, 52%. The anatomic failures were attributed to restenosis (12 patients), occlusion (8 patients), and restenosis with disease progression (6 patients). One patient suffered anatomical failure at the time the procedure was performed. Eighteen patients had clinical failure despite anatomical patency, for a rate or 40%. Specifically, the clinical failure in this group resulted from progression of disease in the treated vessel (12 patients), iliac disease (3 patients), tibial disease (2 patients), and bypass graft failure (1 patient). Successful treatment using supplemental percutaneous procedures was achieved in 50% of the 45 clinical failures.

Conclusion.—Focal disease of the superficial femoral and popliteal arteries can be successfully treated by PTA. Clinical failures resulted from anatomical failure in most cases, but a significant number occurred even when the PTA was patent. Surgical bypass graft success rates are superior to those achieved with PTA, but supplemental PTA could be performed in 50% of patients. Surgical bypass graft procedures may be avoided by using repeated percutaneous treatments.

▶ The results reported by this experienced group are quite similar to those noted in Abstract 2–39. These authors, however, conclude that this is an acceptable therapeutic option for the treatment of focal occlusive disease. The authors do not give the primary patency rate, but I think it is about 50% at 2 years. I do not consider this to be an acceptable result when we have a surgical option with much better anticipated success. I fear we are coming to a philosophical crux. I consider the best operation for a patient to be the one that gives the highest patency rate with minimal complications and the most reasonable cost. Proponents of repeat angioplasty consider the best operation to be one that allows the quickest and easiest discharge from the hospital after each individual procedure. What we have here is a disagreement.

Acute Occlusion of Popliteal and/or Tibial Arteries: The Value of Percutaneous Treatment

Desgranges P, Kobeiter H, d'Audiffret A, et al (Hôpital Henri Mondor, Créteil, France)
Eur J Vasc Endovasc Surg 20:138-145, 2000   2–41

Objective.—A combination of thromboaspiration, thrombolysis, and percutaneous transluminal angioplasty (PTA) may be beneficial for patients with acute occlusion of the popliteal or tibial arteries or both. Early and intermediate-term results in 33 consecutive patients are retrospectively analyzed.

Methods.—Technical success, survival, and limb salvage at 1, 3, 6, and 12 months were determined for 33 patients (13 women), aged 46 to 95 years, treated with combined therapy for acute ischemia between December 1994 and December 1997 (Table 1 and Table 2). Primary, assisted primary, and secondary patency of the recanalized arteries, and major complications were evaluated at 1, 6, and 12 months.

Results.—Technical success, successful thromboaspiration and thrombolysis, was achieved in 27 (82%) patients. Seven (26%) of these patients later had PTA for stenosis of the popliteal artery, peroneal artery, or both popliteal and tibial vessels (Table 3). Thromboaspiration was successful in 15 (46%) patients. Thromboaspiration followed by thrombolysis was successful in 12 of 18 patients. The remaining 6 (18%) patients required surgical conversion. One patient had a distal bypass. Three patients underwent Fogarty embolectomy, of which 2 were successful. The patient whose embolectomy failed underwent an above-the-knee amputation. Two patients whose vein-patch angioplasty failed had an above-the-knee or below-the-knee amputation. Nine (27%) patients had complications that included 4 groin hematomas (12%), 4 compartment syndromes (12%), and 1 hemoglobinuria (3%). Patients were followed up for a mean of 15.3 months. Kaplan-Meier survival rates at 1 month and 1 year were 100% and 94%, respectively. The cumulative limb salvage rates at the same points were both 91%. The cumulative 1-month and 1-year primary patency, assisted primary patency, and secondary patency rates were 81%

TABLE 1.—Clinical Classification of Ischemia

Classification	Patients (%)
I-variable	6 (18)
II-threatened	
IIa	18 (55)
IIb	9 (27)
III-irreversible	0 (0)
Total	33 (100)

TABLE 2.—Etiologies of Occlusions

Aetiologies	Patients (%)
Emboli	23 (70)
Atrial fibrillation	8
Other cardiogenic	1
Abdominal aneurysm	4
Iatrogenic (after PTA)	4
Proximal atherosclerotic plaque	3
Unknown	3
Thrombosis	10 (30)
Total	33 (100)

and 66%, 81% and 72%, and 86% and 77%, respectively. Four patients required reoperation.

Conclusion.—A combination of thromboaspiration, thrombolysis, and PTA provides good early and intermediate-term results in selected patients with acute occlusion of the popliteal or tibial arteries.

▶ I find this French article almost indecipherable. The authors are probably presenting their results of the treatment of acute thrombotic occlusion of popliteal and tibial arteries treated with thromboaspiration; thrombolysis; and, in many cases, other procedures as well. I have no problem with catheter-based thrombolysis, as this procedure is well-established and has an obvious role in selected patients. I suppose if you want to do thromboaspiration, that is acceptable, although I don't see the advantage. The use of the adjunct procedures makes this article practically indecipherable.

TABLE 3.—Location of Thrombosis/Emboli

Location of Occlusion	Thrombosis	Emboli
Popliteal vessel only	3	7
Peroneal/tibial vessel only	2	6
Both	5	10
Total	10	23

Renal Artery

The Effect of Balloon Angioplasty on Hypertension in Atherosclerotic Renal-Artery Stenosis

van Jaarsveld BC, for the Dutch Renal Artery Stenosis Intervention Cooperative Study Group (Eramsus Univ, Rotterdam, The Netherlands; Univ Hosp, Nijmegen, The Netherlands; Ikazia Hosp, Rotterdam, The Netherlands; et al)
N Engl J Med 343:1007-1014, 2000   2–42

Background.—Because renal artery stenosis can cause hypertension, surgical revascularization was developed to treat the stenosis and relieve the hypertension. This first surgical approach gave way to percutaneous transluminal balloon angioplasty with or without stent placement. Few patients had blood pressure return to normal, but improvement was seen. Today's antihypertensive drug therapy also produces good results, and this study compared the medical approach with the surgical approach.

Methods.—The 106 patients studied had atherosclerotic renal artery stenosis, a serum creatinine concentration of 2.3 mg/dL or less or one that increased at least 0.2 mg/dL while taking an angiotensin-converting enzyme inhibitor, and a diastolic blood pressure of 95 mm Hg or higher despite antihypertensive drug treatment. They were randomly assigned to receive either medical therapy (50 patients) or percutaneous transluminal renal angioplasty (56 patients). Assessment points were at 3 and 12 months, when blood pressure, antihypertensive drug dose, and renal function were evaluated. Renal artery patency was also assessed as 12 months.

Results.—At 3 months, mean systolic and diastolic blood pressure values were essentially the same: the angioplasty group's systolic mean was at 169 mm Hg and the diastolic mean was at 99 mm Hg, and the drug group's systolic mean was at 176 mm Hg and their diastolic mean was at 101 mm Hg. Intention-to-treat analysis at 12 months showed no significant differences in systolic and diastolic pressure, daily drug doses, or renal function. Twenty-two of the drug-only group underwent angioplasty after 3 months for persistent hypertension, and these patients received considerably smaller doses of antihypertensive agents than those who had only medical therapy at 3 months, but the difference was not significant at 12 months.

Conclusions.—Only a small advantage is achieved by treating hypertension with angioplasty over the results with antihypertensive drug therapy. Thus, it is recommended that angioplasty be reserved for patients who have taken 3 or more drugs and still have hypertension or have progression of their renovascular disease.

▶ This is an article with potentially profound clinical implications. We have all been hearing for years that surgical repair of stenotic renal arteries in patients with hypertension results in a cure of hypertension in a moderate number of patients and improvement in the large majority. In recent years, similar anecdotal claims have been made for angioplasty with or without stent placement. Finally, we come to a properly designed prospective, randomized clinical trial, although the number of patients is small. A group of patients with renal artery stenosis and hypertension receiving drug therapy was randomly assigned to transluminal renal angioplasty generally without stents or continued best medical therapy. Blood pressure in the 2 groups was identical at the beginning of the study, and, with use of the widely accepted intention-to-treat method of analysis, at 12 months, there were no significant differences between the angioplasty and drug therapy groups in systolic or diastolic blood pressure, the number of daily drugs being taken, or renal function. The authors appropriately concluded that, for the treatment of patients with hypertension and renal artery stenosis, angioplasty showed no advantage over antihypertensive drug therapy. I consider this study to be monumentally important, and I commend it to you, although I suspect critics will claim much better results would have occurred with routine stenting. Perhaps data such as these will decrease cardiologists' drive-by renal artery stenting—but that's probably wishful thinking. Science has never been a match for avarice.

Use of Doppler Ultrasonography to Predict the Outcome of Therapy for Renal-Artery Stenosis
Radermacher J, Chavan A, Bleck J, et al (Medizinische Hochschule Hannover, Germany)
N Engl J Med 344:410-417, 2001   2–43

Background.—To date, it has not been possible to prospectively identify patients whose renal function or blood pressure will improve after correcting renal artery stenosis. Whether a high level of resistance to flow in the segmental arteries of both kidneys can help prospectively identify treatment candidates was investigated.

Methods.—The resistance index was measured in 5950 patients with hypertension for renal artery stenosis by means of color Doppler US. Renal angioplasty or surgery was technically successful in 131 of 138 patients with unilateral or bilateral renal artery stenosis of more than 50% of the luminal diameter. Creatinine clearance and 24-hour ambulatory blood pressure were measured before renal artery stenosis correction and 3, 6, and 12 months after the procedure and annually thereafter. Patients were followed-up for a mean of 32 months.

Findings.—In 34 of the 35 patients with resistance index values of 80 or greater before revascularization, the mean arterial pressure did not decline by 10 mm Hg or more after revascularization. Renal function decreased in 80% of the patients. Forty-six percent became dependent on dialysis. Twenty-nine percent died during follow-up. In all but 6 of the 96 patients with a resistance-index value of less than 80, mean arterial pressure declined by at least 10% after revascularization (Fig 2). Renal function worsened in only 3% in this group, all of whom became dialysis dependent. Three percent of this group died.

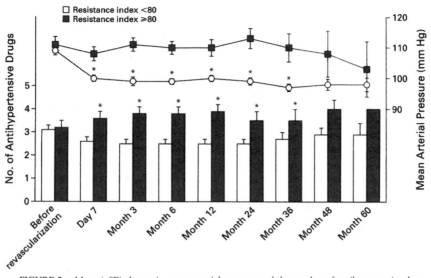

FIGURE 2.—Mean (±SE) change in mean arterial pressure and the number of antihypertensive drugs taken after the correction of renal artery stenosis, according to the resistance index values before revascularization. In the group of patients with a resistance index of less than 80 before revascularization, mean (±SE) blood pressure was 150 ± 22/89 ± 12 mm Hg initially and 135 ± 14/80 ± 10 mm Hg at the last follow-up visit (P < .001); the respective values in the group of patients with a resistance index of at least 80 before revascularization were 164 ± 21/83 ± 16 mm Hg and 163 ± 19/86 ± 10 mm Hg (P = .73)/ The antihypertensive drugs included angiotensin-converting enzyme inhibitors, angiotensin II-receptor blockers, β-blockers, calcium antagonists, α-blockers, direct vasodilators, diuretics, and nitrates. *Asterisks* indicate a significant difference (P < .05) between the 2 groups with use of an unpaired t-test with Bonferroni's adjustment. (Reprinted by permission of *The New England Journal of Medicine* from Radermacher J, Chavan A, Bleck J, et al: Use of Doppler ultrasonography to predict the outcome of therapy for renal-artery stenosis. *N Engl J Med* 344:410-417, 2001. Copyright 2001, Massachusetts Medical Society. All rights reserved.)

Conclusion.—A renal resistance index value of 80 or greater reliably predicts which patients with renal artery stenosis will not have improved renal function, blood pressure, or kidney survival after angioplasty or surgery. Thus, patients with renal resistance index values of at least 80 should not undergo such interventions.

▶ The renal artery resistance index has been around for years as a way to predict the extent of renal parenchymal disease. These authors calculated a very simple resistance index (basically based on the magnitude of diastolic velocity elevation) and found in a noncontrolled study that almost no patients who had a high renal artery resistance did well with either surgery or angioplasty of the renal artery, while a large majority who had a low renal artery resistance did quite well. It certainly appears from this information that if we are determined to intervene upon renal artery stenosis, a preoperative knowledge of the renal artery resistance index may be very helpful. I believe this article is correct, important, and restates previous information in a succinct fashion.

Thoracic Aorta

Treatment of Stanford Type B Aortic Dissection With Stent-Grafts: Preliminary Results

Czermak BV, Waldenberger P, Fraedrich G, et al (Univ Hosp Innsbruck, Austria)

Radiology 217:544-550, 2000   2–44

Background.—A tear within the aortic wall is the initiating event in aortic dissection, resulting in the separation of the aortic wall layers. Typically, the dissection propagates distally from the intimal tear, but proximal propagation is also possible. Dissections may arise at any point along the aortic course, but the most common site of origin is the ascending aorta within a few centimeters of the aortic valve or in the descending thoracic aorta just distal to the origin of the left subclavian artery. In the Stanford classification system, all dissections involving the ascending aorta are designated as type A (proximal) dissections, whereas all other dissections are designated as type B (distal) dissections. Hypertension is the most important predisposing condition for development of aortic dissection. A high mortality rate (5%-26%) has been associated with surgery for aortic dissection, and it has therefore been argued that medical therapy is superior to surgery in the treatment of type B dissections. However, in 20% to 50% of survivors of the acute stage of aortic dissection, aneurysms develop within 1 to 5 years of onset. Significant enlargement of the false lumen and a narrowing of the true lumen are also frequent occurrences. The feasibility and safety of endovascular stent-graft placement in treating Stanford type B aortic dissection were evaluated.

Methods.—Endovascular stent-grafts were placed in 7 patients with type B aortic dissection (Table 1). The dissections were acute in 5 patients and chronic in 2 patients. In 5 patients, the proximal entry tear was within 2 cm of the origin of the left subclavian artery, whereas the tear was beyond this site in 2 patients. Placement of the noncovered proximal

TABLE 1.—Patient Characteristics

Patient No./ Age (y)/Sex	Stage of Dissection	Proximity of Entry Site to Subclavian Artery (cm)	Reentry Site	Symptom Severity
1/68/M	Acute	>2	2 cm proximal to AB	++
2/64/M	Acute	>2	1 cm proximal to RRA	++
3/79/F*	Chronic	<2	1 cm proximal to CA	NA
4/63/M	Acute	<2	External iliac artery	+++
5/43/M	Acute	<2	External iliac artery	+++
6/72/M	Chronic	<2	3 cm proximal to CA	+++
7/80/M	Acute	<2	Superior mesenteric artery	+++

*Treatment was performed because of expansion of the false lumen.
Abbreviations: *AB*, Aortic bifurcation; *CA*, celiac artery; *RRA*, right renal artery; ++, moderate, +++, severe.
(Courtesy of Czermak BV, Waldenberger P, Fraedrich G, et al: Treatment of Stanford type B aortic dissection with stent-grafts: Preliminary results. *Radiology* 217:544-550, 2000. Radiological Society of North America.)

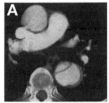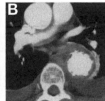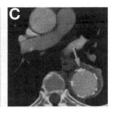

FIGURE 3.—Acute type B dissection in 1 patient. Transverse contrast-enhanced CT scans obtained (**A**) before transfemoral placement of a stent-graft, (**B**) postoperately, and (**C**) 6 months after surgery. After stent-graft implantation, clot formation occurred in the false lumen, and shrinkage of the false lumen was monitored for 6 months. The false lumen is completely obliterated (*arrow* in **C**) at 6-month follow-up. (Courtesy of Czermak BV, Waldenberger P, Fraedrich G, et al: Treatment of Standford type B aortic dissection with stent-grafts: Preliminary results. *Radiology* 217:544-550, 2000. Radiological Society of North America.)

portion of the stent-graft in 3 patients was across the origin of the left subclavian artery. Follow-up studies were conducted at 3, 6, 12, and 24 months after intervention for assessment of the efficacy of the procedure.

Results.—Technical and clinical success were achieved in 6 of 7 patients (86%). The left subclavian artery maintained patency in all patients. In 2 patients who had involvement of aortic branches, the placement of the endovascular stent-graft restored adequate blood flow to the compromised branches. In 1 patient, the dissection extended into the ascending aorta, and the patient was readmitted 1 month later. Closure of the entry tear and thrombosis of the false lumen along the stent-graft were achieved in all the other patients. There was considerable shrinkage in all of the false lumina (Fig 3). The mean time of follow-up was 14 months.

Conclusion.—Endovascular stent-graft placement is a safe and effective procedure for the treatment of type B aortic dissections within and beyond 2 cm of the origin of the left subclavian artery.

► This article presents a detailed review of the use of stent-grafts in 7 patients with type B thoracic aortic dissection. This experience established the feasibility of placing the proximal stent across the subclavian artery without occlusion. An endovascular stent-graft was associated with restoration of normal luminal flow and perfusion of the visceral arteries. A single patient required a fenestration procedure in the left external iliac. A single patient had a retrograde dissection into the arch and required surgery. I believe this article does establish, in a very well documented fashion, the feasibility of using a thoracic stent-graft to cover the origin of the dissection and to compress and obliterate the false lumen. Obviously, coverage of the distal reentry site is not essential. I suspect that stent-graft placement will become the treatment of choice in those patients with an acute type B dissection not adequately treated by drug therapy alone.

Stent Treatment for Coarctation of the Aorta: Intermediate Term Follow up and Technical Considerations
Thanopoulos BD, Hadjinikolaou L, Konstadopoulou GN, et al (Aghia Sophia Children's Hosp, Athens, Greece; Univ Hosp of Thessalia, Larissa, Greece)
Heart 84:65-70, 2000   2–45

Background.—Stenting is an increasingly popular option for the treatment of isolated aortic coarctation. However, there are few data on the intermediate- and long-term rates of recoarctation after stenting. The results of stenting for coarctation of the aorta at an intermediate-term follow-up are reported.

Methods.—From 1992 to 1999, stent implantation was performed in 17 children with aortic coarctation (median age, 11 years). The coarctation was isolated in 6 cases; recurrent in 9 (after either surgical repair or balloon dilatation), and a complex long segment coarctation in 2. A second catheter placed transseptally in the left ventricle or more proximally in the aorta was used to guide the stent implantation procedure. A total of 22 stents were used, and multiple stents were used in the patients

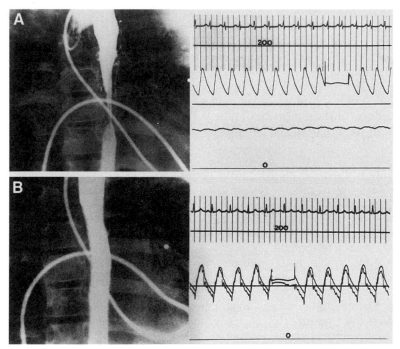

FIGURE 2.—Antegrade ascending aortograms (**left panels**) and simultaneous ascending and descending aortic pressure tracings (**right panels**) obtained from a patient with long segment coarctation before (**A**) and immediately after (**B**) multiple stent implantation. An impressive increase in coarctation diameter and elimination of the pressure gradient across the coarctation is seen after deployment of the stents. (Courtesy of Thanopoulos BD, Hadjinikolaou L, Konstadopoulou GN, et al: Stent treatment for coarctation of the aorta: Intermediate term follow up and technical considerations. *Heart* 84:65-70, 2000, with permission from the BMJ Publishing Group.)

with long-segment coarctation. Stent types were Palmaz 4014 in 11 patients, Palmaz 308 in 5, and Palmaz 154 in 1.

Results.—Stent placement was associated with an immediate drop in the mean peak systolic gradient, from 50.0 to 2.1 mm Hg (Fig 2). Stenting increased the diameter of the stenotic lesion from 5.1 to 13.9 mm. No patient died or experienced procedure-related complications. There were no recurrent clinical or angiographic coarctations through a median follow-up of 33 months.

Conclusions.—This experience demonstrates very low morbidity and mortality in children undergoing stent placement for coarctation of the aorta. At nearly 3 years' follow-up, the results are good. Further studies are needed to determine long-term freedom from recoarctation compared with balloon dilatation.

▶ Overall, this is a remarkable experience. It describes the placement of stents directly across thoracic aortic coarctation, either as initial treatment or after recurrence following surgery or prior balloon angioplasty. The lack of recurrence at 33 months is remarkable, as is the virtual elimination of all gradient. I suspect this may become the procedure of choice in these difficult patients.

Thoracic Aortic Aneurysms: Treatment With Endovascular Self-expandable Stent Grafts
Grabenwöger M, Hutschala D, Ehrlich MP, et al (Univ of Vienna)
Ann Thorac Surg 69:441-445, 2000   2–46

Objective.—Conventional repair of thoracic aortic aneurysms is associated with substantial morbidity. Endovascular stent graft placement has been used successfully to treat abdominal aortic aneurysms. The feasibility and safety of endovascular stent graft placement for repair of thoracic aortic aneurysms was evaluated.

Methods.—Between November 1996 and February 1999, 21 patients (5 women), aged 41 to 87 years, underwent endovascular stent graft repair of a thoracic aortic aneurysm. Underlying medical disorders included hypertension (85.7%), pulmonary hypertension (62%), and coronary artery disease (38.1%). Fifteen patients (71.4%) were not suitable candidates for conventional surgery. Nineteen patients had an aneurysm larger than 6 cm in diameter. Two patients had stent placement for chronic aortic dissection. The Talent endoluminal stent graft system (World Medical Corp, Sunrise, Fla) was used in 16 patients, and the Prograft stent graft system (WL Gore & Associates, Flagstaff, Ariz) was used in 5 patients. Fifteen patients (71.4%) required more than 1 stent.

Results.—Stent deployment was successful in all patients. The average number of stents used was 2.6. Nine patients required subclavian–carotid artery transposition to provide sufficient length to allow safe stent graft deployment. Three patients had leakage into the aneurysmal sac and underwent repeat stenting, 2 during the same procedure and 1 in a second operation. One patient experienced an iliac artery dissection, and an iliac–femoral bypass was performed. Two patients died on postoperative days 1 and 3.

Conclusion.—Endoluminal stent graft repair of thoracic aortic aneurysms is a promising technique that should improve with the technical development of stent grafts and improved patient selection.

▶ It is noteworthy that these authors were generally successful in deploying grafts in the treatment of atherosclerotic descending thoracic aortic aneurysms greater than 6 cm in diameter. Interesting, in a number of these patients, the left subclavian was transposed to the carotid to provide more room for proximal insertion, although one can stent directly across the subclavian ostium with the expectation of continued patency. Several fatal complications occurred in this series, including that of 1 patient with aneurysm rupture and death several days after apparently uneventful stenting. In this patient, the stent migrated into the aneurysmal sac. The second patient died of multiorgan failure presumably related to impaired perfusion of the celiac artery caused by the stent-graft. Overall, these results appear comparable to those of surgery for thoracic aneurysms, and also comparable to those of other endograft series. As in all other things, the information will be revealed by long-term follow-up. We shall see.

Thrombolysis

A Systematic Review of Intra-arterial Thrombolytic Therapy for Lower-Limb Ischaemia
Palfreyman SJ, Booth A, Michaels JA (Northern Gen Hosp NHS Trust, Sheffield, England; Univ of Sheffield, England)
Eur J Vasc Endovasc Surg 19:143-157, 2000   2–47

Background.—Thrombolysis is theoretically effective treatment for acute limb ischemia, but evidence is lacking. Thus, all evidence available regarding the use of thrombolysis to treat acute arterial occlusions of the legs was reviewed, and results were compared with those obtained with surgery.

Methods.—The major databases were searched for randomized controlled trials of thrombolytic therapy used for limb ischemia. Only English language studies or those with a detailed English summary and articles published after 1980 were evaluated. A search of key journals and citations was done by hand, and a random effects meta-analysis was performed.

Results.—Ten reports of randomized controlled trials were found. No significant differences in major amputation or mortality rates were revealed when thrombolysis was compared with surgery. However, thrombolysis carried an increased relative risk of hemorrhaging (2.94). A benefit was noted when thrombolysis was used in cases involving short-duration occlusions and occluded grafts. When the occlusion was present for more than 15 days, especially if it involved native vessels, thrombolysis was contraindicated.

Conclusions.—Only in the case of graft occlusion and ischemia of short duration has the evidence shown thrombolysis to be the preferred treatment over surgery. It can be used as an adjunct to other treatments but should be avoided if ischemia has been present for more than 14 days and involves native vessel occlusions.

▶ A diligent attempt was made to find randomized, controlled trials evaluating intra-arterial thrombolytic therapy in the treatment of limb ischemia. I believe these authors have done about as good a job as one could expect. Their conclusion strikes me as right on the money, namely, that there continues to be insufficient evidence to justify the widespread use of thrombolytic therapy in the treatment of limb ischemia, other than perhaps for certain patients with graft occlusion and some patients with short-duration ischemia.

I might add to this the use of thrombolytic therapy to define an outflow tract in preparation for surgery, as in the case of certain patients with thrombosed popliteal aneurysms. The use of thrombolytic therapy for lower extremity graft occlusion strikes me as wishful thinking. While you may be able to actually open the graft in about 60% to 70% of patients, the 1-year patency rate following such graft opening is in the range of 20% to 30%. In my opinion, such results do not justify the continuing use of the technique for graft thrombosis.

Percutaneous Catheter Thrombus Aspiration for Acute or Subacute Arterial Occlusion of the Legs: How Much Thrombolysis Is Needed?
Zehnder T, Birrer M, Do DD, et al (Univ Hosp Bern, Switzerland)
Eur J Vasc Endovasc Surg 20:41-46, 2000   2–48

Introduction.—The safety and efficacy of percutaneous, catheter-directed thrombolysis continues to be a cause of concern, despite its many years of use in the treatment of acute arterial occlusions of the legs. An ideal catheter-directed method must include the avoidance of hemorrhage along with a marked decrease in the time needed to restore arterial flow comparable to the duration of a surgical procedure. The role of a combined percutaneous endovascular approach, including thrombus aspiration, catheter thrombolysis, and percutaneous transluminal angioplasty (PTA) for treatment of acute and subacute occlusions of native leg arteries was examined retrospectively in 89 consecutive patients (93 legs) in a single institution.

Methods.—The study included 42 men and 47 women ranging in age from 29 to 100 years (mean age, 70.7 years). Major end points were mortality rates, necessity for amputation at 1, 6, and 12 months, and amputation-free survival of the entire patient group at 6 and 12 months after the procedure. Other endpoints included the primary dissolution of occluding thrombus, the number and percentage of secondary reinterventions necessary, and whether secondary procedures were by open surgery or by catheter technique. Patients were observed for 12 months.

Results.—Initial treatment success was 90% of the total legs. Mortality rates at 1 month and 12 months were 8% and 19%, respectively. The amputation-free survival was 78% at 12 months. Aspiration alone was adequate in 31% of cases. The mean dose of urokinase used in 22% of patients was 112,500 IU; PTA was added in 69%. The only major bleeding event was 1 false aneurysm treated by surgically-guided compression. Secondary interventions were needed within 12 months in 30% of cases (14 endovascular, 16 open surgical procedures).

Conclusion.—Catheter thrombus aspiration combined with thrombolysis and/or PTA is very effective. A small number of patients require modest doses of thrombolytics. Serious bleeding complications are rare. This combination procedure is recommended as a first-line treatment for acute or subacute infrainguinal arterial occlusions.

▶ This article reports an institutional experience between 1995 and 1997 of catheter treatment of acute thrombotic occlusion of the lower extremity native arteries in 89 patients. This is a classic potpourri of everything. Some of these were thrombotic, some were embolic, some patients had associated stenoses, some did not, some received only clot aspiration, and some received thrombolytic therapy in addition. I am unable to make any sense out of this study.

Ultrasound Imaging–Guided Noninvasive Ultrasound Thrombolysis: Preclinical Results
Rosenschein U, Furman V, Kerner E, et al (Tel Aviv Sourasky Med Ctr, Israel; Angiosonics Ltd R&D Labs, Tel Aviv, Israel; Meir Med Ctr, Kfar Saba, Israel)
Circulation 102:238-245, 2000   2–49

Introduction.—Catheter-based therapeutic US thrombolysis has recently been shown to be effective and safe. The safety and efficacy of external high-intensity focused US (HIFU) thrombolysis guided by US imaging in experimental settings was investigated.

Methods.—A therapeutic transducer was constructed from an acoustic lens and united with an US imaging transducer. In-vitro clots were introduced into bovine arterial segments and sonicated under real-time ultrasound imaging guidance in a water tank.

Results.—Using pulsed-wave (PW) US, the total sonication time correlated with thrombolysis efficiency ($r^2 = 0.7666$). A thrombolysis efficiency of 91% was observed with optimal PW parameters (1:25 duty cycle, 200-μs pulse length) at a mean intensity (I_{spta}) of more than 35 W/cm². Ultrasound imaging during sonication revealed the cavitation field as a spherical cloud of echo-dense material. Within less than 2 minutes, the vessel lumen evidenced neither residual clot nor damage to the arterial wall

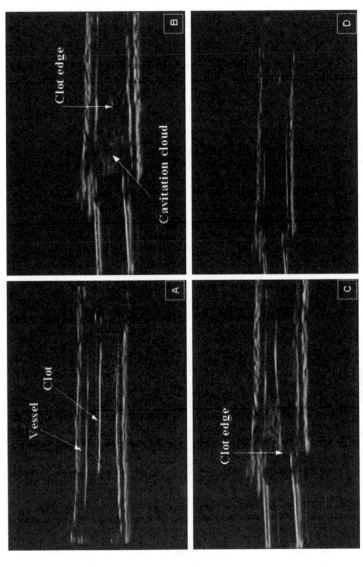

FIGURE 6.—Representative US of experiment using optimal PW parameters. A, Baseline US imaging of thrombotic artery in long-axis view. Thrombus (*dotted box*) could be identified as mildly echo-dense mass occupying vessel lumen. B, During sonication, cavitation was visible as spherical cloud of echo-contrast material. C, When cavitation cloud interacted with clot, it typically shifted to cavitation area (note location of clot edge *vs* its location in baseline image). D, After sonication for 3 minutes, vessel lumen was echolucent, with no sonographic evidence of residual clot or damage to arterial wall. (Courtesy of Rosenschein U, Furman V, Kerner E, et al: Ultrasound imaging-guided noninvasive ultrasound thrombolysis: Preclinical results. *Circulation* 102:238-245, 2000.)

(Fig 6). During serial filtration, 93% of the lysed clot became subcapillary in size (less than 8 µm). In-vitro safety trials demonstrated arterial damage when an I_{spta} of 45 W/cm² was used for periods of 300 or more seconds.

Conclusions.—External HIFU thrombolysis is safe and effective. Its use can be guided by US imaging, allowing the monitoring of therapy.

▶ This remarkable study clearly demonstrates the potential for the use of HIFU to sonicate and break up intravascular thrombi. Interestingly, these preliminary results suggest that over 93% of the thrombus becomes sub-capillary in size (less than 8 µm) after sonication. While these results are obviously preliminary, we may actually be close to the time when we can apply US externally over a thrombosed artery and expect sonication to be therapeutic. I suspect that commercial devices will soon be forthcoming.

3 Vascular Laboratory and Imaging

Carotid

Optimizing Duplex Follow-up in Patients With an Asymptomatic Internal Carotid Artery Stenosis of Less Than 60%
Lovelace TD, Moneta GL, Abou-Zamzam AM Jr, et al (Oregon Health Sciences Univ, Portland)
J Vasc Surg 33:56-61, 2001   3-1

Background.—Carotid endarterectomy has been shown to benefit individuals with 60% to 99% asymptomatic internal carotid artery (ICA) stenosis, but the follow-up intervals yielding the best information concerning progression from less than 60% to the range from 60% to 99% have not been determined. ICAs with stenosis of less than 60% and peak systolic velocities (PSVs) of at least 175 cm/s when evaluated on initial duplex scanning are at high risk of progression to greater degrees of stenosis. This finding was prospectively analyzed, and the optimal follow-up intervals were defined for patients whose stenosis is less than 60% and who are without symptoms.

Methods.—The study population included all patients, regardless of indication, who underwent carotid duplex examination since January 1, 1995 who had at least 1 patent asymptomatic ICA that had not undergone operation and that had less than 60% stenosis. These patients had to have had at least 6 months of follow-up and 1 or more repeated duplex examinations. The initial duplex examination was used to classify ICAs into those with a PSV less than 175 cm/s and those whose PSV exceeded 175 cm/s. Follow-up examinations were performed at various intervals to check for the presence of progression, and Kaplan-Meier curves were prepared to determine the probability of freedom from progression (Fig 2).

Results.—Of the 407 patients undergoing serial duplex scans, symptomatic progression, from 60% to 99% ICA stenosis with transient ischemic attacks occurred in 3 patients, and 4 had occlusion without occurrence of a stroke. None had hemispheric symptoms without ipsilateral progression of the ICA stenosis. At a mean of 18 months, asymptomatic progression was found in 41 patients (46 ICAs). Asymptomatic occlusion occurred in

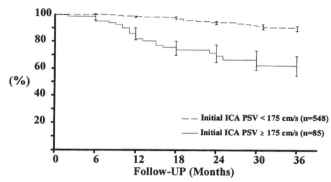

FIGURE 2.—Freedom from progression from less than 60% to 60% to 99% ICA stenosis. $P < .0001$ for all intervals. Excluded are 7 ICAs that became symptomatic and/or progressed to occlusion. *Abbreviation: ICA*, Internal carotid artery. (Courtesy of Lovelace TD, Moneta GL, Abou-Zamzam AM, et al: Optimizing duplex follow-up in patients with an asymptomatic internal carotid artery stenosis of less than 60%. *J Vasc Surg* 33:56-61, 2001.)

3 patients (3 ICAs) at a mean of 16 months, and endarterectomy of 17 ICAs was done for 16 patients. Previous arterial surgery had been performed in 73% of patients who had progression to 60% to 99% stenosis but in only 55% of those who had no progression. These were related to a higher percentage of lower extremity bypass graft procedures previously performed in patients who had progression compared with those who had not had progression. Five hundred forty-eight of 633 patent asymptomatic arteries had initial PSVs less than 175 cm/s, and 24 progressed. For 85 arteries, the PSVs were more than 175 cm/s, and 22 progressed. Freedom from progression was determined to be 95% at 6 months, 83% at 12 months, and 70% at 24 months for ICAs whose initial PSVs were more than 175 cm/s versus 100% at 6 months, 99% at 12 months, and 95% at 24 months for those whose initial PSVs were less than 175 cm/s.

Conclusions.—A greater likelihood of asymptomatic progression to 60% to 99% ICA stenosis was seen in patients who had less than 60% initially and a PSV of more than 175 cm/s. The frequency of this association is enough to dictate repeating duplex studies at intervals of every 6 months. When the ICA stenosis is less than 60% and the initial PSV is less than 175 cm/s, it is safe to perform duplex examinations only after 2 years.

▶ Without question, the Asymptomatic Carotid Atherosclerosis Study (ACAS) and North American Symptomatic Carotid Endarterectomy Trial study have had a profound impact upon practice patterns the world over, at least among vascular surgeons. Studies from my laboratory have established precise criteria for determining which patients are ACAS-positive, namely an ICA PSV greater than 260, and ICA end-diastolic velocity of 70 cm/s or greater. The question being asked in this study is how often a vascular lab carotid exam should be performed in patients who are ACAS-negative on the first exam. The researchers had earlier retrospectively established ICA PSV of 175 as defining the patient group most likely to progress. This number was then prospectively validated in the current study. The study's conclusions are straightforward and probably correct, namely that patients who are ACAS-negative with an ICA PSV greater than 175 should have vascular lab carotid exams at 6-month intervals. Patients who are ACAS-negative with an ICA PSV less than 175 could probably have vascular lab duplex exams performed at 2-year intervals. This would appear to be valid practical advice.

Effect of Contralateral Carotid Artery Stenosis on Carotid Ultrasound Velocity Measurements
Barnett HJM, for the North American Symptomatic Carotid Endarterectomy Trial (NASCET) Group (Univ of Western Ontario, London, Canada; et al)
Stroke 31:2636-2640, 2000   3–2

Background.—It is increasingly common for carotid US to be the only investigation performed before carotid endarterectomy in the investigation of the degree of internal carotid artery (ICA) stenosis on the basis of velocity or frequency measurements. It has been reported in a number of studies that there is a potential source of error in the use of these blood flow measurements; the presence of severe contralateral ICA stenosis or occlusion may result in the artificial elevation of the peak systolic velocity or frequency values used to quantify the degree of stenosis in the artery under investigation. The effects of contralateral ICA stenosis on carotid US measurements of peak systolic velocity were investigated.

Methods.—Symptomatic patients who were participants in the North American Symptomatic Carotid Endarterectomy Trial (NASCET) underwent US before and after carotid endarterectomy. Investigators assessed the mean change in peak systolic velocity in the unoperated artery across all degrees of angiographically defined stenosis and derived a simple theoretical resistance model of the cerebral circulation.

Results.—A total of 386 patients underwent complete bilateral US examination within 90 days of the initial scan. In the presence of a contralateral severe (70% to 99%) stenosis of the ICA, the peak systolic velocity in the unoperated artery was artificially elevated by a mean of 84 cm/s. The mean elevation was less pronounced with lesser degrees of stenosis (11 to 21 cm/s). In contralateral arteries with less than 70% stenosis, small elevations of 3 to 12 cm/s were observed. The patterns of the results were in agreement with the patterns predicted by the theoretic model.

Conclusion.—US peak systolic velocity can be artificially elevated by a severely stenosed contralateral ICA. In this study, the effect was greatest when bilaterally severe stenoses were present, so caution must be used when assessment of the degree of ICA stenosis is based solely on US peak systolic velocity measurements.

▶ Another slice of salami rolls off the great salami roll left over from the NASCET study and frozen in the deep freeze at the University of Western Ontario. The conclusions of this study are actually rather sophomoric, but unarguable. It concludes that the presence of a 70% to 99% contralateral

ICA stenosis will artifactually elevate the peak systolic velocity of the ipsi-lateral ICA by a mean of 84 cm/s, generally related to the amount of contralateral stenosis. This sophomoric information is of little value since it uses mean values and gives us no idea of how to relate the data to an individual patient. The fact that a severe contralateral stenosis can artifactually elevate the velocity on the ipsilateral side has been known for years. I am always pleased when the group at the University of Western Ontario rediscovers the wheel. (See Abstract 3–13.)

Effect of Contralateral Disease on Duplex Measurements of Internal Carotid Artery Stenosis

Ray SA, Lockhart SJM, Dourado R, et al (St Thomas' Hosp, London)
Br J Surg 87:1057-1062, 2000   3–3

Background.—Clinicians are increasingly using duplex US as the only imaging method before carotid endarterectomy. The degree of stenosis in the contralateral carotid artery before and after surgery was investigated.

Methods.—Data on 131 consecutive unilateral endarterectomies were analyzed. Duplex-derived peak systolic velocity (PSV), end-diastolic velocity (EDV), and internal carotid artery/common carotid artery (ICA/CCA) velocity ratios were obtained in the contralateral unoperated ICA before surgery and compared with preoperative angiographic findings. Duplex scans were obtained again 3 months later to document any changes in stenosis severity in the contralateral unoperated artery.

Findings.—Thirty-eight percent of the patients had bilateral ICA disease. US of the 105 unoperated contralateral arteries at 3 months after surgery showed a reduction in mean PSV and EDV that resulted in disease downgrading in 42% of patients to a less severe stenosis category (Table 4). The application of the ICA/CCA velocity ratio prevented overestimation in 8 of the 14 patients who had their stenosis downgraded. Preoperative angiography was used to correctly classify 13 of these 14 patients.

Conclusions.—The use of velocity ratios does not completely correct the reduction in duplex-derived velocity measures after a successful contralat-

---

TABLE 4.—Changes in Internal Carotid Artery Peak Velocities Before and 3 Months After Contralateral Endarterectomy (n = 105)

	Preop.*	3 Months Postop.*	Mean Change (%)†	P
Systolic velocity (m/s)	1·21 (0·83)	1·07 (0·69)	−7 (−11 to −3)	<0·01
Diastolic velocity (m/s)	0·41 (0·29)	0·35 (0·24)	−4 (−12 to +4)	<0·01
Systolic velocity ratio	1·84 (1·54)	1·59 (1·21)	−2 (−9 to +5)	0·01
Diastolic velocity ratio	2·13 (1·78)	2·05 (1·64)	10 (0-20)	0·32

*Values are mean (SD).
†Values in parentheses are confidence intervals.
(Courtesy of Ray SA, Lockhart SJM, Dourado R, et al: Effect of contralateral disease on duplex measurements of internal carotid artery stenosis. *Br J Surg* 87:1057-1062, 2000. Blackwell Science Ltd.)

eral endarterectomy. Reclassification of disease severity often results. Simple modification of velocity thresholds is not likely to resolve this problem.

▶ The conclusion of this study, namely that bilateral carotid artery disease can cause overestimation of the severity of stenosis by duplex US, is unarguable. These authors used the usual model of patients with bilateral disease having unilateral surgery. They found that postoperative measurements indicated that 42% of the patients who apparently had greater than 50% contralateral disease were downgraded postop. This is close to the same one third or so that most centers have found in this area. Clearly, if you are going to do carotid surgery based on duplex alone, you must never do the second side based on duplex obtained before the first side was operated upon At the very least, postoperative duplex must be obtained to confirm that the second side remains in the operative category.

Use of Ultrasound Contrast in the Diagnosis of Carotid Artery Occlusion
Ferrer JME, Samsó JJ, Serrando JR, et al (Vall d'Hebron Hosp, Barcelona)
J Vasc Surg 31:736-741, 2000   3–4

Background.—The reliability of duplex US (DU) in the diagnosis of carotid artery occlusion has been well documented. In initial reports, the accuracy is less than 85%, but more recent publications since the introduction of color duplex scanning have reported the overall accuracy to be between 92% and 100%. However, these reports have been limited by small series and technical difficulties in some patients. In these technically difficult cases, the use of echo-enhancing agents is particularly relevant. In one report, a reduction in uninterpretable cases from 21% to 6% was achieved with the use of echo-enhancing agents. The use of echo-enhancement agents allows a reduction in the number of examinations, an important contribution in light of the incidence of severe complications associated with contrast angiography, which could be as high as 1.2%. The use of an echo-enhancing agent in patients with carotid artery occlusion for improvement of the sensitivity and specificity of carotid color flow ultrasonography was evaluated.

Methods.—A prospective study was conducted between January 1997 and December 1998 that involved 85 cases of carotid artery occlusion in 84 patients. After diagnosis with baseline DU, a second DU study was conducted with the use of echo enhancement US (DUEE) with an enhancement agent, SHU-508-A (Levovist). Contrast angiography was carried out in 82 cases for confirmation of the diagnosis, and surgery was used to confirm the diagnosis in 3 cases.

Results.—Of the 85 occlusions diagnosed at baseline DU examination, there were 7 false occlusions in the examination (2%). The correlation between the DUEE and the contrast angiography in the 82 cases that were compared was 100%. In the 3 cases in which the diagnosis was compared surgically, urgent treatment was required because of severe stenoses observed in the DUEE examination.

Conclusions.—The DUEE study is an effective diagnostic tool that enables differentiation between true occlusions of the carotid artery and pseudo-occlusions.

▶ Just as MR angiography has its enhancing gadolinium, so does vascular US have its enhancing Levovist. This is a compound composed primarily of galactose with a palmitic acid-based agent that generates microbubbles on dissolution in sterile water. It gives echo enhancement for about 4 minutes after a bolus IV injection. These authors contend that the use of this material enhances their ability to differentiate highly stenotic internal carotid arteries from occluded ones. I suspect they are correct, but I am unable to put this agent into perspective. Its use is not benign and is associated with some complications. I am certainly not using it in my vascular lab presently, although perhaps I should be.

The Quest for Early Predictors of Stroke Evolution: Can TCD Be a Guiding Light?

Baracchini C, Manara R, Ermani M, et al (Univ of Padua, Italy)
Stroke 31:2942-2947, 2000   3–5

Background.—Rapid, noninvasive assessment of patients with acute ischemic stroke can be obtained with transcranial Doppler US (TCD). The utility of TCD in the acute phase of ischemic stroke, when major therapeutic decisions are required, was evaluated.

Methods.—Neurologic assessments were conducted in 73 patients with a first-ever ischemic hemispheric stroke. The assessments were conducted according to the Unified Neurological Stroke Scale, with clinical subgrouping according to the criteria of Bamford, and included CT scan, cervical duplex US, and TCD performed within 12 hours of stroke onset. TCD was performed again on days 2 and 7. The patients were followed up for 90 days, during which the fatality rate was calculated and clinical outcome was assessed.

Results.—In 24 cases, emergency TCD revealed absence of flow in the middle cerebral artery (MCA). Emergency TCD also demonstrated MCA asymmetry in 20 subjects. Early MCA recanalization (less than 24 hours) was seen on serial TCD in 6 patients. After 90 days, no patient with MCA occlusion at admission was autonomous, while 17 of 19 patients (89.5%) with a normal baseline TCD were independent. The overall fatality rate at 3 months was 21%, but patients with MCA occlusion had a mortality rate of 46%, and patients without signs of early MCA recanalization had a mortality rate of 61%. Total anterior circulation infarct and abnormal TCD were significantly correlated with a higher mortality rate and a worse outcome; however, early CT ischemic signs and severe carotid disease were not correlated with higher mortality rate and worse outcome. TCD evalu-

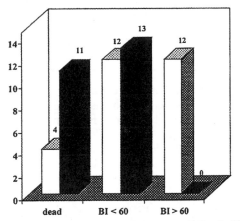

FIGURE 3.—Strong correlation (*P* < .001) between transcriptional Doppler US findings at admission and 90-day outcome in patients with total anterior circulation infarcts. *Black boxes* indicate middle cerebral artery occlusion; *white boxes* indicate middle cerebral artery patency. (Courtesy of Baracchini C, Manara R, Ermani M, et al: The quest for early predictors of stroke evolution: Can TCD be a guiding light? *Stroke* 31:2942-2947, 2000. Reproduced with permission of *Stroke*. Copyright 2000, American Heart Association.)

ation identified 2 prognostic clusters, according to MCA patency at admission, within the total anterior circulation infarct subgroup (Fig 3). On logistic regression analysis, normal baseline TCD was selected as an independent predictor of good long-term outcome, and MCA no-flow was found to be an independent predictor of disability or death.

Conclusion.—Findings on TCD can have an important role in the early prognosis of anterior circulation stroke and may provide possible guidance for therapeutic interventions.

▶ As time passes, more and more uses are being identified for TCD. This study specifically looks at the prognostic value of TCD in the acute phase of ischemic stroke and attempts to evaluate the role of this modality in guiding and monitoring therapeutic intervention. A summary of the information presented indicates that patients with MCA occlusion do worse than those who are not occluded, and that those who recanalize do better than those who do not recanalize. No flow in the MCA on TCD appears as an independent predictor of disability and death. This information is beginning to suggest that TCD in the early phase of ischemic stroke may provide important guidance to direct therapeutic interventions. Perhaps.

Gadopentetate Dimeglumine as a Contrast Agent in Common Carotid Arteriography

Erly WK, Zaetta J, Borders GT, et al (Univ of Arizona, Tucson)
AJNR Am J Neuroradiol 21:964-967, 2000   3–6

Background.—Catheter carotid arteriography is the gold standard for evaluating patients with suspected stenosis of the carotid artery. Nonetheless, carotid angiography is still required for some patients with contraindications to the use of iodine contrast agents. Whether gadopentetate dimeglumine is an acceptable intra-arterial contrast agent for evaluating suspected common carotid artery stenosis was examined.

Methods.—The subjects were 12 adults with suspected carotid artery stenosis. Common carotid arteriograms were obtained in all patients via a standard injection sequence with iohexol and after the administration of gadopentetate dimeglumine. Neurologic status and vital signs were monitored throughout the procedures and for 6 hours thereafter. After each injection, 5 independent observers who were unaware of the contrast agent used evaluated the percentage of carotid stenosis and their degree of

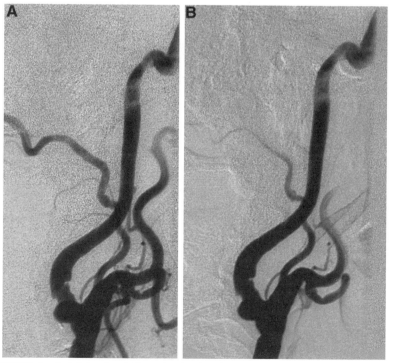

FIGURE 4.—Gadolinium-based (**A**) and iodine-based (**B**) common carotid arteriograms. Lateral injections are nearly identical, except that the gadolinium image has increased graininess because of film contrast. (Courtesy of Erly WK, Zaetta J, Borders GT, et al: Gadopentetate dimeglumine as a contrast agent in common carotid artery arteriography. *AJNR Am J Neuroradiol* 21: 964-967, 2000. Copyright by American Society of Neuroradiology.)

confidence in their rating (6-point scale). The observers also rated the overall quality of the images and, when quality was poor, possible reasons for poor image quality.

Results.—None of the subjects had significant changes in vital signs, and none experienced a neurologic complication. Measurements of common carotid artery stenosis were the same with both imaging agents (mean, 45% with each agent). Observer confidence with gadopentetate dimeglumine was slightly lower than that with iohexol (means, 2.17 and 2.57, respectively; $P = .0009$), but mean values for both agents fell between a grade of 2 ("confident") and 3 ("somewhat confident"). Similarly, overall image quality was slightly lower with gadopentetate dimeglumine than with iohexol (means, 2.95 and 2.53, respectively; $P < .0008$), but means for both agents fell between a grade of 2 ("very good") and 3 ("good"). One of the reasons contributing to the poorer quality of the gadolinium-based images was that gadolinium is less radiopaque than iodine; thus, image contrast had to be increased, which increased the graininess of the image (Fig 4).

Conclusion.—Common carotid arteriography with gadopentetate dimeglumine had slightly poorer image quality compared with iohexol, but measurements of stenosis were identical with the 2 methods. Thus, gadolinium-based contrast agents may represent an alternative to iodine-based agents in selected patients requiring common carotid arteriography. However, because of the decreased radiodensity of gadolinium-based contrast agents, they could lead a reader to mistake a near-total carotid occlusion (string sign) for a total occlusion. Thus, gadolinium should be used cautiously in patients with suspected near-total carotid occlusion.

▶ Gadolinium has been used for years to enhance MR angiography. In recent years, it has also been suggested as an alternative to both iodine and CO_2 in peripheral arteriography. Gadopentetate dimeglumine has an osmolarity greater than that of iodine but is less radiopatent, giving a perception of slightly diminished image quality with arteriography. Nonetheless, it is a contrast agent and can be used quite successfully in arteriography, as shown by this nice study. It is quite expensive and does on occasion cause some focal pain at the site of injection. The ability of this contrast with its slightly diminished image quality to differentiate the subtleties of very high grade stenosis has not been evaluated. Nonetheless, vascular surgeons should keep in mind that we do have an alternative to CO_2 arteriography when iodinated contrast is completely forbidden. Anything would be superior in my opinion to CO_2.

Power Doppler Scanning in the Diagnosis of Carotid Body Tumors

Arslan H, Ünal Ö, Kutluhan A, et al (Yünzüncü Yil Univ, Van, Turkey)
J Ultrasound Med 19:367-370, 2000
3–7

Background.—Carotid body tumors, or chemodectomas, are a slow-growing type of extra-adrenal paraglioma. These are usually benign, hypervascular tumors that, because of their close association with vital structures, are difficult to excise. Sonography is an important screening tool, and angiography makes the diagnosis. The power Doppler findings in a series of patients with carotid body tumors are discussed.

Methods.—The study included 6 patients with carotid body tumors. All were referred for radiologic evaluation of a nontender mass beneath the mandibular angle. Gray scale and power Doppler sonography were performed in all patients, with additional studies as needed. Histopathologic confirmation was obtained in every case.

Results.—Gray scale sonography showed well-defined, solid masses of weak hyperechogenicity in the carotid bifurcation (Fig 1). On power Doppler study, all lesions had abundant flow, appearing as an intense blush throughout the tumor. Doppler sonography also demonstrated the external and internal carotid arteries surrounding the vascularized tumors.

Conclusions.—Gray scale US and power Doppler imaging can demonstrate the key diagnostic features of carotid body tumors. These noninvasive, inexpensive imaging studies are believed to be sufficient to make the primary diagnosis of carotid body tumors, obviating the need for more invasive imaging studies.

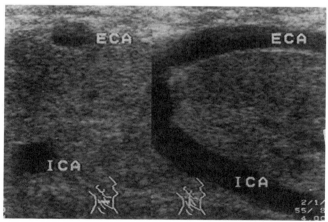

FIGURE 1.—Gray scale US in sagittal and transverse sections. Well-defined, solid masses are seen in the carotid bifurcation. Note the characteristic broadening of the bifurcation with shifting of the internal carotid artery (ICA) posteriorly and of the external carotid artery (ECA) anteriorly and medially. (Courtesy of Arslan H, Ünal Ö, Kutluhan A, et al: Power Doppler scanning in the diagnosis of carotid body tumors. *J Ultrasound Med* 19:367-370, 2000.)

▶ I have never regarded duplex diagnosis of carotid body tumor as rocket science. When the internal and the external are widely spread apart with something that looks like a golf ball between them, it gives you a definite clue that a carotid body tumor may be present. With the modern advent of power Doppler scanning, however, it is inevitable that this modality would be used in the diagnosis of carotid body tumor. As shown in this study, both gray scale US and power Doppler imaging are quite successful in recognizing the splaying of the bifurcation and the perfuse vascularity important in the diagnosis of carotid body tumors. These modalities are certainly appropriate for the primary diagnosis. Whether additional subtle information to support surgery could be obtained from contrast arteriography, CT, or MR angiography is unknown to me. I suspect it would not be necessary.

CT Angiography for the Dectection and Characterization of Carotid Artery Bifurcation Disease
Anderson GB, Ashforth R, Steinke DE, et al (Univ of Alberta, Edmonton, Canada)
Stroke 31:2168-2174, 2000   3–8

Background.—Minimally invasive imaging of the intracranial and extracranial blood vessels can be achieved by CT angiography (CTA). The current gold standard for this purpose is digital subtraction angiography (DSA). This study compared CTA, DSA, and Doppler US for assessment of stenosis at the carotid artery bifurcation.

Methods.—All 3 imaging studies were performed in both carotid arteries of 40 patients with symptomatic transient ischemic attack or stroke. On initial US screening studies, all patients had greater than 50% stenosis of the carotid artery on the involved side. The CTA studies included source axial, maximum intensity projection, and shaded-surface display images. Each imaging study was reviewed for the degree of stenosis quantified and the presence of ulcers, without knowledge of the results of the other 2 studies.

Results.—Of the 3 types of CTA images, the source axial images showed the closest correspondence to DSA, across all degrees of stenosis. The correlation between US and DSA was stronger than that between CTA and DSA. In the detection of mild (0% to 29%) carotid stenosis and carotid occlusion, CTA offered sensitivity, specificity, and accuracy values of nearly 100%. It also performed well in the diagnosis of stenoses greater than 50% (as defined by DSA), with sensitivity of 89%, specificity of 91%, and accuracy of 90%. However, sensitivity dropped to 65% for detection of moderate (50% to 69%) stenosis and to 73% for detection of severe (70% to 99%) stenosis. Similar findings emerged when data from the most clinically relevant symptomatic arteries were analyzed. For the detection of associated ulcers, the results of CTA and DSA were strongly correlated with each other.

Conclusion.—CTA performs very well in the diagnosis of carotid artery occlusion or carotid stenosis of less than 30% or greater than 50%. However, its ability to make the important distinction between moderate and severe stenosis is limited. Thus, CTA is not currently an adequate substitute for DSA.

▶ I find this article very helpful. The short version is that CTA is simply not as good as well-performed arteriography in detecting the subtleties, such as the degree of stenosis in the carotid arteries. Our institutional angiographers reached this conclusion long ago, routinely recommending conventional arteriography over CTA. The seemingly well-constructed data in this study certainly support this position. While CTA may be good for some things, it does not appear especially accurate in detecting significant degrees of carotid stenosis. It may, however, be acceptable for differentiating between 99% stenosis and occlusion. We shall see.

Magnetic Resonance Angiography Is an Accurate Imaging Adjunct to Duplex Ultrasound Scan in Patient Selection for Carotid Endarterectomy

Back MR, Wilson JS, Rushing G, et al (Univ of South Florida, Tampa; James A Haley Veterans Hosp, Tampa, Fla)
J Vasc Surg 32:429-440, 2000   3–9

Background.—The role of MR angiography (MRA) in the assessment of carotid occlusive disease is unclear. The accuracy of MRA for categorizing the severity of carotid disease was compared with that of duplex US scanning and cerebral contrast arteriography (CA) to determine whether MRA obviates the need for cerebral angiography in patients with indeterminate or inadequate duplex scan findings.

Methods.—Forty patients underwent a total of 45 carotid endarterectomies between 1996 and 1998. A total of 74 carotid bifurcations in these patients were imaged with duplex US scanning; MRA; and biplanar, digital subtraction cerebral arteriography.

Findings.—For detecting greater than 50% internal carotid artery (ICA) stenosis, MRA had a sensitivity of 100%, a specificity of 96%, and positive and negative predictive values of 98% and 100%, respectively. For duplex scanning, these values were 100% for sensitivity, 72% for specificity, 88% for the positive predictive value, and 100% for the negative predictive value. For detecting greater than 75% ICA stenosis, MRA had a 100% sensitivity, a 77% specificity, and 76% and 100% positive and negative predictive values, respectively. For duplex US, these values were 90% for sensitivity, 74% for specificity, 72% for the positive predictive value, and 91% for the negative predictive value. Both modalities accurately distinguished greater than 95% stenosis from occlusion. For all patients with 75% to 99% stenosis and in half of those with CA-defined 50% to 74% stenosis, MRA showed short length ICA flow gaps. In

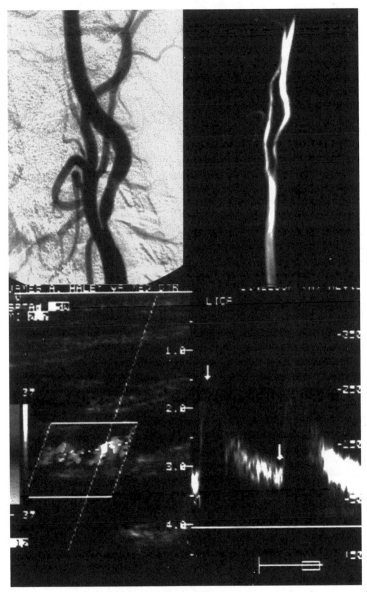

FIGURE 3.—Concordant MRA (**top right**) and duplex scan (**bottom**) confirm the presence of a 65% stenosis at the origin of the ICA with arteriography (**top left**). Lesion has a 66% stenosis measured with MRA and duplex scan velocities of PSV = 267 cm/s, EDV = 120 cm/s, and ICA-CCA ratio = 3.0. *Abbreviations: MRA,* Magnetic resonance angiography; *ICA,* internal carotid artery; *PSV,* peak systolic velocity; *EDV,* end-diastolic velocity; *CCA,* common carotid artery. (Courtesy of Back MR, Wilson JS, Rushing G, et al: Magnetic resonance angiography is an accurate imaging adjunct to duplex ultrasound scan in patient selection for carotid endarterectomy. *J Vasc Surg* 32:429-440, 2000.)

patients with 50% to 74% stenosis, the mean angiographic stenosis was significantly greater when MRA showed a flow gap compared with no flow gap. Overall agreement among duplex US, MRA, and CA was noted in 73% of the carotid vessels (Fig 3). Among the 24% discordant findings between MRA and duplex US, MRA correctly predicted the disease severity in all patients. Inaccurate duplex US scan findings resulted from overestimation in 83%. Findings on CA changed the operative plan in only 1 patient after duplex US and MRA.

Conclusions.—MRA can accurately classify the severity of carotid occlusive disease. Duplex US scanning can usually facilitate patient selection for a carotid endarterectomy. Adjunct use of MRA improves the diagnostic accuracy for greater than 75% stenoses and may obviate the need for CA in patients with duplex scan findings that are inconclusive or that suggest borderline disease severity.

▶ I don't quite know what to make of this article. The authors are trying to convince us that MRA is perfectly adequate in support of duplex US to permit carotid surgery without angiography. It seems clear to me that while MR is marginally better than US, it certainly is not as good as carotid arteriography. As long as we are blessed in our institution with an angiography department that gets excellent results and practically no complications, I will continue to request arteriography in preference to MRA. Interestingly, there is not very much charge differential between the 2 exams. On balance, I have considered the proposal put forth by the authors of this article, and I reject it.

Contrast Agents

Prevention of Radiographic-Contrast-Agent–Induced Reductions in Renal Function by Acetylcysteine

Tepel M, van der Giet M, Schwarzfeld C, et al (Ruhr-Universität Bochum, Herne, Germany)
N Engl J Med 343:180-184, 2000   3–10

Background.—An acute reduction in renal function often results from the administration of radiographic contrast agents. This reduction in renal function can cause significant morbidity and mortality during hospitalization and can lead to chronic end-stage renal disease. There are a number of significant risk factors for contrast agent–induced reductions in renal function, including preexisting renal dysfunction, particularly caused by diabetic nephropathy; reduced effective arterial volume; concomitant administration of drugs that interfere with the regulation of renal perfusion, such as angiotensin-converting enzyme inhibitors; and a higher volume of contrast agent administered. Hydration has been reported to have an ameliorating effect on contrast agent–induced reductions in renal function in patients with chronic renal insufficiency. However, the administration of drugs such as calcium antagonists, theophylline, dopamine, and atrial natriuretic peptide does not prevent the reduction. However, there is increasing evidence that reactive oxygen species play a role in the renal damage caused by contrast agents. Contrast agents increased lipid peroxidation in rats in one study. In another study, superoxide dismutase, a scavenger of reactive oxygen species, preserved renal function. The possibility that the reduction in renal function caused by radiographic contrast agents can be prevented by antioxidants was evaluated.

Methods.—Eighty-three patients with chronic renal insufficiency were prospectively studied. All were undergoing CT with iopromide, a nonionic low-osmolality contrast agent. Patients were randomly assigned to either the antioxidant acetylcysteine and 0.45% saline intravenously before and after contrast agent administration, or placebo and saline.

Results.—In 10 (12%) of 83 patients, there was an increase of at least 0.5 mg/dL in the serum creatinine concentration 48 hours after administration of the contrast agent. Of these 10 patients, 1 of 41 was in the acetylcysteine group and 9 of 41 were in the control group. There was a significant decrease in mean serum creatinine concentration 48 hours after administration of contrast medium in the acetylcysteine group, from 2.5 ± 1.3 to 2.1 ± 1.3 mg/dL. In contrast, a nonsignificant increase in mean serum creatinine concentration was observed in the control group.

Conclusions.—For patients with chronic renal insufficiency, the antioxidant acetylcysteine, when administered orally with hydration, can prevent the reduction in renal function that is induced by iopromide, a nonionic, low-osmolality contrast agent.

▶ I am ambivalent about this article. I have a healthy disrespect for reports of any beneficial effect of antioxidants in clinical medicine. This entire study looks like a fishing expedition to me. However, the results appear quite significant, and I do believe the *New England Journal of Medicine* was correct in publishing the prospective randomized study showing very significant benefit in renal function after the use of acetylcysteine in patients undergoing angiography using the nonionic, low-osmolality contrast agent iopromide. Both the study group and the control group were well-hydrated with similar amounts of saline. I note that the results of this study have already had a profound impact on my practice. All of my patients with elevated creatinine undergoing arteriography are now receiving acetylcysteine first. I look forward to additional confirmatory evidence surrounding the use of this agent. I suspect that if it does indeed prove beneficial, these effects will not reside in any antioxidant properties of the compound.

Randomized Trial of Contrast Media Utilization in High-Risk PTCA: The COURT Trial

Davidson CJ, Laskey WK, Hermiller JB, et al (Northwestern Mem Hosp, Chicago; Univ of Maryland Hosp, Baltimore; The Care Group, Indianapolis, Ind; et al)
Circulation 101:2172-2177, 2000   3–11

Introduction.—In vitro and in vivo trials have previously indicated that a relationship exists between thrombus-related events and type of contrast media. Low osmolar contrast agents seem to improve the safety of the diagnostic and coronary artery interventional procedures. No data are available regarding percutaneous transluminal coronary angioplasty (PTCA) outcomes using an isosmolar contrast agent. The isosmolar non-ionic dimer iodixanol was compared with the low osmolar ionic agent ioxaglate (in 405 and 410 procedures, respectively) in a multicenter, phase IV, prospective, randomized, double-blind trial including 856 high-risk patients undergoing coronary artery intervention.

Methods.—Patients were randomly assigned to receive either iodixanol or ioxaglate. All patients received aspirin 325 mg before and after undergoing PTCA. All patients receiving stent implantation received ticlopidine twice daily. Heparin was given as a weight-adjusted dose using prespecified guidelines. Abciximab was used at the discretion of the surgeon. The major end point was a composite variable of in-hospital major adverse clinical events (MACE). Major angiographic and procedural events during and after PTCA were assessed.

Results.—The composite in-house primary end point was less common in patients who received iodixanol than in those who received ioxaglate (5.4% and 9.5%, respectively). Core laboratory-defined angiographic success was significantly more common for patients who received iodixanol (92.2% vs 85.9%). A significant trend toward fewer total clinical events at 30 days was observed in patients who were randomly assigned to iodixanol versus ioxaglate (9.1% vs 13.2%, respectively). Significant multivariate predictors of in-hospital MACE were use of ioxaglate versus iodixanol

TABLE 6.—Secondary In-Hospital Clinical Outcomes: Adjudicated Assessments

	Iodixanol (N=405)		Ioxaglate (N=410)		
	n	%	n	%	P
Noncardiac death	0	0.0	0	0.0	...
Arrhythmia requiring therapy	6	1.5	9	2.2	0.45
Angina with ECG changes	15	3.7	21	5.1	0.33
Hypotension with intervention	34	8.4	41	10.0	0.43
Renal failure requiring medication	2	0.5	2	0.5	0.99
Post PTCA bleeding	17	4.2	16	3.9	0.83
Composite outcome	63	15.6	73	17.8	0.39

(Courtesy of Davidson CJ, Laskey WK, Hermiller JB, et al: Randomized trial of contrast media utilization in high-risk PTCA: The COURT Trial. *Circulation* 101:2172-2177, 2000.)

and treatment of a de novo lesion. Both groups were similar in secondary in-hospital complications (Table 6).

Conclusion.—Both iodixanol and ioxaglate had a similar low rate of in-hospital clinical events. Patients who received iodixanol had a 45% decrease of in-hospital MACE, compared with patients who received ioxaglate.

▶ As you all know, there has been a quiet revolution in angiography in recent years surrounding the choice of contrast media. Despite cost, the choice has usually come down to one between a nonionic, low-osmolar agent and an ionic low-osmolar agent. In the current study, the results of coronary angiography clearly came down on the side of the nonionic iso osmolar agent iodixanol being superior to the iso osmolar ionic agent ioxaglate. Assuming this information can be exported beyond coronary arteries, perhaps we have some evidence here for the use of iodixanol in peripheral arteriography. The theoretic differences in promoting coagulation between these 2 agents was not born out in this study, as the theory predicted that the ionic agent conveyed greater anticoagulant properties. While it may, that fact certainly did not appear relevant in this study.

Femoral Pseudoaneurysm

Treatment of Iatrogenic Femoral Arterial Pseudoaneurysms: Comparison of US-Guided Thrombin Injection With Compression Repair
Paulson EK, Sheafor DH, Kliewer MA, et al (Duke Univ, Durham, NC)
Radiology 215:403-408, 2000   3–12

Background.—The traditional treatment of pseudoaneurysms is surgery so that rupture can be avoided. However, in the last 10 years, US-guided compression has become the initial therapy for iatrogenic femoral arterial pseudoaneurysms in many institutions. Compression is relatively safe and effective, but the procedure has significant limitations. Compression must be applied for a considerable time, the procedures are painful and must be performed with the patient under conscious sedation, and the success rate for US-guided compression is only 75% (lower when patients undergo anticoagulation). In addition, compression is not effective on some pseudoaneurysms, including those in which flow in the aneurysm cannot be halted, those associated with exquisite tenderness, and those that arise above the inguinal ligament. An alternative to compression, US-guided percutaneous thrombin injection directly into the pseudoaneurysm flow lumen, has recently been reported. This alternative was evaluated in conjunction with US-guided compression repair.

Methods.—Direct thrombin injection was performed with continuous color Doppler US guidance in 26 patients with iatrogenic femoral arterial pseudoaneurysms. The demographics, clinical variables, pseudoaneurysm characteristics, and results in these patients were compared with those parameters in 281 consecutive patients who underwent US-guided compression repair.

TABLE 3.—Success Rates of Thrombin Injection Versus Compression

Therapy	Thrombin Injection (N = 26)	Compression (N = 281)	P Value
Initial			.006
Success	20 (100)*	203 (72.2)	
Failure	0	78	
Final			.013
Success	25 (96)	209 (74.3)	
Failure	1	72	

Note.—Data in parentheses are percentages. P values are based on results of the Pearson χ^2 test.
*The denominator in this case is 20 (the number of patients who underwent thrombin injection as initial therapy.)
(Courtesy of Paulson EK, Sheafor DH, Kliewer MA, et al: Treatment of iatrogenic femoral arterial pseudoaneurysms: Comparison of US-guided thrombin injection with compression repair. *Radiology* 215:403-408, 2000. Radiological Society of North America.)

Results.—US-guided direct thrombin injection was successful in 25 of 26 patients, for a success rate of 96%. This was significantly higher than the success rate for the patients treated with compression (74%) (Table 3). The mean thrombosis time for thrombin injection was 6 seconds compared with 41.5 minutes for compression. No complications occurred in the patients treated with thrombin injection, there were no changes in foot pulses, and none of the patients required conscious sedation. No recurrent pseudoaneurysms were seen on follow-up US at 24 hours.

Conclusions.—US-guided thrombin injection appeared to be superior to compression repair in the treatment of iatrogenic femoral arterial pseudoaneurysm.

▶ If treat we must, virtually all comparative information is coming down on the side of thrombin injection in femoral pseudoaneurysms in preference to manual compression. Of course, the real issue is how many of these aneurysms really require treatment. A number of these patients appear to do quite well with simple follow-up.[1]

Reference

1. Toursarkissian B, Allan BT, Petrinee D, et al: Spontaneous closure of selected iatrogenic pseudoaneurysms in arteriovenous fistulae. *J Vasc Surg* 25:803-809, 1997.

Duplex-Guided Thrombin Injection for Iatrogenic Femoral Artery Pseudoaneurysm Is Effective Even in Anticoagulated Patients
Lennox AF, Delis KT, Szendro G, et al (St Mary's Hosp, London)
Br J Surg 87:796-801, 2000
3–13

Background.—The most popular site for radiologic access has been the femoral artery. However, the incidence of iatrogenic pseudoaneurysm is on the increase and has been found to be as high as 1% to 2% in some studies.

This higher incidence would appear to be a result of the use of larger catheters for stenting and endovascular grafting. In addition, the rising incidence of false aneurysms at the puncture site has been linked to the increased use of anticoagulants after interventional procedures. Treatment of iatrogenic pseudoaneurysm has traditionally included observation, surgical repair, or US-guided compression repair (UGCR). The success rate of UGCR has ranged from 33% to 95%, depending on the size, site, and age of the false aneurysm, the number of treatments that have been attempted, and the presence of concurrent anticoagulation.

UGCR is widely used as the primary treatment for iatrogenic pseudoaneurysm of the femoral artery, but it is a time-consuming and painful procedure, and the results are variable. An alternative technique, percutaneous thrombin injection, was evaluated for its safety and efficacy in the treatment of postcatheterization femoral artery pseudoaneurysm in both anticoagulated and nonanticoagulated patients.

Methods.—The study group comprised 30 consecutive patients with a femoral artery pseudoaneurysm resulting from radiologic catheterization. The pseudoaneurysm was confirmed in all patients with duplex imaging. Under duplex US guidance, thrombin of 200 to 2000 units (1000 units/mL) in a titrating dose was injected into the center of the cavity. None of the patients required sedation. Thrombosis was assessed in real time with B mode and color flow. Distal pulses and ankle pressures were evaluated before and immediately after the injection, so that propagation of thrombus into the femoral artery could be excluded.

Results.—For all 30 patients, rapid thrombosis of the false cavity was successfully induced. No immediate or midterm procedure-related complications or recurrences were observed at 6-week follow-up. Anticoagulation with heparin or warfarin was required in 18 patients at the time of the procedure and post procedure.

Conclusion.—Percutaneous thrombin injection was shown to be a simple, efficacious, and safe technique and would be particularly useful in treating patients who are taking anticoagulants.

▶ In the days of yore (a mythical time our residents frequently unsuccessfully ask me to define), we believed that manual compression of femoral pseudoaneurysms was much less likely to succeed in anticoagulated patients. In fact, a general recommendation of that era was to temporarily stop anticoagulation while performing femoral aneurysm compression. Abundant evidence, including this article, confirms that percutaneous thrombin injection is a simple and effective technique for achieving pseudoaneurysm thrombosis, even in patients taking anticoagulants. (See also Abstract 3–12). Now, one needs to ask the haunting question of whether these aneurysms require any sort of manual therapy.

Lower Extremity

Lower Ankle/Brachial Index, as Calculated by Averaging the Dorsalis Pedis and Posterior Tibial Arterial Pressures, and Association With Leg Functioning in Peripheral Arterial Disease

McDermott MM, Criqui MH, Liu K, et al (Northwestern Univ, Chicago; Univ of California, San Diego; Natl Inst on Aging, Bethesda, Md)
J Vasc Surg 32:1164-1171, 2000   3–14

Background.—For patients with lower extremity peripheral arterial disease (PAD), the ankle/brachial index (ABI) is a key noninvasive measure. However, methods of calculating the ABI value vary among studies, and it is unknown which method provides the best indication of PAD prevalence and leg functioning. Three different methods of calculating ABI were compared in a group of patients with PAD.

Methods.—The cross-sectional study included 244 patients aged 55 years or older, some with and some without PAD. The 3 methods of calculating ABI were as follows: method 1, highest arterial pressure in each leg; method 2, lowest arterial pressure in each leg; and method 3, average of dorsalis pedis and posterior tibial pressures in each leg. The prevalence of PAD was assessed with use of each of these methods. The ABI measures

TABLE 3.—Within-Leg Comparisons*

	Method #1	P Value	Method #3	P Value
All study participants (n =244)				
Six-min walk				
Feet/1 unit ABI (model A)	805.4	< .001	811.5	< .001
Feet/1 unit ABI (model B)	112.6	.817	701.5	.149
Four-m walk: usual pace				
Meters per second/1 unit ABI (model A)	0.348	< .001	0.353	< .001
Meters per second/1 unit ABI (model B)	0.032	.315	0.322	.309
Four-m walk: fastest pace				
Meters per second/1 unit ABI (model A)	0.432	< .001	0.462	< .001
Meters per second/1 unit ABI (model B)	−0.580	.193	1.031	.021
PAD patients only (n = 115)				
Six-min walk				
Feet/1 unit ABI (model A)	659.0	.005	832.4	< .001
Feet/1 unit ABI (model B)	−312.6	.642	1044.0	.126
Four-m walk: usual pace				
Meters per second/1 unit ABI (model A)	0.353	.016	0.464	< .001
Meters per second/1 unit ABI (model B)	0.086	.836	0.284	0.500
Four-m walk: fastest pace				
Meters per second/1 unit ABI (model A)	0.572	.1	0.703	< .001
Meters per second/1 unit ABI (model B)	−0.380	.537	1.020	.101

Note: All analyses were performed within leg with lower ABI, defined by averaging dorsalis pedis and posterior tibial arterial pressures in each leg.

*Comparison of average ABI (method #3) versus highest ABI (method #1) as measures of lower extremity functioning among men and women aged 55 years and older.

Abbreviations: ABI, Ankle/brachial index; *PAD,* peripheral arterial disease.

(Courtesy of McDermott MM, Criqui MH, Li K, et al: Lower ankle/brachial index, as calculated by averaging the dorsalis pedis and posterior tibial arterial pressures, and association with leg functioning in peripheral arterial disease. *J Vasc Surg* 32:1164-1171, 2000.)

were also correlated with objective indicators of leg function (ie, 4-m walking speed and 6-minute walking distance).

Results.—The prevalence of PAD was 47% with method 1, 59% with method 2, and 52% with method 3. The leg with the lower ABI measurement, as assessed by method 3, was most closely related to measures of leg function. On the basis of regression coefficients and the level of statistical significance, method 3 was most closely related to both measures of leg functioning (Table 3).

Conclusions.—For patients with PAD, the lower ABI of the 2 legs—on averaging of the dorsalis pedis and posterior tibial artery pressures in each leg—is the best predictor of leg function. Method 3 is the preferred method of ABI measurement in clinical and research settings.

▶ As many of you may know, vascular medicine centers are beginning to blossom, much like dandelions. The group at Northwestern in Chicago is a good example. As far as claudication is concerned, it is heavily into functional outcome and the patient's assessment of disease. The study presented here, however, addresses a very basic variable in vascular surgery lab testing. Namely, is the ABI calculated from the highest pressure at the ankle the one we should be obtaining? In other words, does this pressure correlate most closely with the other parameters of atherosclerotic disease in our patients? From the results presented here, the answer is a resounding no. If we wish to relate the ABI to the speed and distance of treadmill walking, we are forced to conclude that taking the average of the dorsalis pedis and posterior tibial pressures within each leg correlates the most closely. I am fascinated by these results, as they challenge basic tenets. I had always considered it an absolute article of faith that the highest pressure in the foot should be used to calculate ABI. Have we been wrong all these years?

Duplex Scan Surveillance During the First Year After Infrainguinal Autologous Vein Bypass Grafting Surgery: Costs and Clinical Outcomes Compared With Other Surveillance Programs

Visser K, Idu MM, Buth J, et al (Erasmus Univ, Rotterdam, The Netherlands; Harvard School of Public Health, Boston; Catharina Hosp, Eindhaven, The Netherlands; et al)
J Vasc Surg 33:123-130, 2001   3–15

Background.—Early occlusions of infrainguinal autologous vein bypass grafts are most often caused by thrombosis in the first few weeks postoperatively, whereas late occlusions most often are a result of stenotic lesions. These late occlusions have been found to occur in 20% to 30% of vein grafts in the first postoperative year. Vein graft surveillance is increasingly being used for the identification of failing grafts in the first postoperative year. In this study, the costs and clinical outcomes of duplex scan surveillance during the first year after infrainguinal autologous vein bypass

TABLE 5.—Mean Costs and Number of Major Amputations per 1000 Patients Across Various Surveillance Programs for Infrainguinal Autologous Vein Bypass Graft Surgery, Including Induced Costs During 1-Year Follow-up

Surveillance Program	Critical Limb Ischemia (n = 215)			Intermittent Claudication (n = 78)		
	Mean Cost*	Major Amputations†	Incremental Cost‡	Mean Cost*	Major Amputations†	Incremental Cost‡
Duplex scan	2974	19	S	2404	13	D
ABI	6664	100	D	1959	13	D
Clinical follow-up	6340	100	D	1577	13	S

*Costs are in 1995 United States dollars.
†Major amputations per 1000 patients.
‡Incremental cost per major amputation per patient avoided during the first preoperative year.
Abbreviations: ABI, Ankle-brachial index; *D*, inferior by dominance; *S*, superior, meaning that the strategy is both more effective and less costly than the other strategies.
(Courtesy of Visser K, Idu MM, Buth J, et al: Duplex scan surveillance during the first year after infrainguinal autologous vein bypass grafting surgery: Costs and clinical outcomes compared with other surveillance programs. *J Vasc Surg* 33:123-130, 2001.)

grafting surgery were assessed, and duplex scan surveillance, ankle-brachial index surveillance, and clinical follow-up were compared.

Methods.—A group of 293 patients with peripheral arterial disease were observed in a duplex scan surveillance program after they underwent infrainguinal autologous vein bypass grafting surgery. Health care costs were calculated for surveillance and subsequent interventions from 30 days to 1 year postoperatively. Costs were presented in 1995 United States dollars per patient. A simulation model was used to estimate the costs and amputations of duplex scan surveillance, ankle-brachial index surveillance, and clinical follow-up conditional on the indications for surgery. The primary outcome measure was the incremental cost per major amputation per patient avoided in the first postoperative year.

Results.—The least expensive modality was duplex scan surveillance ($2823), which also resulted in the fewest amputations (17 per 1000 patients), compared with ankle-brachial index ($5411 and 77 amputations per 1000 patients) and clinical follow-up ($5072 and 77 amputations per 1000 patients). In patients treated for critical limb ischemia, duplex scan surveillance was the least expensive at $2974 and resulted in the fewest major amputations (19 per 1000 patients). Considering all surveillance programs, 13 major amputations per 1000 patients were performed for intermittent claudication, and clinical follow up had the lowest cost ($1577) (Table 5). A sensitivity analysis for patients treated for intermittent claudication assumed that duplex scan surveillance could have avoided 6 major amputations per 1000 patients. The results indicated that duplex scan surveillance had an incremental cost of $80,708 per major amputation per patient avoided, compared with clinical follow-up.

Conclusion.—These findings indicated that duplex scan surveillance has a high degree of effectiveness for patients treated for critical limb ischemia, which leads to a reduction of major amputations and a reduction in costs in comparison with other surveillance programs. The evidence in support of the effectiveness of duplex scan surveillance for patients with intermittent claudication is less clear, but it would appear that the incremental costs are justified if duplex scan surveillance can avoid 6 major amputations per 1000 patients examined.

▶ I am unable to understand the furor surrounding the use of duplex surveillance in postoperative vein grafting. We consistently find that about 20% of patients require surgical revision. We have now followed the patients undergoing surgical revision out to 10 years, and there is remarkable long-term patency in these patients, approaching 90% at 5 years, and actually approaching 80% at 10 years. Since this is an infinitely superior patency to our primary patency for similar operations, I simply do not understand the basis for continued discussion. I note, however, that in England, the matter is so contentious that a hugely funded prospective, randomized study is under way to attempt to address this problem. I consider this akin to devoting considerable research money to attempting to prove that the wheel is really round. Nonetheless, the investigators from The Netherlands have labored mightily and concluded that duplex scan surveillance is generally a good thing. Amen and amen. For assaulting us with this piece of drivel, I hereby present these investigators with the Honorable Mention CDA Award. With further effort along these lines, I am sure we will able to remove the Honorable Mention portion in the future.

Noninvasive Evaluation Before and After Percutaneous Therapy of Iliac Artery Stenoses: The Value of the Bernoulli-Predicted Pressure Gradient

de Smet AAEA, Tetteroo E, Moll FL, et al (Univ Hosp Utrecht, The Netherlands; St Antonius Hosp Nieuwegein, The Netherlands)
J Vasc Surg 32:153-159, 2000   3–16

Background.—Information on intra-arterial pressure gradients can aid in assessing the hemodynamic importance of an iliac artery stenosis, as well as in measuring the impact of treatment. Duplex scanning velocity data can be used in a modified Bernoulli equation to predict the peak pressure gradient. This noninvasive technique was assessed in a group of patients undergoing iliac percutaneous transluminal angioplasty (PTA) or stent placement and compared with intra-arterial pressure measurements as a reference.

Methods.—A total of 333 stent placement or PTA procedures were performed in 261 patients in whom iliac artery stenoses were causing intermittent claudication. Before and after the procedures, pressure gradients across the lesion were measured with an intra-arterial catheter. If the mean pressure gradient after the procedure was 10 mm Hg or less at rest and during vasodilatation, the procedure was considered a hemodynamic success. Noninvasive measurements, including the pressure gradient according to the Bernoulli equation, the peak systolic velocity ratio, and the ankle-brachial pressure index, were also obtained before and after the procedures.

Results.—On pretreatment assessment, useful information on the hemodynamic significance of the stenoses was provided by both intra-arterially measured and Bernoulli-predicted pressure gradients. In addition, both techniques showed significant improvement in the gradient across the stenosis after treatment. However, there was only a weak correlation between the intra-arterial measurement and the Bernoulli-predicted gradient (Fig 2). Of the 3 noninvasive techniques, none could distinguish between an optimal and a suboptimal result of treatment, as defined by intra-arterial measurements.

Conclusions.—Noninvasive measures based on duplex velocity data are poorly correlated with intra-arterial measurements of pressure gradients in the iliac artery. The reason for this finding is unknown; it may involve errors in pressure or velocity measurements or the situations in which these measurements are obtained. None of the noninvasive techniques evaluated can determine the residual pressure gradient after PTA or stent placement in the iliac artery.

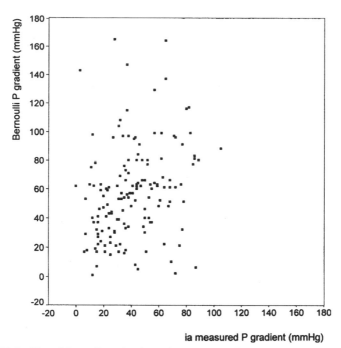

FIGURE 2.—Plot of Bernoulli-predicted systolic pressure gradient versus intra-arterial–measured systolic pressure gradient across iliac artery stenoses. (Courtesy of de Smet AAEA, Tetteroo E, Moll FL, et al: Noninvasive evaluation before and after percutaneous therapy of iliac artery stenoses: The value of the Bernoulli-predicted pressure gradient. *J Vasc Surg* 32:153-159, 2000.)

▶ The Bernoulli-calculated iliac artery pressure gradient in this study is about as worthless as a Bernoulli-calculated gradient elsewhere in the body. The actual correlation between catheter-measured pressure and Bernoulli-calculated pressure was extremely poor. Perhaps a significant part of the error is related to the angle of insonation, although this is uncertain. At any rate, after reading the approximately 10 pages of discussion accompanying this article explaining why the Bernoulli-derived pressure gradient was inaccurate, I needed to take a break to get over my headache.

Skin Perfusion Pressure of the Foot Is a Good Substitute for Toe Pressure in the Assessment of Limb Ischemia

Tsai FW, Tulsyan N, Jones DN, et al (Morristown Mem Hosp, NJ; Univ of Colorado, Denver; Univ of Manitoba, Winnipeg)
J Vasc Surg 32:32-36, 2000   3–17

Background.—Patients with peripheral arterial disease commonly undergo noninvasive measurements of limb systolic pressures for grading of severity and determination of critical limb ischemia. However, certain conditions can make it difficult to achieve reliable measurements of ankle or toe pressures, particularly for patients with diabetes. Skin perfusion

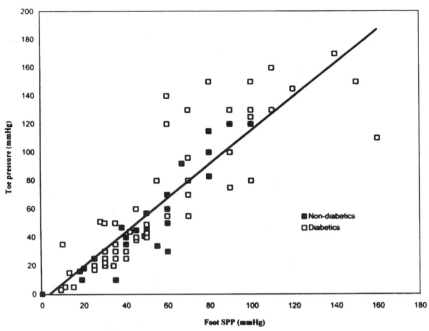

FIGURE.—The relationship of toe pressure to SPP of the foot. ($r = 0.87$, N = 85 limbs, toe pressure = 1.20 [SPP] −4.26). (Courtesy of Tsai FW, Tuslyan N, Jones DN, et al: Skin perfusion pressure of the foot is a good substitute for toe pressure in the assessment of limb ischemia. *J Vasc Surg* 32:32-36, 2000.)

pressure (SPP) measurements are not subject to the same limitations. The correlation between toe pressures and foot SPP measurements was assessed.

Methods.—Seventy-one patients were evaluated in a vascular laboratory for peripheral arterial disease. Forty-three had diabetes. Foot SPP and toe pressure measurements were obtained in a total of 85 limbs, and the 2 measurements were correlated. Toe pressures measured with photoplethysmography were correlated with foot SPP measured with laser Doppler.

Results.—The SPP and toe pressure measurements were strongly correlated with each other in linear fashion (Figure). This correlation was significant for patients with and without diabetes mellitus.

Conclusions.—In a population of patients with peripheral arterial disease, measurements of foot SPP are strongly correlated with toe pressures. When reliable toe pressure measurements cannot be obtained clinically, foot SPP measurements provide a good substitute.

▶ SPP is probably an inappropriately underused method of pressure detection in our vascular laboratories. These investigators make a strong case that SPP in the forefoot is very close to toe pressure and, in fact, can be substituted. Methodology for the determination of SPP is well-standardized and generally accepted. Perhaps we should begin to use this diagnostic modality more widely, although it still seems in the final analysis that the only real way to determine whether, for example, an ischemic amputation is going to heal is to go ahead and do the amputation and observe the outcome.

Near-Infrared Spectroscopy Grades the Severity of Intermittent Claudication in Diabetics More Accurately Than Ankle Pressure Measurement

Komiyama T, Shigematsu H, Yasuhara H, et al (Univ of Tokyo)
Br J Surg 87:459-466, 2000   3–18

Background.—Near-infrared spectroscopy (NIRS), combined with a treadmill-walking test, offers a potentially valuable noninvasive technique for assessment of muscle oxygenation in patients with peripheral vascular disease. The effectiveness of the NIRS-treadmill test for assessment of intermittent claudication (IC) in patients with diabetes, including a comparison with the ankle:brachial pressure index (ABPI) was investigated.

Methods.—The study included a total of 208 symptomatic legs of 153 consecutive patients (142 men, 11 women; mean age, 66 years) with IC caused by peripheral atherosclerosis. Sixty-two of the patients were diabetic. All patients underwent an NIRS-treadmill test and evaluation of resting ABPI, the findings of which were compared. The repeatability of the NIRS-treadmill test was also assessed.

Results.—The NIRS-treadmill test showed good measurement reproducibility. The results distinguished 3 distinct types of IC (Fig 1). Among patients without diabetes these 3 types were associated with significant differences in ABPI. However, ABPI could not grade IC severity in patients with diabetes. The distinction between severe and moderate claudication was more accurately made by recovery time (RT) of muscle oxygenation only in patients with diabetes. For patients without diabetes RT and ABPI offered similar accuracy. In patients without diabetes and for those with diabetes for less than 10 years, RT was significantly correlated with ABPI. These 2 measures were not significantly correlated in patients with longer-term diabetes.

Conclusions.—The NIRS-treadmill test provides a noninvasive measure of measuring muscle oxygenation during exercise. For patients with diabetes with IC, the NIRS-treadmill test provides a more accurate assessment of the severity of IC than conventional ABPI measurement. This test can provide objective information on the presence of IC in patients with diabetes.

▶ The authors report on a promising technology to evaluate muscle ischemia and IC. They compared this method with the ABPI and found NIRS to be more accurate in diabetic patients. Since the usual concern in these patients is evaluating skin blood flow in cases of rest pain or tissue loss, this technology is of no value in such situations since it measures muscle blood

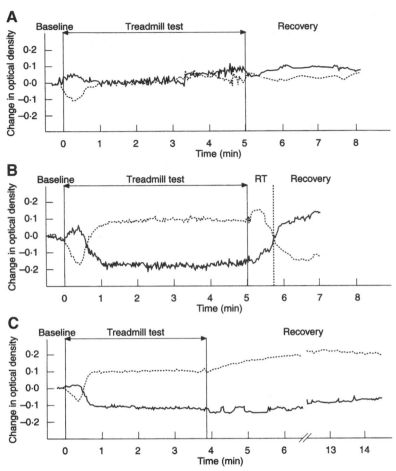

FIGURE 1.—A, Typical type 0, **B**, type 1, and **C**, type 2 tracings of oxygenated hemoglobin (*solid line*) and deoxygenated hemoglobin (*dotted line*) during a near-infrared spectroscopy-treadmill-walking test. The solid vertical lines indicate the beginning and the end of walking; the dotted vertical line indicates the crossing point of the two curves. *Abbreviation: RT*, Recovery time. (Courtesy of Komiyama T, Shigematsu H, Yasuhara H, et al: Near-infrared spectroscopy grades the severity of intermittent claudication in diabetes more accurately than ankle pressure measurement. *Br J Surg* 87:459-466, 2000, Blackwell Sciences, Ltd.)

flow. It would be interesting to compare this method with others that evaluate skin ischemia such as transcutaneous oxygen pressure in an attempt to correlate the degree of muscular blood flow with that of the skin.

A. N. Sidawy, MD

Pneumatic Compression

Improving Walking Ability and Ankle Brachial Pressure Indices in Symptomatic Peripheral Vascular Disease With Intermittent Pneumatic Foot Compression: A Prospective Controlled Study With One-Year Follow-up
Delis KT, Nicolaides AN, Wolfe JHN, et al (St Mary's Hosp, London)
J Vasc Surg 31:650-661, 2000   3–19

Objective.—Mechanical methods are increasingly being used for augmenting arterial flow in legs of patients with peripheral vascular disease (PVD). The effect of (IPC$_{foot}$) intermittent pneumatic foot compression (IPC$_{foot}$) applied daily for a few months, on the claudication distance and leg arterial hemodynamics was prospectively tested in a controlled study in patients with stable intermittent claudication.

Methods.—The long-term effect of IPC$_{foot}$ was tested in 25 patients (group 1). Twelve patients who received no mechanical support served as a control group. Both groups were told to exercise for 1 hour daily and to take 75 mg of aspirin daily for 4.5 months. Initial claudication distance (ICD), absolute claudication distance (ACD), resting ankle brachial index (r-ABI), ankle brachial pressure index after exercise (p-eABI), and popliteal artery volume were measured at baseline, at 2 weeks, and at 1, 2, 3, 4.5, and 12 months.

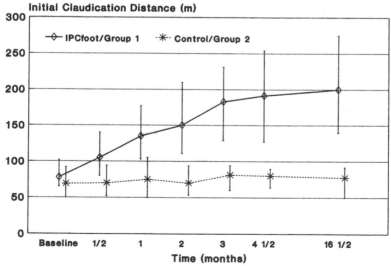

FIGURE 2.—ICD in meters (median and interquartile range) in groups 1 (*IPC$_{foot}$*) and 2 (*control subjects*) over the time points of the study. ICD in group 1 was better than in group 2 as early as the end of month 1 (*P* = .0004; 95% CI: 30, 100 m). *Abbreviations: ICD,* Initial claudication distance; *CI,* confidence interval. (Courtesy of Delis KT, Nicolaides AN, Wolfe JHN, et al: Improving walking ability and ankle brachial pressure indices in symptomatic peripheral vascular disease with intermittent pneumatic foot compression: A prospective controlled study with one-year follow-up. *J Vasc Surg* 31:650-661, 2000.)

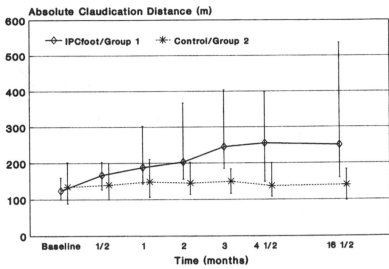

FIGURE 3.—ACD in meters (median and interquartile range) in groups 1 (IPC_{foot}) and 2 (*control subjects*) over the time points of the study. ACD in group 1 was better than in group 2 as early as month 2 ($P < .02$; 95% CI: 9, 196 m). *Abbreviations:* ACD, Absolute claudication distance; CI, confidence interval. (Courtesy of Delis KT, Nicolaides AN, Wolfe JHN, et al: Improving walking ability and ankle brachial pressure indices in symptomatic peripheral vascular disease with intermittent pneumatic foot compression: A prospective controlled study with one-year follow-up. *J Vasc Surg* 31:650-661, 2000.)

Results.—The median ICD and ACD in group 1 were significantly better than in group 2 at 4.5 months (Fig 2, Fig 3). At 4.5 months, group 1 median r-ABI improved significantly from 0.57 to 0.67, median p-eABI from 0.21 to 0.44, and the median popliteal artery volume flow from 100 to 136 mL, whereas measurements in group 2 were unchanged. Results at 12 months were similar for both groups.

Conclusion.—Regular use of intermittent pneumatic foot compression for 4.5 months results in significant improvement of circulatory parameters. Improvements are sustained at 1 year.

▶ This is an absolutely fascinating study. These investigators have shown in a prospective controlled manner that IPC_{foot} significantly improved the initial and absolute claudication distances. In addition, IPC_{foot} significantly improved the resting and postexercise ankle brachial index and popliteal artery blood flow. Therefore, this study suggests that not only was a subjective criterion (claudication pain) improved by IPC_{foot} but that objective, physiologic parameters improved, too. Interestingly, this effect is maintained after IPC_{foot} is stopped at 4.5 months of the study. What is perplexing is how IPC_{foot} exerts its effect. The investigators provided a few possible theories. I am sure we will see further work exploring the physiology of this effect.

A. N. Sidawy, MD

Enhancing Venous Outflow in the Lower Limb With Intermittent Pneumatic Compression: A Comparative Haemodynamic Analysis on the Effect of Foot vs. Calf vs. Foot and Calf Compression

Delis KT, Slimani G, Hafez HM, et al (St Mary's Hosp, London)
Eur J Vasc Endovasc Surg 19:250-260, 2000   3–20

Background.—Intermittent pneumatic compression (IPC) delivered to the foot or to the foot and calf simultaneously improves lower limb hemodynamics in patients with claudication. But which mode of IPC— foot alone, calf alone, or foot and calf simultaneously—is more efficacious? Duplex US was used to compare the hemodynamic effects of 4 different IPC modes in normal subjects and in patients with claudication.

Methods.—The participants were 20 normal subjects (group 1) and 25 patients with intermittent claudication caused by peripheral vascular disease (group 2). The 2 groups were matched for sex and age (mean ages, 59 years in group 1, 63 years in group 2). Participants rested in the sitting

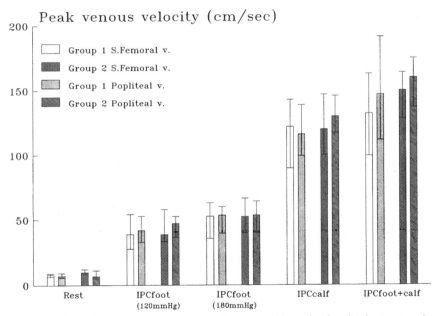

FIGURE 1.—Peak venous velocity generated in the superficial femoral and popliteal veins on application of intermittent pneumatic compression of the foot at 120 mm Hg (IPC$_{foot/120 mm Hg}$), IPC of the foot at 180 mm Hg (IPC$_{foot/180 mm Hg}$), IPC$_{calf}$, and IPC$_{foot+calf}$ in 20 healthy limbs (group 1) and 25 limbs of patients with claudication (group 2). There was no difference ($P > .1$) in the peak velocities between groups 1 and 2 and between the superficial femoral and popliteal veins for all IPC modes. Peak velocities with IPC$_{foot+calf}$ were significantly higher than those with IPC$_{calf}$ ($P < .01$), and the latter were significantly higher than that with IPC$_{foot/180 mm Hg}$ ($P < .001$). Peak velocities with IPC$_{foot/180 mm Hg}$ were higher than those with IPC$_{foot/120 mm Hg}$ ($P < .01$), which on average were at least 3 times higher than the peak velocities at rest ($P < .001$). (Reprinted from the *European Journal of Vascular and Endovascular Surgery* courtesy of Delis KT, Slimani G, Hafez HM, et al: Enhancing venous outflow in the lower limb with intermittent pneumatic compression: A comparative haemodynamic analysis on the effect of foot vs. calf vs. foot and calf compression. *Eur J Vasc Endovasc Surg* 19: 250-260, 2000. Copyright 2000, by permission of the publisher W B Saunders Company Limited London.)

position for 20 minutes, then 4 modes of IPC were tested: IPC of the foot at 120 mm Hg (IPC$_{foot/120 \text{ mm Hg}}$) at 180 mm Hg (IPC$_{foot/180 \text{ mm Hg}}$), IPC of the calf at 120 mm Hg (IPC$_{calf}$), and IPC of the foot and calf (foot impulse 0.5 seconds before the calf impulse) at 120 mm Hg (IPC$_{foot+calf}$). Impulses were delivered with a deflation pressure of 0 mm Hg and an inflation time of 3 seconds, at a frequency of 3 impulses per minute. Duplex US was used to measure venous velocity, volume flow, pulsatility index, and expelled venous volume ratios at baseline and during IPC in the superficial femoral and popliteal veins.

Results.—All measured parameters were significantly increased during all modes of IPC compared with baseline. Increases in groups 1 and 2 were of the same magnitude, as were increases in either the superficial femoral or popliteal veins. The enhancements with IPC$_{foot+calf}$ were significantly greater than those with IPC$_{calf}$, and the latter were significantly greater than either IPC$_{foot/120 \text{ mm Hg}}$ or IPC$_{foot/180 \text{ mm Hg}}$ (Fig 1). The enhancements with IPC$_{foot/180 \text{ mm Hg}}$ were statistically significantly greater than those with IPC$_{foot/120 \text{ mm Hg}}$, but actual differences were minor. Specifically, expelled venous volumes during IPC$_{foot+calf}$ and IPC$_{calf}$ were, respectively, 2-2.5 and 3-3.5 times that during IPC$_{foot/180 \text{ mm Hg}}$.

Conclusion.—IPC is an effective means of improving lower limb hemodynamics in patients with intermittent claudication. The greatest enhancements in venous outflow were seen when IPC was delivered simultaneously to the foot and calf. This is caused in large part by the higher venous volumes expelled with this mode compared with the other modes. Additionally, IPC delivered to the calf alone was superior to IPC delivered to the foot alone. Furthermore, IPC improved venous hemodynamics to a similar extent in both the patients and the normal subjects, which suggests that venous refilling is not attenuated in patients with intermittent claudication.

▶ Pneumatic limb compression has emerged as a reasonably effective venous thrombosis prophylaxis modality. A debate has been raised in recent years as to whether foot compression alone is as effective as calf compression. The experimental data produced here suggest that calf and foot compression together is more effective than either alone. However, recent clinical studies have strongly suggested that foot compression is inadequate in venous thrombosis prophylaxis.[1] For the time being, I consider the matter established. I am unwilling to use foot compression alone as venous thrombosis prophylaxis.

Reference

1. 2001 YEAR BOOK OF VASCULAR SURGERY, p 456.

4 Nonatherosclerotic Conditions

HIV

Clinical Profile of HIV-Related Aneurysms

Nair R, Robbs JV, Naidoo NG, et al (Univ of Natal, Durban, South Africa)
Eur J Vasc Endovasc Surg 20:235-240, 2000   4–1

Background.—The authors previously reported a series of 10 HIV-infected patients with atypical arterial aneurysms. With this report, that experience is expanded to 28 patients.

Methods.—The patients were seen at a South African university teaching hospital over a 6-year period. Clinical records and laboratory findings were reviewed, and microbiological and histologic examinations of surgical specimens were performed.

Results.—The patients were 21 men and 7 women (median age, 30 years). They had a total of 92 aneurysms, with up to 10 per patient. Advanced HIV infection was present in 19 patients. The aneurysms were not found in the typical locations; 24 involved the carotid arteries, 21 the superficial femoral arteries, and 9 the popliteal arteries (Fig 2). Of 31 symptomatic aneurysms, 25 were treated operatively, including arterial reconstruction in 19 cases. The remaining 22 aneurysms were resected and ligated. On histologic examination, the surgical specimens showed distinctive findings of arteritis. There were 2 treatment-related deaths; otherwise, the short-term postoperative outcomes were good.

Conclusion.—Affected patients with HIV-related aneurysms tend to be young. The aneurysms are remarkable for their unusual locations and distinctive histologic findings. Areas with a high prevalence of HIV tend to have a growing number of HIV-related aneurysms.

▶ This abstract and the next (Abstract 4–2) present sobering information about the vascular profile of HIV infections. These surgeons in South Africa have encountered 28 HIV patients with arterial aneurysms apparently caused by HIV. The aneurysms tended to be multiple and were frequently in atypical locations. The histology of the resected aneurysms reveals distinctive fea-

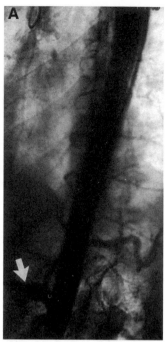

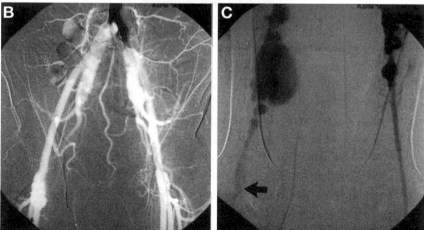

FIGURE 2.—Intra-arterial digital subtraction angiogram of a 30-year-old male showing (A) celiac, (B) right common iliac, bilateral internal iliac, and common femoral, (C) bilateral superficial femoral and right popliteal (*arrow*) aneurysms. In addition, duplex sonography revealed bilateral internal carotid artery aneurysms. (Reprinted from Nair R, Robbs JV, Naidoo NG, et al: Clinical profile of HIV-related aneurysms. *Eur J Vasc Endovasc Surg* 20:235-240, 2000. Copyright 2000, by permission of the publisher, WB Saunders Company Limited London.)

tures of arteritis. This information convinces me that HIV can cause aneurysms and that vascular surgeons should be on the lookout for this affliction.

Occlusive Arterial Disease in HIV-Infected Patients: A Preliminary Report

Nair R, Robbs JV, Chetty R, et al (Univ of Natal, Durban, South Africa)
Eur J Vasc Endovasc Surg 20:353-357, 2000   4–2

Objective.—The first series of HIV-associated arteriopathy with large-vessel occlusive disease is presented.

Methods.—Twenty HIV-positive patients (18 men), aged 17 to 53 years, with symptomatic large-vessel arterial occlusion were treated at a tertiary vascular referral service from 1997 to 1999. Nineteen patients were black and 1 was of Asian ancestry. Twelve had advanced disease, 4 had a history of pulmonary tuberculosis, and 4 had active pulmonary tuberculosis. All had Fontaine III-IV ischemia. Four had upper limb disease, 16 had lower limb disease, and 7 had unilateral disease. Two patients had hyperfibrinogenemia. Angiography, performed in 16 patients, showed occlusive disease. Treatment results were analyzed retrospectively.

Results.—Surgery was performed in 18 patients, and 2 were treated nonoperatively. Eight patients had major amputation. Arterial walls were macroscopically normal with no evidence of plaque. Vessels were occluded with organized thrombus in 7 patients. Four of these patients were successfully treated with balloon catheter embolectomy, and 2 had bypass procedures. Biopsies of arteries from 5 patients revealed normal wall architecture, vessel lumen occluded with bland organizing thrombus, no evidence of intimal atherosclerosis, chronic inflammatory cells in the media and adventitia, focal loss of medial muscle and elastic fibers, no caseous necrosis or features of Takayasu's arteritis, a prominent proliferation of slit-like vascular channels, and a leukocytoclastic vasculitis of the vasa vasora.

Conclusion.—Occlusive arterial disease in HIV patients does not demonstrate features of atherosclerosis but shows characteristics of arteritis. Additional studies are needed to determine whether HIV-related arterial occlusion is a distinct entity.

▶ The authors attempted to study arterial occlusive disease in HIV-infected patients. Although others have shown increased hypercoagulability in HIV-infected patients, in the 11 patients in this group in whom coagulation studies were performed, only 2 had positive results. Without a population-matched control group, it is difficult to know whether the prevalence of hypercoagulability in this group is significant. And, finally, it is surprising that a study of arterial occlusive disease fails to include the usual risk factors of atherosclerosis (smoking, diabetes, hypertension) in the group studied. The authors attempted to show a correlation between HIV infection and arterial occlusive disease, but, unfortunately, they fell short of achieving their goal.

A. N. Sidawy, MD

Reflex Sympathetic Dystrophy

Spinal Cord Stimulation in Patients With Chronic Reflex Sympathetic Dystrophy

Kemler MA, Barendse GAM, van Kleef M, et al (Maastricht Univ, The Netherlands)
N Engl J Med 343:618-624, 2000   4–3

Introduction.—Chronic reflex sympathetic dystrophy (RSD) (also known as the complex regional pain syndrome) is painful and disabling. There is no known treatment, but spinal cord stimulation has been shown to diminish the pain associated with this disorder. The treatment of chronic RSD with spinal cord stimulation and physical therapy was compared with physical therapy alone to determine the effectiveness of spinal cord stimulation in a prospective, randomized, controlled trial.

Methods.—All patients had RSD for at least 6 months. Thirty-six patients were assigned to spinal cord stimulation plus physical therapy, and 18 were assigned to physical therapy alone. The spinal cord stimulator was implanted only in patients for whom a test stimulation was successful. The influence of treatment on the intensity of pain, as determined by a visual analog scale (0 cm, no pain to 10 cm, very severe pain), functional status, and the health-related quality of life, was assessed.

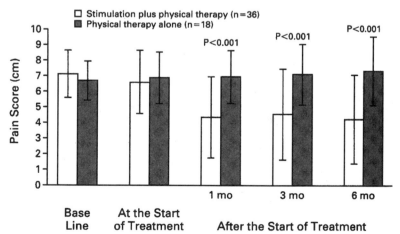

FIGURE 1.—Mean (±SD) scores for pain intensity in patients with reflex sympathetic dystrophy who were assigned to spinal cord stimulation plus physical therapy or to physical therapy alone. The intensity of pain was measured on a visual analog scale from 0 cm (no pain) to 10 cm (very severe pain). Data are from the intention-to-treat analysis. (Courtesy of Kemler MA, Barendse GAM, van Kleef M, et al: Spinal cord stimulation in patients with chronic reflex sympathetic dystrophy. *N Engl J Med* 343:618-624, 2000. Reprinted by permission of *The New England Journal of Medicine* copyright 2000, Massachusetts Medical Society. All rights reserved.)

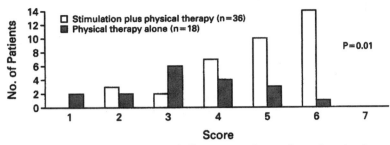

FIGURE 2.—Scores for the global perceived effect at six months according to the assigned treatment. A score of 1 denotes worst ever; 2, much worse; 3, worse; 4, not improved and not worse; 5, improved; 6, much improved; and 7, best ever. Data are from the intention-to-treat analysis. (Courtesy of Kemler MA, Barendse GAM, van Kleef M, et al: Spinal cord stimulation in patients with chronic reflex sympathetic dystrophy. *N Engl J Med* 343:618-624, 2000. Reprinted by permission of *The New England Journal of Medicine* copyright 2000, Massachusetts Medical Society. All rights reserved.)

Results.—The test stimulation of the spinal cord was successful in 24 patients; 12 patients did not receive an implanted stimulator. An intention-to-treat analysis revealed that the group assigned to receive spinal cord stimulation plus physical therapy had a significant mean decrease on the visual analog scale of 2.4 cm, compared with a reduction of only 0.2 cm in the group receiving physical therapy alone (Fig 1). The proportion of patients with a score of 6 (much improved) for the global perceived effect was significantly higher for the spinal cord stimulation group, compared to the control group (39% vs 6%) (Fig 2). Functional status showed no clinically important improvement. Health-related quality of life improved only in the 24 patients who received implants of spinal cord stimulators. Six of these patients had complications that necessitated additional procedures, including removal of the device in 1 patient.

Conclusion.—Electrical stimulation of the spinal cord can significantly diminish pain and improve health-related quality of life in carefully selected patients with RSD.

▶ Over the years, I have found few conditions more confusing and more difficult to analyze than the mystical condition termed reflex sympathetic dystrophy. Anyone who thinks this is a simple sympathetic-mediated pain fiber problem that can be totally and permanently relieved by surgical sympathectomy is either a very noncritical observer or has had very little clinical experience in this area. My experience is that these patients invariably seem to have a completely different reaction to chronic pain than to normal pain. They become victims of pain, continually shopping from doctor to doctor.

Of course, the advocates among us attribute this behavior to the failure of medicine to provide proper care for these patients. Admittedly, that is 1 viewpoint. My viewpoint is that these people had a different makeup to start with and when they experienced chronic pain, they dealt with it in a very different fashion from the usual person who goes on about daily activities despite the presence of pain. At any rate, using the very suspect methods of pain assessment, the investigators attempt to convince us that electric spinal cord stimulation can reduce pain and improve health-related quality of life in these patients.

I note that, disappointingly, the follow-up data on these patients extended for only 6 months. It is fair to say I am totally unconvinced.

Vascular Abnormalities in Reflex Sympathetic Dystrophy (CRPS I): Mechanisms and Diagnostic Value

Wasner G, Schattschneider J, Heckmann K, et al (Christian-Albrechts-Universität, Kiel, Germany)
Brain 124:587-599, 2001   4–4

Objective.—Complex regional pain syndrome type I (CRPS I) may develop as a result of minor limb trauma, stroke, or myocardial infarction. The pain spreads and may be accompanied by abnormal cutaneous vascular and sudomotor function. The pathophysiologic mechanisms of vascular abnormalities were investigated, and the incidence, sensitivity, specificity, and diagnostic value of vascular abnormalities that occur under controlled thermoregulatory conditions in patients with CRPS I were compared with those of healthy control subjects and patients with extremity pain of a different origin.

Methods.—Skin perfusion and extremity skin temperature were measured bilaterally at regular intervals by continuous laser Doppler flowmetry and infrared thermometry in 25 CRPS I patients (18 women; age, 27 to 66 years), in 15 patients (8 women; age, 18 to 57 years) with different chronic pain of 1 limb, and in 20 healthy control subjects (11 women; age, 23 to 45 years). Whole-body temperature changes were accomplished using a thermal suit circulating hot or cold water. Absolute maximal side differences in skin temperature during the entire thermoregulatory cycle were determined, and bilateral plasma noradrenaline levels were measured in 5 CRPS I patients and compared for the 3 groups.

Results.—Twenty CRPS I patients had resting pain of average intensity 3.3 on a 0 to 10 scale. Control patients had a resting unilateral extremity pain of average intensity of 5.0. CRPS I patients showed 3 vascular regulation patterns. In the warm type of regulation, skin temperature and perfusion level of the affected limb were higher than those of the contralateral limb during the entire cycle. In the intermediate type of regulation, the affected side was warmer or colder than the contralateral side. In the cold type of regulation, skin temperature and perfusion level were lower on the affected side during the entire cycle. Healthy control subjects and patients with a different type of extremity pain showed no or little side-to-side skin temperature and perfusion differences. The type of vascular regulation and disease duration were significantly related, and the duration of the disease showed a significant negative correlation with the maximal temperature difference between the affected and unaffected sides (Fig 5). Noradrenaline levels were lower on the affected side than on the unaffected side.

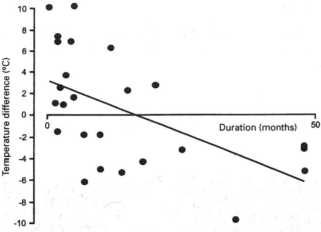

FIGURE 5.—Relationship between vascular abnormalities and duration of CRPS I. Asymmetries in individual maximal skin temperature are plotted against individual duration of CRPS. There was a significant negative correlation ($P < .001$) between the maximal temperature difference between the affected and unaffected sides (no absolute values) achieved during the thermoregulatory cycle and the duration of the disease in months. (Courtesy of Wasner G, Schattschneider J, Heckmann K, et al: Vascular abnormalities in reflex sympathetic dystrophy (CRPS I): Mechanisms and diagnostic value. *Brain* 124:587-599, 2001, by permission of Oxford University Press.)

Conclusion.—Cutaneous sympathetic vasoconstrictor neurones are inhibited in CRPS I patients. Differences in skin temperature during the thermoregulatory cycle is a reliable method of distinguishing CRPS I patients from those with different extremity pain.

▶ Be informed that reflex sympathetic dystrophy is now called complex regional pain syndrome. That kind of gets you where you live, doesn't it? The rather complicated attempts to assess skin temperature responses published here are mildly interesting, but quite unconvincing. I suggest an alternative explanation. It has been my experience that in all patients who maintain a body part in a position of disuse—be it voluntary or perhaps with some neurologic affliction—eventually a cold limb develops. We have come to expect this in patients referred to us with presumed chronic neurogenic thoracic outlet syndrome who have been doctor shopping. The affected arm is held close to the body, frequently in a sling, and is invariably quite cool to the touch. To me, this proves nothing but disuse. While I admire clinical investigative efforts to further elucidate reflex sympathetic dystrophy, I have to confess to a certain disappointment with the results available to date.

Takayasu's Arteritis

Aortic Aneurysms in Patients With Takayasu's Arteritis: CT Evaluation
Sueyoshi E, Sakamoto I, Hayashi K (Omura Municipal Hosp, Japan; Nagasaki Univ, Japan)
AJR 175:1727-1733, 2000   4–5

Background.—Takayasu's arteritis is a primary arteritis of unknown etiology. The aorta and its major branches are commonly affected, as is the

FIGURE 2

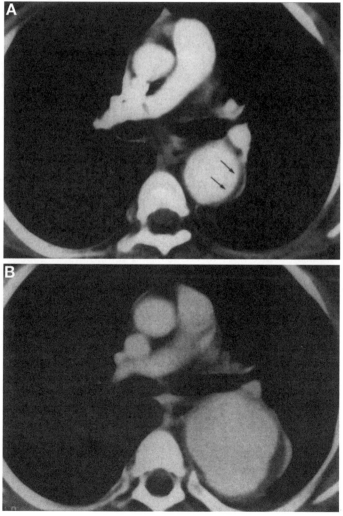

(*Continued*)

pulmonary artery. Takayasu's arteritis is more common in Asia but has been reported worldwide, usually in young women. The vessel walls are involved, resulting in luminal abnormalities including stenosis, occlusion, and aneurysm formation. The prognosis for patients with this disease is relatively good, but the formation of an aneurysm can progress to heart failure because of aortic valve regurgitation and rupture of the aneurysm, leading to a fatal outcome. This is the most frequent fatal course in Takayasu's arteritis. A review of patients with Takayasu's arteritis was conducted for evaluation of the incidence, development, and outcome of aortic aneurysm by CT.

Methods.—The files of 31 patients with Takayasu's arteritis between January 1990 and March 1999 were reviewed. All of the patients were followed up with CT for more than 6 months; the mean follow-up period was 52.9 months. Initial CT in all patients was performed within 6 months of diagnosis. The patient group was composed of 24 female and 7 male patients. The age at first CT examination ranged from 8 to 72 years (mean, 42.6 ± 16.5 years).

Results.—A total of 17 aneurysms in 14 of 31 patients were identified (45.2%). Patients with severe calcification of the aorta demonstrated a significantly lower incidence of aneurysm formation than patients who did not have severe calcification. Three of the 17 aneurysms were not present on the initial CT and appeared in the follow-up period. A rapid increase in size during the follow-up period was noted in 9 of 17 aneurysms; 3 of these

FIGURE 2 (cont.)

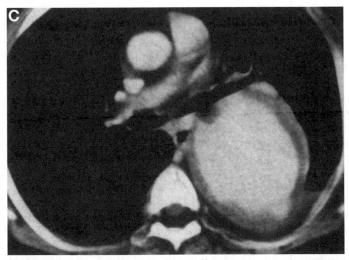

FIGURE 2.—An 8-year-old girl with Takayasu's arteritis. **A,** Initial contrast-enhanced CT image shows fusiform aneurysm and wall thickening of descending thoracic aorta (*arrows*). This finding suggests an active inflammatory process. **B** and **C,** Contrast-enhanced CT images obtained 2 months (**B**) and 4 months (**C**) after **A** show that fusiform aneurysm had rapidly increased in size and wall thickness, in spite of early steroid treatment. (Courtesy of Sueyoshi E, Sakamoto I, Hayashi K: Aortic aneurysms in patients with Takayasu's arteritis: CT evaluation. *AJR* 175:1727-1733, 2000.)

aneurysms ruptured during follow-up. Wall thickening was identified on CT in all 3 ruptured aneurysms (Fig 2). The remaining 6 aneurysms increased in size but did not rupture.

Conclusion.—Aortic aneurysm is not a rare finding in association with Takayasu's arteritis. The possibility of aneurysm formation in an aorta with little calcification is greater in patients with Takayasu's arteritis, and aortic aneurysms accompanied by thickening of the wall can be fatal.

▶ This interesting article from Japan calls our attention to the coexistence of aortic aneurysms in patients with Takayasu's arteritis. In the present group, 45% were found to have aortic aneurysms, with 3 being in the ascending aorta and the arch, 2 being in the distal arch, and 4 in the abdominal aorta. The mean age of the patients with aneurysms was 42 years. As expected, a significant majority were females. I suppose the real take-away message is that we should not get so focused on occlusive aspects of Takayasu's disease that we fail to consider the aneurysmal aspects. I do believe a patient with a diagnosis of Takayasu's disease should have a complete contrast-enhanced CT scan of the entire aorta. These aneurysms clearly have significant rupture potential and must be sought with diligence.

Takayasu's Arteritis: Assessment of Disease Activity With Contrast-Enhanced MR Imaging

Choe YH, Han B-K, Koh E-M, et al (Sunkyunkwan Univ, Seoul, Korea)
AJR 175:505-511, 2000   4–6

Objective.—Because MRI can be used to differentiate between flowing blood and a stationary aortic wall, it has the potential for evaluation of arterial steno-occlusive changes or aneurysms in Takayasu's arteritis. The role of contrast-enhanced MRI for determining the activity of Takayasu's arteritis was assessed in a prospective study.

Methods.—Electrocardiography-gated, contrast-enhanced, T1-weighted spin-echo axial images were obtained with or without fat saturation for the thoracic and abdominal aorta using a 1.5-T scanner in 26 patients (2 males), aged 4 to 65 years, and in 16 control subjects. For better visualization of changes in aortic vessel walls, thin slices (4-5 mm) and smaller fields of view (14 × 14 to 20 × 20 cm) were used.

Results.—High-resolution MRI revealed aortic wall structures (Fig 3). The images suggested Takayasu's arteritis in 16 patients. The aortic wall was enhanced less than the myocardium in 10 patients. MRI findings agreed with clinical results in 23 (88.5%) patients, with erythrocyte sedimentation rates in 24 (92.3%) patients, and with C-reactive protein levels in 22 (84.6%) patients. On early phase contrast-enhanced images, the signal intensity ratio of the aortic wall to the myocardium correlated well

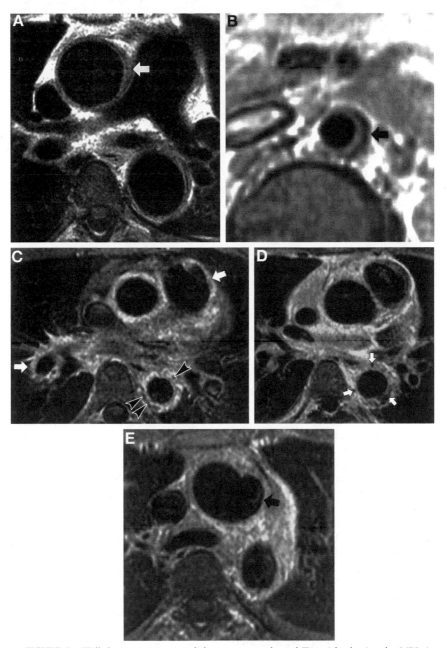

FIGURE 3.—Wall-change patterns revealed on contrast-enhanced T1-weighted spin-echo MRIs in patients with active Takayasu's arteritis. **A,** Type A lesion is revealed at ascending aorta (*arrow*) of 20-year-old woman. **B,** Type B lesion (*arrow*) is revealed in abdominal aorta of 34-year-old woman. **C,** Type C lesions with homogeneously bright walls of ascending and descending thoracic aorta are revealed on this fat-saturated image of 15-year-old girl. Also, note dilated vessels (*arrowheads*) in thickened aortic wall and thick walls (*arrows*) of main and right lower lobe branch pulmonary arteries. **D,** Type D lesion with dilated neovessels (*arrows*) is revealed in thick aortic wall of 25-year-old woman. **E,** Type F lesion with aneurysm (*arrow*) is seen at ascending aorta of 15-year-old girl (same patient as in C). (Courtesy of Choe YH, Han B-K, Koh E-M, et al: Takayasu's arteritis: Assessment of disease activity with contrast-enhanced MR imaging. *AJR* 175:505-511, 2000.)

with the erythrocyte sedimentation rates ($r = 0.78$) and with the C-reactive protein levels ($r = 0.63$).

Conclusion.—Contrast-enhanced MRI provides useful diagnostic information about Takayasu's arteritis and may be helpful for tracking treatment results.

▶ These authors feel they have shown that a ring-like or crescent-like aortic wall thickening of more than 3 mm during contrast enhancement is compatible with active Takayasu's arteritis. The images they publish in this article are reasonably convincing. If there is any doubt about Takayasu's activity in an individual patient, perhaps enhanced MRI of the entire aorta may be beneficial in the differential analysis.

Venous

Endovascular Surgery in the Treatment of Chronic Primary and Postthrombotic Iliac Vein Obstruction

Neglén P, Berry MA, Raju S (River Oaks Hosp, Jackson, Miss)
Eur J Vasc Endovasc Surg 20:560-571, 2000   4–7

Background.—Venous outflow obstruction is thought to be an important contributing factor to venous insufficiency of the lower extremity. An experience with endovascular therapy for chronic iliac venous obstruction—including postthrombotic and nonthrombotic disease—was reported.

Methods.—Over a 12-year period, percutaneous balloon dilation and stenting were performed in 139 consecutive limbs of 137 patients with chronic iliac vein obstruction. The patients were 105 men and 34 women (median age, 48 years). Seventy-eight patients had verified postthrombotic disease (PTS) while 61 had primary disease, ie, May-Thurner syndrome (MTS). The endovascular management and outcomes of the 2 groups were described.

Results.—There was no mortality, and the nonthrombotic complication rate was 3%. Only patients in the postthrombotic group experienced occlusion, with an 8% rate of postoperative occlusion and a late occlusion rate of 3%. The 2-year primary patency rate was 52% in the PTS group and 60% in the MTS group. The primary-assisted patency rate was 88% in the PTS group and 100% in the MTS group; secondary patency rates were 90% and 100%, respectively. Patients in both groups had reductions in pain and swelling after the endovascular interventions. About one half of active venous ulcers were healed.

Conclusion.—Endovascular therapy appears safe and effective for patients with chronic iliac vein obstruction, whether primary or secondary. Both groups benefit from treatment, but patients with postthrombotic obstruction have greater neointimal hyperplasia and are at higher risk for early and late reocclusion. The authors underscore the value of intravascular US in both diagnosis and treatment (Fig 1). Other technical recom-

FIGURE 1

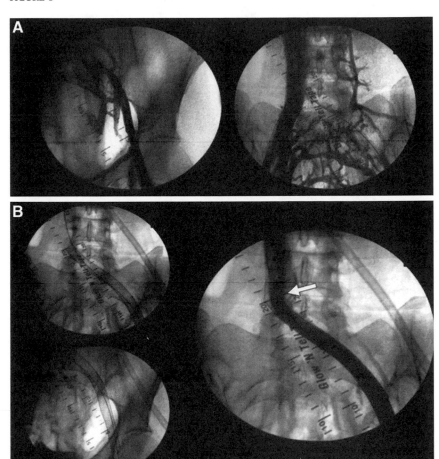

(*Continued*)

mendations include stent placement after balloon dilation; a wide-diameter stent that covers the entire lesion should be selected.

▶ As I have stated on occasions previously, I am fascinated by reports such as this. Despite my preconceived prejudices, it appears quite correct to state that some patients who have chronic iliac vein obstruction can undergo balloon dilatation and stenting, with or without thrombolysis, following which they enjoy prolonged venous patency. I would have predicted that this was impossible and a violation of basic surgical principles. That shows what I know. Dr Michael Dake at Stanford has achieved results very similar to this on a number of occasions. Based on these articles, I have to conclude that not only is such therapy plausible, but it is quite likely to be successful. I do

FIGURE 1 (cont.)

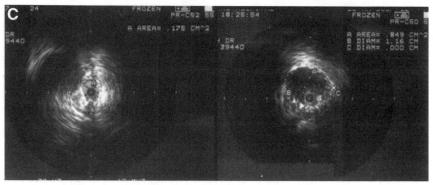

FIGURE 1.—A, Intraoperative transfemoral ascending phlebogram prior to balloon dilation and stenting in a patient with PTS disease and common iliac vein near-occlusion and external iliac vein stenosis. Note the filling of the ascending lumbar vein and the marked transpelvic collateral circulation. B, Status following insertion of 2 overlapping stents (diameter, 12 mm) placed well into the inferior vena cava (IVC) and covering the entire left iliac vein (**left**). Repeated phlebogram shows an uninterrupted flow through the iliac vein into the IVC (proximal end of stent at *arrow*). No collateral circulation is visualized (**right**). C, Intravascular US investigation before (**left**) and after (**right**) insertion of stent. Note area increase from 0.175 to 0.849 cm² and the surrounding high echogenicity indicating phlebosclerosis. (Courtesy of Neglén P, Berry MA, Raju S: Endovascular surgery in the treatment of chronic primary and post-thrombotic iliac vein obstruction. *Eur J Vasc Endovasc Surg* 20:560-571, 2000. Copyright 2000, by permission of the publisher WB Saunders Company Limited London.)

note that the primary patency appears to drop off rather quickly, but the primary assisted and secondary patency—obviously the results of repeated interventions—continue to keep the overall patency rate at a very acceptable level.

Endovenous Management of Saphenous Vein Reflux

Chandler JG, for the Endovenous Reflux Management Study Group (Univ of Colorado, Boulder; et al)
J Vasc Surg 32:330-342, 2000   4–8

Background.—The clinical outcomes of 2 catheter-based endovenous procedures for the elimination or reduction of saphenous vein reflux were evaluated.

Methods.—Through the use of a computer-controlled, dedicated generator and 2 catheter designs, the Closure catheter and the Restore catheter, 210 patients were treated at 16 private clinics and university centers throughout Europe. Resistive heating was applied with the Closure catheter over long vein lengths, prompting maximum wall contraction for permanent obliteration. The Restore catheter was used for induction of a short subvalvular constriction for improvement of the competence of mobile but nonmeeting leaflets (Fig 3).

Results.—Treatment with the Closure catheter caused obliteration in 141 of 151 limbs (93%) (Fig 9). The Restore catheter treatment, used in

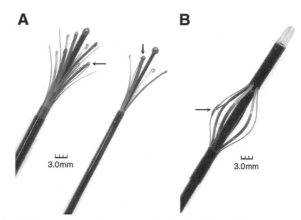

FIGURE 3.—A, Closure catheters (note cupped, uninsulated electrode tips). B, Restore catheter (note central 9-mm uninsulated electrode areas). *Arrows* indicate microthermocouples. (Courtesy of Chandler JG, for the Endovenous Reflux Management Study Group: Endovenous management of saphenous vein reflux. *J Vasc Surg* 32:330-342, 2000.)

shrinkage of 1 or more valves, resulted in acute reduction of reflux to less than 1 second in 41 of 68 limbs (60%). Complications associated with Closure treatments included early recanalization (6%), paresthesias (thigh, 9%; leg, 51%), skin burns (3%), and deep vein thrombus extensions

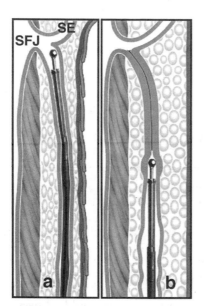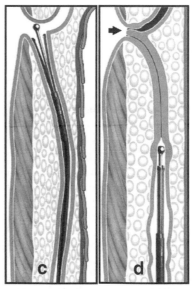

FIGURE 9.—Closure catheter positioning near saphenofemoral junction (*SFJ*). a, Compression wrap around thigh and electrodes expanded just below superficial epigastric vein (*SE*) orifice. b, Treatment in progress (wrap omitted to show undistorted treatment anatomy). c and d, Comparable views show catheter positioned as close to SFJ as possible; in d, note cul-de-sac (*arrow*) and lack of superficial epigastric vein washout. (Courtesy of Chandler JG, for the Endovenous Reflux Management Study Group: Endovenous management of saphenous vein reflux. *J Vasc Surg* 32:330-342, 2000.)

(3%), with 1 embolism. Thrombogenesis occurred in 16% of Restore treatments, despite prophylactic anticoagulation, and treated valves enlarged over 6 weeks and became less competent. The Clinical Efficacy Assessment Project clinical class was improved significantly after both treatments for up to 1 year. Among the Closure patients, 87% of 53 were class 0 or 1 at 6 months; 75% were symptom free, and 96% of 55 treated limbs were free of reflux. Among the Restore patients, 14 of 31 (45%) had no symptoms at 6 months; 55% were rated at class 2 or lower. Only 19% of patients had less than 1-second reflux.

Conclusion.—Despite offsetting complications and early failures, Closure treatment is clinically effective. Procedural modifications are being implemented to address the complications and early failures. Restore valve shrinking is conceptually attractive, but it is too problematic a procedure and does not compare favorably with Closure treatment of saphenectomy.

▶ Oh what we do in the name of progress! The Closure treatment described in this article requires placement of a percutaneous (uncommonly) or cutdown (commonly) catheter into the saphenous vein followed by the application of radiofrequency, which generates heat and obliterates the vein. The idea is to eliminate saphenous vein reflux. The procedure has complications of early recanalization, paraesthesias, skin burns, and occasional deep vein thrombosis. Nonetheless, in a significant number of patients, saphenous vein patency can be eliminated by this procedure. I point out that a 1.5-cm incision under local anesthesia followed by a tie around the saphenous vein will also eliminate saphenous vein reflux. This procedure strikes me as akin to using a sharpshooter with a 30.06 rifle to kill a housefly. With patience and dedication, you may indeed kill the fly with the bullet, but a flyswatter is cheaper and simpler.

Transcatheter Embolization of Complex Pelvic Vascular Malformations: Results and Long-term Follow-up
Jacobowitz GR, Rosen RJ, Rockman CB, et al (New York Univ)
J Vasc Surg 33:51-55, 2001   4–9

Background.—Vascular malformations of the pelvis are rare and difficult to treat. Outcomes of transcatheter embolization therapy for symptomatic complex pelvic vascular malformations were analyzed.

Methods and Findings.—Thirty-five patients were included in the retrospective analysis. Ages ranged from 16 months to 66 years. Fifty-one percent were male. Initial symptoms were pain in 59%, a visible or palpable lesion in 62%, associated palpable pulsation or thrill in 44%, hemorrhage in 27%, congestive heart failure in 18%, and symptoms from mass effect in 35%. Thirty-two percent of the patients had had previous, unsuccessful surgeries of the lesion. The most common lesion type on arteriography was arteriovenous shunting, present in 89%.

A mean of 2.4 embolization procedures were required over a mean of 23.3 months. Rapidly polymerizing acrylic adhesives were the most commonly used agents. The branches of the hypogastric artery were the most common vessels involved and treated, present in 82%. Adjunctive surgery was done after embolization therapy in 15% of patients. At a mean of 84 months' follow-up, 83% of patients were asymptomatic or significantly improved.

Conclusion.—Completely eradicating pelvic vascular malformations is difficult. Recurrences are common, and multiple interventions are needed in many patients. However, in the long term, most of these patients have good outcomes. Transcatheter embolization may be the treatment of choice for symptomatic pelvic vascular malformations.

▶ I suppose if there is one thing we have learned it is that complex pelvic vascular malformations are best treated with catheter embolization and not primary surgery. The excellent and experienced group at New York University presents a recent review of their work in this area, and it is indeed impressive. Their most frequently used embolic material was a polymerizing acrylic adhesive. I find this an interesting, up-to-the-minute, state-of-the-art report on transcatheter embolization for the treatment of symptomatic complex pelvic vascular malformations. While few of these can be eradicated completely, clinical control can be achieved in a large majority by transcatheter embolization. I am impressed with these results.

Miscellaneous

Clinical and Genetic Features of Ehlers-Danlos Syndrome Type IV, the Vascular Type

Pepin M, Schwarze U, Superti-Furga A, et al (Univ of Washington, Seattle; Univ of Zurich, Switzerland)

N Engl J Med 342:673-680, 2000   4–10

Introduction.—Ehlers-Danlos syndrome type IV, a rare autosomal dominant disorder, results from mutations in the gene for type III procollagen (*COL3A1*). Patients with this vascular type of the syndrome are at risk of rupture of arteries, uterus, or intestines. To better understand the course of this disorder, investigators studied the clinical records of 220 index patients and 199 of their affected relatives.

Methods.—In all index patients, the diagnosis of Ehlers-Danlos syndrome type IV was confirmed by biochemical analysis. Relatives were identified as having the syndrome by fulfilling 1 of 3 criteria: cultures of dermal fibroblasts synthesized abnormal type III procollagen molecules, a familial molecular genetic abnormality was identified in their DNA, or a known complication of the disorder had occurred by the age of 50 years. The records of index patients and affected relatives were reviewed for clinical and family histories and medical and surgical complications. Dermal fibroblasts obtained from study subjects underwent biochemical and molecular investigations.

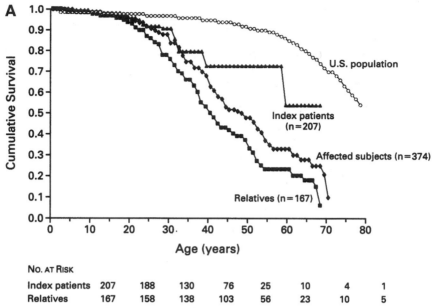

FIGURE 1.—A, Kaplan-Meier estimates of overall survival among 374 research subjects with Ehlers-Danlos syndrome type IV. **A** also includes a curve derived from a 1994 abridged life-table for individuals born in the United States. (Reprinted by permission of *The New England Journal of Medicine*, from Pepin M, Schwarze U, Superti-Furga A, et al: Clinical and genetic features of Ehlers-Danlos syndrome type IV, the vascular type. *N Engl J Med* 342:673-680. Copyright 2000, Massachusetts Medical Society. All rights reserved.)

Results.—The patients had been evaluated between 1976 and 1998. Twenty-six index patients and 105 relatives died; the median survival for the entire cohort was 48 years (Fig 1A). Arterial dissection or rupture was the cause of most deaths. A single complication (ie, arterial dissection or rupture, spontaneous bowel perforation, or organ rupture) had occurred in 68% of the entire cohort. Among index patients, the risk of a medical or surgical complication was 25% by age 20 years and greater than 80% by age 40 years. In the entire cohort of 419 index patients and affected relatives, 272 arterial complications and 87 bowel complications were identified. Arterial ruptures accounted for most deaths, whereas bowel ruptures rarely led to death. Twelve of the 81 women who became pregnant died of complications of pregnancy. There was no apparent relationship between the specific mutation and the type of complication.

Conclusion.—Causative mutations in the *COL3A1* gene were identified in 135 of 220 index patients with Ehlers-Danlos syndrome type IV. The shortened life span in affected individuals was largely a result of vascular ruptures. A diagnosis of this rare syndrome should be considered in young people with unexplained bowel or arterial ruptures.

▶ We are slowly learning more about the inherited arteriopathies. For example, Ehlers-Danlos syndrome type IV, the vascular type, is associated with a mutation in the gene for type III procollagen. Patients with type IV Ehlers-Danlos syndrome usually begin to have some kind of rupture at about the age of 20 years, whether it be the uterus, intestines, or blood vessels. The average age at the time of death is 48 years. Most deaths appear to result from arterial dissection or rupture. Pregnancy appears to be especially hazardous. This article very nicely puts the entire spectrum of type IV Ehlers-Danlos syndrome into very sharp perspective. I recommend it for anyone looking for an up-to-date overview on this subject.

Suppression of Inflammation in Primary Systemic Vasculitis Restores Vascular Endothelial Function: Lessons for Atherosclerotic Disease?
Raza K, Thambyrajah J, Townend JN, et al (Univ of Birmingham, England)
Circulation 102:1470-1472, 2000   4–11

Introduction.—Chronic inflammatory rheumatic disorders are correlated with excess cardiovascular mortality rates. This may be caused by arteriosclerosis following inflammatory damage to the vessel wall by vasculitis. Patients with primary systemic necrotizing vasculitis (SNV) were evaluated to determine whether they had impaired endothelial function.

Methods.—Endothelial function was evaluated in cross-sectional and longitudinal trials of patients with primary SNV by determining flow-mediated, endothelium-dependent brachial artery vasodilatation.

Results.—Patients with primary SNV had significantly impaired endothelial function, compared with normal control subjects. Endothelial function was restored in patients with primary SNV in whom remission was induced.

Conclusion.—Endothelial function was significantly impaired in patients with primary SNV. Thus, it is likely that premature arteriosclerosis in chronic inflammatory disorders results from endothelial dysfunction secondary to vasculitis. Normalization of endothelial function after treatment of primary SNV indicates that early suppression of disease activity in chronic inflammatory rheumatic disorders may decrease long-term vascular damage.

▶ The hypothesis put forward by these investigators is a bit circuitous, but interesting. They point out appropriately that women with lupus and other inflammatory diseases, such as rheumatoid arthritis, have a 50-fold higher rate of myocardial infarction compared with women without these diseases. They show in this study that endothelial function is abnormal in patients with rheumatic disorders and can be normalized by vigorous anti-inflammatory treatment. They suggest that the endothelial inflammation accompanying rheumatic disorders leads to early arteriosclerosis, with its attendant complications including myocardial infarction. Perhaps. While this argument is circuitous, it just may be correct. If so, we may be on the verge of a new generation of extremely vigorous treatment of inflammatory arteritides in the early stages.

5 Perioperative Considerations

Anticoagulation

Oral Anticoagulation Treatment in the Elderly: A Nested, Prospective, Case-Control Study
Palareti G, Hirsh J, Legnani C, et al (Univ Hosp S Orsola-Malpighi, Bologna, Italy; McMaster Univ, Hamilton, Ontario, Canada; Ospedale Regionale Parma, Italy; et al)
Arch Intern Med 160:470-478, 2000

5-1

Background.—It is not clear that oral anticoagulant treatment (OAT) produces more complications in the elderly, but it has been shown that OAT is effective in treating and preventing thromboembolic complications in patients who have cardiovascular disease, many of whom are elderly. The complication rates of OAT were investigated among elderly patients, and the modifiable factors contributing to risk were determined.

Methods.—Two groups of patients were evaluated: 461 patients who were 75 years or older when OAT was begun and 461 patients younger than 70 years with the same indications for OAT and matched for sex and treatment site. Each group was assessed for bleeding and thrombotic events that occurred during OAT.

Results.—Among elderly patients, the bleeding rate was 9.9% patients-years; among younger patients it was 6.6% patient-years. Major bleeding rates were 2.1% for elderly and 1.1% for younger patients. Fatal bleeding occurred in 6 elderly patients and 1 younger patient. When the international normalized ratio (INR) was between 2.0 and 2.9, the bleeding rate was lower (4.5%) for elderly individuals. Higher rates occurred in the first 90 days of treatment and when the indication for treatment was arterial vascular disease. Elderly patients had a 4.2% thrombosis rate, whereas that for younger patients was 2.5%. Thirteen elderly patients and 5 younger patients had fatal thrombotic events. INRs of 2.0 to 2.9 were associated with a thrombosis rate of 1.5%; when the INR was lower than 2.0, 6 of 7 venous events occurred. The thrombosis rate was increased during the first 90 days of treatment.

Conclusions.—When elderly and younger patients were compared, the elderly had a higher rate of both bleeding and thrombotic complications, and significant increases in the number of intracranial bleeding and fatal thrombotic events occurred. INRs less than 2.0 do not protect from thrombotic events or eliminate the bleeding risk. Anticoagulation in the moderate range of 2.0 to 3.0 INR produced the best results with the fewest complications.

▶ These findings confirm those of several previous studies in that (1) fatal or serious hemorrhage is more common in the elderly patient receiving OAT and (2) the highest incidence of bleeding in this elderly cohort occurred in patients whose main indication for OAT was the presence of cerebral vascular disease or peripheral arteriopathy. The risk for bleeding in elderly patients is highest in the first 90 days of treatment, reflecting perhaps difficulty in establishing a steady-state dose, possible interactions with additional medication which are more common in an elderly population, or the "unmasking" of underlying conditions predisposing to hemorrhage following anticoagulation that occur more commonly in the elderly. Despite these problems, the risk for fatal thrombotic events was also significantly higher in the elderly population in this series, and more than one half of these events for which a time-related INR was available occurred when the INR was less than 2.

This finding seriously undermines the commonly held assumption that "light" OAT (maintaining an INR of less than 2) is somehow more effective in preventing thrombotic episodes in elderly patients while minimizing bleeding risk. The bottom line: elderly patients need an effective therapeutic OAT range (INR, 2.0 to 3.0) to prevent fatal thrombotic events just as younger patients do. Unfortunately, these same patients (especially those with peripheral arterial disease) are at greater risk for fatal bleeding events. Since these events seem to occur with greater frequency in the first 90 days of treatment, careful attention to the initiation of therapy (achieving and maintaining the target INR), concomitant drug interactions, and the possibility of predisposing underlying prohemorrhagic events are the most effective means of minimizing risk in this challenging patient population.

R. L. Dalman, MD

Coronary Disease

Peripheral Arterial Disease in Randomized Trial of Estrogen With Progestin in Women With Coronary Heart Disease: The Heart and Estrogen/Progestin Replacement Study
Hsia J, for the HERS Investigators (George Washington Univ, Washington, DC; Univ of California, San Francisco; Wake Forest Univ, Winston-Salem, NC; et al)
Circulation 102:2228-2232, 2000   5–2

Background.—There is evidence that postmenopausal women taking estrogen therapy have reduced carotid atherosclerosis. However, this observation has not been confirmed, and little is known about the effects of estrogen on atherosclerosis in other peripheral arteries. Data from the Heart and Estrogen/Progestin Replacement Study were used to assess the effects of estrogen therapy on peripheral arterial disease in women with coronary heart disease.

Methods.—The randomized, secondary prevention trial included 2763 women with coronary heart disease who were postmenopausal but who had an intact uterus. They were assigned to receive conjugated equine estrogens, 0.625 mg/d, plus medroxyprogesterone acetate, 2.5 mg/d, or placebo. As a specified secondary outcome, the 2 groups were compared for their rates of peripheral arterial procedures or deaths. The mean follow-up was 4.1 years.

Results.—Two hundred thirteen patients had a total of 311 peripheral arterial events during follow-up, which was an incidence of 2.9%/y. There were more events in the placebo group than in the active hormone replacement group, but the difference was not significant: relative hazard, 0.87; 95% CI, 0.66 to 1.14. The rate of peripheral arterial events in the placebo group was higher for women with hypertension and diabetes mellitus; plasma high-density lipoprotein cholesterol and body mass index were negative predictors. In the active treatment group, current smoking status and diabetes mellitus were both independent predictors. Peripheral arterial disease did not significantly increase the risk of death caused by coronary, cardiovascular, or all causes.

Conclusions.—Hormone replacement therapy with estrogen/progestin does not reduce the risk of peripheral arterial disease in postmenopausal women with coronary heart disease. However, the predictors of peripheral arterial events may differ between women receiving estrogen/progestin versus placebo. Findings in this cohort suggest that women with coronary atherosclerosis have up to a 10-fold increase in the risk of lower extremity arterial disease leading to revascularization procedures or amputation.

▶ Established orthodoxies die hard. One wonders how many postmenopausal women in the United States are currently receiving conjugated estrogen and medroxyprogesterone in the belief that such therapy confers protection against morbid cardiovascular events. This late report from the HERS study clearly demonstrates that such therapy does not protect against peripheral vascular events, at least at 4.1 years after initiation of therapy. The HERS investigators had previously reported a similar lack of efficacy in reducing coronary events in this cohort of elderly women.

Yet women do have vascular disease at later ages than men. How can the failure of the HERS trial be reconciled with the recognized predilection of peripheral vascular disease for younger men versus older women? An alternative (and equally satisfactory) explanation may lie in the consequences of 40+ years of menstruation rather than the hormonal influences themselves—specifically the likelihood that menstruating women in the United States (presumable consuming a "Western diet") have much lower levels of total-body iron stores than men at a comparable age. This difference narrows considerably after menopause.

Iron is tightly conserved in healthy subjects, and it is not uncommon for older men to have 10 times the amount of total-body iron stores (as measured via serum ferritin levels) compared with that present in 20-somethings. There is no known biological advantage associated with such high levels of iron. Rather than the lack of cycling estrogen or progesterone, it may be the lack of regular menstrual blood loss and the consequent accumulation of iron itself, with its strong oxidative potential that accelerates the progression of vascular disease in men (at earlier ages) and in women after menopause.

This intriguing hypothesis is currently being tested by the Department of Veterans Affairs Cooperative Study No. 410, the Iron and Atherosclerosis Trial. This study will complete enrollment in 2002 and should conclusively address the possibility that differential cardiovascular morbidity risk between the sexes is not hormonal but rather elemental.

R. L. Dalman, MD

Alcohol Consumption and Risk of Intermittent Claudication in the Framingham Heart Study
Djoussé L, Levy D, Murabito JM, et al (Boston Univ; Framingham Heart Study/NHLBI, Mass)
Circulation 102:3092-3097, 2000   5–3

Objective.—The association between intermittent claudication (IC) and alcohol consumption is controversial. The effects of different types of alcohol on IC risk have not been thoroughly studied. The relation of total alcohol consumption and consumption of different types of alcohol to IC among participants in the Framingham Heart Study were investigated.

Methods.—Data on weekly alcohol consumption were collected at examinations 2, 7, 12, 13, 14, 15, and 17, and at all subsequent examinations for all 5209 individuals, aged 28 to 62 years, in the original cohort that began the study in 1948. At each examination, individuals were asked about exertional leg discomfort, calf cramping, and smoking. Individuals were stratified by alcohol consumption and by sex. Patients were followed for an average of 6.8 years.

Results.—IC developed in 229 men and 185 women. The age-adjusted IC rates for the lowest to highest alcohol intake were 5.27, 4.09, 4.18, 3.20, and 4.56 for men and 3.40, 2.52, 1.50, 1.91, and 2.48 for women. The trend suggested an inverse relationship between alcohol intake and IC incidence mostly for men younger than 65 and for women at all ages. Alcohol intake was associated with a greater reduction in IC incidence among smokers than among nonsmokers. The inverse relationship held when individuals with diabetes and coronary heart disease were controlled for. The hazard ratios for men who drank 13 to 24 g/d and for women who drank 7 to 12 g/d were 0.67 and 0.44, respectively. The protective effect was most apparent with beer and wine.

Conclusion.—Moderate alcohol consumption confers a protective effect against IC for men having 1 to 2 drinks per day and for women having 0.5 to 1 drink per day.

▶ Although the data from this study suggest that alcohol consumption is associated with a decrease risk for IC, some of the conclusions must be taken with a grain of salt. For example, these data suggest that patients who do not smoke and consume alcohol moderately have a higher risk for IC compared with current smokers who drink moderate amounts of alcohol. The hazards ratio for these 2 groups were 1.58 and 0.70, respectively. Does this mean that we should recommend smoking to those patients who consume alcohol moderately? Currently, I have no desire to begin smoking to lower my risk for IC, considering my moderate alcohol consumption.

Nevertheless, the article does speak to the powers of alcohol, primarily beer and wine. The discussion gives a nice summary as to the possible pathophysiology mechanisms of alcohol and its prevention of atherosclerosis. Alcohol has been shown to raise high-density lipoprotein cholesterol, prevent thrombogenesis or improve fibrinolysis, and lower platelet aggregation. Additionally, beer and wine contain polyphenol with antioxidant properties that may delay the onset of atherosclerosis by preventing oxidation of low-density lipoprotein cholesterol. Lastly, on the miracles of wine, grape-skin has been shown to have the antifungal compound, phytoalexin, a compound that may raise high-density lipoprotein cholesterol and reduce platelet aggregation.

R. B. McLafferty, MD

Relation of Consumption of Vitamin E, Vitamin C, and Carotenoids to Risk for Stroke Among Men in the United States
Ascherio A, Rimm EB, Hernán MA, et al (Harvard School of Public Health, Boston; Harvard Med School, Boston; Brigham and Women's Hosp, Boston)
Ann Intern Med 130:963-970, 1999   5–4

Objective.—Vitamin E reduces the risk of atherosclerosis and so might reduce the risk of ischemic stroke. However, there are few firm data on the effects of vitamin E on ischemic stroke risk. Vitamin C and carotenoids also have antioxidant effects. Data from the Health Professionals Follow-up Study were used to assess the relationship between intake of vitamin E, vitamin C, and carotenoids and risk of stroke, including ischemic stroke.

Methods.—In 1986, 51,529 men aged 40 to 75 years enrolled in the study. At baseline and at biannual follow-ups, the men completed a food frequency questionnaire, including information on the use of vitamin supplements. A total of 43,738 men were followed up for stroke through 8 years.

Results.—Of the 328 strokes occurring during follow-up, 210 were ischemic, 70 hemorrhagic, and 48 unclassified. The relationship between antioxidant intake and stroke was adjusted for age, smoking, hypertension, hypercholesterolemia, body mass index, physical activity, parental myocardial infarction, alcohol consumption, and total energy intake. For men in the top quintile of vitamin E intake, the relative risk of ischemic stroke was 1.18 (95% confidence interval, 0.77 to 1.82), compared with the bottom quintile. The median dosages were 411 and 5.4 IU/d, respectively. A vitamin C intake in the top quintile compared with the bottom quintile was associated with a relative risk for ischemic stroke of 1.03 (95% confidence interval, 0.66 to 1.59). The median dosages were 1167 and 95 mg/d, respectively. The effects of vitamin E and C intake on total stroke risk were similar; the effects on hemorrhagic stroke risk were also nonsignificant, with wide confidence intervals. No vitamin dose or duration of use was significantly related to total or ischemic stroke risk. For men taking vitamin E supplementation of 250 IU/d or greater, the relative risk of ischemic stroke was 1.16 (95% confidence interval, 0.81 to 1.67) compared with those taking no vitamin E supplements and 0.93 (95% confidence interval, 0.60 to 1.45) compared with those taking vitamin C supplementation of 700 mg/d or greater. Lutein intake was inversely related to ischemic stroke risk, although this relationship was affected by other dietary factors.

Conclusion.—No significant effect of vitamin E or C supplementation on total or ischemic stroke risk was found. Recent results suggesting that vitamin E increases hemorrhagic stroke risk were not confirmed. Dietary interventions to reduce stroke risk should emphasize increased intake of fruits and vegetables rather than vitamin supplements.

▶ Antioxidants are believed to diminish the risk of atherosclerosis by reducing oxidation of low-density lipoprotein. This study evaluated the relationship between vitamin E, vitamin C, and carotenoid intake and stroke among over 43,000 men in the Health Professionals Follow-up Study. The conclusions are that, in this group of men without cardiovascular disease or diabetes, the risk for stroke was unaffected by antioxidants. It is difficult to garner enthusiasm for vitamin E, as it was also recently shown to have no benefit for cardiovascular events in high-risk patients.[1] As investigations such as this continue to report, we may eventually learn how to minimize our atherosclerotic risks. A more interesting arena may be the relationship between folate and hyperhomocysteinemia.

A. M. Abou-Zamzam, Jr, MD

Reference

1. 2001 YEAR BOOK OF VASCULAR SURGERY, pp 230-231.

Physical Activity and Coronary Heart Disease Risk in Men: Does the Duratlon of Exercise Episodes Predict Risk?
Lee I-M, Sesso HD, Paffenbarger RS Jr (Harvard School of Public Health, Boston; Harvard Med School, Boston)
Circulation 102:981-986, 2000   5–5

Background.—The risk of coronary heart disease (CHD) declines in patients who undertake physical activity, and it is recommended that each adult in the United States accumulate a minimum of 30 minutes of activity most days each week. Whether the duration of exercise influences its effects was assessed; specifically, it was assessed whether a series of short sessions produces the same benefit as longer sessions when the same amount of energy is expended.

Methods.—From 1988 through 1993, 7307 Harvard University alumni (mean age, 66.1 years) were followed up prospectively. Baseline levels of walking, stair climbing, and participation in sports or recreational activities were self-reported, and the duration and frequency for the latter were estimated. CHD developed in 482 men during follow-up. The relative risk of CHD related to the maximum average duration per episode of sports was estimated.

Results.—More than 35% of men engaged in activities for more than an hour each week, including playing tennis, golfing, gardening and yard work, and skiing. When men expended the same amount of energy in physical activity, a longer duration of activity per episode did not diminish CHD risk further. In addition, engaging in sports or recreational activities did not lower the risk of CHD more than did engaging in walking or climbing stairs if the total energy output was equal. When adjustment was made for added risk factors, the duration per episode still showed no correlation with decreased CHD risk.

Conclusions.—Physical activity decreases CHD risk, but accumulating energy expenditure over short sessions has the same positive effect as a longer, continuous exercise session when an equal amount of energy is expended. Thus, sedentary individuals can be encouraged to become more active and can decrease their CHD risk.

▶ Studies such as these are obviously only as good as the data that go into them. Quantifying the duration and intensity of exercise can be a difficult thing to do, and although this is a prospective study, the key data points are based upon each respondent's own recollection of how much exercise he or she had done. How can you quantify and compare gardening with playing tennis? How do you differentiate a casual game of tennis from a competitive game of tennis? The study somewhat makes up for this inherent weakness with sheer numbers (over 7000 respondents), and it is clear from the findings that exercisers have a decreased incidence of coronary artery events compared with nonexercisers. Additionally, it appears that total energy expenditure, rather than the duration of an individual exercise session, is more closely associated with decreased CHD risk. The message to our patients with vascular disease is to focus less on time of exercise and more on frequency.

G. J. Landry, MD

Demographics

Projected Workload for a Vascular Service in 2020
Heikkinen M, Salenius JP, Auvinen O (Univ Hosp, Tampere, Finland)
Eur J Vasc Endovasc Surg 19:351-355, 2000   5–6

Background.—As peripheral vascular disease (PVD) primarily affects older adults, it is expected to be increasingly prevalent in the future with the aging of the population. Extrapolating from data on population trends, the workload of a vascular service in Finland during the next 2 decades was analyzed.

Methods.—Registry data from a university hospital vascular service, along with population data on the region of Finland served by that hospital, were analyzed. The service's current workload was 1420 vascular procedures per million population per year, including 951 surgical and 207 endovascular procedures. Sixty-five percent of these procedures were done on patients older than 65 years. In the region served, the percentage of the population in this age group was expected to increase from 15.6% to 22.9% by 2020.

Results.—On the basis of these data, a 40.5% increase in the total number of vascular procedures was estimated, including a 39.2% increase in endovascular procedures and a 43.5% increase in surgical procedures (Fig 2). The percentage of patients aged 65 years or older was projected to increase to 70.5%. Analysis of numbers of patients with specific indications suggested increases of 35.4% in claudication, 44.2% in critical limb

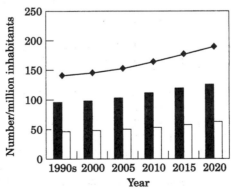

FIGURE 2.—Number of vascular procedures per million inhabitants until the year 2020. *Black bars*, surgical procedures; *white bars*, endovascular procedures; *diamonds*, total number of procedures. (Courtesy of Heikkinen M, Salenius JP, Auvinen O: Projected workload for a vascular service in 2020. *Eur J Vasc Endovasc Surg* 19:351-355, 2000. Copyright 2000, by permission of the publisher WB Saunders Company Limited London.)

ischemia, 34.0% in carotid surgery, 40.7% in abdominal aortic aneurysms, 45.0% in acute limb ischemia, and 27.4% in access surgery.

Conclusions.—The aging of the population is likely to increase the demand for vascular procedures. Even if current trends in the incidence and prevalence of PVD are altered, the rise in the elderly population will be so rapid that vascular services will inevitably see an increase in workload during the next 2 decades.

▶ Workload issues in vascular surgery are timely and important. In the United States, the number of unmatched categorical surgical residency positions is increasing rapidly every year. Thus far, this has not translated to unmatched vascular fellowship positions, but the implication is clear. Ample data exist that the majority of recent general surgery graduates do minimal vascular surgery outside of dialysis access. As the population ages, the number of procedures needed annually is going to increase. Who is going to provide this care? Despite turf concerns regarding interventional radiology and cardiology, it appears that our profession is going to have its hands full providing surgical care for an increasingly aging population. In the coming years, elderly patients with vascular disease are likely to be increasingly cared for surgically in larger referral centers. Those patients in rural environments will have to accept travel and inconvenience as a part of receiving vascular surgical care.

M. R. Nehler, MD

Clinical Governance and the Vascular Surgeon
Irvine CD, Grayson D, Lusby RJ (Univ of Sydney, Australia)
Br J Surg 87:766-770, 2000   5–7

Background.—As a result of recent inquiries into the outcomes of pediatric cardiac surgery in the United Kingdom, attention has been focused on the maintenance of an acceptable standard of surgical outcomes. A perceived inadequacy in the maintenance of standards has resulted in a suggestion for clinical governance, or "audit with teeth" from administrative bodies. Under the clinical governance protocol, consultant surgeons would be evaluated every 2 years, and consultant physicians would be evaluated annually. It has also been recommended that all physicians in the United Kingdom be required to prove competence. However, few data regarding the exact process of this audit and its feasibility are available. In an effort to determine the validity of the clinical governance hypothesis, statistical modeling was applied to 2 indicative vascular procedures—elective abdominal aortic aneurysm and carotid endarterectomy—with accepted rates of adverse outcome.

Methods.—Binomial statistical models were constructed to determine various adverse event rates. A power calculation was then used for prediction of the number of cases required to determine substandard results for individual surgeons and vascular units. Two different scenarios were assumed: The first scenario involved a base adverse event rate of 6% and surgical practice with 9%, 12%, and 24% morbidity rates; the second scenario involved a base adverse event rate of 3% and surgical practice with 6%, 9%, and 12% morbidity rates.

Results.—The mean number of elective abdominal aortic aneurysm repairs yearly was 57, and there were 70 carotid endarterectomies performed each year. The power calculation demonstrated that 130 patients would be necessary for detection of a surgeon with a rate of adverse events twice 6%, and 280 patients would be needed for detection of a surgeon with an adverse event rate twice 3%. To gather this number of patients, it would be necessary to gather 2 years of unit data and 3 to 22 years of individual data to determine a base adverse event rate of 6%. For a base rate of 3%, 7 to 47 years of individual data and 4 to 65 years of unit data would be required; however, detection of widely variant surgical practice (defined as 4 times the morbidity rate as a base) requires only 21 procedures.

Conclusion.—Assumptions regarding accepted practice adverse event rates, confidence criteria, and the definition of substandard results are required for statistical modeling, and data from large patient populations are needed even for common procedures with accepted adverse event rates. These findings call into question the feasibility of clinical governance based solely on morbidity and mortality event rates.

Determinants of Peripheral Arterial Disease in the Elderly: The Rotterdam Study

Meijer WT, Grobbee DE, Hunink MGM, et al (Erasmus Univ, Rotterdam, The Netherlands; Univ Med Ctr Utrecht, The Netherlands; Harvard School of Public Health, Boston)
Arch Intern Med 160:2934-2938, 2000   5–8

Objective.—The etiology of peripheral arterial disease (PAD) is unclear. The ankle-arm systolic blood pressure index (AAI), a measure of PAD, may be a marker of atherosclerosis. Determinants of atherosclerosis involved in the etiology of PAD, and the extent to which atherosclerotic risk factors are involved, were prospectively investigated in a large, population-based setting as part of the Rotterdam Study.

Methods.—PAD was detected by AAI. Possible determinants of PAD—hypertension, diabetes, smoking status, alcohol intake, serum cholesterol level—plasma fibrinogen, and total homocysteine level—were recorded for 6450 patients (3861 women) aged 55 years or older, and were used to calculate age- and sex-adjusted odds ratios (ORs).

Results.—If PAD was defined as AAI of less than 0.90, 19% of patients had the disease. If it was defined as less than 0.70, 8% of patients had PAD. Potential determinants of PAD, according to age- and sex-adjusted ORs and multivariate analysis ORs, were at least 75 years (OR, 1.22 and 1.74), systolic blood pressure (OR, 1.18 and 1.30), hypertension (OR,

1.92 and 1.32), total cholesterol (OR, 1.13 and 1.19), high-density lipo-protein cholesterol (OR, 0.65 and 0.58), plasma fibrinogen (OR, 1.49 and 1.46), current smoking (OR, 2.84 and 2.69), former smoking (OR, 1.14 and 1.15), alcohol intake at least 20 g/d (OR, 1.24 and 1.00), and diabetes (OR, 2.00 and 1.89). Reversible risk factors account for 58% of PAD, and irreversible risk factors account for 11%. That leaves 31% of the risk for PAD unaccounted for.

Conclusion.—Sixty-nine percent of the risk of occurrence of PAD is accounted for by the cardiovascular factors evaluated in this study, with smoking alone being responsible for 18.1%, but 31% is not accounted for. Efforts need to target the 58% of risk factors that are reversible.

▶ This is a large prospective follow-up study designed to investigate deter-minants of the occurrence and progression of chronic disease in the elderly. It is no surprise that the most important determinants of PAD are cigarette smoking and diabetes.

R. A. Yeager, MD

Sympathetic Autoregulation in Peripheral Vascular Disease
Delis KT, Lennox AF, Nicolaides AN, et al (St Mary's Hosp, London)
Br J Surg 88:523-528, 2001   5–9

Objective.—The venoarteriolar response (VAR) moderates the rise in capillary pressure when posture changes from lying to sitting. VAR is

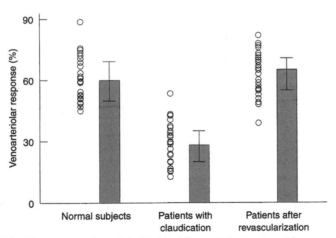

FIGURE 2.—The percentage decrease in skin blood flux on sitting (venoarteriolar response; VAR) in normal subjects, patients with stable intermittent claudication, and patients after successful infrainguinal bypass grafting for severe peripheral vascular disease. Data are presented as combined scattergrams and error bars (median and interquartile range). The VAR was significantly lower in claudicants than in either normal control subjects or grafted subjects ($P < .0001$; Mann-Whitney U test). There was no significant difference between normal and surgical patients ($P = .09$) (Courtesy of Delis KT, Lennox AF, Nicolaides AN, et al: Sympathetic autoregulation in peripheral vascular disease. *Br J Surg* 88:523-528, 2001; publisher, Blackwell Science Ltd.)

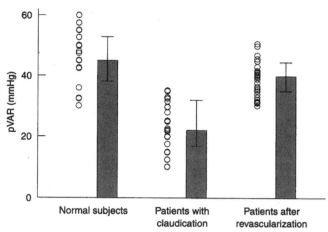

FIGURE 3.—Pressure that elicits the venoarteriolar response (pVAR) in normal subjects, patients with stable intermittent claudication, and patients after successful bypass grafting for severe peripheral vascular disease. Data are presented as combined scattergrams and error bars (median and interquartile range). The pVAR was higher in both normal and grafted subjects than in claudicants ($P < .001$; Mann-Whitney U test). The pVAR in normal subjects was higher than that in patients who underwent surgery ($P = .04$), but the differences failed the corrected (Bonferroni) significance threshold. (Courtesy of Delis KT, Lennox AF, Nicolaides AN, et al: Sympathetic autoregulation in peripheral vascular disease. *Br J Surg* 88:523-528, 2001; publisher, Blackwell Science Ltd.)

impaired in chronic venous insufficiency, diabetic autonomic neuropathy, nifedipine administration, premenstrual syndrome, and aging. The status of peripheral sympathetic autoregulation and its sensitivity were examined in advanced atherosclerosis and after flow reconstruction for ischemia.

Methods.—Foot skin blood flow (flux) was measured using Doppler fluxmetry in 30 control subjects, aged 66 to 74 years; 30 patients, aged 60 to 75 years, with stable intermittent claudication as a result of infrainguinal peripheral vascular disease (PVD) caused by superficial femoral artery occlusion; and 30 patients, aged 55 to 72 years, with infrainguinal PVD who had undergone femoropopliteal or femorodistal bypass grafting. Blood flow was measured in all patients while they were in the horizontal (HBF) and sitting (SBF) positions. VAR was calculated as (HBF−SBF)/HBF × 100%.

Results.—HBF was similar for all groups. In the sitting position, skin flux was significantly higher in claudication patients than in the other 2 groups. The decrease in skin blood flux on sitting was significantly higher in the normal group and the revascularization group than in the claudication group (Fig 2). The pressure that released the VAR was significantly lower in claudication patients than in either of the other 2 groups (Fig 3).

Conclusion.—Claudication patients have an impaired VAR that returns to normal after revascularization. Localized blood flow reduction and chronic tissue ischemia cause the impairment.

▶ Impairment of the VAR has been implicated in a wide variety of conditions including venous insufficiency, diabetic autonomic neuropathy, and aging. In this study, laser Doppler fluxmetry was used as a marker of the VAR. It is accepted that patients with critical limb ischemia have impairment of the VAR, but the results in claudication have been less clear. The authors conclude that the VAR is impaired in patients with claudication but returns to normal after revascularization and is not dependent on the severity of the underlying atherosclerosis. Additionally, they suggest measurement of VAR impairment as a noninvasive means of quantifying the severity of limb ischemia in claudicators. Since for the most part, I treat patients with claudication on the basis of their complaints and lifestyle limitations without regard to the severity of the underlying ischemia, I doubt that I will be using this test, except for research.

J. M. Edwards, MD

Intravascular Sonotherapy Decreases Neointimal Hyperplasia After Stent Implantation in Swine
Fitzgerald PJ, Takagi A, Moore MP, et al (Stanford Univ, Calif; PharmaSonics Inc, Sunnyvale, Calif; Armed Forces Inst of Pathology, Washington, DC)
Circulation 103:1828-1831, 2001   5–10

Background.—The effectiveness of stent implantation is limited by intimal hyperplasia leading to in-stent restenosis. Smooth-muscle cell culture studies have suggested that US energy has the potential to limit neointimal growth after stenting. A swine model was used to assess the effects of intravascular sonotherapy on intimal hyperplasia after stenting.

Methods.—Fourteen swine underwent balloon injury of the femoral arteries, followed by stent placement at 48 sites. The sites were randomized to undergo intravascular sonotherapy (with 700 KHz of US energy applied for up to 5 minutes) or sham treatment. Sonotherapy was applied by means of a custom-built, 8F catheter system. In all 28 stented sites, bromodeoxyuridine histology preparation was used to assess smooth-muscle cell proliferation after 7 days. Twenty sites underwent histomorphometric studies to assess neointimal thickness and percentage stenosis after 28 days.

Results.—Seven-day bromodeoxyuridine staining was 24% at the US-treated sites versus 31% at the sham-treated sites. By 28 days, the percentage stenosis was 36% in the sonotherapy group and 44% in the sham treatment group. The mean neointimal thicknesses were 417 and 643 µm, respectively.

Conclusion.—Intravascular sonotherapy may reduce smooth-muscle cell proliferation and reduce hyperplasia in peripheral vascular stents. This may provide a useful new approach to reducing in-stent restenosis without radiation.

▶ Here is yet another article in a large group of studies designed to identify methods to reduce neointimal hyperplasia following arterial injury—in this case, with stents. Although such methods as antibiotic use and ionizing radiation appear to have some effect, clinical application has yet to catch on. Although porcine studies are a start, there is still a long way to go.

W. K. Williamson, MD

Drugs

Longitudinal Assessment of Neurocognitive Function After Coronary-Artery Bypass Surgery

Newman MF, and the Cardiothoracic Anesthesiology Research Endeavors Investigators (Duke Univ, Durham, NC)

N Engl J Med 344:395-402, 2001   5–11

Background.—Cognitive decline is a potential complication of coronary artery bypass grafting (CABG). Evidence of reduced cognitive function may be found at discharge in up to three fourths of patients and at 6 months' follow-up for one third. A 5-year follow-up study evaluated the course of cognitive change after CABG.

Methods.—The study sample comprised 261 patients undergoing elective CABG. All underwent a battery of neurocognitive tests before surgery; before hospital discharge; and at 6 weeks, 6 months, and 5 years postop-

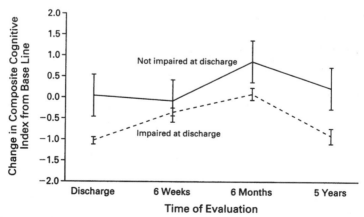

FIGURE 2.—Composite cognitive index as a function of cognitive impairment at discharge. The composite cognitive index is the sum of the scores for the 4 domains and includes cognitive decline as well as increases in scores as a result of learning. Positive change represents an overall improvement (learning), whereas negative values indicate overall decline. The *I bars* represent the standard error. (Reprinted by permission of *The New England Journal of Medicine* from Newman MF, and the Cardiothoracic Anesthesiology Research Endeavors Investigators: Longitudinal assessment of neurocognitive function after coronary-artery bypass surgery. *N Engl J Med* 344:395-402, 2001. Copyright 2001, Massachusetts Medical Society. All rights reserved.)

eratively. A decline of at least 1 standard deviation (about 20%) in any of 4 cognitive function domains was considered significant. A composite cognitive index score was compiled as an overall assessment of neurocognitive status, and factors associated with long-term cognitive decline were evaluated.

Results.—Compared with baseline, 53% of patients met the study definition of cognitive decline at the time of discharge. This percentage decreased to 36% at 6 weeks' follow-up and 24% at 6 months. At 5 years, 42% of patients had evidence of cognitive decline. The presence of cognitive decline at baseline was a significant predictor of long-term cognitive status (Fig 2).

Conclusion.—Cognitive decline is a common finding for post-CABG patients and is persistent for many. Patients show a pattern of improvement in cognitive function in the weeks and months after surgery, with a later decline at long-term follow-up. Cognitive decline in the early postoperative period is a significant predictor of long-term decline. Effective measures to prevent cognitive decline after cardiac surgery are needed.

▶ The family observation that "Uncle Jerry just hasn't been the same since his open-heart surgery" appears to have a basis in fact. While numerous studies have documented a frequent decline in neurocognitive function after CABG, this is the first with clear evidence that the deficits persist over the long term, being present in 42% at 5 years postoperatively. Who could disagree with the author's conclusion that ". . . further investigation . . . is essential."

L. M. Taylor, Jr, MD

The Effect of Previous Coronary-Artery Bypass Surgery on the Prognosis of Patients With Diabetes Who Have Acute Myocardial Infarction
Detre KM, for the Bypass Angioplasty Revascularization Investigation Investigators (Univ of Pittsburgh, Pa; NIH, Bethesda, Md; Mayo Clinic Found, Rochester, Minn; et al)
N Engl J Med 342:989-997, 2000   5–12

Background.—The mortality rate among patients with diabetes who experience acute myocardial infarction is high. The mechanisms responsible for different clinical courses among patients with diabetes according to the type of revascularization they received were investigated. The prognoses of diabetic patients who underwent percutaneous transluminal coronary angiography (PTCA) were compared with those of diabetic patients who underwent coronary artery bypass grafting (CABG) after acute myocardial infarction.

Methods.—The study group was based on classification of patients who were eligible for the Bypass Angioplasty Revascularization Investigation who underwent coronary revascularization within 3 months after entry into the study. Patients were classified as to whether they had undergone

Patients with Q-Wave Myocardial Infarction

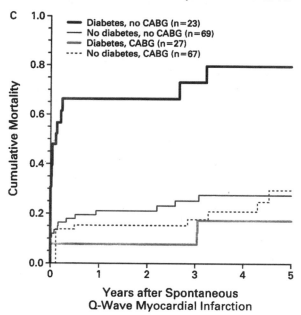

FIGURE 2C.—Mortality after the initial revascularization procedure. Kaplan-Meier estimates of the cumulative mortality in patients with spontaneous Q-wave myocardial infarction according to diabetes status and coronary artery bypass grafting (*CABG*) status (the *numbers in parentheses* refer to the 186 spontaneous Q-wave myocardial infarctions that occurred in 176 patients). Patients who did not undergo CABG were treated only with percutaneous transluminal coronary angioplasty. (Reprinted by permission of *The New England Journal of Medicine* from Detre KM, for the Bypass Angioplasty Revascularization Investigation Investigators: The effect of previous coronary-artery bypass surgery on the prognosis of patients with diabetes who have acute myocardial infarction. *N Engl J Med* 342:989-997. Copyright 2000, Massachusetts Medical Society. All rights reserved.)

PTCA or CABG. Cox regression models were used to estimate the protective effect of CABG with regard to mortality in the presence or absence of subsequent spontaneous Q-wave myocardial infarction.

Results.—The cumulative 5-year rate of death for the 641 patients with diabetes was 20%, compared with the cumulative 5-year death rate of 8% for the 2962 patients who did not have diabetes. Five-year rates of spontaneous Q-wave myocardial infarction were 8% for patients with diabetes and 4% for patients without diabetes. The risk of death after spontaneous Q-wave myocardial infarction in patients with diabetes was significantly reduced by CABG (relative risk, 0.09; 95% confidence interval, 0.03-0.29). The relative risk of death for patients with diabetes who underwent CABG but did not have spontaneous Q-wave myocardial infarction was 0.65 (95% confidence interval, 0.45-0.94). There was no evidence of a protective benefit from CABG among patients without diabetes (Fig 2).

Conclusions.—For patients with diabetes, previous CABG affords a significant beneficial effect on prognosis as compared with angioplasty. A smaller beneficial effect is seen in patients who do not experience infarction. These findings should influence the decision regarding the type of coronary revascularization procedure selected for patients with diabetes who have coronary artery disease affecting several vessels.

▶ Diabetic patients were much less likely to die from a late myocardial infarction (as defined as a new Q wave on ECG) after CABG versus PTCA. The differential likelihood of mortality following late myocardial infarction after the 2 interventions was dramatic (17% vs 80%). With a Cox regression model used to estimate the reduction in mortality conferred by CABG in diabetic patients, the protective effect was approximately 7 times as great after spontaneous Q-wave myocardial infarction as in the absence of such an event. Among patients without diabetes, no significant protective effect of CABG was evident. The protective effect of CABG was further enhanced when internal thoracic artery grafts were employed, suggesting that a good proportion of the benefit was directly attributable to long-term increases in myocardial perfusion.

The authors speculate that since diabetic patients typically have more extensive disease, focal "lesion therapy" offered via PTCA leaves more myocardium at risk for future ischemic events than definitive revascularization, increasing the magnitude of ischemia and subsequent mortality after future coronary occlusions. Although there are many caveats to the data provided in this study, it is clear that a revascularization strategy that uniformly calls for PTCA first, followed by CABG later (after symptomatic recurrence or secondary events) may not provide optimal survival benefit for diabetic patients.

Furthermore, the inherently focal nature of catheter-guided dilation may not be well suited to treatment of diffuse and distal lesions associated with diabetic coronary arteriopathy. Definitive revascularization means (apparently in the diabetic patient, at least) just that.

R. L. Dalman, MD

Cardioprotective Effect of Prior β-Blocker Therapy in Reducing Creatine Kinase-MB Elevation After Coronary Intervention: Benefit Is Extended to Improvement in Intermediate-term Survival
Sharma SK, Kini A, Marmur JD, et al (Mount Sinai Hosp, New York)
Circulation 102:166-172, 2000   5–13

Background.—Studies have found that creatine kinase myocardial bound (CK-MB) isoenzymes are elevated after 6% to 30% of percutaneous coronary interventions. The clinical relevance of this finding and the effects of periprocedural CK-MB elevation after coronary intervention on intermediate and long-term survival have been hotly debated. In numerous earlier studies, most of which involved balloon angioplasty, CK-MB elevation was shown to be associated with increases in subsequent cardiac events and mortality. A higher incidence of postprocedure CK-MB elevation but no definitive increase in intermediate-term mortality were ob-

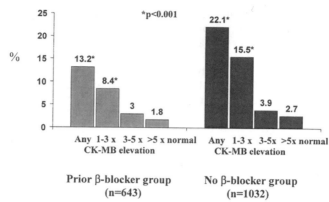

FIGURE 1.—Incidence and magnitude of CK-MB elevation in prior β-blocker therapy versus no β-block therapy groups. (Courtesy of Sharma SK, Kini A, Marmur JD, et al: Cardioprotective effect of prior β-blocker therapy in reducing creatine kinase-MB elevation after coronary intervention: Benefit is extended to improvement in intermediate-term survival. *Circulation* 102:166-172, 2000.)

served in recent trials of newer devices. There are a number of causes of CK-MB elevation after otherwise successful coronary intervention; however, retrospective studies and prospective randomized trials have indicated that improved survival and reduced risk of reinfarction in patients with myocardial infarction can be obtained with β-blockers. The potential for β-blockers to exert similar protective benefits during and after coronary intervention was evaluated by studying the incidence of postprocedure CK-MB elevation in patients with and without previous β-blocker therapy and the effects of β-blocker therapy on intermediate-term survival.

Methods.—A prospective analysis was conducted of 1675 consecutive patients undergoing coronary intervention. β-Blocker therapy was administered to 643 (38.4%) of these patients before the intervention. Intermediate-term survival was considered approximately 1 year (15 ± 3 months).

Results.—CK-MB elevation after coronary intervention occurred in 13.2% of patients receiving β-blocker therapy before intervention and in 22.1% of patients not receiving β-blockers (Fig 1). Patients who received prior β-blocker therapy had lower rates of persistent or recurrent postprocedure chest pain and lower preprocedure and postprocedure heart rates and blood pressures compared with patients who were not receiving β-blocker therapy. In multiple linear regression analysis, β-blocker therapy was shown to be the lone independent factor for lower CK-MB release after coronary intervention. Mortality rates were lower during intermediate follow-up for patients receiving β-blocker therapy compared with patients not receiving β-blockers, but this benefit was found to be independent of reduced CK-MB release.

Conclusions.—These data suggest that a cardioprotective effect is provided by prior β-blocker therapy through the limitation of CK-MB release after coronary intervention. It is also suggested that β-blocker therapy is associated with a lower mortality at intermediate follow-up.

▶ This article represents yet another testimony to the wonders of β-blocker therapy in the prevention of coronary events. Although CK-MB isoenzyme elevation was not correlated with long-term mortality, patients receiving β-blocker therapy before intervention did have a lower mortality rate in follow-up. Not evident in this article is whether patients had a prior intervention or contact with a cardiologist for care.

This fact remains important because only one third of patients were receiving β-blockers prior to intervention. Other literature has shown that less than one third of patients with known coronary artery disease are taking β-blockers. This is certainly confirmed in my own practice where I routinely give patients β-blockers prior to arterial surgery.

It seems that in the large majority of patients with known coronary artery disease, β-blocker therapy should be as common as aspirin therapy. Indeed, I continue patients on β-blockers for life after arterial surgery. Most importantly, education of primary care physicians is needed to increase the use of β-blocker therapy to decrease cardiac events and, more importantly, sudden death.

R. B. McLafferty, MD

Dipyridamole-Thallium/Sestamibi Before Vascular Surgery: A Prospective Blinded Study in Moderate-Risk Patients
de Virgilio C, Toosie K, Ephraim L, et al (Harbor-Univ of California Los Angeles)
J Vasc Surg 32:77-89, 2000   5–14

Background.—Dipyridamole-thallium (DTHAL) and sestamibi (DMIBI) have both proved useful in the detection of coronary artery disease. However, controversy continues regarding to the predictive value of both of both of these agents for adverse cardiac events after vascular surgery. In a prospective, blinded study, the predictive ability of a reversible defect on DTHAL/DMIBI for adverse cardiac events was evaluated in patients with one or more clinical risk factors who underwent elective vascular surgery.

Methods.—In 80 consecutive patients, a preoperative blinded DTHAL/DMIBI was performed. Patients who had recently had congestive heart failure or myocardial infarction or who had severe or unstable angina were excluded from the study. The patient group was 78% male and had a mean age of 65 years.

Results.—The most frequently found clinical risk factor was diabetes mellitus (73%). After diabetes, the most significant risk factors were age older than 70 years (41%), angina (29%), Q wave on electrocardiogram (26%), history of congestive heart failure (7%), and ventricular ectopy (3%). DTHAL/DMIBI results were normal in 36 patients (45%); a reversible plus or minus fixed event was found in 28 patients (36%), whereas a fixed defect was demonstrated in 15 patients (19%) (Table 3). There were 9 adverse cardiac events (11%), including 3 cases of congestive heart failure and 1 case each of unstable angina, Q-wave myocardial infarction,

TABLE 3.—Adverse Cardiac Event Rate With DTHAL/DMIBI Results

DTHAL/DMIBI Result	Cardiac Event Rate
Normal	3/36 (8.3%)
Normal or fixed	5/51 (9.8%)
Fixed alone	2/15 (13.3%)
Reversible defect ± fixed	4/29 (13.8%)
≥ 2 reversible defects	1/8 (12.5%)
≥ 3 reversible defects	0.1 (0%)

(Courtesy of de Virgilio C, Toosie K, Ephraim L, et al: Dipyridamole-thallium/sestamibi before vascular surgery: a prospective blinded study in moderate-risk patients. *J Vasc Surg* 32:77-89, 2000.)

non-Q-wave myocardial infarction, and cardiac arrest, which was successfully resuscitated. There were 2 cardiac deaths (2%). For reversible defects, the cardiac event rate was 14%; the cardiac event rate without reversible defects was 9.8%. For more than 2 reversible defects, the cardiac event rate was 12.5%, and for less than 2 reversible defects, the cardiac event rate was 11.1%. The sensitivity rate of 2 or more areas of redistribution was 11% and the specificity rate was 90%, with positive and negative predictive values of 12.5% and 89%, respectively.

Conclusions.—No association was demonstrated in this study between reversible defects on DTHAL/DMIBI and adverse cardiac events in patients at moderate risk for coronary disease who were undergoing elective vascular surgery.

▶ This is a very well-done piece of clinical research regarding preoperative cardiac evaluation. The authors demonstrated that blinded preoperative cardiac evaluation with nuclear imaging (either DTHAL or DMIBI) was not helpful in predicting adverse coronary events in patients with at least 1 clinical risk factor from the Eagle criteria. Enthusiasm for extensive preoperative cardiac evaluation is clearly waning in the eyes of many vascular surgeons and cardiologists. This is particularly true considering the recent data on perioperative β-blockade in high-risk groups.

However, it is less clear that this message is being received by physicians in anesthesia and internal medicine, both important components in the cooperative effort to prepare a patient for major vascular surgery. Hopefully, the ongoing VA Coronary Artery Revascularization Prophylaxis trial will further our understanding in this important area. I highly recommend this article from the UCLA-Harbor group. The discussion is very well written and nicely summarizes the enormous database on the topic of preoperative cardiac evaluation.

M. R. Nehler, MD

Coronary Stenting Plus Platelet Glycoprotein IIb/IIIa Blockade Compared With Tissue Plasminogen Activator in Acute Myocardial Infarction

Schömig A, for the Stent Versus Thrombolysis for Occluded Coronary Arteries in Patients With Acute Myocardial Infarction Study Investigators (Technische Universität, Munich)

N Engl J Med 343:385-391, 2000   5–15

Background.—The objective of reperfusion therapy after acute myocardial infarction is to prevent myocardial damage. Studies comparing the efficacy of various reperfusion strategies are ongoing. Previous reports have indicated that a combination of coronary stenting plus platelet glycoprotein IIb/IIIa receptor blockade with abciximab may improve myocardial salvage. This strategy and the accelerated infusion of the tissue plasminogen activator alteplase were compared.

Methods.—The randomized controlled trial included 140 patients with acute myocardial infarction seen within 12 hours after symptom onset. One group received IV fibrinolysis with alteplase in a bolus dose of 15 mg, followed by an infusion of 0.75 mg/kg over 30 minutes, then an infusion of 0.5 mg/kg over 60 minutes. The other group underwent coronary stent placement, followed by abciximab, in a bolus dose of 0.25 mg/kg, followed by a continuous infusion of 10 μg/min for 12 hours. Both groups received aspirin and heparin. Serial technetium ^{99m}Tc-sestamibi studies

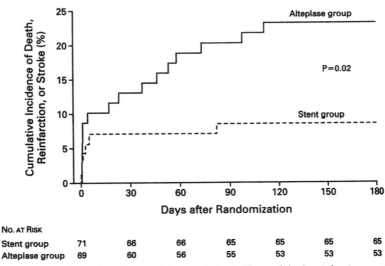

FIGURE 1.—Kaplan-Meier estimates of the cumulative incidence of death, reinfarction, or stroke during the first 6 months after randomization. The log-rank test was used to calculate the *P* value. (Reprinted by permission of *The New England Journal of Medicine* from Schömig A, for the Stent Versus Thrombolysis for Occluded Coronary Arteries in Patients With Acute Myocardial Infarction Study Investigators. *N Engl J Med* 343:385-391, 2000. Copyright 2000, Massachusetts Medical Society. All rights reserved.)

were performed to assess myocardial salvage. Other assessments included a composite end point of death, reinfarction, and stroke within 6 months.

Results.—The median final infarct size was 14.3% of the left ventricle in the stenting-plus-abciximab group compared with 19.4% in the alteplase group. The salvage index (defined as the percentage of left ventricle salvaged divided by the percentage compromised by the initial perfusion defect) was 0.57 for stenting plus abciximab and 0.26 for alteplase. The percentage of patients meeting the composite end point by 6 months was 8.5% with stenting plus abciximab versus 23.2% with alteplase. The corresponding relative risk was 0.34, with a 95% CI of 0.13 to 0.88 (Fig 1).

Conclusion.—A strategy of stenting plus platelet glycoprotein IIb/IIIa blockade with abciximab improves myocardial salvage after acute infarction, compared with accelerated alteplase infusion. Stenting plus abciximab also improves relevant clinical outcomes. It is unknown how much of the observed benefit can be attributed to fibrinogen receptor blockade; further studies of the combined strategy versus fibrinolytic therapy alone are needed.

▶ Glycoprotein IIb/IIIa inhibitors are beginning to emerge as critical adjunctive therapy for patients undergoing thrombolysis, both coronary and peripheral. The Thrombolysis in Myocardial Infarction 14 trial showed that the glycoprotein IIb/IIIa inhibitor, abciximab, increased the success of reestablishment of coronary flow with thrombolysis using tTa.[1] In this key study, abciximab treatment following percutaneous transluminal coronary angioplasty and stenting improved myocardial salvage over thrombolysis alone.

There is also a suggestion that clinical outcome—as measured by death, reinfarction, or stroke—was also improved in the stent/abciximab group, although the statistical power of this study will not allow a firm conclusion on these end points. Nevertheless, it appears that rapid myocardial reperfusion with angioplasty and stenting, followed by a glycoprotein IIb/IIIa inhibitor to prevent rethrombosis of the stent site, will most effectively salvage myocardium at risk during a myocardial infarction. I am sure this study will generate renewed interest in peripheral angioplasty and stenting with the addition of a glycoprotein IIb/IIIa inhibitor, as well it should.

E. J. Harris, Jr, MD

Reference

1. Antman EM, Giugliano RP, Gibson CM, et al: Abciximab facilitates the rate and extent of thrombolysis: Results of the Thrombolysis in Myocardial Infarction (TIMI) 14 trial. *Circulation* 99:2720-2732, 1999.

6 Thoracic Aorta

Ruptured Thoracoabdominal Aortic Aneurysm Repaired With Minimal Aortic Occlusion Time and Continuous Visceral Perfusion—A New Technique
Lord RSA, Chao A, Sim E, et al (Univ of South Wales, Sydney, Australia; Natl Univ Hosp, Singapore; Tan Tock Seng Hosp, Singapore; et al)
Cardiovasc Surg 8:173-180, 2000   6–1

Objective.—Ninety-four percent of abdominal aortic aneurysms can be treated by infrarenal grafting, but those involving the upper abdominal aorta or extending to the thoracic aorta require more complex reconstruction. The modified Crawford reconstruction technique for 2 urgent cases is described.

Case 1.—Asian woman, 71, with crushing central chest pain and a pulling sensation in the left side of the chest, was found to have a pulsatile abdominal mass about 4 cm in diameter. A CT scan and aortogram revealed a leaking thoracoabdominal aortic aneurysm of 7 cm in diameter extending from the diaphragm to below the celiac axis. Urgent surgery was performed. A 20- × 10-mm bifurcated gelatin-impregnated Dacron graft was anastomosed end to side to the proximal end of a 18-mm tube graft, and a Pruitt–Inahara shunt was attached to each side arm (Fig 2). Postoperatively she experienced transient azotemia, which resolved by discharge on day 10.

Case 2.—Asian man, 59, with severe left hypochondrial radiating chest and back pain, was found to have a 7-cm pulsatile mass in the upper abdomen. Helical CT revealed a dissecting aneurysm at the T10 level extending to the origin of the renal arteries. A 22-mm gelatin-impregnated Dacron graft with a 20- × 10-mm bifurcated graft was used to repair the descending thoracic aorta; the distal end was anastomosed to the left common iliac artery, and the aneurysm was excluded between the proximal and distal clamps. One arm of the side arm was anastomosed to the origin of the celiac artery. Postoperative subendocardial myocardial infarction, a mild chest infection, a superficial wound infection, and mild weakness of the hip extensors developed, but the patient recovered and was discharged after rehabilitation.

FIGURE 2

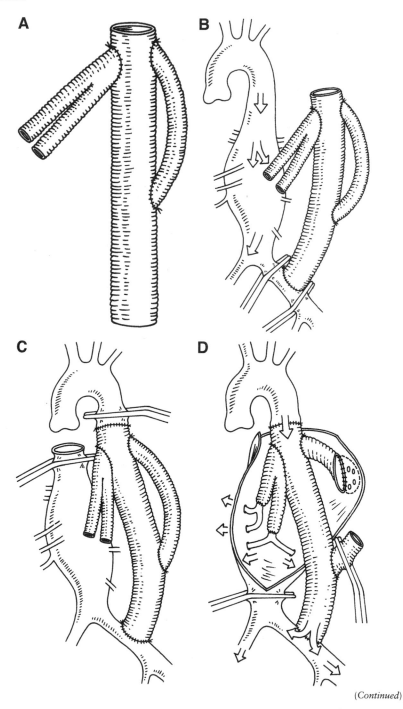

(Continued)

FIGURE 2 (cont.)

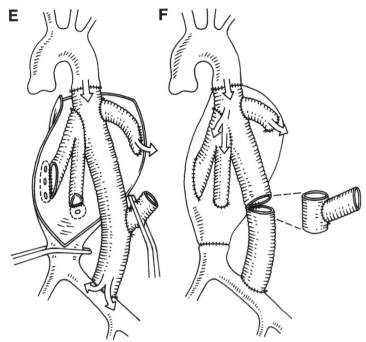

FIGURE 2.—Technique of graft preparation and implantation (see also text). **A,** Side grafts for later anastomosis to visceral and intercostal orifices are attached to a long straight tube graft. **B,** The distal graft—left common iliac anastomosis is fashioned first, after which left iliac flow is restored. **C,** The proximal aorta to graft anastomosis is completed. After clamp release, flow is restored antegrade to the lower limbs and retrograde to the abdominal viscera and spinal cord. **D,** Before the aneurysm is opened fully, Pruitt–Inahara shunts are connected to the bifurcated graft limbs. These shunts perfuse the celiac, superior mesenteric and renal arteries while the intercostal arteries are implanted to the posterior graft. **E,** The intercostal arteries are perfused before visceral and renal implantation. **F,** If necessary, a redundant section of the main graft is removed to avoid kinking or redundancy. (Courtesy of Lord RSA, Chao A, Sim E, et al: Ruptured thoracoabdominal aortic aneurysm repaired with minimal aortic occlusion time and continuous visceral perfusion—a new technique. *Cardiovasc Surg* 8:173-180, 2000. Reproduced with permission from *Cardiovascular Surgery*. Copyright 2000 Elsevier Science Inc.)

Conclusion.—The new technique is simple and inexpensive, requires no complex equipment, minimizes ischemic times, and avoids dissection and axillofemoral bypass, thereby lessening the period of left ventricular strain.

▶ In recent years, there has been a growing consensus that prolonged periods of visceral ischemia are the source of many of the complications of thoracoabdominal aneurysm repair. This article describes a clever technique of maintaining visceral perfusion during surgery for thoracoabdominal aneurysm without the use of extracorporeal shunts or extra-anatomical bypass. There is no doubt that Dr Stanley Crawford's development of the inclusion/ clamp-and-go technique of thoracoabdominal aneurysm repair was a major advance. However, most surgeons cannot duplicate Dr Crawford's technical expertise. The technique detailed in this article is essentially a variant of the old pick-off operation for thoracoabdominal aneurysm repair. For many surgeons, techniques such as this will be more appropriate than the Crawford inclusion technique for thoracoabdominal aneurysm.

G. L. Moneta, MD

Aortic Fenestration for Acute or Chronic Aortic Dissection: An Uncommon but Effective Procedure

Panneton JM, Teh SH, Cherry KJ Jr, et al (Mayo Clinic and Mayo Found, Rochester, Minn)

J Vasc Surg 32:711-721, 2000   6–2

Objective.—Aortic fenestration is rarely performed because of renal complications; it may aid management of vascular complications after aortic dissection. How often and under what circumstances aortic fenestration is indicated in these patients, its safety and efficacy at relieving organ or limb malperfusion, and its long-term durability and the risk for late aortic complications were retrospectively reviewed.

Methods.—From January 1, 1979, to December 31, 1999, 321 of 857 patients with aortic dissection underwent surgical intervention. Fourteen patients (12 men), aged 43 to 81 years, of 81 patients (25%) with malperfusion had aortic fenestration. All patients had hypertension and a smoking history. There were 3 Stanford type A dissections and 11 type B dissections. There were 7 patients with acute dissection and 7 with chronic dissection. In the acute dissection group, 6 patients had malperfusion including ischemia of the lower limb (n = 4, bilateral in 3), renal ischemia (n = 5, anuria in 2), and bowel ischemia (n = 3). Four patients had abdominal aortic fenestration performed at the infrarenal level and 3 at the pararenal level (Fig 2). In the chronic dissection group, 3 patients had infrarenal abdominal aortic aneurysms (AAAs) (2 symptomatic and 1 enlarging), 1 had an enlarging pararenal AAA, 1 had a symptomatic thoracoabdominal aortic aneurysm, 2 had bilateral lower limb claudication, 1 had left renal ischemia, and 1 had severe refractory renovascular hypertension.

Results.—All 10 patients with malperfusion syndrome had relief, and 11 of 14 patients (79%) survived. Three of 7 acute dissection patients (43%) died 3 to 44 days after surgery. Four chronic dissection patients with malperfusion syndrome had complete relief. Two patients required reoperation because of complications. Patients' status was followed for an average of 5.1 years, and all remained symptom-free. No evidence of aneurysmal formation was evident at follow-up in all 10 patients who underwent imaging studies during follow-up. One patient had a large proximal descending thoracic aneurysm at 12.2 years. Two patients died at 7.8 and 12.4 years, with 1 intraoperatively while undergoing exploration for postoperative bleeding after proximal descending thoracic aneurysm repair at another institution.

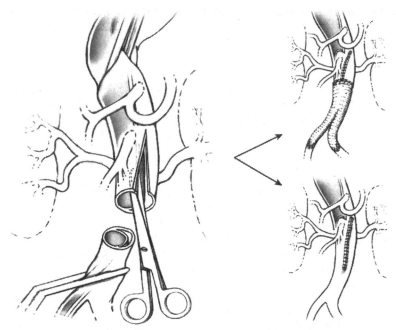

FIGURE 2.—Schematic drawing of aortic fenestration showing infrarenal aortic transection with cephalad pararenal aortotomy and resection of the septum between the false and true lumens (*left*). Pararenal fenestration was followed by infrarenal aortic replacement with an aortobi-iliac graft (*top right*) or primary closure without graft replacement (*bottom right*). (Courtesy of Panneton JM, Teh SH, Cherry KJ Jr, et al: Aortic fenestration for acute or chronic aortic dissection: An uncommon but effective procedure. *J Vasc Surg* 32:711-721, 2000.)

Conclusion.—Aortic fenestration can correct malperfusion syndrome caused by aortic branch vessel compromise after aortic dissection.

▶ While urgent surgical repair of aortic dissection was popular in the late 1960s and early 1970s, enthusiasm for this approach rapidly declined as poor mortality figures were realized. Frequently cited reasons for the high mortality rate include ischemia time and friability of the aortic wall. We now employ endovascular fenestration techniques to deal with ischemic complications of acute and chronic dissection, with lower morbidity and mortality than with operative repair. Whenever possible, we reserve operative intervention for aneurysms; but with the advent of endoaortic stent grafts, operations for dissection-related aneurysms may also decline.

W. K. Williamson, MD

Disappearance of Aortic Intramural Hematoma and Its Significance to the Prognosis

Nishigami K, Tsuchiya T, Shono H, et al (Saiseikai Kumamoto Hosp, Japan)
Circulation 102[suppl III]:III-243–III-247, 2000   6–3

Objective.—An aortic intramural hematoma (IMH), a form of aortic dissection (AD), can progress to a full-fledged AD with fatal consequences. How an IMH progresses and the significance of disappearance of IMH is not known. Short-term changes in an IMH were investigated with the use of transesophageal echocardiography.

Methods.—From January 1993 to December 1996, 44 patients with AD (30 men), aged 48 to 84 years, were treated medically with intravenous and, later, oral antihypertensive agents until systolic blood pressure was less than 120 mm Hg. Transesophageal echocardiography was performed at baseline and at 6 months in 41 patients. The maximum aortic diameter and the maximum size of the IMH were measured at the level of the maximum size of the hematoma. Patients were divided into 2 groups: those in whom IMH disappeared and those in whom it persisted. Patients' status was followed for an average of 1552 days. Survival, occurrence of aortic dissection, and progressive aortic dilatation requiring surgical intervention were compared for the 2 groups.

Results.—IMHs disappeared in 8 patients at 1 month. Three of the remaining 36 patients experienced aortic dissection at 36, 40, and 44 days. An additional 13 IMHs disappeared at 6 months. Patients with IMHs that disappeared were younger than those with persistent IMHs (64 vs 72) and had significantly smaller maximum aortic diameters (33 mm vs 42 mm). IMHs that disappeared did not recur, and surgery was not required. AD occurred in 2 patients at 7 and 11 months, necessitating surgery, and progressive dilatation occurred in 2 additional patients at 12 and 24 months. Cardiovascular event-free rates in the disappearance and persistence groups were 100% and 80% at 3 years.

Conclusion.—The IMH disappearance rate at 6 months was 48%. These patients appear to have a good prognosis.

▶ IMH is a form of AD that is benign in some patients but progresses to frank AD in others. Determining in which patients IMH can be safely treated medically remains unclear. This study gives us some guidance in this matter. Patients in whom the IMH resolved within a month and whose aorta was less than 45 mm in diameter were less likely to have later development of AD. Interestingly, this was true in both type A and B dissections. In patients with large aortas and those with IMHs that persisted past 1 month, overt dissection or progressive AD developed.

J. M. Edwards, MD

Mycotic Aneurysms of the Thoracic and Abdominal Aorta and Iliac Arteries: Experience With Anatomic and Extra-anatomic Repair in 33 Cases

Müller BT, Wegener OR, Grabitz K, et al (Heinrich-Heine Univ, Düsseldorf, Germany)
J Vasc Surg 33:106-113, 2001   6–4

Background.—The term "mycotic aneurysm" applies to any type of infected aneurysm. Treatment of life-threatening mycotic aneurysms of the aorta and adjacent arteries poses challenging problems, whether through in situ replacement or extra-anatomical reconstruction. Patient outcomes may be poor even when the repair is successful. An 18-year experience with treatment of mycotic aneurysms was reported.

Methods.—Of 2520 patients undergoing surgical replacement for aneurysms of the thoracic/abdominal aorta and iliac arteries from 1983 through 1999, 33 had mycotic aneurysms, a rate of 1.31%. The patients' mean age was 64.3 years. The aneurysms involved the lower descending and thoracoabdominal aorta for 13 patients, the suprarenal aorta for 4, and the infrarenal aorta for 10 (Table 2). The iliac arteries were involved for 6 cases. Sixty-one percent of patients had various septic diseases, although no cause was apparent for the remaining 39%. Twenty-four percent of the aneurysms had ruptured by the time of surgery, while 61% had penetrated the periaortic tissues. Only 15% were completely intact. The most common infecting organisms were *Staphylococcus aureus* and *Salmonella* spp.

Each patient underwent careful debridement of infected tissue. In situ reconstruction in the infrarenal aortic and iliac vascular bed was done only for patients with "low-grade" infection. Eight of 16 such cases were managed with extra-anatomical reconstructions. In situ repair was performed in all suprarenal and thoracoabdominal aortic aneurysms. All patients received antibiotics preoperatively and for an extended period after repair.

TABLE 2.—Location of Mycotic Aneurysm

Location	No. of Patients	%
Iliac artery	6	18.2
Aorta abdominal	14	42.4
Infrarenal	10	
Suprarenal	4	
Aorta thoracoabdominal	13	39.4
TAA I	4	
TAA II	1	
TAA III	1	
TAA IV	7	

Abbreviation: TAA, thoracic aortic aneurysm.
(Courtesy of Müller BT, Wegener OR, Grabitz K, et al: Mycotic aneurysms of the thoracic and abdominal aorta and iliac arteries: Experience with anatomic and extra-anatomic repair in 33 cases. *J Vasc Surg* 33:106-113, 2001.)

Survival Function

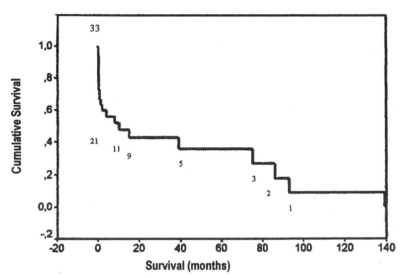

FIGURE 3.—Kaplan-Meier survival analysis. (Courtesy of Müller BT, Wegener OR, Grabitz K, et al: Mycotic aneurysms of the thoracic and abdominal aorta and iliac arteries: Experience with anatomic and extra-anatomic repair in 33 cases. *J Vasc Surg* 33:106-113, 2001.)

Results.—Thirty-six percent of the patients died in the hospital. The small size of the sample precluded analysis of the prognostic importance of aneurysm type or location or type of reconstruction. Patients with ruptured aneurysms were clearly at a higher risk of death. At a mean follow-up of 30 months, 10 of the 21 surviving patients had died. However, only one of these deaths was thought to result from the mycotic aneurysm. Eleven patients were alive and free of signs of persistent or recurrent infection (Fig 3).

Conclusion.—This experience highlights the seriousness of mycotic aneurysms of the aortic iliac region. The outlook is particularly bad for patients with ruptured aneurysms. Despite the septic content of the aneurysmal sac, in situ reconstruction is feasible for most patients, even for aneurysms in the suprarenal and thoracoabdominal aorta. Diagnosing myotic aneurysms before rupture would likely reduce the high operative mortality rate.

▶ This article contains an especially challenging subgroup of 13 patients with thoracoabdominal mycotic aneurysms. All patients were treated by aneurysm resection and in situ prosthetic grafting (9 by tube, 4 by patch). The overall operative mortality rate in this subgroup was 38%, which is high but still respectable considering the serious nature of the surgical problem and the fact that prosthetic graft material was used in an infected field. Of note is the fact that the surgeons soaked their gelatin-sealed Dacron grafts in rifampin and also utilized gentamicin-soaked gauze to tamponade the pseudoaneurysm cavity. The authors also recommend extensive debridement of all infected tissue and the use of culture-specific antibiotics for at least 3 months. These results, as well as others in the literature, provide some basis for hope of recovery when surgeons are required to use prosthetic graft material in an infected field.

R. A. Yeager, MD

Distal Thoracic Aorta as Inflow for the Treatment of Chronic Mesenteric Ischemia

Farber MA, Carlin RE, Marston WA, et al (Univ of North Carolina, Chapel Hill)
J Vasc Surg 33:281-288, 2001   6–5

Background.—Traditionally, revascularization for chronic mesenteric ischemia (CMI) involves a transabdominal approach with antegrade or retrograde bypass grafts originating from the supraceliac or infrarenal aorta. However, for patients with abdominal disease or prior surgery that would complicate transperitoneal exposure, a better inflow source may be the distal thoracic aorta (DTA). The outcomes of patients undergoing CMI

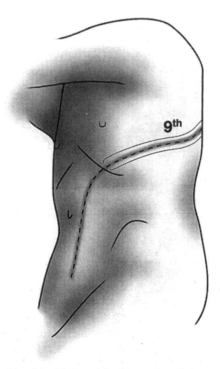

FIGURE 1.—Patient positioned in right lateral decubitus position before undergoing thoracomesenteric bypass grafting. *Dashed line* shows intended location of incision. (Courtesy of Farber MA, Carlin RE, Marston WA, et al: Distal thoracic aorta as inflow for the treatment of chronic mesenteric ischemia. *J Vasc Surg* 33:281-288, 2001.)

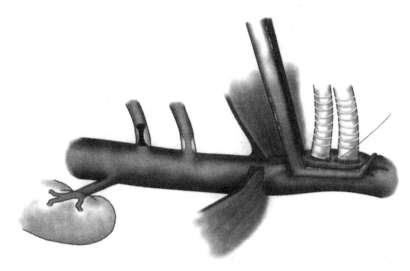

FIGURE 3.—Partial occlusion clamp placed on distal thoracic artery. Proximal graft anastomoses of individual grafts depicted. (Courtesy of Farber MA, Carlin RE, Marston WA, et al. Distal thoracic aorta as inflow for the treatment of chronic mesenteric ischemia. *J Vasc Surg* 33: 281-288, 2001.)

in which the DTA was used as the inflow source were retrospectively evaluated.

Methods.—Medical records for 1990 to 1999 were used to identify all patients with CMI who underwent mesenteric revascularization with a graft originating from the DTA. Presenting symptoms and outcomes were evaluated. The procedure used for thoracomesenteric bypass grafting with the DTA as inflow, in brief, is as follows. With the patient in the right lateral decubitus position, the thoracic and upper abdominal aorta were exposed via a ninth interspace thoracoretroperitoneal incision (Fig 1). The peritoneum and its contents were mobilized bluntly, and the diaphragm was incised to preserve innervation.

The inferior pulmonary ligament and the crus of the diaphragm were divided, and the celiac and superior mesenteric vessels were exposed to identify a suitable bypass graft site. The left kidney was left undisturbed, and distal aortic blood flow to the kidney and the spinal cord was maintained via a partial occlusion clamp technique (Fig 3). To minimize repeated trauma to the thoracic aorta, a single clamp was used for proximal anastomoses. Antegrade flow was established by routing prosthetic bypass graft conduits through the diaphragmatic hiatus to their respective vessels and performing end-to-side anastomoses. Duplex sonography was performed at regular intervals during follow-up to assess graft patency.

Results.—The 18 patients identified included 17 men and 1 woman ranging from 36 to 79 years of age (mean age, 64.4 years). At admission, all patients had chronic abdominal pain or weight loss; 2 patients with acute exacerbation of symptoms required urgent revascularization. All but 3 of the patients (83%) were smokers, and all but 3 (83%) had hypertension. A total of 33 vessels were reconstructed, including the superior mesenteric artery in all patients and the celiac artery as well in 3 patients (17%). During surgery, 1 patient died of multiorgan failure; both bypass grafts were patent. Three other patients (17%) also had a major complication, including 2 cases of myocardial infarction and 1 case of respiratory failure requiring intubation. However, none of the patients experienced kidney failure, spinal cord ischemia, or mesenteric infarction. During a mean follow-up of 34.8 months, all patients remained free of symptoms, and graft patency was 100%. Life-table survival rates at 1, 3, and 5 years were 89%, 89%, and 76%, respectively.

Conclusion.—Antegrade mesenteric revascularization of CMI using the DTA as inflow was associated with low morbidity and mortality rates. Midterm graft patency was excellent, with no thrombolytic complications. Survival was also excellent and was limited by other comorbid conditions. Thus, this technique should be considered a primary approach for the surgical treatment of CMI.

▶ These authors present excellent results for visceral revascularization utilizing the DTA as inflow. This approach seems quite reasonable for those familiar with the thoracoabdominal approach and is an extension of this group's experience with thoracobifemoral bypass. A mortality rate of 6% and long-term objective patency of 100% in this small series compare favorably with results from other groups. The thoracic aorta should be kept in mind as an inflow site, and grafts similar to these have been employed for visceral revascularization during repair of thoracoabdominal aortic aneurysms.[1] Dr Porter's group recently reported their isolated superior mesenteric artery bypass series with predominately retrograde grafts with results similar to this current report.[2] In visceral revascularization, antegrade versus retrograde and single versus multiple bypasses continue to be dealer's choice.

A. M. Abou-Zamzam, Jr, MD

References

1. 2000 YEAR BOOK OF VASCULAR SURGERY, pp 271-273.
2. Foley MI, Moneta GL, Abou-Zamzam AM Jr, et al: Revascularization of the superior mesenteric artery alone for treatment of intestinal ischemia. *J Vasc Surg* 32:37-47, 2000.

7 Aortic Aneurysm

Aneurysm Screening

Psychological Consequences of Screening for Abdominal Aortic Aneurysm and Conservative Treatment of Small Abdominal Aortic Aneurysms
Lindholt JS, Vammen S, Fasting H, et al (Hosp of Viborg, Denmark)
Eur J Vasc Endovasc Surg 20:79-83, 2000   7–1

Background.—Medical screening programs are associated with certain disadvantages, including reduction in quality of life, personal economic costs, and psychological consequences. This study assessed the possible psychological impact of a screening program for abdominal aortic aneurysms (AAAs).

Methods.—The case-control study included a random sample of elderly men participating in a randomized trial of AAA screening. A quality-of-life questionnaire was completed by 168 subjects who did not respond to screening (response rate, 48%); 271 attenders before screening was carried out (response rate, 81%); 286 attenders after screening was performed (response rate, 85%); 127 subjects with a diagnosis of a small AAA at screening (response rate, 85%); and 231 control subjects who were randomly assigned to the nonscreening group (response rate, 66%).

Results.—Compared with controls, the men with small AAAs had an initial 5% reduction in quality-of-life score, largely resulting from a perception of poorer health. During conservative therapy, there was a further decline to 7% below control scores, mainly related to changes in scores for perceived health and psychosomatic distress. For 29 men who underwent surgery, all scores improved to control levels. For attending men, quality-of-life scores before screening were significantly lower than for control men and lower than for attending men after screening.

Conclusions.—Men invited to a screening program who turn out not to have AAA show a temporary increase in psychological distress. For patients with a diagnosis of AAA, conservative treatment is associated with a persistent and progressive reduction in quality of life. This impairment may be reversed after surgery. The psychological impact should be considered in evaluations of screening and treatment for AAA.

▶ I continue to be amazed with the multiple factors that may be involved with the natural history of AAAs. In this small series of patients with aneurysms less than 5 cm, follow-up revealed that the growth rate of thrombus area was the most predictive factor of whether the aneurysm ruptured. More interestingly, those patients without thrombus did not have aneurysmal rupture during follow-up. The authors allude to possible patho-physiologic mechanisms including the possibility that plasminogen, which is bound to clot, could be activated to plasmin, which then activates matrix metalloproteinases. These enzymes have been associated with possible increased proteolytic activity and aneurysm rupture. Other mechanisms include the possibility of thrombus causing arterial wall anoxia or increased turbulent flow, which then causes aneurysm wall weakening. An improvement in determining whether thrombus load is truly associated with an increased incidence of rupture would be to use 3-dimensional reconstructions of CT scans. The increased use of endografting for aneurysm repair has led to computer software that could allow for this calculation. Furthermore, a larger series is needed with the specific goal of following up these parameters of aneurysm morphology and their association with growth rates and rupture.

R. B. McLafferty, MD

Yield of Repeated Screening for Abdominal Aortic Aneurysm After a 4-Year Interval

Lederle FA, and the Aneurysm Detection and Management Veterans Affairs Cooperative Study Investigators (Veterans Affairs Med Ctr, Minneapolis; et al)
Arch Intern Med 160:1117-1121, 2000   7–2

Objective.—Most studies of US screening for abdominal aortic aneurysms (AAAs) have found a cost benefit, but the optimal design of a screening program has not been determined. The yield of a second US screening for AAAs in a screening population was investigated.

Methods.—A subset (n = 5151) of 16,643 initially screened veterans, aged 50 to 80 years, with no history of AAA, was invited for a second screening 4 years later, between December 1996 and July 1997. Records and databases were searched for deaths and diagnoses of AAA for all those who were not rescreened.

Results.—There were 598 deaths (11.6%). Of 558 death records located, none listed AAA as the cause of death. A second screening was performed on 2622 (50.9%), 20 (0.4%) of whom had an interim diagnosis of AAA. Of those rescreened, 58 had new AAAs. Three were 4.0 to 4.9 cm, 10 were 3.5 to 3.9 cm, and 45 were 3.0 to 3.4 cm. Univariate predictors of a new AAA were a history of smoking (odds ratio, [OR], 2.20), number of years smoking (OR, 1.26), current smoker at initial screening (OR, 3.31), and coronary artery disease (OR, 1.73). When the model was reanalyzed to include any atherosclerosis, this variable was also a significant predictor (OR, 1.93). Mutivariate predictors included current smoking (OR, 3.09) and coronary artery disease (OR, 1.81). Atherosclerosis was predictive in all models (OR, 1.97). Combining the initial and re-screening diagnosis rates gives a 4-year AAA incidence rate of 2.6%.

Conclusion.—A second rescreening is of little value after 4 years. Re-screening only those with AAAs of 2.5 cm or larger would have missed more than two thirds of new AAAs.

▶ The fruit is continuing to ripen in the VA Aneurysm Detection and Management (ADAM) study. This study looks at the results of aneurysm re-screening after an initial negative duplex examination. At 4 years after an initial negative screening evaluation, the incidence of subsequent aneurysm formation was 2.6%, slightly greater than half of the 4.6% incidence at the time of initial screening. All of the aneurysms detected at the time of the second examination were small (< 4.9 cm), suggesting that rescreening at 4 years is likely not cost effective. However, subjects with an initial negative screening examination clearly cannot be given a lifelong bill of health, and screening at longer intervals may be warranted. The ADAM study was extremely well designed and run and will continue to provide us with valuable information about AAAs in the years to come.

G. J. Landry, MD

The Aneurysm Detection and Management Study Screening Program: Validation Cohort and Final Results
Lederle FA, and the Aneurysm Detection and Management Veterans Affairs Cooperative Study Investigators (Veterans Affairs Med Ctr, Minneapolis; et al)
Arch Intern Med 160:1425-1430, 2000   7–3

Objective.—The prevalence and associations of abdominal aortic aneurysms (AAAs) in 73,451 veterans, aged 50 to 79 years, who underwent US screening were previously reported. The final results of the Aneurysm Detection and Management (ADAM) study screening program of the Department of Veterans Affairs have been reported, and previous findings have been validated by comparing them with those obtained from patients undergoing screening after the first report.

Methods.—US screening was performed on a second cohort of 52,745 veterans, aged 50 to 79 years, with no history of AAA. Most had a history of smoking.

Results.—AAA was diagnosed in 1917 (3.6%) veterans. The AAA diameter was 4.0 cm or larger in 613 (1.2%) of the subjects. According to multivariate analysis, the odds ratios for factors associated with an AAA diameter of at least 4.0 cm versus a normal infrarenal aortic diameter for the combined group compared with the second cohort were respectively, age (1.71 vs 1.81), female sex (0.18 vs 0.12), black race (0.53 vs 0.59), family history (1.94 vs 1.94), smoking (5.07 vs 4.45), high cholesterol level (1.44 vs 1.29), hypertension (1.15 vs 1.14), diabetes (0.52 vs 0.50), and atherosclerosis (1.66 vs 0.60). Associations for AAAs smaller than 4.0 cm were weaker but similar.

Conclusion.—The AAA prevalences were lower in the second cohort than in the first, but the magnitude and direction of the associations were similar with age, male sex, and smoking being the strongest associations.

▶ The ADAM investigators have compiled 2 cohorts of veterans with AAA to give a database of 126,196 patients with AAA. The authors point out that combining these cohorts may yield misleading data, as the prevalence of AAA between the two are different, perhaps because of changes in screening practices. However, even when disregarding the combined results, a clear association between age, male sex, and family history of AAA and detection of AAA on screening is seen. Interestingly, a previously thought association between chronic obstructive pulmonary disease and AAA does not appear in this study. The data presented provide an important framework for designing AAA screening programs, an issue of important national health care concern.

W. K. Williamson, MD

Population Screening Reduces Mortality Rate From Aortic Aneurysm in Men
Heather BP, Poskitt KR, Earnshaw JJ, et al (Gloucestershire Royal Hosp, Gloucester, England; Cheltenham Gen Hosp, England)
Br J Surg 87:750-753, 2000   7–4

Background.—A significant cause of death in men older than 65 years is rupture of an abdominal aortic aneurysm (AAA). AAA rupture is estimated to account for 1.4% of all deaths among men in this age group and is thought to be responsible for about 6000 deaths annually in England and Wales. Overall mortality rates for AAA rupture range from 80% to 94%, but many surgical units have reported mortality rates for elective AAA repair of less than 5%. This striking difference between the elective surgical mortality rate and the outcome for AAA rupture strongly suggests that only a policy of screening for asymptomatic aneurysm and an increased rate of elective aneurysm repair will bring about a reduction in the overall mortality rate from AAA rupture. The results of a screening program in 1 county in the United Kingdom were presented.

Methods.—A screening program for unsuspected abdominal aortic aneurysm has been conducted since 1990 in Gloucestershire, England among men aged 65 years and older. Changes in the mortality rate from aortic aneurysm in the screened portion of the population were investigated. From computerized death certificate records and hospital and postmortem records, the total number of deaths from all AAA-related causes in the county were calculated for the years 1994 to 1998. The overall number of deaths related to aneurysm in men aged 65 to 73 years and who have been

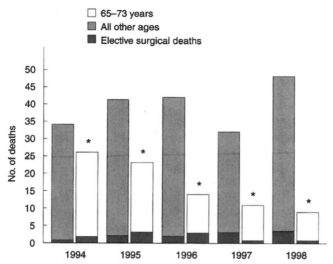

FIGURE 2.—Total number of aneurysm-related deaths in men in Gloucestershire, 1994 to 1998. *Asterisk* indicates $P < 0.001$ (χ^2 test for trend). (Courtesy of Heather BP, Poskitt KR, Earnshaw JJ, et al: Population screening reduces mortality rate from aortic aneurysm in men. *Br J Surg* 87:750-753, 2000. Blackwell Science Ltd.)

participants in the screening program was compared with the number of aneurysm-related deaths for men of all other ages.

Results.—There was a progressive annual reduction in the total number of aneurysm-related deaths in men from 65 to 73 years of age between 1994 and 1998 (Fig 2). The reduction was statistically significant. No such reduction in aneurysm-related deaths was seen in the unscreened portion of the population.

Conclusion.—The screening of men 65 years of age and older for asymptomatic AAA rupture has resulted in a significant reduction in the mortality from all aneurysm-related causes in the portion of the male population in whom the screening was conducted.

▶ Screening for AAAs in patients at risk seems like a good idea. After all, rupture of AAA is a significant cause of death among elderly men. Screening is, however, controversial. One must always ask when screening an elderly population whether the number of years of life saved is worth the cost. In addition, a screening program will only be effective if treatment can be done with minimum morbidity and mortality. It is important to keep in mind that most patients with AAAs do not die of their aneurysms. Finally, patients who come in for screening may be the ones least likely to have the problem in the first place. This is likely to reduce the overall effect of the screening program. Screening programs for relatively low-prevalence conditions in elderly populations will remain controversial. Given the concerns regarding such programs, I suspect that despite the data presented in this article, the fiscal authorities will remain reluctant to provide reimbursement for purely screening examinations.

G. L. Moneta, MD

Management

Management of Synchronous Renal Neoplasm and Abdominal Aortic Aneurysm
Hafez KS, El Fettouh HA, Novick AC, et al (Cleveland Clinic Found, Ohio)
J Vasc Surg 32:1102-1110, 2000   7–5

Background.—Sometimes a patient will be seen with a renal neoplasm (RN) and an abdominal aortic aneurysm (AAA) at the same time. The debate regarding how best to manage these synchronous problems is ongoing. An experience of 50 patients with concurrent RNs, and AAAs is reviewed.

Methods.—The patients were treated at 1 center over an 18-year period. Twenty-three patients had small, asymptomatic AAAs or metastatic renal involvement, for which they received conservative management. The remaining 27 patients underwent staged or simultaneous surgery for both problems.

Results.—The mean AAA diameter in the surgical group was 6.0 cm. Forty-one percent of patients underwent radical nephrectomies and 37% had partial nephrectomies. In 22% of patients, both radical and partial nephrectomies were performed because of bilateral renal tumors. The timing of AAA surgery was at the same time as the renal surgery in 41% of patients, before in 48%, and after in 11%. In 89% of patients, AAA repair was carried out through an open approach, although 3 patients in the latter part of the series underwent endovascular AAA repair with staged partial nephrectomies.

There was a 23% rate of major complications, including 3 cases of acute renal failure, 2 cases of acute respiratory failure, and 1 case each of a pulmonary embolism and a stroke. At 5 years' follow-up, the overall survival rate was 62%, and the cancer-specific survival rate was 81%. The cancer-specific survival rate was significantly better for patients undergoing simultaneous versus staged surgery: 80% versus 35%, respectively.

Conclusions.—This experience encourages simultaneous treatment of synchronous RNs and AAAs. Many patients undergoing simultaneous surgery will be long-term survivors. Endovascular AAA repair is a promising new option for these patients.

▶ In my practice, we find 1 or 2 renal neoplasms in the course of evaluating patients for atherosclerotic disease. Deciding the sequence of treatment can be difficult, and I rarely elect to treat them simultaneously. The Cleveland Clinic has elected to perform simultaneous repair of AAAs and partial or radical nephrectomies in just fewer than one half of patients who had both AAAs they felt were large enough to fix and resectable renal tumors. The incidence of complications was similar in patients with staged and combined operations. The authors also note that recently they have begun using endovascular AAA repair for staged procedures. They fail to convince me that a combined operation is preferable to a staged operation, and I think I will continue to recommend separate operations.

J. M. Edwards, MD

Watchful Waiting in Cases of Small Abdominal Aortic Aneurysms—Appropriate for All Patients?

Valentine RJ, DeCaprio JD, Castillo JM, et al (Univ of Texas Southwestern Med Ctr, Dallas; Dept of Veterans Affairs North Texas Health Care System, Dallas)
J Vasc Surg 32:441-450, 2000   7–6

Background.—The low risk of rupture for abdominal aortic aneurysms (AAAs) smaller than 5 cm have prompted many clinicians to adopt a watchful waiting program (WWP) approach for such patients, using serial radiologic measures until the AAA meets size or growth criteria for repair. However, in clinical settings, follow-up of patients with such AAAs may not be complete. The impact of incomplete follow-up in WWPs has not been assessed. The effect of patient compliance with WWPs was investigated.

Methods.—One hundred one men at a regional Veterans Medical Center were studied. All had AAAs of less than 5 cm and no medical contraindications to operative repair. The mean follow-up was 34 months.

Findings.—Sixty-nine percent of the patients were fully compliant with the WWP, undergoing a mean 4.5 radiologic tests. In this subgroup, no AAA ruptures occurred. Thirty-six percent of these patients had indications for AAA repair, and 41% did not meet criteria for repair. Prohibitive medical risks developed in 23% of the compliant patients during follow-up. Half of these patients died, all from causes unrelated to AAA. Of the 32 noncompliant patients, 84% did not keep any scheduled appointments, and 16% were lost to follow-up after 1 or 2 examinations. AAA ruptures were documented in 3 noncompliant patients, and a rupture was suspected in a fourth. Compliant and noncompliant patients did not differ in mean age, distance from home to the hospital, or AAA size at initial detection.

Conclusions.—WWPs rely heavily on patient compliance. Among compliant patients, WWPs are feasible, as fewer than half of the patients will meet criteria for intervention within a mean of 3 years. In this series, however, one third of the candidates for WWPs are unable to participate and are at risk of ruptures.

▶ It seems that the so-called noncompliant patients and their primary care physicians require some education concerning the natural history of small aneurysms. The authors suggest that perhaps a phone call to the patient might help. I support that idea. On the other hand, considering the disappointing 8.3% perioperative mortality rate associated with elective aneurysm repair in this small series, maybe the "noncompliant" patients are better informed than we think.

R. A. Yeager, MD

Endoleaks Following Conventional Open Abdominal Aortic Aneurysm Repair
Chan CLH, Ray SA, Taylor PR, et al (Guy's & St Thomas' NHS Trust, London; King's College Hosp, London)
Eur J Vasc Endovasc Surg 19:313-317, 2000   7–7

Background.—Many patients with infrarenal abdominal aortic aneurysm undergo the endovascular implantation of a stent-graft prosthesis. However, leakage of contrast material outside the graft but within the aneurysmal sac is a well-documented complication of this approach. The case of 6 patients with endoleaks after conventional open repair of abdominal aortic aneurysm were reported, and their treatment and outcomes were described.

Case Reports.—The 6 patients (all men) ranged in age from 58 to 80 years. All underwent successful elective or emergent open repair of abdominal aortic aneurysm. Primary repair was accomplished with woven Dacron polyester fabric grafts secured with 3'0' Prolene sutures at both the proximal and distal ends. Then, from 1 to 18 months later, the patients returned with back or abdominal pain or hypotension. CT and digital subtraction angiography identified contrast material leaks at the distal anastomosis in 5 patients (Fig 2) and at the proximal anastomosis in 1. Surgical repair was successful and involved resuturing the defect in 4 cases and replacing the Dacron graft in 2. There was no evidence of infection. None of the patients had further complications during 6 months to 5 years of follow-up.

Conclusion.—Endoleaks can occur after open repair as well as stent grafting in patients with abdominal aortic aneurysm. Patients in whom back or abdominal pain develops within 18 months of open repair should be evaluated for an endoleak by CT and digital subtraction angiography.

▶ Endoleaks? These authors describe what sounds like 6 cases of anastomotic pseudoaneurysms after open abdominal aortic aneurysm repair. The pseudoaneurysms just happened to be contained within the old aneurysm sac. (For the claim that such pseudoaneurysms have not been previously described, I suspect J.P. would present these authors the CDA.)

A. M. Abou-Zamzam, Jr, MD

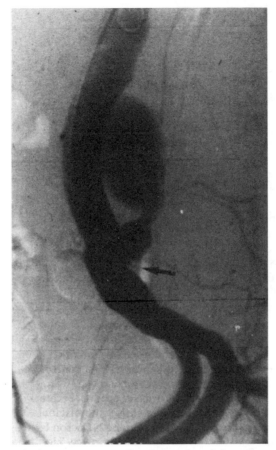

FIGURE 2.—Digital subtraction angiogram (lateral view) shows leakage of contrast from the anastomotic suture line (*black arrow*). (Reprinted from the *European Journal of Vascular and Endovascular Surgery* courtesy of Chan CLH, Ray SA, Taylor PR, et al: Endoleaks following conventional open abdominal aortic aneurysm repair. *Eur J Vasc Endovasc Surg* 19:313-317, 2000. Copyright 2000, by permission of the publisher, WB Saunders Company Limited London.)

Ruptured Aneurysm

Aneurysm Rupture Is Independently Associated With Increased Late Mortality in Those Surviving Abdominal Aortic Aneurysm Repair

Kazmers A, Perkins AJ, Jacobs LA (Wayne State Univ, Detroit; Dept of Veterans Affairs, Ann Arbor, Mich; Univ of Michigan, Ann Arbor)
J Surg Res 95:50-53, 2001   7–8

Introduction.—Survival improvements after elective abdominal aortic aneurysm (AAA) repair justify an increasingly aggressive approach in patients with intact AAAs. Similar improvements in survival have not been observed for patients undergoing repair of ruptured AAAs. Most trials analyzing survival after AAA repair have been restricted to the immediate postoperative period. Late survival was compared in patients who survived repair of intact AAAs versus those who had repair of ruptured AAAs.

Methods.—The VA Patient Treatment File (PTF) was used to identify all patients who underwent AAA repair in diagnosis related groups 110 and 111 at all Veterans Affairs Medical Centers during fiscal 1991-1995. Late mortality was determined using VA administration databases. Illness severity and patient complexity were determined using PTF discharge data that were further assessed via patient management software. Follow-up was as long as 6 years after AAA repair. Operative mortality was considered death within 30 days of surgery or during the hospitalization in which the AAA was repaired.

Results.—Elective and ruptured AAAs were repaired in 5833 and 427 patients, respectively. For patients undergoing elective AAA repair, the operative mortality rate was 4.5% (265/5833); for patients with ruptured AAAs, it was 46% (195/427). Overall mortality during a mean of 2.62 years of follow-up, including operative mortality, was 22% (1282/5833) and 65% (260/427), respectively, for patients with intact and ruptured AAAs (*P* < .001). In patients who survived AAA repair and lived 30 days or more after surgery, 28% (65/232) who initially survived repair of rupture and 18% (1017/5568) of those who survived intact repair died during follow-up (*P* < .001). Stepwise logistic regression revealed that increasing age, illness severity, patient complexity, and AAA rupture and graft complications were increasingly and independently correlated with late mortality in patients who initially survived AAA repair. The mean

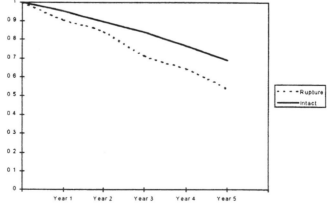

FIGURE 1.—In those who initially survived abdominal aortic aneurysm repair, overall mortality was related to aneurysm rupture. Mean survival time was 1681 days for those who survived 30 or more days after surgery and who were discharged alive after repair of ruptured AAA versus 1821 days for those who initially survived repair of intact AAA (*P* < .001). (Courtesy of Kazmers A, Perkins AJ, Jacobs LA: Aneurysm rupture is independently associated with increased late mortality in those surviving abdominal aortic aneurysm repair. *J Surg Res* 95:50-53, 2001.)

survival time was 1681 versus 1821 days, respectively, in patients who survived more than 30 days and who were discharged alive after repair of ruptured versus intact AAAs (*P* < .001) (Fig 1).

Conclusion.—Patients with repair of ruptured AAAs have higher mortality postoperatively and during long-term follow-up than those who undergo intact repairs.

▶ Despite the advances in information technology, our global understanding of many relevant clinical issues remains marginal. The current database consists of either more detailed aspects of care from selected centers, or global snapshots from large databases (Medicare, VA) that suffer from modest detail (usually *ICD-9* codes and mortality data) but are more representative of populations. With the advent of electronic medical records, this could potentially change. However, current pilot versions (at the Denver VA, for example) have most of the data in text format, which is completely useless for data query and analysis. In this regard, medicine lags far behind other major industries.

The above editorial aside, this study by Kazmers et al details the mortality outcomes of patients undergoing repair of ruptured AAAs from the multicenter VA database. Important findings were roughly a 50% operative mortality rate and approximately a 30% long-term mortality rate in the 1.6 mean years of follow-up. In addition, these patients had a 5% to 6% incidence of significant graft-related complications during the follow-up period. All of these values were markedly greater than observed in the elective AAA repair group. These data have implications on decision analysis models for risk-benefit of AAA repair. These data also imply a significant negative functional impact of repair of a ruptured AAA.

M. R. Nehler, MD

Randomized, Multicentre, Double-blind, Placebo-controlled Trial of the Use of Aprotinin in the Repair of Ruptured Abdominal Aortic Aneurysm
Robinson J, for the Joint Vascular Research Group (Northern Gen Hosp, Sheffield, England)
Br J Surg 87:754-757, 2000   7–9

Background.—Repair of ruptured abdominal aortic aneurysm (AAA) has typical associated operative mortality rates of 41% to 57%. The mortality rate for this procedure has remained high despite a higher proportion of operations being performed by vascular surgeons and improvements in intensive care facilities. The survival of patients undergoing repair of AAA rupture is affected by comorbidity, postoperative complications, excessive blood loss, and the need for multiple blood products. Of the patients who die in intensive care, most do so after coagulopathy and after initiation of the systemic inflammatory response initiates a downward spiral of multiple-organ failure.

TABLE 3.—Blood Products Transfused During and After Surgery for Ruptured Abdominal Aortic Aneurysm

	Aprotinin	Placebo	P
Perioperative transfusion (units)			
Blood	7 (0-20)	10 (2-32)	n.s.
FFP	2 (0-40)	4 (0-12)	n.s.
Platelets	0 (0-12)	0 (0-10)	n.s.
Postoperative transfusion (units)			
Blood	1 (0-14)	3 (0-13)	0·02
FFP	2 (0-22)	0 (0-10)	n.s.
Platelets	0 (0-24)	0 (0-12)	n.s.
Total transfusion (units)			
Blood	10 (2-29)	14 (4-38)	0·053
FFP	4 (0-69)	4 (0-19)	n.s.
Platelets	0 (0-36)	6 (0-18)	n.s.

Note: Values are median (range). Statistical test used: Kruskal-Wallis.
Abbreviations: FFP, Fresh frozen plasma; *n.s.*, not significant.
(Courtesy of Robinson J, for the Joint Vascular Research Group: Randomized, multicentre, double-blind, placebo-controlled trial of the use of aprotinin in the repair of ruptured abdominal aortic aneurysm. *Br J Surg* 87:754-757, 2000. Publisher, Blackwell Science Ltd.)

Aprotonin has been shown to preserve platelet function, inhibit plasmin and kallikrein, and reduce the activation of neutrophils and complement, thereby inhibiting fibrinolysis. Aprotonin has also been used in the reduction of perioperative bleeding, and use of aprotonin has been associated with a significant decrease in blood transfusions during reoperative cardiac surgery. In elective repair of AAA, the use of aprotonin has been shown to reduce the blood loss in suction drains without reducing the total blood loss or transfusion requirement. The effects of aprotonin on morbidity and mortality rates and blood product requirements in patients undergoing emergency repair of a ruptured AAA were evaluated.

Methods.—In a prospective randomized trial involving 9 centers, 77 patients with a ruptured AAA received aprotonin (38 patients) or placebo (39 patients). The quantity of blood products transfused during operative repair and in the first 12 hours post surgery, the incidence of complications, the length of hospital stay, and mortality rates were noted.

Results.—There were 17 deaths among the 38 patients who received aprotonin and 17 deaths among the 39 patients who received placebo within the first 30 days post surgery, for an overall mortality rate of 44%. In the aprotonin group, the median amount of blood transfused after surgery was 1 unit; the placebo group required a median of 3 units (Table 3). The total number of units of blood transfused ranged from 2 to 29 for the aprotonin group compared with a range of 4 to 38 units for the placebo group. The difference was not statistically significant.

Conclusion.—High-dose aprotonin during operative repair of a ruptured AAA reduced blood transfusion requirements in the first 12 hours after surgery, but there was no significant reduction in the overall blood transfusion requirement.

▶ All vascular surgeons have had the misfortune of repairing a ruptured aneurysm with prompt hemorrhage control and graft insertion, only to be frustrated by profound and diffuse blood loss from the ensuing coagulopathy associated with a ruptured AAA. We have all craved a systemic treatment that can arrest this coagulopathy, allow prompt closure of the abdomen, and a prompt return to the ICU for ongoing resuscitation. Aprotinin, a nonspecific protease inhibitor, decreased perioperative bleeding in elective AAA repair and decreased transfusion requirements for reoperative cardiac surgery. The Joint Vascular Research Group hoped aprotinin would prove useful for treatment of ruptured AAA. Unfortunately, no significant decrease in overall blood transfusion requirements was realized, and this expensive agent cannot be routinely recommended in the treatment of ruptured AAA. It appears that early recognition and prompt intervention for ruptured AAA remain the best method of diminishing coagulopathy and hemorrhage from AAA. Perhaps the emerging use of endovascular stent-grafting for ruptured AAA will demonstrate a role in diminishing the perioperative coagulopathy associated with open repair of ruptured AAA.

E. J. Harris, Jr, MD

Miscellaneous

The Inflammatory Response Following Treatment of Abdominal Aortic Aneurysms: A Comparison Between Open Surgery and Endovascular Repair

Ødegård A, Lundbom J, Myhre HO, et al (Univ of Tromsø, Norway)
Eur J Vasc Endovasc Surg 19:536-544, 2000   7–10

Background.—Treatment for infrarenal abdominal aortic aneurysms (AAAs) is followed by a systemic inflammatory response. Endovascular AAA repair would be expected to produce a lesser inflammatory response than open surgical repair. Indicators of inflammatory response in patients undergoing endovascular AAA repair were compared with those in patients undergoing open surgical repair.

Methods.—The study included 20 patients undergoing AAA repair, 10 by open surgery and 10 by endovascular technique. Blood samples were obtained before, during, and after the procedure for measurement of various inflammatory markers.

Results.—The open surgery group had a longer hospital stay and were more likely to require blood transfusion than the endovascular group. Postoperative increases in interleukin-6 and C-reactive protein were greater in the open surgery group. Reductions in platelet count were noted after initial angiography in the endovascular group, and a greater reduction was noted before aortic cross-clamping in the open surgery group. The endovascular group also had a significant reduction in leukocyte count after initial angiography, but, thereafter, the count showed an increase. In the open surgery group, a similar increase in leukocyte count occurred after declamping. After initial angiography in the endovascular group and after declamping in the open surgery group, leukocyte and platelet degranulation products increased significantly. The were no or only small changes in complement activation products and in tumor necrosis factor-α.

Conclusions.—Endovascular AAA repair is less traumatic than open surgical repair, yet significant leukocyte and platelet activation still occurs. These effects may be related to administration of radiographic contrast material. Other potential contributors to the inflammatory response after endovascular AAA repair remain to be assessed.

▶ The study purports to show that operative stress (as measured by plasma levels of a variety of nonspecific acute-phase reactants) is similar between contemporary, nonrandomized cohorts of endovascularly excluded (ENDO) and open aortic aneurysm repair patients (OPEN). The timing of the rise in plasma markers in the ENDO group suggests a relationship to contrast infusion during the imaging portion of the procedure. The reproducibility and significance of these results are highly suspect, however, for the following reasons: (1) the volume of contrast used per procedure was twice that reported in large US series (300 mL); (2) although the hospital stay of the ENDO group was half that of the OPEN group, it still averaged 6 days, suggesting that issues other than 2 simple 2-inch transverse inguinal incisions were present in many if not most of the ENDO patients to prolong their hospital stays; and (3) considerably more patients in the OPEN group required periprocedural blood transfusion, suggesting if nothing else more hemodynamic insufficiency or instability during open repair. Since most contemporary endovascular AAA exclusions studies report mean hospital stays on the order of 1 to 3 days, the significance of elevated serum or plasma acute-phase reactants on the ultimate outcome of the exclusion procedure days, weeks, or months later is uncertain and probably trivial. Attempting to claim that the ENDO patient and the OPEN patient are equally stressed after standard procedures of comparable scale is a dubious and patently futile exercise—the real and enduring question regarding the ENDO patients is not how they recover from their procedure, but whether the aneurysm is in fact definitively treated by the initial procedure.

R. L. Dalman, MD

Incidence of Femoral and Popliteal Artery Aneurysms in Patients With Abdominal Aortic Aneurysms

Diwan A, Sarkar R, Stanley JC, et al (Univ of Michigan, Ann Arbor)
J Vasc Surg 31:863-869, 2000   7–11

Background.—Many patients with femoral or popliteal artery aneurysms are also found to have aortic abdominal aneurysms (AAAs). The incidence of extremity aneurysms in a group of patients with AAAs, and the etiologic implications of such a relationship were analyzed.

Methods.—During a 3-year period, 313 consecutive patients (251 men, 62 women), aged from 50 to 93 years, with AAAs underwent US scanning

TABLE 1.—Distribution of Aortic, Femoral, or Popliteal Aneurysms
(University of Michigan Series)

Aneurysm	No. of Patients
Aortic aneurysms	313
Femoral or popliteal artery aneurysms	36
Unilateral femoral artery aneurysms	11
Bilateral femoral artery aneurysm	1
Unilateral popliteal artery aneurysms	15
Bilateral popliteal artery aneurysms	4
Unilateral femoral + unilateral popliteal artery aneurysm	1
Unilateral femoral + bilateral popliteal artery aneurysms	2
Bilateral femoral + unilateral popliteal artery aneurysms	1
Bilateral femoral + bilateral popliteal artery aneurysms	1

(Courtesy of Diwan A, Sarkar R, Stanley JC, et al: Incidence of femoral and popliteal artery aneurysms in patients with abdominal aortic aneurysms. *J Vasc Surg* 31:863-869, 2000.)

to look for femoral and popliteal aneurysms. Etiologic risk factors for AAA patients with associated extremity aneurysms were compared with those without such extremity aneurysms as well as for a statewide series of AAA patients.

Results.—Fifty-one aneurysms of the femoral and popliteal arteries were found among 36 (14%) AAA patients, all of whom were men (Table 1). The incidence of such extremity aneurysms among men was 14%, compared with 0% among women. Only 1 (3%) of the 36 men with femoral or popliteal artery aneurysms had a family history of aneurysms compared with 23% of female patients. Thirty-nine percent of the men with extremity aneurysms had peripheral arterial occlusive disease compared with 9% of men without extremity aneurysms. Otherwise, the various groups of patients were similar in their etiologic risk factors.

Conclusions.—A high rate of femoral and popliteal aneurysms exists among patients with AAA. For unknown reason, this association appears stronger in men. Few etiologic differences were noted between male AAA patients with extremity aneurysms and those without such aneurysms. These femoral and popliteal aneurysms are usually clinically undetectable, suggesting that US screening may be appropriate for men diagnosed as having AAAs.

▶ This study from the University of Michigan documents an increased incidence of femoral and popliteal aneurysms detected by US in patients with known AAAs. I am not sure that the conclusion of this article can be generalized, since patients referred to the University of Michigan may differ from those encountered in primary practice and may be more likely to have arteriomegaly or multiple arterial aneurysms. We do not screen patients with normal body habitus, who have AAAs, for femoral or popliteal aneurysm. We rely on physical examination alone, since very small aneurysms or arteriomegaly detected by ultrasound would not alter patient management.

J. L. Mills, Sr, MD

Oral Health of Patients Scheduled for Elective Abdominal Aortic Correction With Prosthesis

Häyrinen-Immonen R, Ikonen TS, Lepäntalo M, et al (Univ of Helsinki)
Eur J Vasc Endovasc Surg 19:294-298, 2000   7–12

Background.—A high mortality rate (17% to 40%) is associated with perioperative prosthetic infection in infrarenal aortic surgery, which is generally otherwise successful. The source of infection is not always found, but oral infections of which the patient is unaware may be a contributing factor. How frequently oral infections serve as foci of infection was prospectively evaluated among patients scheduled for elective abdominal aortic surgery.

Methods.—Fifty patients were examined and underwent an evaluation of oral health and dentures before undergoing aortic surgery. Radiographic and clinical examinations were performed to detect acute and chronic oral and ontogenic conditions that may have contributed to infection of an aortic prosthesis.

Results.—A degree of oral infection foci was found in 82% of patients. Among the patients studied, the mean number of teeth remaining was 9.3; potential infectious foci were found in 21%. Oral *Candida* infection was found in 26% of the patients. Dental condition was poor: 74% of patients had total or partial dentures, of which 45% did not fit well and were in need of repair.

Conclusions.—Oral infectious foci that could contribute to infection in an aortic prosthesis were found frequently in patients who required aortic surgery. Recommendations for this group include both preoperative oral evaluation and the elimination of any intraoral infections before abdominal aortic repair is undertaken.

▶ These authors found foci of abnormal oral infection in 82% of patients scheduled for unspecified aortic surgery. While they speculate that this may serve as a source of perioperative or prosthetic infection, this uncontrolled study does not refute or support this speculation. Likewise, they provide no evidence that this prevalence of dental ill health is more or less than one would find in the general age- and gender-matched population. Some food for thought, none for conclusion.

L. M. Taylor, Jr, MD

8 Aortoiliac Disease

Effect of Left Renal Vein Division During Aortic Surgery on Renal Function

Elsharawy MA, Cheatle TR, Clarke JMF, et al (Norfolk and Norwich Hosp, England)

Ann R Coll Surg Engl 82:417-420, 2000   8–1

Objective.—Left renal vein division (LRVD) is sometimes necessary to facilitate exposure of the juxtarenal part of the abdominal aorta when operating on an aneurysm or occlusive disease of the aorta. Whether LRVD is a useful adjunct that minimizes long-term sequelae or impairs renal function is controversial. The effect of LRVD on mortality rate and renal function was examined retrospectively.

Methods.—Between December 1994 and October 1998, 398 patients (61 male) had aortic surgery with LRVD (n = 40) or left renal vein intact (LRVI) (n = 230). Renal function was assessed with preoperative, perioperative, postoperative, and long-term postoperative creatinine measurements.

Results.—Compared with LRVI, there was no significant effect of LRVD on mortality rate (0% vs 2.2%), elective aneurysm surgery (8% vs 11%), urgent aneurysm surgery (29% vs 18%), ruptured aneurysm (58% vs 77%), or overall aortic surgery (31% vs 32%). There were no significant differences in creatinine levels between the 2 groups regardless of surgical indication (Table 6). Three LRVD patients and 6 LRVI patients had elevated creatinine levels at 3 months, but none required dialysis. Creatinine levels normalized within 2 to 9 months in the 8 survivors.

TABLE 6.—Mean Serum Creatinine (µmol/L ± SD) Levels in Patients Who Survived Surgery for Aortic Aneurysm

	LRVD (*n* = 40)	LRVI (*n* = 230)	P Value
Pre-operative	107 ± 21	103 ± 29	0.14
Peri-operative (1 week)	111 ± 21	107 ± 31	0.05
Peri-operative (predischarge or 30 days)	106 ± 16	105 ± 29	0.20

(Courtesy of Elsharawy MA, Cheatle TR, Clarke JMF, et al: Effect of left renal vein division during aortic surgery on renal function. *Ann R Coll Surg Engl* 82:417-420, 2000.)

Conclusion.—LRVD is a safe procedure during aortic surgery and does not result in long-term elevated creatinine levels.

▶ Additional important data gained from this article included that patients having LRVD had no significant increase in mortality when operated on because of aortic occlusive disease, elective aneurysm surgery, urgent aneurysm surgery, or ruptured aneurysm surgery. I believe, as taught by my mentor, Dr Porter, that LRVD occasionally may be necessary to gain safe access to the infrarenal aortic neck of the aneurysm. The data in this report would have been much stronger if the authors also had reported the status of the renal arteries from preoperative arteriograms. The authors could have also brought the patients back for split renal function testing. Obviously, the contralateral kidney may be masking any deleterious effects of LRVD. I have always thought that the worsening of renal function with LRVD is from the clamp being placed closer to the renal arteries, thereby increasing the susceptibility to intimal flap and atheroembolism. I suspect this view is shared by many, and the left renal vein may be divided in difficult cases to obtain proximal aortic control.

R. B. McLafferty, MD

---

pHi Monitoring of the Sigmoid Colon After Aortoiliac Surgery: A Five-Year Prospective Study
Björck M, Lindberg F, Broman G, et al (Umeå Univ, Sweden; Uppsala Univ, Sweden)
Eur J Vasc Endovasc Surg 20:273-280, 2000   8–2

Introduction.—Attempts to improve survival in patients who have undergone abdominal aortoiliac surgery have been discouraging. Earlier trials have shown that a prolonged sigmoid colon pHi less than 6.86 is diagnostic for bowel gangrene after aortoiliac surgery. Also, low-grade sigmoid colon ischemia (defined as pHi <7.1 for >2 hours) is predictive for all major complications and death, and a pHi less than 7.0 is associated with higher concentrations of endotoxins and cytokines and signs of organ dysfunction. Even low-grade intestinal ischemia may impact outcome after aortoiliac surgery. In a single-center, nonrandomized prospective study the effectiveness of sigmoid pHi to diagnose colon ischemia in patients who have undergone aortoiliac surgery was assessed.

Methods.—Between 1994 and 1998, 83 patients underwent surgery for aortoiliac disease. Of 31 patients who were operated on for ruptured abdominal aortic aneurysm (rAAA), 24 were in shock, 3 were on anticoagulation therapy, and 5 were pulseless without measurable blood pressure. Forty-one patients with risk factors for development of colon ischemia were monitored by means of sigmoid-pHi perioperatively and/or postoperatively. Thirty-five postoperative colonoscopies were done. A postmortem examination was performed on all patients who died.

TABLE 3.—The Six Patients With Colon Ischemia

Age	Sex	Indication for Surgery	Duration of pHi<7.10	Lowest pHi-Value	Depth of Lesion	Outcome
63 y	M	rAAA, shock	80 h	6.70	Mucosal	Ischaemia spinal cord injury. Recovery
52 y	M	AAA, dissection, Ehlers-Danlos' syndrome	25 h	6.82	Muscular	Sigmoid stricture recovery
72 y	M	rAAA, shock	50 h	6.95	Mucosal	Recovery
80 y	M*	rAAA, shock	16 h*	6.70*	Mucosal*	Died after 24 h*
67 y	M	rAAA, shock	21 h†	6.50	Gangrene	Colectomy. Recovery
62 y	M	rAAA, shock	24 h	6.50	Gangrene	Sigmoid resection. Recovery

*Treatment was withheld 16 hours after surgery.
†At relaparotomy at 21 hours total colectomy was performed.
Abbreviation: rAAA, Ruptured abdominal aortic aneurysm.
(Reprinted from Björck M, Lindberg F, Broman G, et al: pHi monitoring of the sigmoid colon after aortoiliac surgery: A five-year prospective study. *Eur J Vasc Endovasc Surg* 20:273-280, 2000. Copyright 2000, by permission of the publisher W B Saunders Company Limited London.)

Results.—The perioperative mortality was 26% (8/31) for patients with rAAA and 0% for nonruptured AAA. Five of the 6 patients who developed colon ischemia had emergency surgery. All 6 patients had pHi values less than 7.1 for 16 to 80 hours (Table 3). Two patients had transmural gangrene and pHi values less than 6.6. The pHi monitoring allowed early diagnosis, colectomy, and recovery. Three patients developed mucosal gangrene. They were treated conservatively and recovered. Nine patients who had no ischemic lesions had pHi values of less than 7.1 for 1 to 5 hours without adverse outcome. The risk of colon ischemia was significantly increased with bilateral ligation of the internal iliac arteries.

Conclusion.—The use of pHi monitoring was helpful in diagnosing colon ischemia. Mucosal and transmural gangrene could be distinguished. The importance of the internal iliac circulation was shown. The low mortality rate and the fact that no patients died from bowel ischemia indicate that pHi monitoring may improve survival after rAAA.

▶ We are all aware that postoperative colon ischemia is an uncommon but potentially lethal problem in vascular surgery patients. This study attempts to define whether selective sigmoid pHi monitoring can improve results after aortoiliac surgery. In addition, the authors wanted to investigate whether this method could be diagnostic for colon ischemia and whether transmural gangrene could be distinguished from mucosal ischemic lesions. I do not believe the authors achieved their stated objectives with this article. Without question, they have demonstrated that the mucosal pH can be measured. They can identify some patients who have a significant decrease in the mucosal pH. Although they state that the level of the pH and the duration of a low level of pH correlate with clinical results, I feel that it is difficult to reach this conclusion with the data in this report. Of the 6 patients who did develop colon ischemia, it is difficult for me to draw a conclusion that outcome and duration of lowest pH are corrected. In addition, they state that a combination of pH monitoring and colonoscopy can help them distinguish between mucosal ischemia and transmural gangrene, but it is unclear to me how one could make that distinction in our patients. As with other publications on this subject, this report is interesting, but I feel that the data presented are not definitive and offer little help in my practice of deciding which patient has mucosal or transmural gangrene of the colon.

J. O. Menzoian, MD

Localized Dissection and Delayed Rupture of the Abdominal Aorta After Extracorporeal Shock Wave Lithotripsy
Neri E, Capannini G, Diciolla F, et al (Univ of Siena, Italy)
J Vasc Surg 31:1052-1055, 2000   8–3

Introduction.—Extracorporeal shock wave lithotripsy (ESWL) is the preferred treatment of most upper ureteric and renal calculi. Some serious and sometimes fatal complications have been associated with ESWL, in-

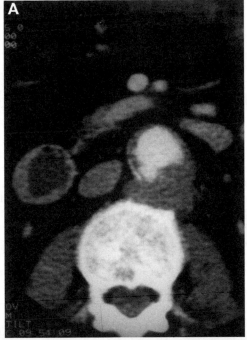

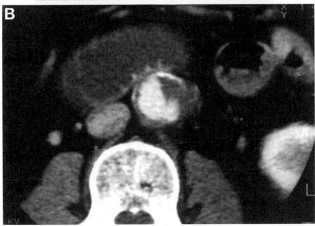

FIGURE 2.—**A,** Abdominal contrast CT scan showing localized disruption of a calcified plaque and limited wall dissection on the left lateral side of the infrarenal aorta, (**B**). (Courtesy of Neri E, Capannini G, Diciolla F, et al: Localized dissection and delayed rupture of the abdominal aorta after extracorporeal shock wave lithotripsy. *J Vasc Surg* 31:1052-1055, 2000.)

cluding kidney rupture, psoas abscess formation, subcapsular hematoma of the spleen, portal and iliac vein thrombosis, and abdominal aortic aneurysm rupture. Reported is a patient who experienced rupture of a severely calcified abdominal aorta 3 months after undergoing ESWL for treatment of renal calculi.

Case Report.—Man, 65, underwent 3 sessions of ESWL during a 3-month period. At 3 months after the final ESWL, he experienced abdominal and left flank pain associated with difficulty in walking. An abdominal duplex scan echography revealed a severely calcified abdominal aorta with a diameter of 18 mm. Thoracic and abdominal contrast CT scan revealed the presence of localized disruption of a calcified plaque. Limited wall dissection was observed on the left lateral side of the infrarenal aorta (Fig 2). The left ileopsoas muscle was found to be infiltrated by organized blood, and an immediate longitudinal laparotomy was performed. The aorta was opened, and a mobile calcified plaque was observed. Underneath the plaque, the aortic wall seemed disrupted, and a fistulous tract gave access to a cavity in the left ileopsoas muscle. An old mural thrombus in this cavity was indicative of a primary-contained rupture in the left ileopsoas muscle soon after plaque disruption, followed by a delayed rupture in the retroperitoneum 3 months after the final procedure. An abdominal aortic resection was done, and an aorto-aortic 16-mm graft was placed. The patient was discharged 6 days later and had an uneventful postoperative course.

Conclusion.—This patient's history and chronologic course of events strongly indicate that ESWL played a role in the genesis of the abdominal aorta rupture.

▶ A frightening case report, as ESWL has become the treatment of choice for most patients with renal calculi. Previous case reports have documented ESWL-associated rupture of abdominal aortic aneurysms, but this case report suggests that heavily calcified aortas are also at risk. I have had several aortic reconstructions for occlusive disease where I had wished ESWL or dynamite might have helped me with a severely calcified aorta. Perhaps a few minutes of ESWL on call to the OR will become a standard order for aortic reconstruction in our future. (Just kidding!)

E. J. Harris, Jr, MD

Axillofemoral Bypass for Aortoiliac Occlusive Disease
Martin D, Katz SG (Huntington Mem Hosp, Pasadena, Calif; Univ of Southern California, Pasadena)
Am J Surg 180:100-103, 2000   8–4

Objective.—Aortobifemoral bypass is the treatment of choice for aortoiliac occlusive disease and carries excellent patency rates at 5 years, but it also leads to a risk of significant morbidity in high-risk and elderly patients. Axillofemoral bypass has been reported to be effective, but patency rates vary widely. The role of axillofemoral bypass in the manage-

TABLE 1.—Life Table Analysis for Time of Patency for All Grafts (n = 61)

Interval (Year)	Number of Grafts at Risk at Start	Number of Occluded Grafts	Withdrawn	Number of Deaths	Interval Patent Rate	Cumulative Patent Rate (%)	Standard Error (%)
0-0.5	61	7	11	8	0.86	100	0.0
0.5-1	35	3	9	3	0.90	86	4.8
1-2	20	1	7	2	0.94	77	6.5
2-3	10	1	5	0	0.87	72	7.8
3-4	4	0	1	0	1.00	63	11.2
4-5	3	0	2	0	1.00	63	11.2

(Courtesy of Martin D, Katz SG: Axillofemoral bypass for aortoiliac occlusive disease. *Am J Surg* 180:100-103, copyright 2000, with permission from Excerpta Medica Inc.)

ment of elderly and poor-risk patients with severe aortoiliac occlusive disease was retrospectively reviewed.

Methods.—Records were reviewed of 60 consecutive patients (30 men), aged 50 to 92, with chronic aortoiliac occlusive disease who underwent 61 axillofemoral bypass grafting procedures (8 axillounifemoral) from January 1984 to December 1997. Patients' status was followed at 3-month intervals for the first year and at 6-month intervals thereafter. Follow-up averaged 13 months and ranged from 1 to 61 months. The outcome measure was graft failure. Patency survival curves were calculated using the Kaplan-Meier method.

Results.—At an average of 6.5 months, occlusions developed in 10 grafts, all in patients with axillobifemoral grafts. Six occlusions occurred in the femorofemoral limb with continued patency in the axillofemoral component. Five were repaired, and 1 patient died before a revision could be attempted. Of 4 patients with an axillobifemoral occlusion, 3 were treated successfully and 1 died before intervention. No axillounifemoral graft patients experienced an occlusion. One patient underwent lower extremity amputation. The 30-day mortality rate was 4.9%. No predictors of long-term patency were found. Cumulative patency rates were excellent and reproducible (Table 1).

Conclusion.—Long-term patency rates for elderly patients having axillofemoral bypass for aortoiliac occlusive disease were excellent and reproducible. The procedure is an option for elderly patients with other chronic diseases.

▶ Referencing the late Dr Porter's own methods, these authors describe a cumulative graft patency rate of 72% at the 36-month interval after axillofemoral bypass for occlusive disease. Not surprisingly, these results are similar to those previously published by the Oregon group. How many of these patients would have been candidates for aortofemoral bypass grafting or percutaneous catheter-based iliac angioplasty/recanalization/stenting in other practice settings is unknown. Clearly, catheter and guide wire technology and technical options for percutaneous management of advanced iliac occlusive disease have undergone dramatic evolutionary refinements in the past 10 years. In our own practice, most if not all such patients can be offered in-line, anatomic reconstruction with confidence that intermediate and late primary and secondary patency rates are comparable or better than the results reported herein. It is reassuring to remember, however, that should the need arise, the "extra-anatomic" option is available, reasonably durable, and still being used with some frequency and confidence (in Los Angeles and Portland, Oregon, at least. . .).

R. L. Dalman, MD

Severe Aortic Thrombosis in the Neonate—Successful Treatment With Low-Molecular-Weight Heparin: Two Case Reports and Review of the Literature

Klinger G, Hellmann J, Daneman A (Univ of Toronto)
Am J Perinatol 17:151-158, 2000   8–5

Background.—Newborns may have aortic thrombosis, most often as a complication of umbilical arterial catheter (UAC) use. The reported prognosis varies widely because of delays in diagnosis, differences in treatment, and variations in severity. The use of low molecular weight heparin (LMWH) to treat 2 cases of severe aortic thrombosis in newborns is reported.

Patients.—The patients were 2 baby boys born at term, 1 requiring vacuum extraction and 1 requiring emergency cesarean section. The latter patient had a UAC placed in the course of management of seizures and apneic episodes; the former patient, who was being evaluated for tachypnea of pallor of the lower limbs, did not undergo UAC placement. Both infants had signs of decreased lower limb perfusion soon after birth. US showed aortic occlusion by an infrarenal thrombus in each. Both patients were treated with LMWH, and the dosage was increased to achieve antifactor Xa levels in the therapeutic range. In both cases, the infant's condition improved, and femoral pulses became palpable within 24 to 48 hours after the start of LMWH treatment. Follow-up US showed resolution of the thrombi, and no treatment complications occurred. Both patients continued receiving LMWH treatment for 3 months after discharge.

Conclusions.—The authors review the clinical features of neonatal aortic thrombosis, including 63 cases from the literature. This problem is associated with the triad of UAC, hypertension, and decreased lower limb perfusion, although not all patients have a UAC in place. The authors' experience suggests that LMWH is a treatment option; if medical management fails or is contraindicated, surgical management is indicated.

▶ As a young staff doctor, there is nothing that tightens my sphincter more than bad vascular problems in pediatric patients. As a general rule, most neonatal vascular problems can be managed nonoperatively. However, as the parents, grandparents, aunts, uncles, cousins, friends, and family dog glare at you wondering why you can't just "fix" their child's purple legs, it is nice to have some data to back yourself up. The authors reviewed their own and the medical literature's experience with severe aortic thrombosis in the neonate. The treatment algorithm runs in the following order: (1) anticoagulation, (2) thrombolysis, and (3) surgery. While thrombus resolution is the rule, the mortality rate in all reported cases was a sobering 29%, with half of survivors having complications. I suspect that promptness of recognition and appropriate treatment is the key. As the authors point out, aortic coarctation is frequently misdiagnosed in these patients, leading to treatment delays.

G. J. Landry, MD

Idiopathic Pedunculated Mural Thrombus of the Nonaneurysmal Infrarenal Aorta Presenting With Popliteal Embolization: Two Cases Treated With Thrombolytic Therapy
Dougherty MJ, Calligaro KD, Rua I, et al (Pennsylvania Hosp, Philadelphia)
J Vasc Surg 32:383-387, 2000   8–6

Background.—The finding of a large pedunculated infrarenal aortic mural thrombus associated with only trivial atherosclerotic plaque has been observed in several patients seen with peripheral large-vessel embolism. The successful treatment of 2 such patients with a combination of catheter-directed thrombolytic therapy and anticoagulation was reported.

Case 1.—Woman, 71, with no history of or risk factors for atherosclerotic disease was seen with abrupt onset of claudication in the left calf and intermittent rest pain. Physical examination revealed a pallid left foot with absence of pedal pulses; the pulse was normal elsewhere. The only significant finding on laboratory study was a mildly elevated hemoglobin level. Arteriography revealed a pedunculated thrombus (2 cm) in the infrarenal aorta and a 1-cm embolus in the popliteal artery but no significant changes elsewhere. Urokinase therapy was intitiated by means of an infusion catheter positioned in the popliteal embolus. After 12 hours, the popliteal lesion had lysed completely. Pedal pules returned, but there was no change in the aortic lesion. Surgical removal of the aortic lesion was initially declined by the patient, who was anticoagulated with heparin. No aortic thrombus was visible on US and MRI 5 days later. The patient was treated with warfarin therapy for 6 months, followed by aspirin; she remained free of abnormality on duplex surveillance through 54 months of follow-up. Although initial hypercoagulability profiles were normal, the patient was ultimately given a diagnosis of polycythemia vera.

Case 2.—Woman, 59, a smoker with no other atherosclerotic risk factors, was seen with a 3-day history of intermittent left foot rest pain 6 weeks after sigmoid colectomy for colon cancer. She had been hospitalized for treatment of chemotherapy-related dehydration and granulocytopenic colitis 1 week before presentation.

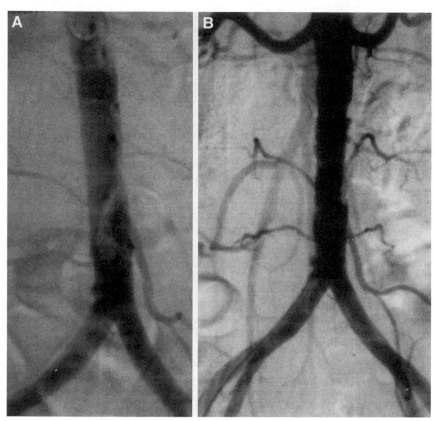

FIGURE 2.—A, Pedunculated mural thrombus arising from infrarenal aorta. **B,** Nearly complete resolution of filling defect after thrombolytic therapy. (Courtesy of Dougherty MJ, Calligaro KD, Rua I, et al: Idiopathic pedunculated mural thrombus of the nonaneurysmal infrarenal aorta presenting with popliteal embolization: Two cases treated with thrombolytic therapy. *J Vasc Surg* 32:383-387, 2000.)

Physical examination revealed an ischemic left foot, with absent pedal pulses; other pulses were normal, as were laboratory studies. Arteriography showed a 1.5-cm teardrop-shaped filling defect in the infrarenal aorta as well as a popliteal embolus (Fig 2). A minimally invasive approach to therapy was chosen in light of the patient's recent surgery and complications. Urokinase therapy was directed to the aortic thrombus, which resolved within 12 hours. However, additional embolization at the popliteal and tibial level necessitated repositioning of the catheter in the popliteal artery and further thrombolysis. This treatment was successful, but massive colonic bleeding, that was presumed to be secondary to her recent colitis, developed. The bleeding continued after cessation of urokinase infusion but was controlled with intra-arterial infusion of pitressin. No additional treatment was necessary.

Conclusion.—The incidence of aortic mural thrombus is more common than previously appreciated, and the optimal treatment of incidentally found lesions is unknown. However, thrombolytic therapy may have an important role in the treatment of patients who experience peripheral embolization.

▶ Thrombosis involving the wall of the thoracic and abdominal aorta in the absence of gross atherosclerotic degeneration of the aortic wall is now well recognized. The etiologies for the occurrence of such a thrombus appear to be multifactorial, and no consistent underlying risk factors are reported. The article emphasizes that an aortic mural thrombus should be considered even in patients without overt atherosclerosis when such patients are seen with peripheral embolization and a negative cardiac workup.

G. L. Moneta, MD

9 Visceral Renal Artery Disease

Mesenteric-Celiac Repair

Revascularization of the Superior Mesenteric Artery Alone for Treatment of Intestinal Ischemia

Foley MI, Moneta GL, Abou-Zamzam AM Jr, et al (Oregon Health Sciences Univ, Portland; Portland Dept of Veterans Affairs Med Ctr, Ore)
J Vasc Surg 32:37-47, 2000   9–1

Background.—Autopsy studies have demonstrated a high prevalence of atherosclerosis involving the mesenteric arteries (6%-10%), but symptomatic splanchnic artery occlusive disease is uncommon; less than 0.5% of all peripheral vascular reconstructions involve mesenteric revascularization procedures. Nevertheless, the mortality associated with acute mesenteric ischemia is high. Many authors have recommended complete revascularization for the treatment of intestinal ischemia. However, observations that postprandial intestinal hyperemia is limited to the superior mesenteric artery (SMA) have suggested to these authors that SMA revascularization by itself should be an adequate treatment. The results of a management approach in which intestinal ischemia is treated with a single bypass graft to the SMA were reported.

Methods.—From a prospectively established vascular surgical registry, 49 patients were identified. Patients were assessed for acute versus chronic intestinal ischemia, preoperative angiographic findings, type of operation used, perioperative morbidity and mortality, late symptomatic relief, cause of death, and survival and graft patency as determined by life table analysis. Follow-up angiography or duplex scanning was used in determination of graft patency.

Results.—Fifty grafts to the SMA alone were performed in 49 patients for treatment of intestinal ischemia (Fig 1). Additional splanchnic arteries were available for bypass grafting in all patients. Perioperative mortality was 3% among patients with chronic symptoms and 12% overall. Symptomatic improvement was obtained in all patients. Assisted primary graft patency at 9 years was 79%, and patient survival at 5 years was 61%

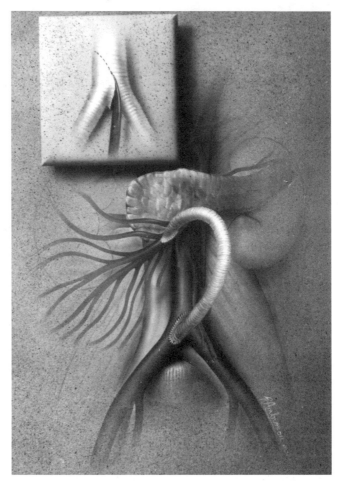

FIGURE 1.—Retrograde bypass graft from the right common iliac artery to the SMA in the C-loop configuration. The *inset* demonstrates the creation of a flange for the proximal anastomosis as described by Wylie et al. (Courtesy of Foley MI, Moneta GL, Abou-Zamzam AM Jr, et al: Revascularization of the superior mesenteric artery alone for treatment of intestinal ischemia. *J Vasc Surg* 32:37-47, 2000.)

(Table 2). There were two late deaths in patients with recurrent intestinal ischemia that resulted from graft occlusion.

Conclusions.—It would appear that bypass grafting to the SMA alone is an effective and durable procedure for the treatment of intestinal ischemia. These results appear to be equal to those reported for "complete" revascularization for intestinal ischemia. In patients in whom the SMA is a suitable recipient vessel, multiple bypass grafts to other splanchnic vessels are unnecessary.

TABLE 2.—Life Table–Determined Assisted Primary Graft Patency

Interval	At Risk	Occlusions	Withdrawn	Interval Patency	Cumulative Patency	SE
0-1 mo	50	3	8	0.935	0.935	0.0364
1 y	39	1	9	0.971	0.908	0.0443
2 y	29	1	5	0.962	0.873	0.0543
3 y	23	0	6	1	0.873	0.0543
4 y	17	0	4	1	0.873	0.0543
5 y	13	1	5	0.905	0.79	0.093
6 y	7	0	1	1	0.79	0.093
7 y	6	0	2	1	0.79	0.093
8 y	4	0	1	1	0.79	0.093
9 y	3	0	2	1	0.79	0.093

(Courtesy of Foley MI, Moneta GL, Abou-Zamzam AM Jr, et al: Revascularization of the superior mesenteric artery alone for treatment of intestinal ischemia. *J Vasc Surg* 32:37-47, 2000.)

▶ The Oregon group has long maintained that isolated reconstruction of the SMA is sufficient for long-term relief of intestinal ischemia. It is hard to argue with their results. The anatomic picture shown in the article is very clear and should be reviewed by the reader. In patients in whom one's preference is to originate the mesenteric bypass from the infrarenal aorta or a previously placed aortofemoral bypass graft, I would recommend this technique.

J. L. Mills, Sr, MD

Chronic Mesenteric Ischemia: Open Surgery Versus Percutaneous Angioplasty and Stenting

Kasirajan K, O'Hara PJ, Gray BH, et al (Cleveland Clinic Found, Ohio)
J Vasc Surg 33:63-71, 2001   9–2

Background.—Atherosclerotic occlusive disease of the mesenteric circulation is an uncommon disorder. If not detected and treated, it may culminate in fatal intestinal gangrene. Reports have indicated that open surgical (OS) revascularization provides an excellent, long-lasting symptomatic cure. However, this technique has been associated with perioperative complications ranging from 19% to 54%, and mortality rates have ranged from 0% to 17%. Recent interest in the use of minimally invasive endovascular therapy for atherosclerotic short-segment occlusive disease has spread to the management of chronic mesenteric ischemia. Studies by proponents of percutaneous angioplasty and stenting (PAS) have reported lower complication rates ranging from 0% to 25% with this procedure, as well as a low periprocedural mortality rate of 0% to 13%. The safety and efficacy of PAS was evaluated in comparison with traditional OS revascularization for the treatment of chronic mesenteric ischemia.

Methods.—PAS was performed in 28 patients and 32 vessels over a 3.5-year period for symptoms of chronic mesenteric ischemia. Five of 28 patients (18%) underwent balloon angioplasty alone, and 23 of 28 (82%) underwent angioplasty and stenting. Results in these patients were com-

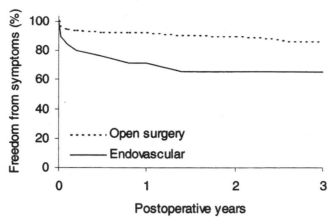

FIGURE 3.—Cumulative freedom from recurrent symptoms comparing open surgical treatment group with endovascular treatment group ($P = .001$; SE < 10 for all values). (Courtesy of Kasirajan K, O'Hara PJ, Gray BH, et al: Chronic mesenteric ischemia: Open surgery versus percutaneous angioplasty and stenting. *J Vasc Surg* 33:63-71, 2001.)

pared with those in a previously published series of 85 patients and 130 vessels treated with OS revascularization.

Results.—Findings were similar in the PAS and OS groups in terms of baseline comorbidities, duration of symptoms, and the number of vessels involved, but the patients differed in their age at presentation; patients in the PAS group were seen at a median of 72 years, whereas patients in the OS group were seen at a median of 65 years. Patients in the PAS group had fewer vessels revascularized (1.1 ± 0.4) compared with the OS group (1.5 ± 0.6). Overall, 85.7% of patients in the PAS group had 1 vessel revascularized, and 14.3% had 2 vessels revascularized. In comparison, 48.2% of the patients in the OS group had 1 vessel revascularized, and 47.1% had 2 vessels revascularized. There were no differences noted between the 2 groups in terms of early in-hospital complications or the mortality rate. The PAS group had a reduced length of hospital stay (median, 5 days) compared with the OS group (median, 13 days), but the difference was not statistically significant. No significant difference was found between the 2 groups in the 3-year cumulative recurrent stenosis rate or the mortality rate, but the PAS group had a higher incidence of recurrent symptoms (Fig 3).

Conclusions.—The PAS and OS groups had similar findings in the areas of morbidity, death, and recurrent stenosis, but an association was noted between PAS and a significantly higher incidence of recurrent symptoms. On the basis of these findings, it is suggested that OS should be preferentially offered to patients who are considered fit for open revascularization.

▶ The authors have examined the results of treatment of chronic mesenteric ischemia, and have compared open surgical repair with endovascular repair. They compare 2 series performed over different times and have accumulated a significant number of patients for their analysis. They con-

clude that open surgical repair yields a preferable result with greater durability. I agree with the authors' conclusions, but note that the endovascular
results reported here, in agreement with reports in the literature, indicate
that acceptable results can be obtained with endovascular treatment of
chronic mesenteric ischemia. This should certainly be remembered when
deciding how to treat a patient with chronic mesenteric ischemia who is a
poor risk for open major surgery.

M. A. Golden, MD

**Laparoscopic Release of Celiac Artery Compression Syndrome Facili-
tated by Laparoscopic Ultrasound Scanning to Confirm Restoration
of Flow**
Roayaie S, Jossart G, Gitlitz D, et al (Mount Sinai-New York Univ Med Ctr)
J Vasc Surg 32:814-817, 2000   9–3

Objective.—Surgical exploration of the rare celiac artery compression
syndrome has required an upper midline incision. A laparoscopic approach to treatment of this disorder was described.

> *Case Report.*—Woman, 43, with a 20-year history of intermit-
> tent postprandial pain leading to a 35-pound weight loss, had an
> exploratory laparotomy, sonogram, upper and lower endoscopies,
> CT scan, and a small-bowel series. None of these revealed the
> source of the problem. An MR angiogram revealed a short segment

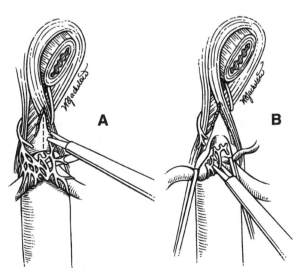

FIGURE 4.—**A,** Laparoscopic division of the median arcuate ligament. **B,** Laparoscopic excision of the
celiac plexus. (Courtesy of Roayaie S, Jossart G, Gitlitz D, et al: Laparoscopic release of celiac artery
compression syndrome facilitated by laparoscopic ultrasound scanning to confirm restoration of flow. *J
Vasc Surg* 32:814-817, 2000.)

of high-grade stenosis of the anterior wall of the celiac artery and led to a diagnosis of celiac artery compression syndrome. The patient underwent laparoscopic division of the median arcuate ligament and resection of all neural and lymphatic tissue with the use of a 10-mm laparoscopic 7.5-MHz US scanning probe with a flexible head and Doppler US scanning at 60° (Fig 4). The patient was discharged 15 hours after surgery. Her symptoms had been completely resolved at the time of her 3-month follow-up visit, and no celiac artery stenosis was detected on MR angiography.

Conclusion.—The laparoscopic approach to treating celiac artery compression avoids laparotomy and results in less postoperative pain, a shorter hospital stay, and a faster recovery. Longer follow-up is required before this procedure can be validated.

► This is innovative therapy for a nondisease.

G. L. Moneta, MD

Renal Artery Reconstruction

Long-term Results After Surgical Reconstruction for Renal Artery Fibromuscular Dysplasia

Reiher L, Pfeiffer T, Sandmann W (Heinrich Heine Univ, Duesseldorf, Germany)

Eur J Vasc Endovasc Surg 20:556-559, 2000   9–4

Background.—There is continued uncertainty over the optimal treatment for renovascular hypertension caused by fibromuscular dysplasia. Angiography has largely replaced surgical reconstruction, but randomized trials comparing the 2 techniques are lacking. The short- and long-term results of surgical reconstruction for renal artery fibromuscular dysplasia (RFMD) in 101 patients were reviewed.

TABLE 1.—Preoperative Renal Artery Angiographic Morphology in 101 Patients

	Patients	Kidneys	Arteries	
RAA	11	13	23	13/10*
RAS	58	81	89	84/5*
RAO	6	6	10	
RAA and RAS	26	40	67	39/28*
	101	140	189	

*Mainstem/segmental arteries.

Abbreviations: RAA, Renal artery aneurysm; *RAS,* renal artery stenosis; *RAO,* renal artery occlusion.

(Reprinted from the *European Journal of Vascular and Endovascular Surgery* courtesy of Reiher L, Pfeiffer T, Sandmann W: Long-term results after surgical reconstruction for renal artery fibromuscular dysplasia. *Eur J Vasc Endovasc Surg* 20:556-559, 2000. Copyright 2000, by permission of the publisher W B Saunders Company Limited London.)

TABLE 2.—Methods of Renal Artery Reconstruction in 101 Patients

	Initial Procedures	Secondary Procedures
Saphenous vein interposition	68	10
Resection and reanastomosis	21	
Dilatation with probes	17	
Saphenous vein bridging bypass	9	
Interposition of hypogastric artery	9	1
Aneurysm resection and direct suture	9	1
Splenic artery transposition	1	
Nephrectomy	1	
PTFE bypass		2
PTRA		1

(Reprinted from the *European Journal of Vascular and Endovascular Surgery* courtesy of Reiher L, Pfeiffer T, Sandmann W: Long-term results after surgical reconstruction for renal artery fibromuscular dysplasia. *Eur J Vasc Endovasc Surg* 20:556-559, 2000. Copyright 2000, by permission of the publisher W B Saunders Company Limited London.)

Methods.—The patients (80 women and 21 men; mean age, 43 years) underwent renal artery reconstruction (RAR) between 1980 and 1997 (Tables 1 and 2). Initial results in all patients were assessed. Survivors were recalled for clinical examination, including color duplex US of the renal arteries.

Results.—Initial postoperative success was evaluated by angiography in 90 patients and renal scintigraphy in 3; the technical success rate in this group was 89%. The reoperation rate was 5%, with 4 patients having early occlusion and 1 having stenosis. The mortality rate at 30 days was 2%, with morbidity of 12%. The 5-year primary patency rate was 74%. Restenosis led to repeat surgery for 15 patients at a mean of 33 months, for

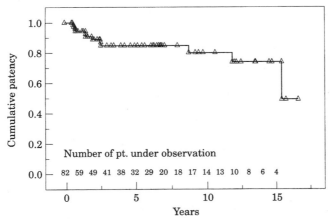

FIGURE 1.—Cumulative secondary patency after surgical reconstruction for renal artery fibromuscular dysplasia according to Kaplan-Meier. *Numbers below grafts* are patients at risk. Standard error exceeds 5% after 8.7 years. (Reprinted from the *European Journal of Vascular and Endovascular Surgery* courtesy of Reiher L, Pfeiffer T, Sandmann W: Long-term results after surgical reconstruction for renal artery fibromuscular dysplasia. *Eur J Vasc Endovasc Surg* 20:556-559, 2000. Copyright 2000, by permission of the publisher W B Saunders Company Limited London.)

a 5-year secondary patency rate of 85% (Fig 1). Sixty-one patients had patent RARs at the time of clinical reexamination. Hypertension was considered cured in only 36% of this group, but was improved in another 31%.

Conclusion.—Surgical reconstruction for RFMD achieves a good long-term patency rate, with good renal perfusion and function. These patients need close US follow-up. Even among patients with patent RARs, the cure rate of hypertension is disappointingly low.

▶ This relatively large series of patients undergoing surgical reconstruction for fibromuscular dysplasia documents technical success rates of 90% and a 5-year primary patency rate of 74%. The hypertension cure rate was only 36% during long term follow-up.

In our practice, the majority of these patients are treated with percutaneous transluminal angioplasty (PTA), a procedure that is much less invasive. As the authors acknowledge in their discussion, the results of PTA appear to be equivalent to their own results for surgical reconstruction.

J. L. Mills, Sr, MD

Management of Ischemic Nephropathy: Dialysis-Free Survival After Surgical Repair
Hansen KJ, Cherr GS, Craven TE, et al (Wake Forest Univ, Winston-Salem, NC)
J Vasc Surg 32:472-482, 2000   9–5

Background.—Authorities disagree on the best renal artery intervention. The outcomes of surgical management of severe hypertension and ischemic nephropathy from atherosclerotic renovascular disease at one center were reviewed.

Methods.—In 1997 and 1998, 590 patients underwent surgical renal artery repair. Of these, 232 had hypertension, atherosclerotic renovascular disease, and preoperative serum creatinine concentrations of 1.8 mg/dL or greater. Eighty-three patients underwent unilateral renal artery repair, and 149 underwent bilateral repair. A total of 332 renal arteries were reconstructed. Thirty-two nephrectomies were performed.

Findings.—Seventeen patients died within 30 days of surgery, which yielded a mortality rate of 7.3%. Factors that were significantly, independently associated with perioperative mortality were advanced patient age and congestive heart failure. Fifty-eight percent of the patients had improved renal function postoperatively. Functioning was unchanged in 35% and worse in 7%. During follow-up, death from all causes or progression to dialysis dependence was significantly, independently associated with the early renal function response (Figs 2A and 3). Diabetes mellitus was also significantly, independently associated with death or need for dialysis during follow-up.

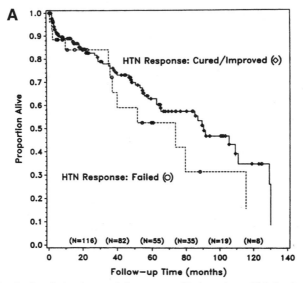

FIGURE 2A.—Product-limit estimates of all-cause mortality for patients with ischemic nephropathy as a function of hypertension (HTN) response to operation. (Courtsey of Hansen KJ, Cherr GS, Craven TE, et al: Management of ischemic nephropathy: Dialysis-free survival after surgical repair. *J Vasc Surg* 32:472-482, 2000.)

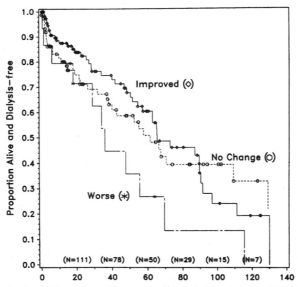

FIGURE 3.—Product-limit estimates of time to death or dialysis for patients with ischemic nephropathy according to renal function response after operation. (Courtsey of Hansen KJ, Cherr GS, Craven TE, et al: Management of ischemic nephropathy: Dialysis-free survival after surgical repair. *J Vasc Surg* 32:472-482, 2000.)

Conclusions.—Surgery for atherosclerotic renovascular disease can restore excretory renal function in select patients with hypertension with ischemic nephropathy. Patients with improved renal functioning had a significant, independent increase in their dialysis-free survival rate compared with those whose functioning was unchanged or worse after surgery.

▶ These authors report a large experience with renal artery reconstruction in patients with severe hypertension and ischemic nephropathy. The goal of therapy in this setting is to improve dialysis-free survival. While 87% of patients had improvement or cure of their hypertension, this did not predict improved long-term dialysis-free survival. A postoperative improvement in renal function was seen in 58% of patients, and 27 dialysis-dependent patients (75%) became dialysis free. Not surprisingly, an early improvement in renal function was a significant predictor of improved long-term dialysis-free survival. What we don't know is whether the patients with unchanged or worsened renal function would have been better off without surgery. It is clear that surgical renal revascularization helps a subgroup of patients with ischemic nephropathy, but the challenge is to optimize the selection of these patients before intervention. As the authors note, a prospective, randomized trial is clearly needed.

A. M. Abou-Zamzam, Jr, MD

Outcome of Renal Artery Reconstruction: Analysis of 687 Procedures
Darling RC III, Kreienberg PB, Chang BB, et al (Albany Med College, NY)
Ann Surg 230:524–532, 1999   9–6

Introduction.—Reconstruction of the renal arteries for either primary renal indications or a concomitant procedure with aortic reconstruction has changed during the past 40 years. There is concern that renal artery reconstructions are associated with significant rates of morbidity and mortality and that they may compare poorly with less-invasive procedures. The short- and long-term results of surgical reconstruction of the renal arteries in 687 procedures performed during a 12-year period (1986-1998) were retrospectively analyzed.

Methods.—Of 687 renal artery reconstructions performed, 105 patients had simultaneous bilateral renal artery reconstructions. The cohort was 56% male, 11% had diabetes, and 35% admitted to smoking at the time of surgery. The mean patient age was 67 years (range, 1-92 years). One hundred fifty-six (23%) reconstructions were primary procedures, and the remainder were adjunctive procedures with aortic reconstructions; 406 (76%) were abdominal aortic aneurysms and 125 (24%) were aortoiliac occlusive disease. Five hundred, 108, 72, and 7 procedures were bypasses, endarterectomies, reimplantations, and patch angioplasties, respectively. The surgical (elective and emergent) mortality rate for the entire group was 5.5% (31 deaths). Predictors for increased risk of death of patients were aortoiliac occlusive disease and bilateral simultaneous renal artery revascularization. The most common cause of death was cardiac related. Other nonfatal complications included bleeding and wound infection in 9 and 3 patients, respectively. Immediate and late occlusions occurred in 9 (1.3%) and 10 (1.5%) patients, respectively. Thirty-three (4.8%) patients experienced temporary worsening of their renal function after surgery.

Conclusion.—Renal artery revascularization is a safe and durable procedure that may be performed in selected patients for primary renovascular pathology. It may also be used as an adjunct to aortic reconstruction with acceptable mortality and morbidity rates.

▶ This large clinical series of renal revascularization is from a center of established excellence. Despite the results, a few interesting points arise. In many areas of the country, renal angioplasty/stenting has largely displaced renal revascularization. It seems the authors had selective amnesia in largely omitting this from the discussion. Renal angioplasty series demonstrate minimal procedural mortality (an advantage compared with the surgical series), but do have restenosis rates of 10% to 50% (a distinct disadvantage compared with the patency rates reported for surgery). However, it is not clear how much upfront misery is acceptable to achieve a 5-year patency rate that is markedly superior to your survival rate at the same interval. Vascular surgeons need to ask the question, does it really make sense to accept significant morbidity/mortality to provide an operation that is markedly more durable than the patients you are working on? In addition, the authors failed to mention the report by Williamson et al describing fairly benign clinical consequences (creatinine/blood pressure) of a nonoperative approach to patients with combined aortic/renal pathology discovered on a preoperative aortogram.

M. R. Nehler, MD

10 Leg Ischemia

Alternate Leg Revascularization

Autogenous Arterial Bypass Grafts: Durable Patency and Limb Salvage in Patients With Inframalleolar Occlusive Disease and End-Stage Renal Disease

Treiman GS, Lawrence PF, Rockwell WB (Univ of Utah, Salt Lake City)
J Vasc Surg 32:13-22, 2000   10–1

Background.—Autogenous vein grafts (AVGs) to inframalleolar arteries have been associated with excellent patency and limb salvage in most patients. However, in patients with end-stage renal disease (ESRD), the results have been significantly less gratifying. In these patients, arterial occlusive disease distal to the malleolus and affecting arteries within the foot may result in inadequate perfusion to ischemic or infected areas. Technical limitations to more distal revascularization are size disparity when the outflow artery is less then 1 mm in diameter, and limited runoff, which results in very low graft velocities and AVG thrombosis. In an attempt to provide sufficient revascularization and successful wound healing in patients with ESRD, autogenous arterial grafts (AAGs) to distal pedal or plantar arteries placed under microscopic visualization have been used. The effectiveness of the use of AAGs to distal pedal arteries in improving the patency of grafts and limb salvage in patients with ESRD and nonhealing ischemic wounds was evaluated, and indications for use of AAGs were more clearly defined.

Methods.—A review of consecutive patients with ESRD undergoing AAGs from 1994 through 1999 was conducted at a university hospital. In all 11 patients evaluated, noninvasive studies confirmed inadequate perfusion pressures. On prebypass arteriography, no patent major arteries were identified at the level of the malleolus, with reconstitution of only a distal or branch pedal or plantar vessel with a diameter of less than 1 mm. Bypass surgery with AAG alone was performed in 5 patients with patent tibial vessels to just above the ankle. Six patients also had proximal occlusive disease that required grafts that were longer than the AAGs alone. In these patients, an AVG proximal to the AAG was placed by using a composite technique. The conduit was the subscapular artery in 4 patients, the deep inferior epigastric artery in 4 patients, the superficial inferior epigastric artery in 2 patients, and the radial artery was used in 1

TABLE.—Life Table Data for 11 Patients With Renal Failure Undergoing
Autogenous Arterial Bypass Grafting

Interval (Mo)	No. of Patients			Patency	
	At Risk	Failed	Withdrawn	Interval	Cumulative
0-1	11	2	0	0.82	1.00
1-3	9	0	0	1.00	0.82
4-6	9	0	1	1.00	0.82
7-9	8	0	2	1.00	0.82
10-12	6	0	0	1.00	0.82
13-18	6	0	3	1.00	0.82
19-24	3	0	0	1.00	0.82
25-30	3	0	2	1.00	0.82
31-36	1	0	0	1.00	0.82
37-42	1	0	0	1.00	0.82
43-48	1	0	0	1.00	0.82
49-60	1	0	0	1.00	0.82
61-72	1	0	1	1.00	0.82

(Courtesy of Treiman GS, Lawrence PF, Rockwell WB: Autogenous arterial bypass grafts: Durable patency and limb salvage in patients with inframalleolar occlusive disease and end-stage renal disease. *J Vasc Surg* 32:13-22, 2000.)

patient. Main outcome measures included assisted primary graft patency and functional limb salvage rate.

Results.—Follow-up for these patients ranged from 6 to 63 months, with a mean of 20 months. Duplex scanning was used in determination of graft patency. At this writing, all 11 patients are alive, with 9 patent grafts, including 3 after revision for graft stenosis. At 3 years, assisted primary patency was 82% (Table). The 9 patients with patent grafts remained ambulatory and had either healed wounds or limited forefoot amputations.

Conclusions.—AAGs were found to be effective in the treatment of limb-threatening ischemia in patients with ESRD and inframalleolar arterial insufficiency. Graft patency and the rates of limb salvage were higher than the rates reported for AVGs in these patients. Thus, AAGs may be an effective alternative to autogenous vein grafting in selected patients.

▶ These vascular surgeons, working in conjunction with their colleagues from plastic surgery, are performing autogenous arterial bypass grafts for limb salvage to small (<1 mm in diameter), distal outflow arteries in the foot. The distal anastomoses are performed with the aid of a microscope by using interrupted 9-0 or 10-0 monofilament suture. Preliminary results, in 11 highly selected patients with ESRD, appear promising.

R. A. Yeager, MD

Remote Superficial Femoral Artery Endarterectomy: Medium-term Results

Galland RB, Whiteley MS, Gibson M, et al (Royal Berkshire Hosp, Reading, England)

Eur J Vasc Endovasc Surg 19:278-282, 2000   10–2

Background.—Remote superficial femoral artery endarterectomy (RSFE) provides a minimally invasive alternative to superficial femoral artery bypass with a synthetic graft. The medium-term results of RSFE in 25 limbs are discussed.

Methods.—The RSFE was performed in closed fashion through a single incision over the origin of the superficial femoral artery, using a stent to secure the cut end of distal atheroma. The RSFE technique was successful in 25 of 32 limbs in which it was done. Follow-up of these limbs included quarterly duplex scans of the superficial femoral artery, with digital subtraction angiography when any abnormality was detected. All patients had intermittent claudication, accompanied by pain at rest in 3 cases and ulceration/gangrene in 3. An atheromatous core length of 10 to 30 cm was removed during the RSFE procedure. All patients were followed up for at least 1 year.

Results.—During follow-up, a total of 14 stenoses developed in 11 arteries. Nine of the stenoses were noted within 9 months after the procedure. Cumulative stenosis risk in a patent artery increased from 24% at 6 months to 63% at 12 months. Percutaneous transluminal angioplasty was performed in 11 stenoses, 9 of which remained patent at a median 12 months' follow-up. Primary patency rate was 40% at 1 year and 29% at 2 years; primary-assisted patency rate was 72% and 57% at 1 and 2 years,

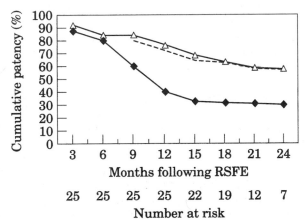

Number at risk

FIGURE 2.—Cumulative primary, primary-assisted and secondary patency after remote superficial femoral artery endarterectomy, *Diamonds*, primary; *dashed line*, primary-assisted; *triangles*, secondary. (Reprinted from Galland RB, Whiteley MS, Gibson M, et al: Remote superficial femoral artery endarterectomy: Medium-term results. *Eur J Vasc Endovasc Surg* 19:278-282, 2000. Copyright 2000 by permission of the publisher W B Saunders Company Limited London.)

respectively, and secondary patency rate was 76% and 57%, at 1 and 2 years, respectively (Fig 2).

Conclusions.—The RSFE technique provides a new option for patients with superficial femoral artery occlusion, particularly high-risk patients with no appropriate vein and limited life expectancy. However, problems with restenosis will limit the use of this procedure.

▶ Superficial femoral artery (SFA) endarterectomy is back. The authors describe a remote semiclosed technique involving a small groin incision. The results are predictably poor, but are still better than those of long segment SFA angioplasty. I don't think I am going to learn the technique though. If I am going to try to minimize operative time, I'll perform an above-knee bypass, maybe even with prosthetic.

J. M. Edwards, MD

Femorodistal PTFE Bypass Grafting for Severe Limb Ischaemia: Results of a Prospective Clinical Study Using a New Distal Anastomotic Technique

Rückert RI, Settmacher U, Krüger U, et al (Humboldt Univ, Berlin; Queen Elisabeth Hosp Herzberge, Berlin)
Eur J Vasc Endovasc Surg 20:51-56, 2000   10–3

Background.—Arterial bypass for restoration of blood flow to a patent distal artery is the most appropriate treatment for occlusive arterial disease of the lower extremity. The greater saphenous vein is the conduit of choice for infrainguinal femorodistal bypass procedures, but there continues to be a significant segment of patients who do not have sufficient length or quality of autologous vein. Expanded polytetrafluoroethylene (ePTFE) has been used as an alternative bypass graft material in these patients. However, the patency rates of heterologous grafts are inferior to those of autologous vein grafts. Several techniques, including venous cuff techniques and arteriovenous fistula, have been used to improve the patency of below-knee ePTFE arterial grafts.

In 1992 a new type of distal end-to-side anastomosis was developed by Scholz to address the importance of hemodynamics for the development of myointimal hyperplasia. This technique is characterized by a bifurcated double bulb and is termed femorocrural patch prosthesis (FCPP). In vitro flow visualization studies and color-coded Doppler sonography, as well as numerical simulation of the complex flow field, have demonstrated improved hemodynamics within the FCPP in comparison with other types of end-to-side anastomosis. Graft patency and limb salvage after femorodistal bypass with ePTFE with the use of this new anastomotic technique were evaluated.

Methods.—In a prospective nonrandomized study, 129 patients underwent 135 operations for severe limb ischemia. The mean age of the patient groups was 65.2 ± 10 years. The new ePTFE anastomosis was attached to

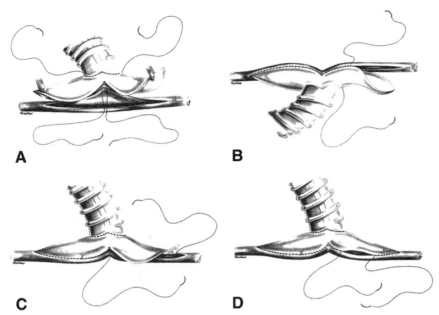

FIGURE 2.—Schematic representation of the surgical technique used to perform the distal femoro-crural patch prosthesis (FCPP) anastomosis. The expanded polytetrafluoroethylene (ePTFE) prosthesis is prepared at its distal end by suturing it to a patch, also made from ePTFE, which is especially configured as a double bulb. The suture line starts from the center of the posterior wall (**A**) and runs first to the proximal corner and thereafter back to the center of the anterior wall (**B**). A second running suture is performed to create the distal part of the FCPP anastomosis (**C**), with the 2 sutures meeting to be tied on the anterior wall (**D**). (Reprinted from the *European Journal of Vascular and Endovascular Surgery* courtesy of Rückert RI, Settmacher U, Krüger U, et al: Femorodistal PTFE bypass grafting for severe limb ischaemia: Results of a prospective clinical study using a new distal anastomotic technique. *Eur J Vasc Endovasc Surg* 20:51-56, 2000. Copyright 2000, by permission of the publisher W B Saunders Company Limited London.)

the popliteal (21 patients), anterior (46), posterior (52), and tibial and peroneal (16) arteries (Fig 2). Kaplan-Meier analyses were performed for evaluation of cumulative primary and secondary patency rates and limb salvage and survival rates.

Results.—Follow up ranged from 6 to 72 months, with a median of 45 months. No perioperative mortality occurred. At 1, 2, 3, 4, and 5 years the cumulative primary patency rates were 63%, 44.9%, 35.7%, 33.1%, and 27.6% respectively, and the secondary patency rates were 74.5%, 55.2%, 44.8%, 43%, and 37.6%, respectively (Fig 4a). Cumulative limb salvage rates at 1, 3, and 5 years were 86.4%, 78.7%, and 73.2%, respectively.

Conclusion.—The new FCPP anastomotic design was shown to be feasible and effective in producing long-term acceptable results in patients with severe limb ischemia.

▶ Do vein cuffs improve the patency of prosthetic bypasses because they are vein, or is it because of their shape and the resulting change in flow characteristics? This article seems to indicate that it is the shape and not the

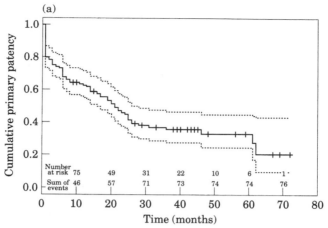

(a)

FIGURE 4.—Cumulative primary (a) patency rate according to Kaplan-Meier in 135 expanded polytetrafluoroethylene bypass grafts with distal femorocrural patch prosthesis anastomosis. The *dotted lines* indicate the 95% confidence intervals. The *numbers* at each point give the number of grafts at risk and the number of censored events at the beginning of the interval. (Reprinted from the *European Journal of Vascular and Endovascular Surgery* courtesy of Rückert RI, Settmacher U, Krüger U, et al: Femorodistal PTFE bypass grafting for severe limb ischaemia: Results of a prospective clinical study using a new distal anastomotic technique. *Eur J Vasc Endovasc Surg* 20:51-56, 2000. Copyright 2000, by permission of the publisher W B Saunders Company Limited London.)

material. This finding is not too surprising given other studies that show areas of hyperplasia are distributed dependent on hemodynamic profiles. In vitro flow studies of the "double bulb" configuration have shown it to be one configuration of the end-to-side anastomosis that minimizes flow phenomena associated with hyperplasia. However, just because a finding supports our preconceptions or biases does not mean it is true. The 3-year primary and secondary patency rates of 36% and 45% deserve further study of this technique.

J. M. Edwards, MD

Claudication

Outcome Events in Patients With Claudication: A 15-Year Study in 2777 Patients
Muluk SC, Muluk VS, Kelley ME, et al (Univ of Pittsburgh, Pa)
J Vasc Surg 33:251-258, 2001   10–4

Background.—Intermittent claudication may affect a minimum of 10% of individuals older than 70 years and leads to gangrene and amputation on rare occasions. Systemic atherosclerosis often has such dire outcomes, and the rates are higher among those who experience intermittent claudication. The long-term outcomes for 2777 men with claudication were analyzed, and the risk factors that may predict mortality rates for this population were determined.

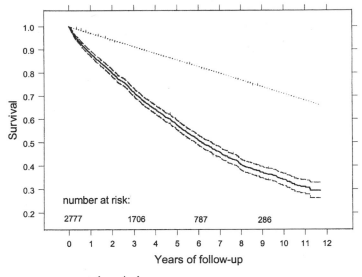

FIGURE 1.—Kaplan-Meier survival curves for study cohort (*solid line*) and for age-adjusted healthy US male population (*dotted line*). A 95% CI is shown for study cohort survival curve. (Courtesy of Muluk SC, Muluk VS, Kelley ME, et al: Outcome events in patients with claudication: A 15-year study in 2777 patients. *J Vasc Surg* 33:251-258, 2001.)

Methods.—The principal outcomes were identified as death, revascularization, or amputation for the patients studied. All had both clinical and noninvasive laboratory confirmation of their claudication; those with pain on resting or ulcers were excluded. Expected survival rates were computed (Fig 1).

Results.—Follow-up extended for a mean of 47 months, over which time the cohort mortality rate was 12% per year, which is significantly greater than among the age-matched US male population. Heart disease accounted for 66% of the deaths for which a cause was known. Among the baseline risk factors found, the significant independent predictors of death were older age, lower ankle-brachial index, diabetes that required medication for control, and having a stroke. No significant predictive associations were noted with either a history of angina or myocardial infarction. Those who had major or minor amputations had a 10-year cumulative rate less than 10%, whereas the rate for revascularization was 18% (Fig 2).

Conclusions.—The risk factors predicting death were older age, lower ankle-brachial index, diabetes sufficiently severe to require medication, and having a stroke. Those with these risk factors had a significantly higher mortality rate. Factors that were not significantly predictive of death included a history of angina and myocardial infarction. The risk for a major amputation at a 10-year follow-up among these patients was low.

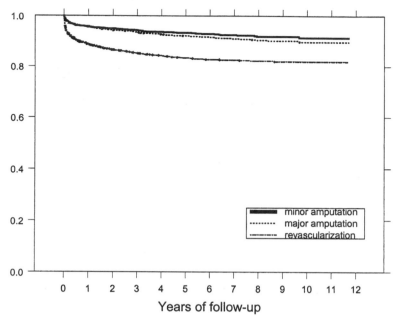

FIGURE 2.—Kaplan-Meier curves showing probability of freedom from selected limb-related events: minor amputation, major amputation, and surgical revascularization. (Courtesy of Muluk SC, Muluk VS, Kelley ME, et al: Outcome events in patients with claudication: A 15-year study in 2777 patients. *J Vasc Surg* 33:251-258, 2001.)

▶ A carefully studied group of male claudicants forms the basis for this report. Not surprisingly, limb loss was exceedingly low, but the annual mortality risk was 12% of the at-risk group. Clinical factors predictive of death included older age, lower ankle-brachial index, diabetes, and a history of stroke. Statistically, smoking was not predictive of death because virtually all patients (94%) had a smoking history. Curiously, a history of myocardial infarction or angina was not predictive of death for unclear reasons. Nonetheless, from this study and others the message is clear: claudicants are more at risk for cardiovascular death than they are for amputation.

R. A. Yeager, MD

Quality of Life in Patients With Intermittent Claudication Using the World Health Organisation (WHO) Questionnaire
Breek JC, Hamming JF, De Vries J, et al (St Elisabeth Hosp, Tilburg, The Netherlands; Martini Hosp, Groningen, The Netherlands; Tilburg Univ, The Netherlands)
Eur J Vasc Endovasc Surg 21:118-122, 2001   10–5

Background.—Intermittent claudication severity is typically assessed by treadmill walking distance or ankle brachial pressure index, neither of which correlates well with patient-reported functional impairment. Quality of life (QOL) was investigated in patients with intermittent claudication.

Methods and Findings.—One hundred fifty-one consecutive patients with claudication and 161 healthy persons completed a revised version of the World Health Organization Quality of Life Assessment Instrument-100. Scores on the physical health and levels of independence domains were significantly worse in the patient group than in the control group. Patients also scored lower on facets of pain and discomfort, energy and fatigue, mobility, activities of daily living, dependence on medication and treatments, working capacity, negative feelings, recreation and leisure, and overall QOL and general health. Increasing disease to incapacitating claudication affected only the mobility facet and the level of independence domain.

Conclusion.—Patients with intermittent claudication had a reduced QOL in many aspects. Comorbidity appears to strongly affect QOL, whereas the effect of walking distance on QOL may be minimal. The findings suggest the need for a reserved attitude toward invasive (even minimally invasive) treatment of such patients.

▶ The measurement of QOL has become increasingly important in vascular surgery. The difficulties inherent in this field lie in the lack of a standardized questionnaire. This article describes the results of the WHOQOL-100 in patients with claudication. Not surprisingly, these patients had a markedly diminished QOL compared with that of healthy controls. Interestingly, walking distance had a small effect on overall QOL, affecting only mobility and level of independence. The authors speculate that comorbidities have a greater effect on QOL than claudication, a reasonable assumption. The key to sorting these variables may be to adopt a questionnaire specific for patients with claudication (such as the Walking Impairment Questionnaire) along with a general QOL questionnaire (MOS-SF36, Nottingham Health Profile). There is a real need for consensus on the optimal surveys to use in our vascular patients.

A. M. Abou-Zamzam, Jr, MD

Influence of Upper- and Lower-Limb Exercise Training on Cardiovascular Function and Walking Distances in Patients With Intermittent Claudication
Walker RD, Nawaz S, Wilkinson CH, et al (Northern Gen Hosp, Sheffield, England)
J Vasc Surg 31:662-669, 2000   10–6

Background.—Exercise improves walking distance in patients with intermittent claudication. However, it is unclear whether this benefit comes from improvements in central cardiovascular function or in localized changes within the lower limb. The effects of upper-extremity exercise was

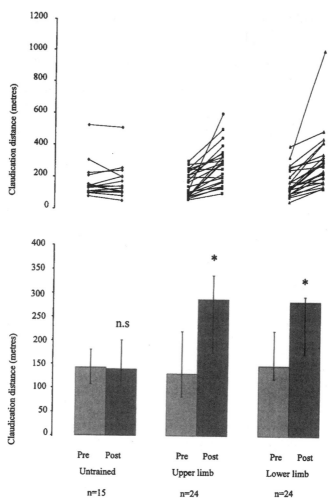

FIGURE 4.—Effects of upper- and lower-limb exercise training on pain-free (claudication) distance in individuals (*upper*) and the group as a whole (*lower*). Data are medians and 25th and 75th quartiles. *P < .001 vs pretraining, Wilcoxon signed rank test. (Courtesy of Walker RD, Nawaz S, Wilkinson CH, et al: Influence of upper- and lower-limb exercise training on cardiovascular function and walking distances in patients with intermittent claudication. *J Vasc Surg* 31:662-669, 2000.)

compared with those of lower-extremity exercise on walking distances in patients with intermittent claudication.

Methods.—The study included 67 patients, aged 33 to 82 years, with moderate to severe intermittent claudication. Upper- and lower-limb ergometric studies were performed to assess the maximum power generated by both forms of exercise, and the shuttle walk test was used to determine pain-free and maximum walking distances. Fifty-two patients were randomized to 6 weeks of arm-cranking or leg-cranking exercise. Exercise sessions were supervised and conducted twice weekly. The remaining 15 patients served as an untrained control group.

Results.—Both exercise groups showed significant gains in maximum power generated during upper- and lower-limb ergometry tests. Furthermore, both forms of exercise were associated with improvement in pain-free walking distance and maximum walking distance. The 2 exercise groups attained similar benefit, compared with no change in the untrained group (Fig 4).

Conclusions.—For patients with intermittent claudication, exercise-induced gains in walking distance appear to result at least partly from improvements in cardiovascular fitness. These patients may gain prompt symptomatic improvement through a carefully prescribed regimen of upper-extremity exercise, while avoiding the discomfort caused by lower-extremity weight-bearing exercise.

▶ This well-controlled study has made the noteworthy observation that an upper limb intermittent exercise program of short duration produced statistically and functionally significant improvement in walking distance in claudicants that was similar in magnitude to the improvement resulting from a lower limb exercise program conducted simultaneously in control claudicants. The authors speculated but did not demonstrate that upper limb exercise programs might be better tolerated in claudicants because of the absence of pain.

L. M. Taylor, Jr, MD

Oral Beraprost Sodium, a Prostaglandin I$_2$ Analogue, for Intermittent Claudication: A Double-blind, Randomized, Multicenter Controlled Trial
Lièvre M, for the Berapost et Claudication Intermittente (BERCI) Research Group (Hôpitaux de Lyon, France; et al)
Circulation 102:426-431, 2000   10–7

Background.—Intermittent claudication is a common lower-limb arterial disease. Among men aged 50 to 75 years, the prevalence of intermittent claudication is estimated to be from 1% to 7%. The goals of medical therapy for patients experiencing intermittent claudication are the improvement of symptoms and the prevention of cardiovascular events. A number of medications, including vasodilators, have been investigated for relief of symptoms, and their outcomes are subject to continuing debate.

Epoprostenol (prostaglandin I$_2$) has demonstrated antiplatelet and vasodilating properties that have made it a theoretically interesting agent in the treatment of intermittent claudication; however, the short half-life and high chemical instability of epoprostenol has precluded its use therapeutically. A number of analogues have been developed including iloprost, which has been shown to provide pain relief and acceleration of ulcer healing in patients with stage III or IV critical leg ischemia. However, an IV infusion of iloprost is required, which precludes its use in the long-term

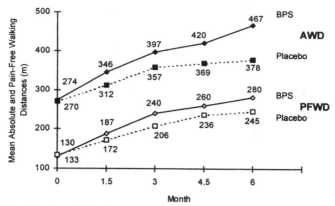

FIGURE 2.—Pain-free and absolute walking distances. Comparison of mean absolute (*AWD*) (*solid symbols*) and mean pain-free (*PFWD*) (*open symbols*) walking distances for beraprost sodium (*BPS*) (*solid lines*) and placebo (*dashed lines*) groups. Distances are in meters. (Courtesy of Lièvre M, for the Berapost et Claudication Intermittente (BERCI) Research Group: Oral beraprost sodium, a prostaglandin I₂ analogue, for intermittent claudication: A double-blind, randomized, multicenter controlled trial. *Circulation* 102:426-431, 2000.)

treatment of intermittent claudication. A recently developed, stable prostaglandin I_2 analogue, beraprost sodium (BPS), is an orally active agent with antiplatelet and vasodilating properties that has been tried in patients with intermittent claudication.

Methods.—A group of 549 patients with intermittent claudication and a pain-free walking distance of 50 to 300 m was enrolled in a 4-week, single-blind, placebo run-in phase. Patients whose pain-free walking distance changed by less than 25% were then randomly assigned to either BPS or placebo in a double-blind phase for 6 months. Treadmill exercise tests were used to measure pain-free and maximum walking distance at baseline and at 1.5, 3, 4.5, and 6 months after randomization. Success was defined as a greater than 50% improvement in pain-free walking distance at 6 months and in 1 or more treadmill tests in the absence of critical cardiovascular events.

Results.—Successful outcomes were achieved in 43.5% of the BPS group and 33.3% of the placebo group. Pain-free walking distances also improved significantly in the BPS group (81.5%) compared with the placebo group (52.5%), while maximum walking distances improved by 60.1% in the BPS group and 35% in the placebo group (Fig 2). The incidence of critical cardiovascular events was 4.8% for patients in the BPS group and 8.9% in the placebo group.

Conclusion.—BPS was shown to be an effective agent in the symptomatic treatment of patients with intermittent claudication. The results of this trial should be confirmed by additional clinical trials.

▶ The current medical therapy for claudication is an interesting paradox. The absolute claudication distance (ACD) is more reliable than the initial claudication distance (ICD). Despite multiple different trials of exercise rehabilitation demonstrating improved ACD efficacy far exceeding that observed in pharmaceutical trials, only recently has a *Current Procedural Terminology (CPT)* code emerged that would allow clinicians to have this care reimbursed. Pharmaceutical trials are carefully designed to exclude patients who cannot consistently perform on the treadmill. Despite this, all trials demonstrate an improvement in ACD over time in the placebo group, attributed to treadmill training or a familiarization effect. If the treadmill is a fixed rate load (as in the current study), debilitated patients with minimal baseline ACD (who theoretically may have the most to benefit from the drug), are excluded because they cannot walk far enough for enrollment. Finally, despite Food and Drug Administration approval, some formularies (VA for example) have been slow to include new claudication drugs because of cost concerns and in their opinion, modest efficacy.

These observations are illustrated in the current trial of beraprost sodium. One of 5 patients enrolled failed to be included in the study because of inconsistent baseline treadmill performance. The treatment group had a 60% improvement in ACD at 6 months, compared with 35% in the placebo arm. This translated to walking an additional 70 m compared with an additional 36 m in the treatment versus placebo arms, respectively. A similar trial in the United States finished enrollment earlier this year, and those results will be crucial to the future of this drug. Whether an expensive TID drug is worth an additional 35 m will clearly be subject to serious debate.

M. R. Nehler, MD

Lower Extremity Vein Grafts

Patency and Characteristics of Lower Extremity Vein Grafts Requiring Multiple Revisions

Landry GJ, Moneta GL, Taylor LM Jr, et al (Oregon Health Sciences Univ, Portland)
J Vasc Surg 32:23-31, 2000   10–8

Introduction.—About 20% of lower-extremity vein grafts (LEVGs) need revision to maintain graft patency. Characteristics of recurrent LEVG lesions and the patency achieved after several revisions have not been highlighted in reports on infrainguinal vein graft stenosis. The patency of multiple revised LEVGs and the timing, location, and angiographic and duplex features of recurrent lesions in patients who underwent LEVGs between January 1990 and December 1998 were assessed in a prospective study.

Methods.—Angiography was performed before all revisions. To characterize recurrent lesions at the time of previous and current graft revision, medical records were reviewed in patients with multiple LEVGs for data regarding the immediate preoperative angiogram and duplex examination findings, angiograms made before the previous revision, and duplex procedures performed after the previous revision. A comparison was made between the patencies of grafts that underwent single revisions and those that underwent multiple revisions.

TABLE 4.—Five-Year Assisted Primary Patency in Grafts Undergoing Single and Multiple Revisions

Interval (Mo)	At Risk	Occluded	Withdrawn	Interval Patency	Cumulative Patency	SE
A. Single revision						
0-1	146	0	0	1.000	1.000	0.0000
2-6	146	2	6	0.986	0.986	0.0099
7-12	138	5	18	0.963	0.948	0.0191
13-24	115	2	29	0.982	0.930	0.0227
25-36	84	1	17	0.988	0.917	0.0256
37-48	66	2	10	0.970	0.886	0.0329
49-60	54	0	15	1.000	0.886	0.0329
B. Multiple revisions						
0-2	37	0	0	1.000	1.000	0.0000
2-6	37	0	0	1.000	1.000	0.0000
7-12	37	1	2	0.972	0.972	0.0274
13-24	34	2	2	0.941	0.913	0.0479
25-36	30	0	7	1.000	0.913	0.0479
37-48	23	0	7	1.000	0.913	0.0479
49-60	16	0	3	1.000	0.913	0.0479

Note: P was not significant between singly and multiply revised grafts.
(Courtesy of Landry GJ, Moneta GL, Taylor LM Jr, et al: Patency and characteristics of lower extremity vein grafts requiring multiple revisions. J Vasc Surg 32:23-31, 2000.)

Results.—Of 233 LEVGs performed, 50 (21%) were repeat revisions. Of grafts needing more than 1 revision, 98% were normal or duplex examinations after initial revision. The 5-year assisted primary patency of multiple revised grafts was similar to those with a single revision (91% vs 89%) (Table 4). Of 60 lesions repaired in the 50 repeat revisions, 29 (48%) were at the previously revised site and 31 (52%) were at new sites. The time between revisions was less when the same site was revised (mean, 11 months), compared with a different site (mean, 20 months). Arteriographic verification of minor (<50% diameter) lesions was present at the time of the initial revision in 23% of the patients for whom revision of the second site was subsequently needed.

Conclusion.—In a series of 233 LEVGs, 21% of those needing initial revision ultimately needed additional revisions. The long-term patency of multiple revised LEVGs is excellent. Lesions occur with the same frequency at the site of prior revision as at new sites. Lesions needing revision at new sites occur significantly later and are infrequently found on prior imaging studies.

▶ Approximately 80% of graft stenoses are isolated, and once repaired, grafts harboring such lesions behave like a normal unrevised vein graft. About 20% of grafts that have been revised, however, as documented in this study, develop subsequent lesions that require re-revision. This article lends support to the concept that vein grafts should be followed up for the patient's life, since they are at ongoing risk for repeat failure, even though the highest risk period is in the first year after implantation.

J. L. Mills, Sr, MD

Infrainguinal Arterial Reconstructions With Vein Grafts in Patients With Prior Aortic Procedures: The Influence of Aneurysm and Occlusive Disease

Upchurch GR Jr, Conte MS, Gerhard-Herman MD, et al (Harvard Med School, Boston)
J Vasc Surg 31:1128-1134, 2000   10–9

Background.—Duplex surveillance has been used to demonstrate that there is an increase over time in the diameter of vein grafts performed for popliteal artery aneurysms, as opposed to vein grafts performed for occlusive disease. The initial diameter of the vein graft was predictive of diameter at final follow-up in a linear regression model. These data suggested that alteration of the remodeling of vein grafts performed in patients with peripheral arterial aneurysms might beneficially affect patency rates. This study investigated whether altered graft patency is present in infrainguinal reconstructions with autogenous vein (IR) in patients with prior abdominal aortic aneurysm (AAA) compared with those grafts performed in patients who have undergone prior aortobifemoral bypass grafting procedures (ABF) for aortoiliac occlusive disease.

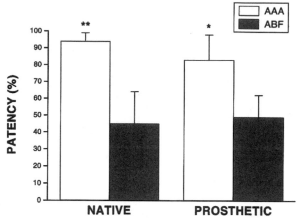

FIGURE 2.—Cumulative 5-year limb primary patency in the abdominal aortic aneurysm (*AAA*) and the aortobifemoral bypass grafting (*ABF*) groups by origin (native or prosthetic) of infrainguinal reconstruction. *Asterisk* indicates $P < .05$, compared with ABF group. *Double asterisk* $P < .007$, compared with ABF group. (Courtesy of Upchurch GR Jr, Conte MS, Gerhard-Herman MD, et al: Infrainguinal arterial reconstructions with vein grafts in patients with prior aortic procedures: The influence of aneurysm and occlusive disease. *J Vasc Surg* 31:1128-1134, 2000.)

Methods.—From 1979 to 1998, 64 autogenous single-segment saphenous IRs solely for infrainguinal occlusive disease were performed in 54 patients with prior aortic reconstructions. Among these patients were 30 IRs with an earlier AAA repair and 34 IRs with an earlier ABF repair. During this same period, 1642 autogenous vein lower-extremity bypass grafting procedures (LEBs) were performed in 1274 patients. Lower-extremity native arterial diameters (AAA, n = 6, ABF, n = 11) and vein graft diameters (AAA, n = 6, ABF, n = 6) were determined by angiography and duplex US. Results for the 3 reconstruction groups—AAA, ABF, and LEP—were compared.

Results.—The cumulative 5-year primary graft patency rate was significantly higher for the AAA group (92% ± 5%) than for the LEB group (63% ± 2%) and the ABF group (44% ± 11%) (Fig 2). In addition, the cumulative 5-year patency rate was decreased in the ABF group compared with the LEB group. Linear regression and a Student's *t* test demonstrated a significant increase in both native arterial and vein graft diameter in the AAA group compared with the ABF group.

Conclusion.—Compared with those in patients without a previous aortic procedure, IRs in patients with prior AAA repairs have substantial improvements in graft patency, while IRs in patients with prior ABF reconstructions for aortoiliac occlusive disease have significantly decreased graft patency. For patients with prior AAA repairs, larger arterial diameter and altered vein graft adaptation may contribute to the superior long-term outcomes of IRs.

▶ These data show that patency of infrarenal arterial reconstructions is superior in patients with prior AAA repair. Figure 2 is impressive in that the cumulative 5-year patency of vein grafts in patients with prior AAA repair is 92%. Moreover, the cumulative 5-year patency of prosthetic grafts in this group was well over 80%. We do know that the vein diameters in patients with prior AAA repair dilate with time, but from these data it is not the only reason for superior patency, given that the prosthetic graft also has a high 5-year patency. Perhaps something systemic is acting on the vein graft and clotting mechanisms in patients with aortic aneurysms leading to superior graft patency or, in contrast, perhaps patients with occlusive disease are more apt to thrombose their grafts. This article does not give any information regarding hypercoagulable states or whether patients were taking warfarin. Although this report is informative in describing what happens over time in these 2 groups of patients, I find that it has stimulated many questions as to why this occurs, and it indirectly proves that patients with aneurysms are very different from those with atherosclerotic occlusive disease. More questions is a good thing.

R. B. McLafferty, MD

Predictors of Outcome When Reoperating for Early Infrainguinal Bypass Occlusion
Lombardi JV, Dougherty MJ, Calligaro KD, et al (Pennsylvania Hosp, Philadelphia)
Ann Vasc Surg 14:350-355, 2000   10–10

Background.—Among patients undergoing infrainguinal bypass grafting, early graft thrombosis is a poor prognostic sign. For many patients, attempts to salvage these failed grafts are unsuccessful and carry high morbidity. Predictors of success or failure of interventions for early infrainguinal graft thrombosis were identified.

Methods.—The retrospective study included 33 patients who experienced thrombosis within 30 days after infrainguinal bypass grafting. Five factors were assessed for their impact on the 12-month patency rate: conduit type (single-segment saphenous vein vs another vein, or composite conduit); type of repair (construction of a new graft at the initial take-back procedure, local revision, or thrombectomy) (Table 2); good versus poor

TABLE 2.—Procedure Performed at Reoperation

Reoperative Modality	n (%)
Thrombectomy alone	3 (9)
Thrombectomy/revision	18 (55)
Graft replacements	
SVG replaced with PTFE	10 (30)
SVG replaced with spliced vein	1 (3)
Spliced vein replaced with PTFE	1 (3)

Abbreviations: SVG, Saphenous vein graft; *PTFE*, polytetrafluoroethylene.
(Courtesy of Lombardi JV, Dougherty MJ, Calligaro KD, et al: Predictors of outcome when reoperating for early infrainguinal bypass occlusion. *Ann Vasc Surg* 14:350-355, 2000.)

TABLE 3.—Life Table for Cumulative Secondary Patency Rate

Interval	Grafts at Risk (n)	Failed Grafts (n)	Withdrawn (n)	Interval Salvage	Cumulative Patency (%)	Standard Error
0-1	33	9	1	0.72	100.0	0.00
1-4	23	0	3	1.00	72.3	7.93
4-8	20	3	1	0.85	72.3	8.51
8-12	16	0	1	1.00	61.2	9.53
12-16	15	1	1	0.93	61.2	9.84
16-20	13	0	2	1.00	57.0	10.36
20-25	11	0	1	1.00	57.0	11.27
25-30	10	2	1	0.79	57.0	11.82
30-35	7	0	2	1.00	45.0	12.61
35-40	5	0	2	1.00	45.0	14.92
40-50	3	0	1	1.00	45.0	19.26
50-55	2	0	1	1.00	45.0	23.59
55-60	1	1	0	1.00	45.0	33.36
60-75	0	1	1	3.00	45.0	33.36

(Courtesy of Lombardi JV, Dougherty MJ, Calligaro KD, et al: Predictors of outcome when reoperating for early infrainguinal bypass occlusion. *Ann Vasc Surg* 14:350-355, 2000.)

run-off; correctable versus noncorrectable problem; and history of previous ipsilateral bypass versus no such history.

Results.—The 30-day mortality rate was 3%, and complications included 9 recurrent graft thromboses and 8 amputations. At 12 months, the limb salvage rate was 65% and the secondary patency rate was 61% (Table 3). All 5 variables studied were significant predictors. On logistic regression, 3 independent predictors of 1-year patency were type of revision, previous bypass, and run-off. One-year patency was only 6% for a patient with thrombectomy/revision, a previous bypass, and poor run-off compared with 99% for a patient with none of these factors.

Conclusions.—Useful predictors of the results of intervention for early infrainguinal bypass occlusion are identified. For a patient with no focal lesion that is clearly causing the occlusion, consideration should be given to complete graft replacement, even if a prosthesis will be required. When poor risk factors are present, primary amputation may be preferable to repeated salvage attempts.

▶ It is well established by all modern series of infrainguinal arterial bypass procedures that an early graft failure rate of 3% to 7% is to be expected. This failure rate reflects technical error, which usually translates to judgmental errors, such as accepting an inferior conduit, accepting a poor runoff target, or true errors in technique, such as tunneling errors, twisting and kinking, and anastomotic errors. What then predicts early graft failure? Bad judgment, which is difficult to quantify, is variable in its expression, and certainly will not be influenced by multivariate analysis. Judgment is often shaped by one's last bad outcome and by one's favorable outcomes. Yet fatigue and stress often influence judgment in negative ways, which I believe accounts for the majority of technical errors leading to early graft failure. Therefore, the only message from this article is that this group of competent vascular surgeons showed poor judgment in 4.5% of the 724 infrainguinal bypass procedures performed during a 7-year period, clearly acceptable results. Attempts to salvage the grafts with better judgment only salvaged 45% of the grafts through 3-year follow-up. To attempt to develop a clinical algorithm from these data would be deserving of the Camel Flatulence Award.

E. J. Harris, Jr, MD

Is Lower Extremity Revascularization Worthwhile in Patients With End-Stage Renal Disease?
Korn P, Hoenig SJ, Skillman JJ, et al (Cornell Univ, New York; Harvard Med School, Boston)
Surgery 128:472-479, 2000   10–11

Background.—The presence of comorbid diseases may complicate treatments for leg ischemia, thus resulting in less favorable outcomes. Therefore, patient subgroups for whom the risk and cost of lower extremity revascularization outweigh the benefits need to be identified. The outcomes of lower extremity revascularization in patients with end-stage renal disease were reported to determine the benefits and costs of an aggressive approach to limb preservation in such patients.

Methods.—Twenty-three patients receiving dialysis who underwent 33 bypass operations on 31 limbs at 1 center during 5 years were studied. Indications for revascularization included limited or extensive tissue loss and ischemia without tissue loss. Femorotibial/pedal bypasses were performed in 22 patients, femoropopliteal bypasses were performed in 10, and an aortobifemoral bypass was performed in 1. Fifty-seven percent of the limbs underwent digital or transmetatarsal amputation.

Findings.—The primary patency rate at 30 days was 100%. At 2 years, the cumulative primary and secondary patency rates were 65% and 79%, respectively. Limb salvage rates were 67% at 1 year and 59% at 2 years. The patient survival rate at 2 years was only 47%. Peritoneal dialysis predicted a short survival duration: 4 of 5 such patients died within 3 months of treatment. In addition, extensive tissue loss predicted a reduced rate of limb salvage. At 1 year, only 39% of limbs with extensive tissue loss were salvaged compared with 78% and 100% of limbs with limited and no tissue loss, respectively (Fig 2). The mean hospital cost was $44,308 per year of limb salvage.

Conclusions.—Revascularization of ischemic limbs in patients receiving dialysis can result in excellent initial graft patency and reasonable limb salvage rates. However, patient survival duration is short, and the cost is high, which indicates that a selective approach to revascularization may be more appropriate for this patient population. Primary amputation may be

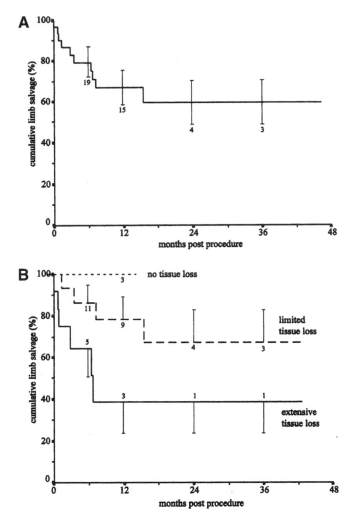

FIGURE 2.—**A**, Cumulative limb salvage for lower extremity revascularization of 31 limbs in 23 patients treated with long-term dialysis. **B**, Impact of tissue loss on limb salvage. Patients who died without having undergone major amputation were censored. *Bars* indicate the SE. *Numbers below the graphs* indicate the number of remaining limbs; initial sample size n = 31 limbs. (Courtesy of Korn P, Hoenig SJ, Skillman JJ, et al: Is lower extremity revascularization worthwhile in patients with end-stage renal disease? *Surgery* 128:472-479, 2000.)

the best treatment for patients receiving peritoneal dialysis and for patients with extensive tissue loss.

▶ The central observation in this and the many other recent series on outcome after limb salvage surgery in patients with end-stage renal disease (ESRD) is the remarkably short life expectancy of this cohort after otherwise successful (in terms of operative mortality and graft patency) revascularization. This is at least the third recent series in the vascular literature to define survival as 2 years or less for most such patients. Added to that is the observation (similar to our own and many others) that limb loss is distressingly frequent despite ongoing graft patency. It is therefore clear that the pathophysiology of limb ischemia in the setting of ESRD is unique and poorly understood. Fortunately, the medical community at large is increasingly aware of the synergistic risks associated with lower limb ischemia and dialysis-dependent renal failure[1]—enough so that the US Department of Veterans Affairs has recently launched a Cooperative Studies program focused on homocysteine metabolism and peripheral vascular disease in patients with ESRD. Hopefully, this and future studies will make meaningful contributions to understanding the pathophysiology and optimizing treatment for this challenging clinical condition.

R. L. Dalman, MD

Reference

1. Reddan DN, Marcus RJ, Owen WF Jr, et al: Long-term outcomes of revascularization for peripheral vascular occlusive disease in end stage renal disease patients. *Am J Kidney Dis* 38:57-63, 2001.

Pedal Branch Artery Bypass: A Viable Limb Salvage Option
Connors JP, Walsh DB, Nelson PR, et al (Dartmouth Med School, Lebanon, NH)
J Vasc Surg 32:1071-1079, 2000   10–12

Background.—The pedal branch arteries (PBAs) have emerged as potential bypass targets for patients requiring distal revascularization. A 10-year experience with the use of PBAs for limb salvage is reviewed, including patient and technical variables associated with favorable outcomes.

Methods.—From 1988 to 1998, the investigators performed a total of 24 vein grafts to PBAs for limb salvage in 23 patients. These cases accounted for 3% of infrainguinal revascularization procedures performed for chronic critical limb ischemia during this time. The patients all lacked adequate tibial, peroneal, or dorsal pedal target arteries. The graft patency and limb salvage results were assessed and compared with the results of 133 perimalleolar posterior tibial grafts—at or below the level of the ankle—or dorsalis pedis bypass grafts performed during the same period.

Results.—Ninety-two percent of patients undergoing PBA bypasses were men compared with 69% of those in the comparison group. The patients in the PBA group were relatively less likely to have overt coronary artery disease or strokes but were more likely to have end-stage renal disease. The anterior lateral malleolar artery, an unconventional bypass target, was used in 17% of PBA cases (Fig 1B). The patients in the PBA group had a 2-year primary patency rate of 70% compared with 78% in the perimalleolar bypass group (Fig 2A). Limb salvage rates were 80% versus 91% for the PBA and perimalleolar bypass groups, respectively. The

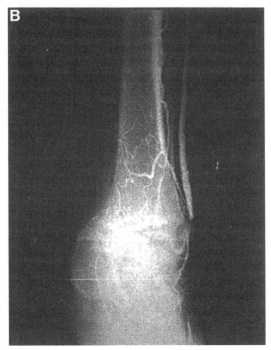

FIGURE 1.—Anterior lateral malleolar bypass. Preoperative lateral (B) arteriogram demonstrating anterior lateral malleolar artery branch of peroneal artery; intraoperative arteriogram demonstrating a patent distal bypass to anterior malleolar artery. (Courtesy of Connors JP, Walsh DB, Nelson PR, et al: Pedal branch artery bypass: A viable limb salvage option. *J Vasc Surg* 32:1071-1079, 2000.)

use of above-knee or below-knee inflow arteries made no difference in terms of the patency rate or limb salvage results.

Conclusions.—For patients lacking more proximal target arteries, an autogenous vein bypass to the PBAs is a potential alternative for salvage of the limb. Patency and salvage rates are similar to those for perimalleolar tibial artery bypasses. The possibility of a PBA bypass should be considered before resorting to amputation.

▶ To my knowledge, no one has yet reported femoral to digital artery bypass for limb salvage. These authors are getting close, and with surprisingly good results. Our arteriograms are necessarily going to have to show us more and more distal detail if we are to truly exhaust all possibilities for limb salvage.

L. M. Taylor, Jr, MD

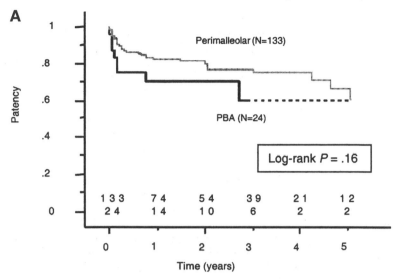

FIGURE 2.—A, Life table analysis for patency for PBA versus perimalleolar bypass. Kaplan-Meier life table plot comparing cumulative graft patency for PBA bypass and perimalleolar bypass. The *numbers* in the table correspond to number of bypasses at risk of failure in each group at beginning of each interval. The *dashed line* indicates where SE exceeds 10% for the PBA bypass group. Statistical comparison performed with Mantel-Cox log-rank analysis. *Abbreviation: PBA*, Pedal branch artery. (Courtesy of Connors JP, Walsh DB, Nelson PR, et al: Pedal branch artery bypass: A viable limb salvage option. *J Vasc Surg* 32:1071-1079, 2000.)

Impact of Increasing Comorbidity on Infrainguinal Reconstruction: A 20-Year Perspective

Conte MS, Belkin M, Upchurch GR, et al (Harvard Med School, Boston)
Ann Surg 233:445-452, 2001   10–13

Background.—During the past 20 years, these authors have noted that more patients are requiring treatment for infrainguinal arterial occlusive disease. These patients seem to have more comorbidities, and demographics appear to have shifted as well (eg, more women are being treated). Changes in demographics and risk factors and their impact on surgical outcomes of patients undergoing lower extremity vascular reconstruction (LER) were reviewed over a 20-year period at Brigham and Women's Hospital in Boston.

Methods.—Medical records were used to identify all patients who had undergone LER by means of an autogenous vein conduit between 1978 and 1997. For analysis, patient data were examined in 4 time frames: 1978-1982 (group 1), 1983-1987 (group 2), 1988-1992 (group 3), and 1993-1997 (group 4). Patient demographics, risk factors, and outcomes were compared among these 4 intervals.

Results.—Between 1978 and 1997, 1274 patients underwent 1642 autogenous vein LER procedures at the authors' institution. Follow-up was complete for 70% of patients overall (mean follow-up, 968 days), including 56%, 68%, 63%, and 82% of patients in groups 1, 2, 3, and 4, respectively. Compared with groups 1 and 2, patients in group 4 were significantly older (median age, 65 and 67 vs 70 years, respectively); more likely to be female (26% and 40% vs 47%); and more likely to have diabetes mellitus (37% and 36% vs 52%), prior coronary artery bypass grafting (6% and 5% vs 21%), and renal insufficiency (6% and 7% vs 21%).

These changes in patient demographics and risk factors were reflected by changes in indications and procedural variables. Comparing groups 1 and 2 to group 4, the proportion of patients undergoing LER for claudication decreased significantly (30% and 31% vs 20%), while the proportions of patients undergoing LER for ulceration (18% and 20% vs 37%) or tissue necrosis (31% and 35% vs 53%) increased significantly. As time passed, the use of nonreversed greater saphenous vein (0% and 5% vs 38%) and ectopic (4% and 3% vs 7%) or composite (0.4% and 2% vs 12%) vein grafts increased significantly. Additionally, the level of outflow used during LER became more distal, with significantly more tibial/pedal outflow sites in the most recent interval (23% and 45% vs 68%).

Yet despite these trends, the surgical mortality rate remained unchanged throughout this period, at 2%. The incidence of complications decreased as well, with a significant decrease in early graft occlusion between groups 1 and 4 (9% vs 5%). The patient survival rate did not differ significantly according to interval (overall 5-year survival, 70%), nor did primary graft patency (overall at 5 years, 63%), secondary graft patency (overall at 5 years, 73%), or limb salvage rates (overall at 5 years, 85%).

However, among LER procedures performed exclusively for limb salvage indications, 5-year limb salvage rates improved significantly between the earliest and latest intervals (75% vs 86%). Finally, the length of hospital stay decreased significantly between groups 3 and 4 (from 15.7 to 11.7 days; a 25% decrease).

Conclusion.—The demographics and risk factors of patients undergoing LER procedures have changed substantially over the past 20 years. The management of these patients is increasingly complex, yet the safety, durability, and effectiveness of LER with autogenous vein grafts has remained consistently excellent.

▶ In this article Dr Conte and associates reflect on 20 years of lower extremity reconstructive surgery. Their results show us not only how things have changed over the past 2 decades, but they also demonstrate trends that are likely to continue over the ensuing years. In general, patients are older and sicker, and revascularization procedures are becoming increasingly complex. Yet even when the deck is stacked against you, the authors demonstrate the excellent results that can be achieved with respect to patency, limb salvage, and perioperative morbidity with an aggressive program of autogenous bypass procedures and postoperative surveillance. Their experience reflects our own in Oregon, and, I suspect, that of many vascular surgeons around the country.

G. J. Landry, MD

Management of Ischemic Heel Ulceration and Gangrene: An Evaluation of Factors Associated With Successful Healing

Treiman GS, Oderich GSC, Ashrafi A, et al (Univ of Utah, Salt Lake City; Hawaii Permanente Med Group, Honolulu)
J Vasc Surg 31:1110-1118, 2000   10–14

Background.—Ulcers and gangrene affecting the heel are difficult problems to treat. Treatment failure commonly leads to amputation of the foot. The response of unhealing heel ulcers and gangrene to treatment interventions was analyzed and the variable associated with successful treatment were identified.

Methods.—The multicenter review included 91 patients at 4 hospitals. All had heel wounds that had not healed for 1 to 12 months because of arterial insufficiency, that is, absent pedal pulses and a decreased ankle/brachial index (ABI). The patients were 57 men and 34 women, mean age, 67 years, with a mean preoperative ABI of 0.51. Thirty-one percent had infected wounds. Risk factors included impaired renal function in 55%, with 24% undergoing dialysis; diabetes in 70%; and smoking in 64%. All patients received topical wound care, and 50% underwent wound debridement. Treatment included infrainguinal bypass in 81 patients, inflow procedures in 4, superficial femoral artery percutaneous transluminal angioplasty in 3, and primary below-knee amputation in 3. The treatment outcomes were assessed, including the effects of patient risk factors, hemodynamic variables, and arteriographic findings.

Results.—Eighty-five percent of patients had in-line flow to the foot with 1 or more patent vessels after surgery. A pedal pulse was present in 66%, and the mean ABI improved from 0.40 to 0.91. At a mean of 21 months' follow-up, 85% were alive. Seventy-three percent of the patients' wounds had healed; the mean healing time was 3 months, and all wounds had healed by 6 months. Sixteen percent did not heal and a below-knee amputation was necessary in 11%. The 3-year limb salvage rate was 86%. Ninety-one percent of infrainguinal bypasses remained patent throughout follow-up, with a 3-year primary assisted patency rate of 87%. The wounds of all patients with graft occlusion did not heal. Significant predictors of successful healing included normal renal function, a palpable pedal pulse, posterior tibial artery patency beyond the ankle, and the number of patent tibial arteries after bypass to the ankle. The success of treatment was unaffected by ABI, infection, diabetes, and other cardiovascular risk factors.

Conclusions.—For patients with unhealing ulcers or gangrene of the heel, complete healing is achievable but may take up to 6 months. Short-term graft patency has a minimal impact on healing. Most wounds will heal with successful arterial reconstruction, particularly when the posterior tibial artery is patent postoperatively. Impaired renal function is a risk factor for treatment failure, but such patients are still candidates for surgical revascularization.

▶ This article supports other data that patients with renal failure have dismal limb salvage rates despite technically successful revascularization. This article is also important in that it addresses the outcome of limb bypass surgery a bit more from the functional standpoint by giving detailed information on wound healing. A current "wave" in vascular research is to better define functional outcomes from various interventions, as there is a large deficit in the vascular literature on adequate descriptions of functional outcomes.

W. K. Williamson, MD

11 Upper Extremity Vascular and Hemoaccess

Hemodialysis

Use of Superficial Femoral Vein for Hemodialysis Arteriovenous Access
Huber TS, Ozaki CK, Flynn TC, et al (Univ of Florida, Gainesville; Gainesville VA Med Ctr, Fla)
J Vasc Surg 31:1038-1041, 2000   11–1

Background.—Maintaining access for hemodialysis in patients with end-stage renal disease is challenging. There are clinical practice guidelines for establishing access in these patients, but there is little consensus on how to maintain access in patients with repeated access failures, veins that are unsuitable for arteriovenous fistula, or relative contraindications to prosthetic materials. Two patients for whom a composite saphenous–superficial femoral vein autogenous access was constructed were described.

Case 1.—Woman, 29, had a 9-year history of end-stage renal disease of unknown etiology. Previous efforts at renal transplantation, peritoneal dialysis, and implantation of prosthetic arteriovenous accesses had failed. At presentation, the patient was dialyzed through a right internal jugular catheter. Arterial studies were performed, and a polytetrafluoroethylene graft was inserted in the right axillary artery–right axillary vein. This graft thrombosed the next day, so it was removed and replaced with a composite autogenous access constructed from the right saphenous and superficial femoral veins. This graft also thrombosed the next day. The autogenous access was removed and used to create a right superficial femoral artery–common femoral vein access (Fig 1). The patient began using this access at 6 weeks postoperatively, and it has been working well for the past 16 months.

Case 2.—Man, 61, had chronic renal insufficiency caused by Wegener's granulomatosis. A Tenckhoff catheter had been inserted

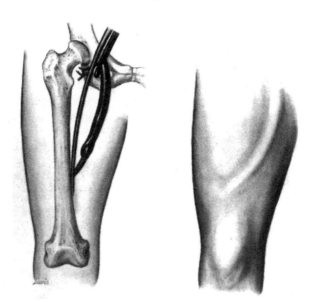

FIGURE 1.—The configuration of the thigh autogenous access and its superficial appearance. A composite saphenous–superficial femoral vein composite graft was constructed. Both vein segments were used in a reversed fashion, and the valves were not lysed. The arterial anastomosis was performed to the distal superficial femoral artery near the level of the adductor canal, and the venous anastomosis was performed to the common femoral vein. (Courtesy of Huber TS, Ozaki CK, Flynn TC, et al: Use of superficial femoral vein for hemodialysis arteriovenous access. *J Vasc Surg* 31:1038-1041, 2000.)

3 years earlier, but had never been used. Arterial studies were performed, and an autogenous access constructed of the saphenous and superficial femoral veins was inserted in the right brachial artery–axillary vein (Fig 2). This access worked for about 8 months, at which time decreased flow through the access was

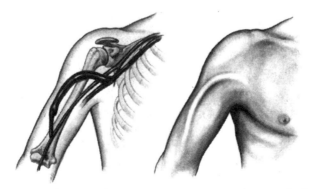

FIGURE 2.—The configuration of the arm autogenous access and its superficial appearance. A composite saphenous–superficial femoral vein composite graft was constructed. Both vein segments were used in a reversed fashion, and the valves were not lysed. The arterial anastomosis was performed to the brachial artery proximal to the antecubital crease, and the venous anastomosis was performed to the axillary vein within the axilla. (Courtesy of Huber TS, Ozaki CK, Flynn TC, et al: Use of superficial femoral vein for hemodialysis arteriovenous access. *J Vasc Surg* 31:1038-1041, 2000.)

noted. A stenosis was identified in the graft near the anastomosis of the superficial femoral vein and the axillary vein. An interposition graft with an additional segment of superficial femoral vein was implanted from the distal aspect of the superficial femoral vein to the more distal axillary vein. Flow through the graft returned to baseline levels, and this access has worked well for the subsequent 5 months.

Conclusion.—The superficial femoral vein is a popular choice for aortic and venous reconstruction and for infrainguinal revascularization, with good long-term results. This is the first report of the use of the superficial femoral vein for providing hemodialysis access. Early results indicate that this access functions like a mature arteriovenous fistula. More follow-up is needed to determine whether this access can withstand repeated cannulations and whether intimal hyperplasia will develop at the venous anastomosis (as occurs with prosthetic accesses). Nonetheless, composite saphenous–superficial femoral vein autogenous access may be useful in maintaining hemodialysis access in patients with limited access options.

▶ The superficial femoral vein (SFV) represents a viable alternative in complicated patients with normal lower extremity arterial and venous circulation. Whether a saphenous vein interposition is necessary to limit flow and potential limb steal and facilitate the transposition of the SFV from a deep to superficial plane remains to be seen. Surprisingly, this appears to be the first published report of SFV-based hemodialysis access—it most certainly will not be the last. For young patients, this should be considered as a further arrow in the quiver of the all-autogenous hemodialysis access revolution that continues to grow in influence and popularity. Adherence to just such a policy in our own practice in the last year has noticeably reduced the number of intermediate and late access failures and infectious complications previously associated with prosthetic devices. Innovations like this bring closer the day when 90% or more of all high-flow fistula or shunt procedures will be performed strictly using autogenous conduit, a goal far surpassing the 1997 expectations of the NKF-DOQI guidelines.

R. L. Dalman, MD

Brachial Arterial Access: Endovascular Treatment of Failing Brescia-Cimino Hemodialysis Fistulas—Initial Success and Long-term Results
Manninen HI, Kaukanen ET, Ikäheimo R, et al (Kuopio Univ, Finland)
Radiology 218:711-718, 2001   11–2

Objective.—Most patients undergoing chronic hemodialysis in European centers are equipped with Brescia-Cimino fistulas. Because the patency of these fistulas is only 65%, there are a number of methods for the treatment of failing grafts. The usefulness and technical performance of endovascular therapy for failing Brescia-Cimino fistulas have not been

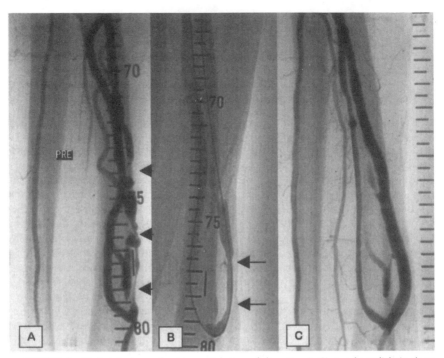

FIGURE 1.—Typical endovascular intervention in a failing Brescia-Cimino hemodialysis shunt through antegrade brachial arterial access. **A,** Angiogram obtained from the frontal view before the intervention (*PRE*) demonstrates multifocal tight stenoses (*arrowheads*) at the efferent antebrachial vein. **B,** Angiogram obtained from the frontal view shows the balloon inflated at the disease segment (*arrows*). **C,** Angiogram obtained from the frontal view after percutaneous transluminal angioplasty shows patency. There is slight spasm at the afferent radial artery because of mechanical handling of the artery during the intervention. The scale is in centimeters on a radiopaque ruler. (Courtesy of Manninen HI, Kaukanen ET, Ikäheimo R, et al: Brachial arterial access: Endovascular treatment of failing Brescia-Cimino hemodialysis fistulas—Initial success and long-term results. *Radiology* 218:711-718, 2001. Radiologcal Society of North America.)

well-documented. The safety and efficacy of endovascular intervention via antegrade brachial artery access in failing Brescia-Cimino hemodialysis fistulas were prospectively evaluated.

Methods.—Beginning in 1994, a prospective trial was begun to evaluate the total life span of antebrachial Brescia-Cimino fistulas. There were 103 interventions performed in 53 Brescia-Cimino shunts in 51 patients (29 men), aged 22 to 80 years. The average functional time before intervention was 10.5 months.

> *Technique.*—Balloon angiography was performed on stenosed or occluded segments, and, in the case of thrombus formation, boluses of urokinase were forcefully injected into the thrombotic segment (Fig 1).

Results.—Twenty fistulas required repeated interventions. In 37 (74%) of the 50 repeated interventions, the site of the stenosis was the same, in 11 interventions additional new segments were involved, and in 2 interventions only new segments were involved. The anatomical and technical success rates were 76% and 92%, respectively. The overall technical success rate for primary and subsequent interventions was 95%. The complication rate was 12% and included 8 minor and 4 major complications, none of which required surgical intervention. During the average 23.3-month follow-up, 14 patients received an allograft kidney, and 2 patients received a new Brescia-Cimino hemodialysis fistula. The 6-month, and 1-, 2-, and 3-year primary clinical patency rates were 58%, 44%, 40%, and 32%, respectively. The corresponding assisted patency rates were 88%, 82%, 77%, and 77%, respectively. Poor outcome was predicted when the main lesion was located at the arteriovenous anastomosis rather than at other segments, and by a small inflow artery rather than a normal-caliber inflow artery.

Conclusion.—Endovascular interventions with antegrade brachial arterial access are effective and can be repeated as necessary to restore function of failing Brescia-Cimino fistulas.

▶ What to do with the "failing" arteriovenous fistula and the "thrombosed" arteriovenous fistula are 2 different kettles of fish. As best gathered from these data, 10 fistulas had thrombosis that required some type of thrombolysis. The remaining 43 were patent, yet either not fully mature or failing because of problems on the dialysis machine. The important question is whether patients who underwent intervention for thrombosis did as well as patients who had interventions for a failing fistula. If the subset of patients with thrombosis had exceedingly poor secondary patency rates, then endovascular intervention should be abandoned. This is certainly true for surgical thrombectomy of autogenous fistulas. Whether surgery or endovascular intervention is best for the "failing" fistula remains an important issue. My gut feeling is surgical repair would be more durable, but there are few data to back that belief. I still believe that if a fistula has a thrombosis, it is time for new hemodialysis access. My hat goes off to the authors for their diligent long-term follow-up. "Long-term" remains a phrase that is often missing in articles addressing hemodialysis access.

R. B. McLafferty, MD

Long-term Results of Arteriovenous Fistulas Using Transposed Autologous Basilic Vein
Murphy GJ, White SA, Knight AJ, et al (Leicester Gen Hosp, England)
Br J Surg 87:819-823, 2000   11–3

Background.—For patients who require long-term hemodialysis, the first choice for vascular access is the radiocephalic arteriovenous fistula. Improvements in hemodialysis and in life expectancy for these patients

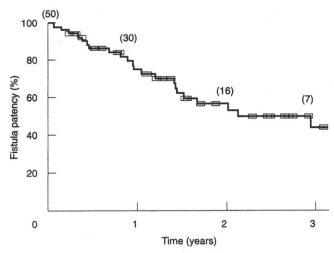

FIGURE 1.—Cumulative secondary patency of 50 brachiobasilic arteriovenous fistulas that were used successfully for dialysis. (Courtesy of Murphy GJ, White SA, Knight AJ, et al: Long-term results of arteriovenous fistulas using transposed autologous basilic vein. *Br J Surg* 87:819-823, 2000. Publisher, Blackwell Science Ltd.)

have led to an increasing number of patients who are in need of secondary or tertiary vascular access procedures. When suitable superficial veins cannot be found in the arm because of previous fistula formation or venipuncture, vascular access is usually obtained by means of a transposed autologous vein or prosthetic graft. More recently, the outcomes with use of polytetrafluoroethylene (PTFE) arteriovenous grafts have improved, 1-year secondary patency rates ranging from 80% to 90% have been reported. In addition, these grafts are always available, and they have a high technical success rate. Earlier cannulation of PTFE grafts compared with autologous veins has also been reported.

However, PTFE grafts have been associated with a high complication rate (60%-100%), and reported complications include infection and thrombosis, requiring an average of 1 operation per graft per year for maintenance of patency. Less attention has been given to the brachial artery to transposed (autologous) basilic vein arteriovenous fistula, but early reports have demonstrated promising results, with primary patency rates of 75% to 90% at 1 year. The long-term patency rate and associated complications of basilic vein arteriovenous fistula for long-term hemodialysis were evaluated.

Methods.—Brachiobasilic fistulas (74) were performed in 65 patients. In 84% of patients, the procedure was a secondary or tertiary access procedure.

Results.—Fifty (68%) of 74 fistulas were successfully used for dialysis and 24 (32%) were never used, including 13 fistulas that failed without being used for dialysis. Failure occurred in 34 of 74 (46%) fistulas. Five patients underwent transplant, and 10 patients died with a functioning fistula. The 30-day secondary patency rate was 73% at 1 year, 53% at 2 years, and 43% at 3 years (Fig 1). Further surgical procedures were performed in 19 patients. Complications developed in 51 (69%) fistulas, the most common complication being arm edema (24%), thrombosis (22%), and bleeding (18%).

Conclusion.—The autologous transposed brachiobasilic fistula demonstrated equivalent patency and lower complication rates compared with the PTFE interposition graft in high-risk patients.

▶ In my practice, I tend to see dialysis patients with multiple failed access sites, usually PTFE bridge grafts. How to provide access for these patients is often problematic. The basilic transposition procedure has been useful for these patients, although it is a more involved procedure than this article suggests. The basilic vein is larger than any other arm vein, and has usually been protected from phlebotomy and venipuncture trauma. The mobilization of the vein and the tunneling of the vein graft without twisting or kinking are more difficult steps than one would expect. Its length is variable among patients, and with a short segment it is sometimes difficult to mobilize enough length to tunnel the vein to the brachial artery. The durability of this fistula is well documented by the results from this series, and my own experience is similar.

E. J. Harris, Jr, MD

Improving Longevity of Prosthetic Dialysis Grafts in Patients With Disadvantaged Venous Outflow
Wladis AR, Mesh CL, White J, et al (Good Samaritan Hosp, Cincinnati, Ohio)
J Vasc Surg 32:997-1005, 2000   11–4

Objective.—The autogenous arteriovenous fistula is the gold standard of access for chronic dialysis hemoaccess. Veins not suitable for fistula creation are accessed by means of a prosthetic arteriovenous bridge graft (AVBG), although these grafts are associated with increased rates of thrombotic and infectious complications. Preoperative venous duplex scanning was used to direct the construction of prosthetic AVBGs to improve the outcome in patients with disadvantaged venous outflow.

Methods.—Between July 1, 1997, and May 31, 1998, 114 patients underwent 115 placements of AVBGs. There were 64 patients with normal venous outflow and an initial arteriovenous bridge graft. Patients with disadvantaged venous outflow (DVO) were divided into those who had a clinical examination (REDO/DVO, 16 patients) and those who had a clinical examination and preoperative duplex scanning (MAP/DVO, 34 patients). Life table primary and secondary patency rates were calculated and compared for the 3 groups.

Results.—Primary patency rates at 6 months were 65.9% for the normal venous outflow group, 66.4% for the MAP/DVO group, and 43.8% for the REDO/DVO group. The corresponding secondary patency rates were 91.9%, 91.1%, and 75.0%.

Conclusion.—Normal venous outflow and MAP/DVO secondary patency rates were significantly better than REDO/DVO secondary patency rates for at least 12 months. Preoperative venous duplex mapping increases the longevity of arteriovenous bridge grafts in patients with disadvantaged outflow.

▶ The authors point out that preoperative venous mapping of upper extremity veins should be routinely performed before placement or revision of an upper extremity arteriovenous dialysis shunt. The old axiom holds true that better outflow equals better patency, and clearly the vascular laboratory provides more accurate and objective measurements of venous outflow in preparation for operations for arteriovenous fistulas. Even the tiniest step forward is welcome in the frustrating world of maintaining hemodialysis access in patients with chronic renal failure.

G. L. Moneta, MD

The Effect of a Venous Anastomosis Tyrell Vein Collar on the Primary Patency of Arteriovenous Grafts in Patients Undergoing Hemodialysis

Gagne PJ, Martinez J, DeMassi R, et al (Naval Med Ctr, Portsmouth, Va; Norfolk Surgical Group, Va)
J Vasc Surg 32:1149-1154, 2000   11–5

Objective.—Failed access is the most frequent cause of hospitalization in patients undergoing hemodialysis for end-stage renal disease. Polytetrafluoroethylene arteriovenous grafts (AVGs) are becoming increasingly more common even though the average patency is only 13 months. Whether a Tyrell collar could improve primary AVG patency by decreasing compliance mismatch and venous outflow tract intimal hyperplasia was investigated in a randomized, prospective study (Fig 1).

Methods.—Between August 1996 and March 1998, 17 patients (8 men), aged 31 to 79 years, were prospectively randomly assigned to undergo conventional end-to-side venous anastomosis (control group = 10) or end-to-side anastomosis with a Tyrell vein collar between the graft and the outflow vein (study group = 7). Graft failure was defined as graft thrombosis, graft removal and ligation, or inadequate graft function requiring revision. The study was terminated early for ethical reasons.

Results.—Outflow vein diameters were significantly smaller in the study group than in the control group (4.4 vs 5.2 mm). Six (86%) study patients and 2 (20%) control patients had graft failure within 9 months. One study patient had a patent graft at 12 months. Four study grafts failed because of stenosis, 1 was ligated for arterial steal, and 1 failed because of hypotension. Four (57%) had graft thrombosis.

Conclusion.—The Tyrell vein collar placed at the venous anastomosis of AVGs led to early graft failure by increasing intimal hyperplasia, venous outflow tract stenosis, and early AVG thrombosis.

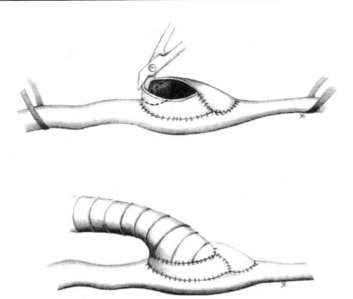

FIGURE 1.—Diagram of a Tyrell vein collar with and without a polytetrafluoroethylene graft. (Courtesy of Gagne PJ, Martinez J, DeMassi R, et al: The effect of a venous anastomosis Tyrell vein collar on the primary patency of arteriovenous grafts in patients undergoing hemodialysis. *J Vasc Surg* 32:1149-1154, 2000.)

▶ Vein collars or vein patches have been suggested to improve the patency of distal lower extremity arterial reconstructions with polytetrafluoroethylene to the below-knee popliteal and tibial vessels. One would think that the same process applied to an arteriovenous fistula would also be effective. These authors, and others, including our own group, have shown that vein patches not only lack benefit when applied to the arteriovenous circulation, but actually may be detrimental. The reasons for this are uncertain, but I would suggest that the hemodynamics of an arteriovenous fistula are much different than those of a distal arterial bypass. A huge pressure drop occurs across the fistula, especially as one gets into the venous outflow tract, and a prophylactic vein patch in this region of the anastomosis may actually aggravate the situation.

J. L. Mills, Sr, MD

Distal Emboli as an Unusual Late Complication of a Thrombosed Arteriovenous Hemodialysis Graft
Yang GP, Lee WA, Olcott C IV (Stanford Univ, Calif)
J Vasc Surg 32:1229-1231, 2000   11–6

Objective.—Because many patients undergoing hemodialysis do not have a suitable conduit for autogenous construction, they require prosthetic or xenograft conduits with a variety of arteriovenous anastomosis. Thromboses frequently develop in these conduits. A rare and never pre-

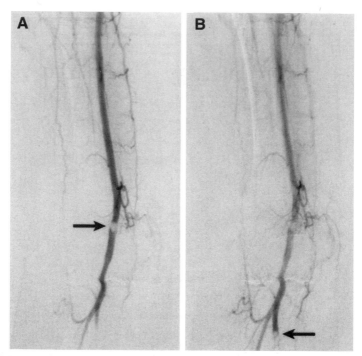

FIGURE 1.—Selective right upper extremity arteriogram. Note the two distinct thromboembolic lesions, one in the above-elbow brachial artery (**A**) and another located in the proximal ulnar artery just beyond the bifurcation (**B**). An exophytic protrusion of chronic thrombus was found on exploration of the proximal brachial artery anastomosis. (Courtesy of Yang GP, Lee WA, Olcott C IV: Distal emboli as an unusual late complication of a thrombosed arteriovenous hemodialysis graft. *J Vasc Surg* 32:1229-1231, 2000.)

viously reported complication of distal embolization from a chronically thrombosed, upper extremity expanded polytetrafluoroethylene (EPTFE) arteriovenous graft is described.

> *Case Report.*—Woman, 44, with end-stage renal disease from Alport's syndrome, reported a 24-hour history of periodic right-hand coolness and pain that was exacerbated by physical activity. She had arteriovenous grafts in both arms that she no longer used because she had received a cadaver kidney. She had received a right forearm brachial-antecubital loop EPTFE graft followed by an upper arm brachial-axillary EPTFE bridge graft, both of which had thrombosed. She had markedly delayed capillary refill on examination, no ulnar pulse, a water-hammer type radial pulse next to the wrist, and Allen test–positive ulnar and radial arteries. A Doppler scan revealed an obstructed radial artery and a weakly monophasic ulnar signal. She received heparin therapy and was given an arch aortogram that revealed 2 thromboembolic lesions (Fig 1). When she failed to improve after receiving catheter-directed recombinant tissue plasminogen activator, she underwent surgery

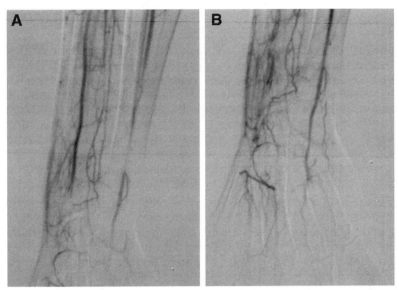

FIGURE 2.—Digital subtraction angiography with delayed images demonstrating occlusion of the radial artery (A), poor filling of the digital artery (B), and early collateralization. (Courtesy of Yang GP, Lee WA, Olcott C IV: Distal emboli as an unusual late complication of a thrombosed arteriovenous hemodialysis graft. *J Vasc Surg* 32:1229-1231, 2000.)

and both arterial grafts were taken down. The arteriotomies were repaired, and she had an uneventful recovery with complete resolution of all symptoms.

Discussion.—The emboli appeared to originate in the upper arm graft, possibly resulting from a thromboembolic process aggravated by extrinsic arm compression while the patient was sleeping (Fig 2).

Conclusion.—Routine removal of thrombosed arteriovenous grafts is not recommended because of the risk of distal thromboembolization, but it should be considered when acute hand or finger ischemia is observed in patients with chronically occluded grafts.

▶ I am not certain whether the vascular community wants to hear about any additional ways dialysis access patients can have complications, but here it is. This article reports embolization from a previously thrombosed proximal arteriovenous access. This phenomenon has been described in thrombosed axillary femoral grafts as well. I am certain we will soon see a report describing extensive asymptomatic digital and forearm arterial occlusions (from presumed embolization) distal to previously thrombosed proximal arteriovenous access in a population of patients with renal failure sent to the vascular laboratory for screening. Indeed, chronic embolization from failed access may be responsible for the distal hand arterial occlusions observed in a subgroup of patients who have distal steal develop after access procedures and require the distal revascularization interval ligation procedure.

M. R. Nehler, MD

Thoracic Outlet

Long-term Functional Outcome of Neurogenic Thoracic Outlet Syndrome in Surgically and Conservatively Treated Patients

Landry GJ, Moneta GL, Taylor LM Jr, et al (Oregon Health Sciences Univ, Portland)

J Vasc Surg 33:312-319, 2001   11–7

Background.—The term "disputed" neurogenic thoracic outlet syndrome (NTOS) refers to those cases with symptoms of upper extremity pain and paresthesia, but without the objective diagnostic findings of bony and electrodiagnostic abnormalities. Most patients undergoing thoracic outlet decompression have the disputed form of NTOS, yet there are few objective data on the effectiveness of such surgery. The long-term functional outcomes of patients with disputed NTOS—with and without surgical treatment—were analyzed.

Methods.—The study included 79 patients with disputed NTOS whose symptoms were severe enough to cause at least temporary inability to work. Patients with electrodiagnostically confirmed NTOS were excluded. The patients with disputed NTOS underwent independent medical examinations over an 8-year period; they were not treated by the investigators performing the evaluations. At a mean follow-up of 4.2 years, the patients' functional outcomes were assessed by means of a standardized telephone interview or patient questionnaire. Outcomes of interest included return to work, current symptoms, and symptom progression.

Results.—Nineteen percent of patients underwent first-rib resection surgery; the rest were managed conservatively. The mean amount of missed work time was 27.6 months for surgically treated patients versus 14.9 months for those not undergoing surgery. Sixty percent of surgically treated patients and 78% of the conservatively managed group were able to return to work; the difference was nonsignificant. Among the surgically treated patients, current symptoms were rated as severe by 7%, moderate by 47%, mild by 40%, and absent by 7%. Similar severity ratings were noted for the conservatively managed group. The 2 management groups also reported similar proportions of symptom resolution, improvement, and worsening (Table 4).

Conclusion.—Most patients with the disputed form of NTOS appear to have symptomatic improvement and the ability to return to work without surgical management. Pending research proof that surgical management offers superior results, the researchers will continue to recommend conservative treatment for patients with disputed NTOS.

▶ The optimal therapy for patients with NTOS in the absence of bony and electrodiagnostic abnormalities remains an issue that polarizes vascular

TABLE 4.–Outcome Based on Treatment Received

	Current Level of Symptoms in Operated and Nonoperated Patients			
	Severe	Moderate	Minimal	Asymptomatic
Operated (n = 15)	1 (7%)	7 (47%)	6 (40%)	1 (7%)
Nonoperated (n = 64)	7 (11%)	35 (55%)	19 (30%)	3 (5%)

	Progression of Symptoms Since Onset in Operated and Nonoperated Patients				
	Resolved	Marked Improvement	Minimal Improvement	No Improvement	Worse
Operated (n = 15)	1 (7%)	4 (27%)	6 (40%)	2 (13%)	2 (13%)
Nonoperated (n = 64)	1 (2%)	19 (30%)	14 (22%)	20 (31%)	10 (16%)

Note: P = NS between the operated and nonoperated group.
(Courtesy of Landry GJ, Moneta GL, Taylor LM Jr, et al: Long-term functional outcome of neurogenic thoracic outlet syndrome in surgically and conservatively treated patients. *J Vasc Surg* 33:312-319, 2001.)

surgeons. The Oregon group suggests that patients with disputed NTOS have long-term outcomes that are similar whether or not surgical decompression is performed. While there are some shortcomings of this article—the treatment was not standardized, the evaluation was by questionnaire alone, and the rate of follow-up was only 59%—the findings are interesting. Patients who underwent surgical decompression missed more work, yet had similar self-reported long-term outcomes. NTOS has so many pretenders that it's hard to appropriately select patients for surgery in the absence of objectively documented findings. The group from Michigan recently reported that depression, nonmarried status, and less than a high school education predicted poor outcome after surgery for TOS.[1] Perhaps searching for underlying depression and treating such disorders should have an expanded role in the treatment of these patients. Interestingly, the overall results of the surgical group in the Michigan series are similar to those of the nonoperated group in the Oregon report. It certainly would be nice to see a randomized trial comparing surgery with nonoperative therapy for TOS.

A. M. Abou-Zamzam, Jr, MD

Reference

1. Axelrod DA, Proctor MC, Geisser ME, et al: Outcomes after surgery for thoracic outlet syndrome. *J Vasc Surg* 33:1220-1225, 2001.

Outcome of Surgery for Thoracic Outlet Syndrome in Washington State Workers' Compensation

Franklin GM, Fulton-Kehoe D, Bradley C, et al (Univ of Washington, Seattle)
Neurology 54:1252-1257, 2000   11–8

Background.—Most patients given diagnoses of and treated for thoracic outlet syndrome (TOS) have a nonspecific neurogenic form of TOS whose diagnosis depends on both the capability of provocative measures to reproduce symptoms and the lack of any other specific diagnosis. Surgical treatment has been peformed, but its outcomes vary. The results of surgery for TOS were studied in cases cared for under workers' compensation; clinical, functional, work disability, and patient satisfaction outcomes were evaluated, and predictors of work disability outcome 1 year after surgery were analyzed.

Methods.—Computerized bill payment records and medical record validation reviews identified 158 injured workers undergoing TOS surgery from 1986 to 1991. At an average of 4.8 years after surgery, functional status and quality-of-life outcomes were assessed via telephone interview; the main outcome measure was work disability status 1 year postoperatively. A comparison group included workers with TOS who did not have surgery.

Results.—Work disability continued for 60% of patients 1 year after surgery. Sustained disability could be predicted based on the degree of work disability present before surgery, increased time between injury and

TOS diagnosis, and older age when injured. The type of surgery, performance of provocative testing, and surgeon's experience showed no association with work disability outcome. In 72.5% of workers, vigorous activity was reportedly limited significantly an average of 4.8 years after surgery. Medical costs for patients who underwent surgery were 50% greater than for those who did not have surgery, and patients who underwent surgery were 3 to 4 times more likely to have a work disability.

Conclusions.—TOS surgery outcomes in this population of workers are dramatically worse than the outcomes of workers with TOS not undergoing surgery. In addition, the outcomes reported here are worse than those found among the general population.

▶ This article demonstrates clearly that nonspecific neurogenic TOS is an indistinct entity. The authors examined all workers' compensation TOS surgical cases in the state of Washington in a certain period and followed them over time retrospectively and with a delayed survey. They also examined a nonoperated group of patients. The retrospective nature of the study, combined with the extreme difficulty of defining the entity itself, makes this a problem. The functional outcomes are also the product of physical and occupational therapy and psychological work, in addition to the use of surgery. These factors were not controlled, and it is likely that case selection bias may have been present in terms of severity of disease. Additional information is needed to clarify the response of nonspecific TOS to therapy and to define the role of surgery, which is not often performed and is therefore potentially more prone to problems.

M. A. Golden, MD

12 Carotid and Cerebrovascular Disease

Carotid Infection

Dacron Carotid Patch Infection: A Report of Eight Cases
Rizzo A, Hertzer NR, O'Hara PJ, et al (Cleveland Clinic Found, Ohio)
J Vasc Surg 32:602-606, 2000   12–1

Objective.—Vein patch angioplasty improves the safety and durability of carotid endarterectomy (CEA), but the infection of Dacron patches has occurred. Charts of 8 patients treated at 1 institution between 1995 and 1999 for infected Dacron patches after CEA were reviewed and discussed.

Methods.—Of the 1258 CEAs performed from 1995 through 1998, 1183 (94%) were repaired with patches. The greater saphenous vein (GSV) was harvested in 843 (67%) patients, Dacron was used in 322 (26%), and polytetrafluoroethylene was used in 18 (1.4%) patients. Primary arteriotomy was performed in 75 patients. All patients were symptomatic. Bacterial cultures were obtained at the time of reoperation.

Results.—Seven patients had *Staphylococcus* or *Streptococcus* species infections. Patches were removed and the surrounding tissue debrided. Arterial repair was affected with a saphenous vein patch in 5 patients or a reversed saphenous vein graft in 3. Patients were treated with oral or IV antibiotics for 2 to 6 weeks. Hospital stay ranged from 3 to 13 days and averaged 7 days. One patient died after a car crash during the follow-up period which averaged 17 months. No late strokes or recurrent infections occurred, and the 4 patients that had duplex scanning or angiography showed patent arterial reconstructions.

Conclusion.—Vein patch infections are rare and may be unavoidable. Additional research needs to be conducted to determine whether there are etiologic mechanisms underlying the infections.

▶ As everyone is patching more carotids, we too are seeing a few of these prosthetic infections. Our results and conclusions agree entirely with the authors. While it is tempting to use this rare occurrence as evidence to prefer vein patching, that material as well is not free of complications of patch rupture, patch aneurysm, or both. It is probably best to conclude that all patch materials have a low but inescapable incidence of complications, and to be ready to manage them. This article clearly provides the recipe for managing infected prosthetic carotid patches.

L. M. Taylor, Jr, MD

Recurrent Carotid Blowout Syndrome: Diagnostic and Therapeutic Challenges in a Newly Recognized Subgroup of Patients
Chaloupka JC, Roth TC, Putman CM, et al (Yale Univ, New Haven, Conn)
AJNR Am J Neuroradiol 20:1069-1077, 1999   12–2

Background.—Rupture of the carotid artery, or carotid blowout syndrome (CBS), is a not uncommon complication of aggressive head and neck surgery. Recurrent episodes of CBS (rCBS) have recently been noted. A retrospective review of rCBS was undertaken to characterize this entity and its management.

Study Design.—The records of the last 46 consecutive patients treated for CBS were reviewed. Of these patients, 12 had rCBS. All were studied emergently with carotid angiography, and intervention was based on these findings.

Findings.—Among the 12 patients with rCBS, there were 32 CBS events, with an interval of 1 day to 6 years. Of the 20 recurrent events, 65% were attributed to progressive disease (PD) and 35% to treatment failure (TF) (Fig 2). In the PD group, 54% of patients had recurrent ipsilateral disease and 46% had recurrent contralateral disease. Of the 32 CBS events in this group, 27 were treated with endovascular therapy. Four of the 6 TFs were also treated successfully with endovascular therapy. Two TFs were managed successfully with surgery. One patient in the PD group died of hemorrhagic complications. There were no permanent neurologic or ophthalmologic complications in this study group.

Conclusion.—Recurrent CBS is a common serious complication for patients who have been previously managed by aggressive endovascular or surgical intervention. Most cases of rCBS appear to be related to PD, but TFs also occur. Most of these patients can be successfully managed with an interdisciplinary approach and endovascular interventions.

▶ Mortality and neurologic morbidity for surgical treatment of CBS is high, averaging approximately 40% in many series. It is now clear that, when possible, blowout of the carotid artery is best treated with endovascular techniques. This article informs us that one quarter of such patients will rebleed, usually within a week of the initial treatment. The authors, however, make a convincing case that episodes of recurrent hemorrhage should also

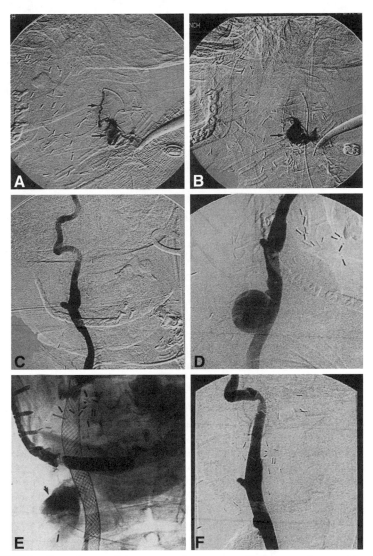

FIGURE 2.—Illustrative case of the spectrum of recurrent carotid blowout syndrome and its management. **A, B,** Sixty-year-old woman initially presented with carotid blowout syndrome (CBS). Lateral views from superselective injection of a facial arterial branch (*short arrow*) in early (**A**) and late (**B**) arterial phases show a ruptured pseudoaneurysm with extensive extravasation (*long arrows*). This was successfully treated with coil embolization. **C,** Twenty-one days later, the patient had a second episode of CBS as the result of a flap dehiscence. Oblique view from right common carotid artery injection shows no evidence of pseudoaneurysm and prior ligation of the external carotid artery. The patient's balloon test occlusion failed at this time, prompting a flap revision. **D,** Seventeen days later, the patient had a third episode of CBS. Oblique view from right common carotid artery injection shows a large pseudoaneurysm of that vessel. Acute hemorrhage initially was arrested by placement of 2 overlapping 8 × 20–mm Wallstents across the rent of the artery (not shown). **E, F,** One day later, a fourth episode of CBS developed as the result of a treatment failure of the previously deployed stents. After inflation of a balloon occlusion catheter across the carotid rent, the pseudoaneurysm was directly punctured and embolized with cyanoacrylate. Fluoroscopic spot film (**E**) and subtracted-control angiography (**F**) from right common carotid artery injection (oblique view) shows complete obliteration of the pseudoaneurysm with cyanoacrylate (*arrow*) and patency of the parent artery. (Courtesy of Chaloupka JC, Roth TC, Putman CM, et al: Recurrent carotid blowout syndrome: Diagnostic and therapeutic challenges in a newly recognized subgroup of patients. *AJNR Am J Neuroradiol* 20:1069-1077, 1999. Copyright by American Society of Neuroradiology.)

be treated endovascularly, and that with persistence, a favorable outcome is likely.

G. L. Moneta, MD

Clinical Reports

Carotid Endarterectomy in Female Patients: Are the Concerns of the Asymptomatic Carotid Atherosclerosis Study Valid?

Rockman CB, Castillo J, Adelman MA, et al (New York Univ)
J Vasc Surg 33:236-241, 2001   12–3

Background.—The results of the Asymptomatic Carotid Atherosclerosis Study (ACAS) clearly demonstrated the benefits of surgical management versus medical management of severe carotid artery stenosis; however, the results for women in particular were less certain. To some extent this was because of the higher perioperative complication rate that was observed in the 281 women (3.6% vs 1.7% in men). Whether the perioperative results in women differ from those in men was determined with a review of an experience with carotid endarterectomy in a large group of female patients.

Methods.—A prospectively compiled database of all carotid endarterectomies performed between 1982 and 1997 was reviewed. The review also involved a comparison between operations performed in 991 female patients and those performed in 1485 male patients.

Results.—There was a significantly lower incidence of diabetes, coronary artery disease, and contralateral carotid artery occlusion in female patients compared with male patients (Table 1). However, female patients had a significantly higher incidence of hypertension. No significant difference was noted between the 2 groups in age, smoking history, anesthetic route, shunt use, or clamp tolerance. Preoperative symptoms were present in 659 of 991 female patients (66.5%), and 332 patients (33.5%) underwent carotid endarterectomy for asymptomatic stenosis (Table 2). Among 1485 male patients, 1041 (70.1%) had symptoms, whereas 444 (29.9%) were symptom free before surgery. No significant differences in the peri-

TABLE 1.—Comparison of Demographics Between Male and Female Patients

	Female Patients (n = 991)	Male Patients (n = 1485)	P Value
Hypertension	62.0% (614)	53.6% (796)	< .001
Diabetes mellitus	19.5% (193)	23.0% (341)	.04
Coronary artery disease	37.5% (372)	49.9% (741)	< .001
Smoking history	36.3% (360)	38.0% (564)	NS
Age (mean)	68.6 years	69.1 years	NS
Contralateral occlusion	9.5% (94)	18.3% (272)	< .001

Note: All P values (except age) are derived by the χ^2 test and are corrected for continuity.
Abbreviation: NS, Not significant.
(Courtesy of Rockman CB, Castillo J, Adelman MA, et al: Carotid endarterectomy in female patients: Are the concerns of the Asymptomatic Carotid Atherosclerosis Study valid? *J Vasc Surg* 33:236-241, 2001.)

mal thickness was similar for the 2 groups. The prevalence of abnormalities was significantly higher in patients aged 30 to 39 years than in patients aged 20 to 29 years.

Conclusion.—The prevalence of asymptomatic carotid artery disease is common in young patients treated with neck irradiation for lymphoma and is similar to that for patients treated with radiation and chemotherapy.

▶ This small but controlled study provides clear evidence of a relationship between early life cervical irradiation and increased thickness/stenosis of the cervical carotid arteries. As the authors fully acknowledge, it is not presently known nor addressed by their study whether this radiation-related abnormality is more or less likely to produce symptoms, occlusions, or both, than are carotid abnormalities resulting from atherosclerosis in patients with no history of radiation exposure.

L. M. Taylor, Jr, MD

Stroke

Immediate Reexploration for the Perioperative Neurologic Event After Carotid Endarterectomy: Is it Worthwhile?

Rockman CB, Jacobowitz GR, Lamparello PJ, et al (New York Univ)
J Vasc Surg 32:1062-1070, 2000   12–21

Background.—Debate over how to manage a patient who has a new neurologic deficit after carotid endarterectomy (CEA) continues. An important question is which of these perioperative neurologic events (PNEs) are likely to improve with surgical reexploration. A series of PNEs was analyzed to determine whether information on the timing and mechanisms of the event can predict the chances of improvement after reoperation.

Methods.—Using a prospective database, the investigators identified 2024 primary CEAs performed over a 12-year period. Thirty-eight patients had new neurologic deficits during the perioperative period, which yielded a rate of 1.9%. Causes were identified through clinical findings, reexploration, and imaging and other tests.

Results.—Causes of the PNEs included thromboembolic events in 63.2% of cases, ischemia related to intraoperative clamping in 13.2%, and intracerebral hemorrhaging in 13.2%. The new deficit was unrelated to the vessel operated on in CEA in 10.5% of cases. Eighty-eight percent of events occurring within the first 24 hours postoperatively were caused by thromboembolic events, whereas later deficits were more likely to result from other causes (Table 5). Immediate reexploration was performed in 18 of 25 patients with PNEs developing in the first 24 hours. Eighty-three percent of these explorations revealed intraluminal thrombi. Reexploration led to complete resolution or significant improvement in the new deficit in 12 of 18 cases.

Conclusions.—When new neurologic deficits occur after CEA, information on the timing and presentation of the PNE can aid in identifying patients likely to benefit from reexploration. Thromboembolic events are

TABLE 2.—Comparison of Preoperative Symptoms and Indications for Surgery Between Male and Female Patients

	Female Patients (n = 991)	Male Patients (n = 1485)	P Value
Asymptomatic	33.5% (332)	29.9% (444)	NS (.064)
Preoperative hemispheric symptoms (TIA or CVA)	66.5% (659)	70.1% (1041)	
Preoperative stroke (CVA)	21.8% (216)	25.9% (384)	.038
Preoperative TIA	44.7% (443)	44.1% (657)	

Note: All *P* values (except age) are derived by the χ^2 test and are corrected for continuity.
Abbreviations: TIA, Transient ischemic attack; *CVA,* cerebrovascular accident; *NS,* not significant.
(Courtesy of Rockman CB, Castillo J, Adelman MA, et al: Carotid endarterectomy in female patients: Are the concerns of the Asymptomatic Carotid Atherosclerosis Study valid? *J Vasc Surg* 33:236-241, 2001.)

operative stroke rate were noted between men and women overall (2.3% vs 2.4%) or when divided into symptomatic (2.5% vs 3.0%) and asymptomatic (2.0% vs 1.2%) patients.

Conclusions.—Perioperative stroke rates were equally low in both symptomatic and asymptomatic men and women who underwent carotid endarterectomy. The lowest overall stroke rate was found among symptom-free female patients. On the basis of these findings, the concerns of the Asymptomatic Carotid Atherosclerosis Study regarding the benefit of carotid endarterectomy in female patients should not prevent the recommendation or performance of carotid endarterectomy in appropriately selected symptom-free female patients.

▶ Including a cohort of women patients larger than that included in ACAS itself, these investigators found in a single-center study no gender-based difference in carotid surgery outcome. The uniform application of patch closure probably eliminates internal carotid artery diameter as a significant risk factor for perioperative thrombotic occlusions and early events. The main drawback of this report is the limited 30-day follow-up, compared with 5 years in ACAS. This series complements our own experience, which suggests that asymptomatic carotid artery surgery can be performed for appropriate indications with equal confidence in women and men.

R. L. Dalman, MD

Carotid Thromboendarterectomy for Recent Total Occlusion of the Internal Carotid Artery
Kasper GC, Wladis AR, Lohr JM, et al (Good Samaritan Hosp, Cincinnati, Ohio)
J Vasc Surg 33:242-250, 2001   12–4

Background.—Questions have been raised regarding the efficacy of emergency carotid thromboendarterectomy (CTEA) for the treatment of acute internal carotid artery (ICA) thrombosis. The use of CTEA in patients with recent ICA occlusion was evaluated.

Methods.—Patients who underwent urgent CTEA for recent ICA thrombosis from August 1989 to December 1999 were retrospectively evaluated. The patient data that was analyzed included age, sex, comorbid risk factors, the diagnostic evaluation, the operative procedure, and long-term follow-up with a clinical assessment and a carotid duplex scan. The Modified Rankin Scale (MRS) was used for the evaluation of patients' neurologic status before and during the procedure and at 3- to 6-months' follow-up.

Results.—Emergency ipsilateral CTEA for acute ICA thrombosis was performed in 29 patients over 10 years. The average age of the patients was 69.9 ± 1.7 years, and 66% of the patients were men. Among the patient risk factors were diabetes (24%), hypertension (72%), coronary artery disease (29%), and a history of tobacco use (69%). Among the presenting symptoms were cerebrovascular accident (24%), stroke in evolution (7%), and amaurosis fugax (10%). Diagnostic modalities used included a CT scan (100%), MRI/MR angiography (14%), a duplex scan evaluation of the carotid arteries (79%), and cerebral angiography (64%). CTEA successfully restored antegrade flow in the ICA in 24 of 29 patients (83%) as confirmed by intraoperative angiography or duplex US. Postoperative morbidity included hematomas (2 patients), transient cranial nerve deficits (4 patients), and conversion to hemorrhagic stroke (1 patient). The conversion to a hemorrhagic stroke was responsible for the only death. The average preoperative MRS score was 3.4 ± 0.2 preoperatively, and improvement or deterioration was defined as a change of ±1 in the MRS score. At the immediate postoperative assessment, 14 patients (48%) had improved, 2 (7%) had deteriorated, and 13 (45%) had no change. At 3- to 6-months' follow-up, 20 of 27 (74%) had improved, 7 (26%) had no change, and none had deteriorated. Twenty-three of 24 patients (96%) with successful CTEA had a patent ICA on follow-up duplex scan evaluation, and no evidence was found of recurrent ipsilateral neurologic events at an average of 49 months.

Conclusions.—These findings are supportive of the use of aggressive early surgical intervention in carefully selected patients with acute ICA thrombosis. In the previous decade, a 46% long-term success rate for establishment of antegrade flow in the ICA was reported. Data from this study indicates a long-term success rate of 79% for the establishment of antegrade flow in all patients undergoing emergency CTEA. Improved outcomes have resulted from new and improved modalities, which have allowed better patient selection.

▶ From the initial experiences with CTEA, it has been clear that operative intervention in symptomatic patients with acute carotid occlusion has yielded inferior results when compared with medical management alone. Few brave souls have risen to challenge this dogma over the last 40 years. One such soul is the senior author of this group from Good Samaritan Hospital in Cincinnati, who reported a series of 24 patients explored between 5 and 21 days after acute internal artery occlusion some 20 years ago. Patency of the ICA was successfully reestablished in 63% of these patients, with no new neurologic deficits and no mortality.[1] In spite of these impressive results, most vascular surgeons continue to treat acute carotid artery occlusions, except those seen after carotid endarterectomy, with medical management, even with ongoing neurologic symptoms. This current series, developed over the last 10 years, again challenges this management scheme. ICA patency was reestablished in 83% of these patients, with 96% patency of the repair through 75 months of follow-up. Tempering any enthusiasm for this result must be 2 unpredicted outcomes: (1) in the one patient who was explored, patency could not be reestablished, and the patient had a new cerebrovascular accident (CVA); and (2) another patient operated on 8 days after ICA occlusion that converted to a hemorrhagic CVA ultimately died. For the present, I will continue to observe acute carotid artery occlusions outside the operating room.

E. J. Harris, Jr, MD

Reference

1. Welling RE, Cranley JJ, Krause RJ, et al: Surgical therapy for recent total occlusion of the internal artery. *J Vasc Surg* 1:57-61, 1984.

Chronic Infections and the Risk of Carotid Atherosclerosis: Prospective Results From a Large Population Study

Kiechl S, Egger G, Mayr M, et al (Univ of Innsbruck, Austria; Univ of Verona, Italy)
Circulation 103:1064-1070, 2001   12–5

Background.—The infection hypothesis has emerged as one of the most compelling hypotheses for atherogenesis, given the high prevalence of this risk factor in the general population and the potential availability of preventive interventions. This hypothesis is older than one might suspect, with roots dating from the 19th century. Only in the past few decades, however, has the bulk of supportive evidence for this hypothesis emerged. Epidemiologic evidence for an infectious risk factor in atherogenesis has been mainly indirect and has been restricted to certain pathogens. The Bruneck Study, a prospective population-based survey, describes the epidemiologic features and pathogenesis of atherosclerosis.

Methods.—In 1990, a group of men and women aged 40 to 79 years in the Italian town of Bruneck were recruited for a study of the pathogenesis of atherosclerosis. Final follow-up was available for 826 participants. High-resolution duplex scanning was used for assessment of 5-year changes in carotid atherosclerosis, and the presence of chronic respiratory, urinary tract, dental, and other infections was determined by standard diagnostic criteria.

Results.—The risk of atherosclerosis development in the carotid arteries was amplified by the presence of chronic infections. This association was found to be most pronounced in participants who were free of carotid atherosclerosis at baseline and was applicable to all types of chronic

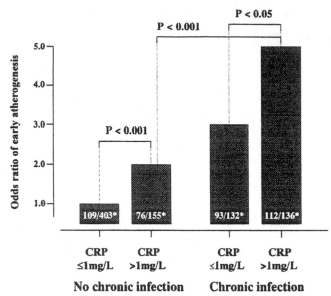

FIGURE 3.—Odds ratios of new carotid plaques according to chronic infection status and level of C-reactive protein. Odds ratios were adjusted for age, sex, and baseline atherosclerosis. *Numbers of research subjects with incident atherosclerosis per number of patients at risk. (Courtesy of Kiechl S, Egger G, Mayr M, et al: Chronic infections and the risk of carotid atherosclerosis: Prospective results from a large population study. *Circulation* 103(8):1064-1070, 2001.)

(bacterial) infections (Fig 3). The association between the increased risk of atherosclerosis development and the presence of chronic infections remained independently significant after adjustment for classic vascular risk attributes and extended to low-risk individuals who were free of conventional risk factors. Among participants who had chronic infections, the risk of atherosclerosis was highest in those with a prominent inflammatory response. Participants with chronic infections had elevated levels of markers of systemic inflammation, such as soluble adhesion molecules and circulating bacterial endotoxin, as well as elevated levels of soluble human heat-shock protein 60 and antibodies to mycobacterial heat-shock protein 65. Elevated levels of these markers were predictive of an increased risk of atherosclerosis.

Conclusions.—Solid evidence for a role for common chronic infections in human atherogenesis was provided by these findings. Potential pathophysiologic links may be provided by the induction of systemic inflammation and immunity.

▶ For many years, the surgical dictum was no acid, no ulcer. We now know that many ulcers are caused by a bacterium, *Helicobacter pylori*, and an antibiotic may cure the ulcer. A long line of data suggests that atherosclerosis may be inflammatory in etiology, and the present study examines the possibility that the inflammation may be the result of chronic infection. I would view this article as suggesting, but not establishing, an association between infection and atherosclerosis. Periodontal disease, for example, has been suggested to correlate with the development of acute coronary events. It is still unclear whether infection is an innocent bystander, perhaps related to the increased susceptibility to infection associated with high-risk behavior, such as cigarette smoking. Wouldn't it be interesting if atherosclerosis is ultimately proven to be an infectious disease?

J. L. Mills, Sr, MD

Improving the Outcomes of Carotid Endarterectomy: Results of a State-wide Quality Improvement Project
Kresowik TF, Hemann RA, Grund SL, et al (Univ of Iowa, Iowa City; Iowa Found for Med Care, Des Moines; Univ of Kansas, Kansas City)
J Vasc Surg 31:918-926, 2000   12–6

Objective.—Patients with symptomatic and asymptomatic carotid occlusive disease who receive a carotid endarterectomy (CEA) have a lower stroke rate than those treated medically. A project was developed to document the statewide outcomes of CEA and to distribute confidential institution-specific outcome and care process reports to surgeons and hospital staff. Results of the quality improvement effort are discussed.

Methods.—The Iowa Foundation for Medical Care (IFMC), a Medicare peer review organization, collected data on demographics, indications, procedure, perioperative care, and postoperative outcomes for all Medicare patients who underwent CEA from January 1994 through December 1994, and from June 1995 through May 1996. Confidential reports were supplied to the 29 and 30 hospitals and to the 78 and 79 surgeons performing CEA procedures during the respective periods.

Results.—During the 2 study periods, the number of statewide CEA-alone procedures performed increased from 798 to 1265, and the number of patients increased from 726 to 1160. Fourteen hospitals performed 74% of the procedures. Statewide, the median age, 74 years, remained the same as did the percentage of male patients (60% and 59%). The percentage of asymptomatic patients increased from 20% to 40%. The combined stroke or mortality rate declined significantly from 7.8% to 4.0%. The individual mortality and nonfatal stroke rates declined significantly from 2.9% and 4.9% to 1.1% and 2.8%, respectively. Among the 14 hospitals performing most of the procedures, the combined stroke or mortality rates decreased significantly from 6.5% (January 1994-December 1994) to 3.7% (June 1995-May 1996) to 1.8% (June 1997 to May 1998). The respective mortality rates declined significantly in the 3 periods from 2.4% to 1.3% to 0.6%. The respective nonfatal stroke rates declined significantly from 4.2% to 2.5% to 1.2%

Conclusion.—Confidential quality intervention feedback has a significant effect on improving processes and outcomes for patients having CEA.

▶ In the search for a classic article exemplifying "evidence-based medicine," this one may represent one Holy Grail. Thankfully, CEA lends itself to the ability to follow-up outcomes with relative reproducibility and reliability. Notwithstanding the inherent flaws of a retrospective study, the data presented in this article make sense. With feedback to surgeons regarding outcomes, the combined stroke and mortality rate declined over time. In addition, intraoperative monitoring for cerebral perfusion, patch placement, and postreconstruction assessment all increased during the 3 periods. What is not stated in the article is whether certain surgeons were identified and requested to stop performing these procedures. It would have been extremely helpful to know how many surgeons in the second or third periods were no longer doing CEAs, and whether the majority of patients were then referred to those surgeons performing these procedures more routinely and with more success. I congratulate the authors in providing the state of Iowa with improved outcomes in CEA through a standardized and confidential program. I hope it stays confidential.

R. B. McLafferty, MD

The Contribution of the External Carotid Artery to Cerebral Perfusion in Carotid Disease

Fearn SJ, Picton AJ, Mortimer AJ, et al (Univ Hosp of South Manchester, England)
J Vasc Surg 31:989-993, 2000   12–7

Background.—While collateral cerebral circulations are recognized for their importance, the extent to which the external carotid artery (ECA) supplies cerebral perfusion has not been fully elaborated. An evaluation was made of the ipsilateral ECA's contribution to cerebral perfusion in patients undergoing carotid endarterectomy to manage significant stenosis of the internal carotid artery (ICA).

Methods.—The patients (108, 72% men) had symptomatic ICA stenosis of 70% or more determined noninvasively by duplex Doppler US. During sequential cross-clamping of the external carotid artery (ECA) and then the ipsilateral ICA while carotid endarterectomy was being done, transcranial Doppler US was used to monitor blood flow velocity in the middle cerebral artery. Near-infrared spectroscopy was used to measure regional cerebral oxygen saturation.

Results.—A 3% median fall in regional cerebral oxygen saturation was noted on the ipsilateral ECA cross-clamp, which fell a further 3% when the ICA cross-clamp was added (Fig 1). Middle cerebral artery blood flow velocity fell 12% during ECA clamping and 48% during ICA clamping (Fig 2). Transcranial Doppler US detected greater falls during ECA clamping, with more severe ipsilateral ICA stenosis. A statistically significant correlation was found between regional cerebral oxygen saturation and transcranial Doppler US values when the ECA was clamped.

Conclusion.—Because the findings on transcranial Doppler US correlated with regional cerebral oxygen saturation, it can be inferred that a fall in cerebral perfusion was present. Thus, during severe stenosis of the

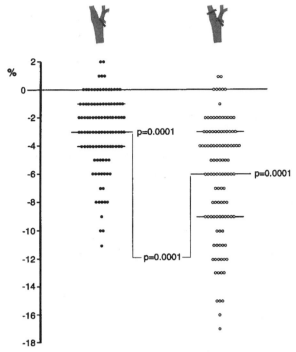

FIGURE 1.—Absolute fall in the percentage of cerebral oxygen saturation on clamping the external carotid artery (ECA) and then on additional clamping of the internal carotid artery (ICA) for each patient. Median and interquartile ranges are shown, and statistical comparison is by the nonparametric Mann-Whitney U test. (Courtesy of Fearn SJ, Picton AJ, Mortimer AJ, et al: The contribution of the external carotid artery to cerebral perfusion in carotid disease. *J Vasc Surg* 31:989-993, 2000.)

carotid arteries, the ipsilateral ECA makes a significant contribution to blood flow to the brain and to oxygen saturation values.

▶ Whereas none would disagree that the ECA contributes to cerebral circulation, most would be hard pressed to quantify this contribution. This article demonstrates that transcranial Doppler velocity in the middle cerebral artery decreases by 12% and regional cerebral oxygen saturation decreases by 3% after ECA clamping in patients undergoing carotid endarterectomy. The clinical significance of this contribution to cerebral perfusion is unclear. A safe stance is to preserve the ECA whenever possible during the performance of carotid surgery. I do note that embolism, not flow, is the usual culprit in extracranial carotid disease.

A. M. Abou-Zamzam, Jr, MD

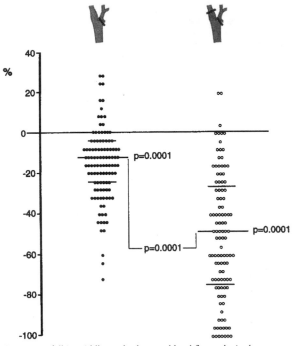

FIGURE 2.—Percentage fall in middle cerebral artery blood flow velocity by transcranial Doppler US on clamping the external carotid artery (ECA) and then on additional clamping of the internal carotid artery (ICA) for each patient. Results are expressed as median and interquartile ranges and demonstrate significant falls in middle cerebral blood flow on both ECA and ICA cross-clamp (Mann-Whitney U test). (Courtesy of Fearn SJ, Picton AJ, Mortimer AJ, et al: The contribution of the external carotid artery to cerebral perfusion in carotid disease. *J Vasc Surg* 31:989-993, 2000.)

Carotid Endarterectomy in the Community Hospital in Patients Age 80 and Older

Maxwell JG, Taylor AJ, Maxwell BG, et al (Univ of North Carolina, Chapel Hill; New Hanover Regional Med Ctr, NC; Coastal Area Health Education Ctr, Wilmington, NC)
Ann Surg 231:781-788, 2000   12–8

Background.—The incidence of stroke increases with age and the population of the United States is aging, with a predicted increase from 8 million people age 80 years or older now to about 70 million octogenarians in 2030. Thus, it seems important to determine whether carotid endarterectomy (CE), performed to prevent stroke, is of benefit to this older population and whether the death and complication rates differ among octogenarians from those seen in younger patients.

Methods.—Chart review was undertaken for all CE procedures done from 1979 through 1998. Procedures were evaluated, not patients, so each CE was counted, whether performed in the same patient or not. Data included demographics, risk factors, surgical descriptions, length of hospital stay, deaths, and complications.

Results.—Of the 2398 CEs performed, 2180 were in 1783 patients under age 80 years and 218 were in 187 octogenarians. Neurologic symptoms occurred in 65% of octogenarians and 67% of younger patients. Stenosis in 89% of asymptomatic patients was 75% or greater. Stroke occurred in 62 (2.8%) of the 2180 procedures involving younger patients and in 7 (3.2%) of the 218 procedures involving octogenarians. Octogenarians' death rate was 0.9%; that of younger patients was 1.4%. The values compare well with those of other studies.

Conclusion.—Octogenarians do well with CE procedures, with outcomes that do not differ significantly from those of younger patients with respect to stroke, complications, and death rates. All rates were within the range deemed necessary for CE to be considered beneficial in preventing stroke.

▶ This is another clinical series demonstrating that vascular surgery can be performed on octogenarian patients, with similar (or slightly greater) morbidity and mortality rates as those for younger populations. This theme has been explored extensively in carotid, aortic, and lower extremity revascularization. All of these clinical series describe the aging of our population, resulting in an explosion in numbers comprising persons older than 80 years. The longevity of 80-year-old patients based on vital statistic data is noted. The current series demonstrated low perioperative stroke rates among a collection of obviously skilled vascular surgeons. The authors are criticized for the fairly weak data presented documenting actual degree of stenosis and lack of follow-up beyond the perioperative period.

Despite these results, I offer some words of caution. Approximately 30% of the octogenarians in this study were operated on for asymptomatic lesions and another 15% for posterior circulation symptoms. Although vital statistic data describe a mean survival of 7 to 9 years for an 80-year-old person, these data are not applicable to all patients with peripheral vascular disease. Available data in the octogenarian vascular population describe much shorter survival. Data from the randomized trials in CE cannot be extrapolated here because patients older than 80 were not enrolled in these trials. The length of stay in the current study was a median of 5 days, which would appear to indicate some sort of functional setback. Finally, despite these good results among vascular surgeons who decided to get together their data, regional surveys of modern CE do not paint such a pretty picture. High stroke rates and large numbers of patients operated on for indications that do not meet current guidelines have caused a serious backlash from the neurology community. The challenge for much of the next decade in vascular surgery will not be can we do this, but rather should we?

M. R. Nehler, MD

Carotid Endarterectomy: Characterization of Recent Increases in Procedure Rates

Morasch MD, Parker MA, Feinglass J, et al (Northwestern Univ, Chicago)
J Vasc Surg 31:901-909, 2000   12–9

Background.—In 1996, 130,000 carotid endarterectomies (CEAs) were performed in the United States, representing a 94% increase from 1991. Hospital administration data from Florida from 1992 to 1996 were studied to characterize the increase in CEA procedure rates and to determine patient outcomes from population-based data.

Methods.—Between 1992 and 1996, 45,744 CEAs were performed in Florida. Hospital administration data were analyzed to characterize trends in patient age, sex, type of admission, size of hospital, ownership of hospital, teaching status of hospital, and annual CEA volume per hospital and surgeon. The incidences of inpatient myocardial infarction, stroke, and death were also examined to identify any trends in complication rates.

Results.—Between 1992 and 1996, the number of CEAs in Florida increased from 63.7 to 110.8 per 100,000 residents per year—a 74% increase. The number of CEAs increased sharply in the last half of 1994 (Fig 1), from 16.6 to 28.8 per 100,000 residents per quarter—a 73.5% increase. This increase coincided with the dissemination of an Asymptomatic Carotid Artery Study advisory regarding the benefits of CEA in asymptomatic patients. Over the period of study, there were significant trends toward fewer emergency admissions for CEAs (from 10.7% in 1992 to 8.2% in 1996) and fewer procedures performed in small hospitals (less

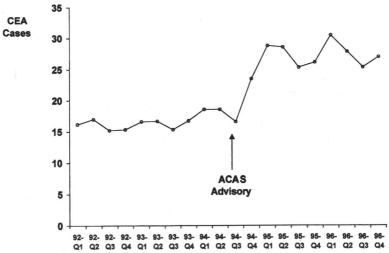

FIGURE 1.—Quarterly Florida carotid endarterectomy (*CEA*) procedures per 100,000 residents between 1992 and 1996. *Abbreviation: ACAS*, Asymptomatic Carotid Artery Study. (Reprinted from the *European Journal of Vascular and Endovascular Surgery* courtesy of Morasch MD, Parker MA, Feinglass J, et al: Carotid endarterectomy: Characterization of recent increases in procedure rates. *J Vasc Surg* 31: 901-909, 2000. Copyright 2000, by permission of the publisher, W B Saunders Company Limited London.)

than 350 beds, from 51.9% to 49.7%) and low-volume hospitals (less than 100 CEA admissions per year, from 74.3% in 1992 to 30.0% in 1996). There were also significant trends toward more CEAs performed in non-teaching hospitals (from 79.0% in 1992 to 81.7% in 1996) and by high-volume surgeons (30 or more CEAs/year; from 31.8% in 1992 to 61.2% in 1996). During this period, procedure rates increased for both sexes and for all ages of patients. The rate of perioperative myocardial infarctions remained constant between 1992 and 1996 (0.07%-0.09%). However, there were significant decreases in the rates of inpatient stroke (from 7.3% to 4.0%) and in-hospital death (from 1.1% to 0.7%). Again, these trends in complications were seen in both sexes and in all ages.

Conclusion.—Based on these data from Florida, more patients of all ages and both sexes are undergoing CEAs by high-volume surgeons at bigger, busier hospitals. Much of this increase can be attributed to the publication of the Asymptomatic Carotid Artery Study results in 1994, even though that report advised caution when applying its results to women, minorities, and very elderly patients. In-hospital deaths and strokes have decreased significantly, which may be related to the trends in referral patterns.

▶ The number of CEAs performed each year in the United States has steadily increased since 1991, with a stepwise increase being noted after each carotid surgery trial. In the 30 months after the report of the Asymptomatic Carotid Artery Study (ACAS), the carotid surgery rate in Florida increased by 74%, with almost all the increase occurring in the initial 6 months after the report. While the ACAS was limited to patients younger than 80 and the results were not significant for women, the increase in procedure rates in CEAs included those older than 80 and women. While the increase in procedure rates in patients who will not clearly benefit from CEA is disturbing, the finding that more procedures are done in high-volume centers by high-volume surgeons with decreased stroke rates is reassuring.

J. M. Edwards, MD

Intraoperative Use of Stents for the Management of Unacceptable Distal Internal Carotid Artery End Points During Carotid Endarterectomy: Short-term and Midterm Results
Ross CB, Ranval TJ (Vanderbilt Univ, Nashville, Tenn; Vascular Specialists, Paducah, Ky)
J Vasc Surg 32:420-428, 2000   12–10

Background.—The management of unacceptable distal internal carotid artery (ICA) end points during a carotid endarterectomy is a challenge. An intraluminal stent may be placed, but limited clinical experience with this approach has been reported. One experience with intraoperative stenting of the ICA for correcting unacceptable distal ICA end points during a carotid endarterectomy was reviewed.

Methods.—Data on 316 consecutive carotid endarterectomies performed from January 1997 to June 1999 were analyzed. The technique, 30-day outcomes, and midterm outcomes were assessed for patients undergoing adjunctive ICA stenting.

Findings.—At 30 days, the overall combined stroke and death rate was 1.9%. Adjunctive distal ICA stents were used in 13 patients (4.1% of the whole group) to correct unacceptable distal ICA end points (Fig 1). This subgroup consisted of men with a mean age of 70 years. None of these patients died or had a stroke or transient ischemic attack within 30 days of the procedure. Their mean length of stay postoperatively was 1.8 days.

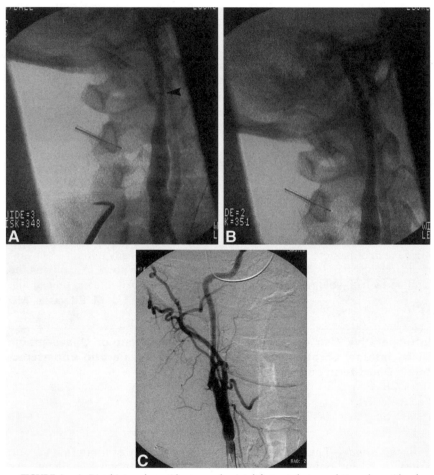

FIGURE 1.—**A,** Distal internal carotid artery end point defect noted at completion of carotid endarterectomy in 59-year-old man. **B,** Completion arteriogram after implantation of 7 × 20-mm Wallstent. **C,** Selective carotid arteriogram obtained 29 months postoperatively. Note minimal narrowing of lumen within stent caused by intimal hyperplasia. (Courtesy of Ross CB, Ranval TJ: Intraoperative use of stents for the management of unacceptable distal internal carotid artery end points during carotid endarterectomy: Short-term and midterm results. *J Vasc Surg* 32:420-428, 2000.)

At an average follow-up of 15 months, none of the patients had died. No significant asymptomatic recurrences were documented, although 1 patient had an isolated episode of amaurosis fugax without demonstrable restenosis 8 months after the procedure.

Conclusions.—The adjunctive use of stents for correcting unacceptable distal ICA end points during a carotid endarterectomy appears to be safe, and has acceptable outcomes in the short term and midterm. Continued follow-up is needed before this method may be considered superior to an expeditious secondary alternative.

▶ The authors describe their excellent results with the use of intraoperative stents to treat unacceptable distal end points during CEAs. They felt obligated to use this strategy in 13 of 316 cases (4.1%). I have 2 problems with this report. The first is that our practice group has not encountered anywhere near this rate of trouble—in the last 10 years we have performed more than 1300 CEAs without this problem. Perhaps this is because we have not aggressively pursued operation in patients with high bifurcations or extensive distal disease, but I doubt it. My other concern is the use of stents in the carotid artery without knowledge of the long-term consequences, particularly when they are placed in surgically inaccessible locations. While we have some intermediate-term results of carotid stenting, I remain concerned about the long-term consequences of carotid stenting, particularly in locations such as the distal carotid artery that are not surgically approachable. I will continue to use other strategies to deal with this problem, including jaw dislocation and vein interposition grafting, and accept the risk of nerve injury in the exceedingly rare cases when dissection has to be carried high into the neck.

J. M. Edwards, MD

Clinical Trials

Long-term Clinical and Angiographic Outcomes in Symptomatic Patients With 70% to 99% Carotid Artery Stenosis

Barnett HJM, for the North American Symptomatic Carotid Endarterectomy Trial (NASCET) Group (Univ of Perugia, Italy; Univ of Western Ontario, London, Canada; Univ Med Centre, Utrecht, The Netherlands; et al)
Stroke 31:2037-2042, 2000   12–11

Background.—Ten years ago, the North American Symptomatic Carotid Endarterectomy Trial (NASCET) demonstrated the benefit of carotid endarterectomy for symptomatic patients with 70% to 99% stenosis. Patients were followed up until 1997. The risks and causes of ipsilateral strokes in the NASCET randomized groups and in patients who had delayed endarterectomy or continued to receive medical treatment were analyzed. The evolution of carotid disease on follow-up imaging was also examined.

Methods and Findings.—Six hundred fifty-nine patients were originally enrolled in the NASCET. By the end of 1997, clinical follow-up data were available for 99% of those patients. The mean follow-up was 3.6 years in the medical group and 7 years for the surgical group. Efficacy analysis indicated that the risk of any ipsilateral stroke at 3 years was 28.3% in the medical group and 8.9% in the surgical group. The risk of a disabling ipsilateral stroke was 14%, and the risk of a fatal ipsilateral stroke was 3.4%. In the medically treated group, more than 80% of initial strokes at 3 years were of large-artery origin. After February 1991, 116 patients in the medical group had endarterectomies within 6 months, and 115 continued to receive medical treatment. At 3 years, the risk of any ipsilateral stroke was 7.9% and 15% in medical and continuing treatment groups, respectively. During follow-up, 81 patients had angiograms similar to the baseline images. Ten percent or more progression was noted in 7 patients, regression was noted in 8, and no change was noted in 39. Twenty-seven patients had occlusion. One fourth of the 247 medically treated patients progressed to occlusion on both angiography and US, including 31.7% who had ipsilateral strokes before or on the day of occlusion.

Conclusions.—Endarterectomy is effective in the long term for patients with 70% to 99% stenosis and recent symptoms. Medically treated patients who underwent delayed endarterectomies had a moderate benefit compared with patients continuing medical therapy. Patients given medical treatment had a high risk of occlusion.

▶ This article contains more useful follow-up information and data from the NASCET Group. In February 1991, NASCET released a clinical alert reporting a clear benefit with carotid endarterectomy for patients with stenosis of more than 70%. After this report, a number of study patients (n = 116) in the medical treatment arm crossed over to surgery. This article reports an improved stroke risk reduction at 3 years in the delayed endarterectomy group compared with the continuing medical group (7.9% vs 15%). Although the risk of stroke in the medically treated group continued to accumulate, the longer patients remained stroke free, the lower was their subsequent risk. If patients in the medical arm remained symptoms free for 2 years, their risk of stroke for the ensuing year was only 3.2%. In addition, when patients in the medical treatment arm underwent additional imaging studies during follow-up, it was noted that fully one quarter of the patients had progressed to occlusion of the study artery. This was over a mean follow-up of only 2 years. One third of patients who progressed to occlusion experienced a stroke around the time of the carotid occlusion.

R. A. Yeager, MD

Carotid Endarterectomy in Octogenarians: Comparison With Patient Characteristics and Outcomes In Younger Patients

Schneider JR, Droste JS, Schindler N, et al (Evanston Hosp, Ill; Glenview Hosp, Ill; Northwestern Univ, Chicago)

J Vasc Surg 31:927-935, 2000   12–12

Background.—Many studies have shown the benefits of carotid endarterectomy (CEA) in selected patients with severe atherosclerotic carotid artery occlusive disease. However, most of these studies have excluded octogenarians. A comparison was made of patient characteristics and outcomes between octogenarians and younger patients after CEA.

Methods.—For 13 years, the same surgical staff performed 582 primary CEAs in 528 patients. All procedures involved conventional surgical techniques, including general anesthesia, selective shunting, and selective patch closure of the carotid arteriotomy. Outcomes (perioperative and late ipsilateral stroke and death) were compared between the octogenarians (90 CEAs in 88 patients; 54 men and 34 women; mean age, 83.2 years) and the younger patients (492 CEAs in 458 patients; 290 men and 168 women; mean age, 69.5 years).

Results.—Between 1985 and 1998, the number of octogenarians undergoing CEA increased significantly, from 6 between 1985 and 1988 to 68 between 1993 and 1998. Compared with the younger patients, the octogenarians were significantly more likely to have a history of congestive heart failure (16% vs 5%) or hypertension (79% vs 68%) and significantly less likely to have a history of smoking (44% vs 62%) or chronic obstructive lung disease (2% vs 9%). Indications for CEA were similar in the 2 groups, and 27% of octogenarians and 33% of the younger patients

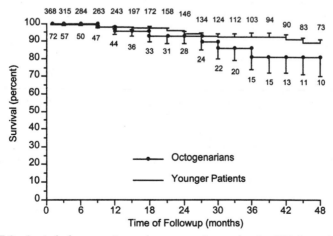

FIGURE 2.—Survival of octogenarians and younger patients undergoing CEA (log-rank, $P = 11$). *Error bars* represent SEM. The number of patients entering the next interval alive is given for octogenarians below survival lines and younger patients above survival lines. (Courtesy of Schneider JR, Droste JS, Schindler N, et al: Carotid endarterectomy in octogenarians: Comparison with patient characteristics and outcomes in younger patients. *J Vasc Surg* 31: 927-935, 2000.)

underwent CEA because of asymptomatic disease. However, octogenarians were significantly more likely to have 80% or more stenosis (90% vs 78%). Nine perioperative strokes occurred (all were ipsilateral), with no significant difference in incidence between octogenarians (1, or 1.1%) and younger patients (8, or 1.6%). Thirty-day mortality rates were also similar in the octogenarians (no deaths) and younger patients (2 deaths). Two octogenarians experienced late stroke (1 ipsilateral), as did 4 younger patients (2 ipsilateral; no significant difference). Life table analysis estimated that 98% of octogenarians and 97% of younger patients would be free of ipsilateral stroke at 2 years. Life table analysis also estimated that 81% of octogenarians and 89% of younger patients would be alive at 4 years after CEA (Fig 2).

Conclusions.—The indications for CEA and comorbidities are similar in octogenarians and younger patients selected for CEA. These groups were also similar in early mortality rates and early and late neurologic outcomes. From a cost-benefit perspective, the length of hospital stay and the direct costs associated with CEA were similar in the 2 patient groups, and more than 80% of patients in both groups would be expected to be alive 4 years postoperatively. Thus, CEA has clear benefits in this population and should be considered for intellectually intact octogenarians without unusually severe comorbidities.

▶ A large number of reports have demonstrated that many if not most vascular operations can be performed in carefully selected patients of advanced age with outcomes comparable to those achieved in much younger age groups. Thus, it bears emphasis that chronologic age *alone* remains at best a crude predictor of the risk of perioperative morbidity and mortality, as well as long-term life expectancy. Our population is aging rapidly, and vigorous older Americans should not be denied treatment on the basis of a simple age cutoff. Nonetheless, in the gray zone of risk-benefit analysis, the decision to advocate a surgical intervention is not always clear-cut. Treatment of an asymptomatic carotid stenosis or, for that matter, a small aortic aneurysm is directed at eliminating the risk of a devastating event that is admittedly infrequent if the disease is managed with medical therapy or left alone. The risk-benefit scale most favors those patients who will otherwise be alive and well for a substantial period after intervention. Perhaps we can look forward to improved tools that will allow us to better select those lesions at greatest risk and patients with long survival times. In the meantime, our recommendations, by necessity, will be largely based on an assessment of individual comorbidities—an inexact science at best.

E. L. Chaikof, MD

Effect of Contralateral Occlusion on Long-term Efficacy of Endarterectomy in the Asymptomatic Carotid Atherosclerosis Study (ACAS)

Howard VJ, for the ACAS Investigators (Loyola Univ, Maywood, Ill; et al)
Stroke 31:2330-2334, 2000   12–13

Objective.—The Asymptomatic Carotid Atherosclerosis Study (ACAS) showed that carotid endarterectomy reduced the long-term risk of stroke in asymptomatic patients with 60% stenosis or greater. Patients with a contralateral carotid occlusion would seem to be at increased risk for stroke. Outcomes of ACAS patients with and without a contralateral internal artery occlusion at baseline were compared in a randomized study.

Methods.—The ACAS randomly allocated 1662 patients with documented significant carotid stenosis to aspirin and risk factor reduction management or to this regimen plus carotid endarterectomy. Baseline Doppler assessment of stenosis was available for 1648 patients. Patients were divided into 4 groups: those with no contralateral occlusion who had medical (748 patients) or surgical treatment (737 patients) and those with contralateral occlusion who had medical (77 patients) or surgical treatment (86 patients). The primary end points were stroke or death during the 30-day perioperative period, ipsilateral stroke during the post–30-day follow-up period, and the 5-year event rate.

Results.—The 5-year estimated event rates were 11.7% for the group without contralateral occlusion and medical management and 5.0% for surgical management. For the group with contralateral occlusion, the estimates were 3.5% for medical management and 5.5% for surgical management. There was a significant difference in the efficacy of surgery versus medical management between patients with and without contralateral occlusion (8.7%). The perioperative event rate was equivalent for surgical patients with and without contralateral occlusion. Surgery increased the event rate by 2% in those who had a contralateral occlusion

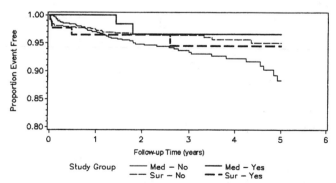

FIGURE 1.—Kaplan-Meier survival estimates for those patients medically managed without contralateral occlusion (*Med–No*), surgically managed without contralateral occlusion (*Sur–No*), medically managed with contralateral occlusion (*Med–Yes*), and surgically managed with contralateral occlusion (*Sur–Yes*). (Courtesy of Howard VJ, for the ACAS Investigators: Effect of contralateral occlusion on long-term efficacy of endarterectomy in the asymptomatic carotid atherosclerosis study (ACAS). *Stroke* 31:2330-2334, 2000. Reproduced with permission of *Stroke*. Copyright 2000, American Heart Association.)

compared with those who did not. The perioperative event rate for medically managed patients with a contralateral occlusion was significantly lower than for those without a contralateral occlusion (3.5% vs 11.0%) (Fig 1).

Conclusion.—Prophylactic carotid endarterectomy does not help prevent stroke and death in asymptomatic patients with a contralateral occlusion. Surgery is associated with a 2.0% increase in risk for these patients.

▶ This is another slice of the pie from ACAS. This post hoc analysis suggests that carotid endarterectomy (CEA) in asymptomatic patients with a contralateral occlusion "provides no long-term benefit (and may be harmful)." A 5-year risk reduction of 6.7% was seen in patients undergoing CEA without contralateral occlusion (very similar to the overall ACAS results), yet there was a 2% absolute increase in risk in the 86 surgical patients with contralateral occlusion. Patients with contralateral occlusions had a similar perioperative event rate as those without occlusions (2.3% vs 2.2%), supporting the concept that CEA can be safely performed regardless of the status of the contralateral carotid. However, the medically treated patients with contralateral occlusion had a 5-year event rate of 3.5%, whereas those medically treated patients without contralateral occlusions had a 5-year event rate of 11.7%. Why would this be? The authors speculate on the protective merits of good collateral circulation. However, intuitively there is no explanation for these findings, and likely this discrepancy represents the vagaries of post hoc analysis. I would agree wholeheartedly with the authors' statement that this analysis "be interpreted with caution." Until further studies examining the effect of contralateral occlusion as a primary end point are available, this information should be kept on the back burner.

A. M. Abou-Zamzam, Jr, MD

Perioperative and Late Stroke Rates of Carotid Endarterectomy Contralateral to Carotid Artery Occlusion: Results From a Randomized Trial
AbuRahma AF, Robinson P, Holt SM, et al (West Virginia Univ, Charleston; Boehringer Ingelheim Pharmaceuticals Inc, Ridgefield, Conn)
Stroke 31:1566-1571, 2000   12–14

Objective.—Patients with a contralateral occluded carotid artery are at high risk for carotid endarterectomy (CEA). Results of surgery for patients with contralateral carotid artery occlusion were analyzed in a prospective randomized trial of closure methods.

Methods.—The study included 357 patients undergoing 399 CEAs who were randomly assigned to primary closure (n = 135), polytetrafluoroethylene patching (n = 134), or vein patch closure (n = 130). Patients were divided into 2 groups: group A (n = 49 CEAs) who underwent CEAs for significant ipsilateral carotid artery (ICA) stenosis and group B (n = 350 CEAs) who underwent CEAs for significant ipsilateral ICA stenosis without contralateral occlusion. The number of perioperative strokes and stroke-free survival were analyzed by means of the Kaplan-Meier method.

Results.—Group A had a significantly higher incidence of contralateral TIAs, contralateral strokes, and combined TIAs/strokes compared with group B. Group A and group B had similar rates (nonsignificant) of perioperative stroke (2% and 2.9%), all strokes (4.1% and 3.4%), perioperative TIAs (0% and 2.6%), all TIAs (14.3% and 6.3%), perioperative neurologic events (2% and 5.4%), and all neurologic events (18.4% and 9.7%), respectively. Perioperative mortality rates and all mortality rates, were also similar for both groups. The 5-year cumulative stroke survival rates were 84% for group A and 77% for group B and were similar for patients with and without symptoms.

Conclusion.—Patients undergoing CEA with an occluded contralateral carotid artery are not at increased risk.

▶ A subgroup analysis from a randomized trial comparing carotid patch repair versus primary closure, this slice of the salami examines the results of surgery for the modest (n = 49) number of patients with a contralateral carotid occlusion, compared with the surgical results of all other patients in the trial. The authors demonstrate that the perioperative and long-term stroke risk in these patients is no different than that of the larger cohort. Other than the obvious potential for type II statistical error with such disparate numbers in the 2 groups, the data are sound and as noted in the discussion, confirmed by several other previous comparative clinical series, including the North American Symptomatic Carotid Endarterectomy Trial.

M. R. Nehler, MD

Dissection

Surgical Treatment of 50 Carotid Dissections: Indications and Results
Müller BT, Luther B, Hort W, et al (Heinrich-Heine-Univ, Düsseldorf, Germany)
J Vasc Surg 31:980-988, 2000   12–15

Background.—Cervical artery dissection is increasingly recognized as a cause of strokes, particularly in younger individuals, whether as a result of a higher incidence or recent advances in neurovascular diagnostic techniques. One report described carotid artery dissection in 2.5% of 1200 patients with a first stroke and in as many as 22% of the patients with strokes who were younger than 30 years. Arterial dissections result either from intramural hemorrhaging, probably because of bleeding from the vasa vasorum, or from penetration of blood into the arterial wall through a primary intimal tear. An intramural medial hematoma may lie in closer proximity to the adventitia, causing aneurysmal dilatation, or may extend toward the intima, causing stenosis. A spontaneous recanalization of the stenosed and even occluded dissected internal carotid and normalization of volume blood flow has been reported in several studies in 47% to 85% of cases within 6 months. Because the rate of spontaneous healing is high,

TABLE 4.—Operative Technique

Technique	No. of Operations (%)
Resection, vein interposition graft	40 (80)
Ligation or clip	5 (10)
Thromboendarterectomy + patch angioplasty	3 (6)
Dilatation	2 (4)

(Courtesy of Müller BT, Luther B, Hort W, et al: Surgical treatment of 50 carotid dissections: Indications and results. *J Vasc Surg* 31:980-988, 2000.)

the current approach to acute carotid dissection is nonsurgical. However, persistent high-grade stenosis and a persistent or newly developed aneurysm of the dissected internal carotid after 6 months of medical treatment may be an indication for surgical revascularization. The course of 49 patients with 50 chronic carotid dissections who underwent surgical treatment is reported.

Methods.—Surgical treatment was provided in 48 patients with 49 chronic carotid dissections after a median anticoagulation period of 9 months because of persistent high-grade stenosis or aneurysms. One other patient was treated with early operative reconstruction 12 hours after onset because of fluctuating neurologic symptoms. A retrospective review of medical and surgical records and imaging studies was performed. Follow-up of 41 patients (85%) after a median of 70 months included an examination of the extracranial vessels in the neck by Doppler US scanning and a questionnaire regarding the patients' medical histories and personal assessments of cranial nerve function.

Results.—Spontaneous dissection had occurred in 70% of patients; the cause of dissection was trauma in 18%. Fibromuscular dysplasia was present in 12% of all patients and in 22% of female patients. In 40 patients (80%), flow restoration was achieved by resection and vein graft placement, whereas thromboendarterectomy and patch angioplasty were performed in 3 patients (6%). Gradual dilatation was effectively performed in 2 patients (4%) (Table 4). In 5 patients (10%), the internal carotid artery had to be clipped because dissection extended into the base of the skull. Recurrent minor strokes occurred in 5 patients (10%). Damage to the cranial nerves was unavoidable in 29 patients (58%), but in most patients, the damage was transient. One patient died of unrelated causes during follow-up, and 1 patient experienced a neurologic event of unknown cause.

Conclusions.—Surgical reconstruction of chronic carotid dissection can be an effective treatment for prevention of further ischemic or thromboembolic complications after 6 months of medical treatment has failed or in the setting of persistent or newly developed high-grade carotid stenosis.

▶ This is a very large series of patients who underwent surgery at one institution for carotid dissection. Nerve injury was relatively common, presumably because these patients required high carotid exposure. In addition, the stroke rate was 10%. The authors recommend surgical reconstruction if the patient has failed medical treatment (anticoagulation for 6 months) or if carotid aneurysms develop. These operations were almost never performed acutely. For the rare patient with dissection who requires surgery, this article would appear to offer some useful hints. I am surprised, with the authors relatively rigid indications for surgery, that they were able to find 48 such patients requiring surgery over a period of only 9 months.

J. L. Mills, Sr, MD

MR Angiography for the Long-term Follow-up of Dissecting Aneurysms of the Extracranial internal Carotid Artery
Djouhri H, Guillon B, Brunereau L, et al (Hôpital Saint-Antoine, Paris)
AJR 174:1137-1140, 2000   12–16

Background.—Dissection of the internal carotid artery (ICA) has emerged as an important cause of stroke in young to middle-aged adults. Few data have been published on the long-term course of these dissecting aneurysms. The long-term changes in dissecting ICA aneurysms were assessed in an MR angiographic follow-up study.

Methods.—The retrospective study included 101 consecutive patients with dissecting aneurysms of the extracranial ICA. Of these, 20 patients (16 men, 4 women; mean age, 51 years) with a total of 26 spontaneously dissecting ICA aneurysms underwent follow-up MR angiography every 1 to 2 years, for a mean follow-up of 41 months. Seventeen of the 20 patients received antiplatelet therapy.

Results.—At last follow-up, 4 aneurysms had decreased in size by a mean of 43%, and 2 had resolved completely (Fig 2). The remaining 20 aneurysms were unchanged throughout follow-up. One patient had a recurrent dissecting ICA aneurysm, which remained asymptomatic. No clinical episodes of thromboembolic stroke or transient ischemic attack were noted.

Conclusions.—For most patients with dissecting aneurysms of the extracranial ICA, MR angiography demonstrates no significant change in size during a follow-up of 3 to 4 years. Some aneurysms resolve or decrease in size, but apparently none increase in size. The results suggest that surgical or endovascular treatment may be unnecessary for this group of patients.

▶ I am impressed by the number of patients in this series, which examines the natural history of dissecting aneurysms of the extracranial ICA. The knowledge of the natural history of this often vexing problem becomes very helpful when deciding what to do with dissecting aneurysms of the carotid. One shortcoming of the study is the classification of small aneurysms— those less than 1 cm. I wonder whether this "aneurysm" is, in fact, just a defect in the wall from the dissection. I say this with some certainty because these aneurysms were the ones most likely to become smaller or resolve

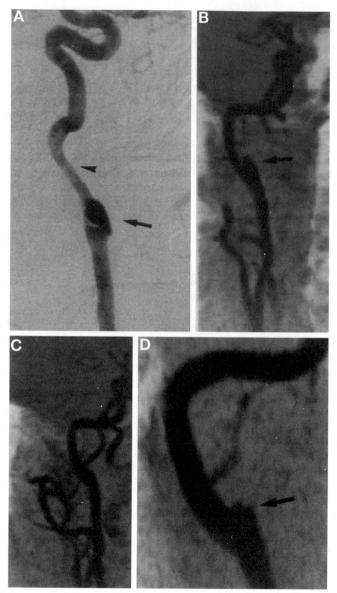

FIGURE 2.—45-year-old man with right-sided painful Horner's syndrome. A, Carotid arteriogram shows aneurysmal type of dissection (*arrow*) with saccular aneurysm located in midcervical segment of right internal carotid artery (ICA). Note luminal stenosis (*arrowhead*). B, Coronal MR angiogram obtained 3 months after A shows unchanged aneurysm (*arrow*). Note good correlation with arteriogram and resolution of luminal stenosis. C, Follow-up MR angiogram obtained 48 months after B. Aneurysm is unclear. D, Follow-up axial MR angiogram centered on dissected ICA shows residual aneurysm (*arrow*) because of higher resolution. This aneurysm decreased in size more than 50%. (Courtesy of Djouhri H, Guillon B, Brunereau L, et al: MR angiography for the long-term follow-up of dissecting aneurysms of the extracranial internal carotid artery. *AJR* 174:1137-1140, 2000.)

completely. Images from MR angiography seem to be good with this disease and probably relates to the large size of these arteries. In contrast, I continue to be underwhelmed with the quality of MR angiography for atherosclerotic occlusive disease of the extracranial cerebral arteries.

R. B. McLafferty, MD

Aneurysmal Forms of Cervical Artery Dissection: Associated Factors and Outcome
Touzé E, Randoux B, Méary E, et al (Hôpital Sainte Anne, Paris)
Stroke 32:418-423, 2001   12–17

Background.—As many as 20% of ischemic strokes in young adults can be attributed to cervical artery dissection (CAD). The exact pathogenesis of CAD has remained unclear, but it has been postulated that CAD is the result of an underlying arteriopathy, which leads to a so-called weakness of the vessel. The clinical and anatomical outcomes of aneurysmal forms of extracranial internal carotid artery (ICA) and vertebral artery (VA) dissections were assessed, as were the factors associated with aneurysmal forms of CAD.

Methods.—The findings in 71 consecutive patients with CAD were reviewed. Using all available angiograms, 2 neuroradiologists identified aneurysmal forms of CAD. A comparison of the frequency of arterial risk factors, multiple vessel dissections, and artery redundancies was performed in patients with and without aneurysms. Patients who were identified as having aneurysms were invited by mail to a final clinical and radiologic evaluation.

Results.—A total of 42 aneurysms were identified in 35 of 71 patients (49.3%). Of these 42 aneurysms, 30 were located on a symptomatic artery (ICA, 23; VA, 7) and 12 were located on an asymptomatic artery (ICA, 10; VA, 2). Multiple dissections of cervical vessels were observed more frequently in patients with aneurysms than in patients without aneurysms, as were arterial redundancies. Patients with aneurysms were also more likely to have histories or migraines and to be tobacco users. Clinical and anatomical follow-up information was available for 35 patients (100%) and 33 patients (94%), respectively. During a mean follow-up period of more than 3 years, none of the patients demonstrated signs of cerebral ischemia, local compression, or a rupture. There was no change at follow-up in 46% of the aneurysms involving symptomatic ICA; however, 36% of this type of aneurysm had disappeared, and 18% had decreased in size (Fig 2). Resolution of the aneurysm was more common in those involving the VA than in aneurysms involving the ICA (83% vs 36%). None of the aneurysms located on an asymptomatic ICA had disappeared.

Conclusions.—It is quite common for aneurysms caused by CAD to persist, but the risk of clinical complications for patients with this type of aneurysm was found to be very low. Clinicians should keep this favorable

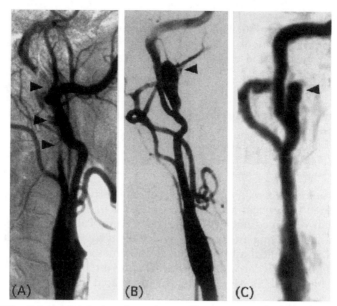

FIGURE 2.—A, Initial digital subtraction angiogram shows severe stenosis of the right internal carotid artery but no obvious aneurysm. **B,** Follow-up digital subtraction angiogram performed 3 months later shows resolution of the stenosis and appearance of a saccular aneurysm. **C,** Follow-up gadolinium-enhanced MR angiogram performed 50 months later shows that the aneurysm decreased in size. (Courtesy of Touzé E, Randoux B, Méary E, et al: Aneurysmal forms of cervical artery dissection: Associated factors and outcome. *Stroke* 32:418-423, 2001. Reproduced with permission from *Stroke*. Copyright 2001 American Heart Association.)

clinical outcome in mind before potentially harmful treatment is considered.

▶ Apparently the intermediate-term natural history of the aneurysmal form of extracranial carotid artery dissection is more benign than previously appreciated. Although a minority of postdissection carotid aneurysms resolved during a mean follow-up of 36.6 months in this consecutive series accruing patients over a 10-year period, more than half decreased or disappeared, and the remaining aneurysms were unchanged. Complete resolution was significantly more frequent for vertebral aneurysms. Importantly, no patient with an aneurysm had a transient ischemic attack, stroke, or clinical symptoms suggestive of compression of surrounding structures or rupture during follow-up, and no new lesions were appreciated on surveillance MRI. Since these results are consistent with previous observations regarding the relatively benign natural history of postdissection extracranial aneurysms, clearly the onus is on those who favor aggressive intervention (either open or catheter based) to demonstrate that expensive, potentially risky and heretofore unproven procedures to resect or exclude such aneurysms will prove necessary or beneficial.

R. L. Dalman, MD

Surgical Treatment of Extracranial Internal Carotid Artery Aneurysms
Rosset E, Albertini J-N, Magnan PE, et al (Hôpital de La Timone, Marseille, France)
J Vasc Surg 31:713-723, 2000   12–18

Background.—Extracranial internal carotid artery (ICA) aneurysms are localized increases of caliber of more than 50% in comparison with reference values. The most frequent identifying symptoms are neurologic manifestations; hemorrhages or compression from giant aneurysms are now rarely seen. With the development of reconstructive surgery of ICA lesions, all lesions, even the most distal, can be treated surgically. An experience with the reconstructive surgical treatment of extracranial ICA lesions, including lesions located at the base of the skull, was reported.

Methods.—Over 18 years, from 1980 to 1997, 25 ICA reconstructions for extracranial ICA aneurysms were performed in 22 men and 3 women (mean age, 54.4 years). The cause of the extracranial ICA aneurysm was atherosclerosis in 9 patients, trauma in 3 patients, dysplasia in 12 patients, and undetermined in 1 patient. For 15 patients, the symptoms were focal, whereas 3 patients had nonfocal symptoms and 1 patient was seen with glossopharyngeal nerve compression. Six patients were asymptomatic, including 3 that were given diagnoses after ICA dissection. The upper limit of the ICA aneurysm extended to the base of the skull in 9 patients. Exposure and control of the ICA was achieved with a combined approach by an ear, nose, and throat surgeon (Fig 2).

Results.—There were 2 transient ischemic attacks, 1 temporary stroke, and 11 cranial nerve palsies (1 with sequelae) after surgery but no deaths. In all but 1 patient, the ICA was patent after the procedure. Two deaths from myocardial infarction occurred during follow-up of a mean of 66 months; there was 1 incident of a focal epileptic seizure at 2 months and 1 incident of a transient ischemic attack at 2 years. Duplex scanning was performed in December 1998 and showed patency of the reconstructed ICA in all but 1 patient.

Conclusions.—Surgical reconstruction can be used successfully in the treatment of extracranial ICA aneurysms, even when the lesion is located at the base of the skull.

▶ As with abdominal aortic aneurysms, the increased use of sophisticated imaging techniques has led to increased detection of extracranial ICA aneurysms, although ICA aneurysms remain rare. By far the majority of such lesions can be approached and replaced by a competent vascular surgeon. Aneurysms extending to the base of the skull can be approached if one has an interested neurosurgeon or otolaryngologist available to resect some bone at the base of the skull, with surprisingly low morbidity if using the approach described in this article. I suspect that no one surgeon will ever develop a large series of such patients, so the information presented in this article must be considered seriously.

E. J. Harris, Jr, MD

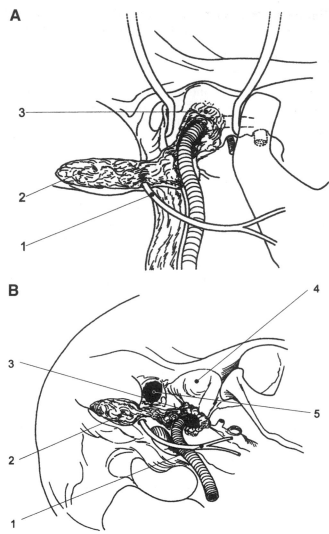

FIGURE 2.—A, An exposure of the distal internal carotid artery after drilling the vaginal process of the tympanal bone and the tip of the mastoid process. A special retractor maintains mandibular subluxation. **B,** An inferior view of the base of the skull, showing the extended bone resection and exposure of the carotid artery. *1,* Facial nerve; *2,* area of mastoid process drilling; *3,* area of vaginal process drilling; *4,* glenoid cavity; *5,* jugular foramen. (Courtesy of Rosset E, Albertini J-N, Magnan PE, et al: Surgical treatment of extracranial internal carotid artery aneurysms. *J Vasc Surg* 31:713-723, 2000.)

Radiation

Carotid Stenosis After Radiotherapy for Nasopharyngeal Carcinoma

Cheng SWK, Ting ACW, Lam LK, et al (Univ of Hong Kong, China)
Arch Otolaryngol Head Neck Surg 126:517-521, 2000   12–19

Background.—A well-known sequela of cervical radiotherapy (RT) is radiation injury to the carotid arteries with resulting stenosis and stroke. However, the incidence of and pattern of radiation-induced carotid stenosis in patients who have been treated with cervical RT have been rarely studied, despite the widespread use of irradiation of the head and neck. Carotid endarterectomy in an irradiated field is often hindered by the presence of adhesions as well as an extensive distribution of disease. Interest in RT-induced carotid stenosis has been rekindled with the introduction of carotid angioplasty and stenting as an alternative treatment of these difficult lesions. Among Chinese patients in Hong Kong, nasopharyngeal carcinoma (NPC) is a common form of malignant neoplasm, with an estimated annual incidence of 18.7 per 100,000 population. The treatment of choice for early NPC is external irradiation, along with adjuvant treatment of local and cervical lymph node recurrences. Improvements in surgical treatment, such as nasopharyngectomy, and the aggressive use of adjuvant RT have resulted in longer survival for more patients. However, in these patients, carotid stenosis represents a threat of stroke, and this should be remembered by surgeons and radiation oncologists. The prevalence and risk factors for RT-induced carotid stenosis in patients treated for malignant neoplasms of the head and neck were investigated.

Methods.—At tertiary oncology and vascular referral center in Hong Kong, 96 consecutive patients were studied. The 75 men and 21 women (mean age, 53.6 years) had undergone cervical RT for nasopharyngeal more than 12 months before enrollment in the study (mean post-RT interval, 79.9 months). Cerebrovascular symptoms were present in 14 patients. A control group of 96 healthy individuals was used for comparison.

Results.—Stenosis of 70% or more of the internal carotid artery was found in 14 arteries in 12 patients, with 6 occlusions. Stenosis of 70% or more of the common carotid artery was found in 11 arteries in 9 patients, with 4 occlusions. Overall, critical stenosis of the common or internal carotid artery was present in 15 patients (16%). Moderate stenosis was found in another 20 (21%) patients. None of the control patients had critical carotid stenosis. Factors associated with severe post-RT carotid stenosis were age, smoking, heart disease, no prior oncological surgery, cerebrovascular symptoms, and interval from RT. Multivariate logistic regression analysis identified smoking, interval from RT, cerebrovascular symptoms, and no prior head and neck surgery as independent predictors for severe carotid stenosis.

Conclusions.—There is a higher risk of significant carotid stenosis after 5 years among patients who undergo irradiation of the head and neck. Routine duplex US screening is recommended for these patients.

▶ Studies like this add numbers to our perceptions. We know that radiation therapy of head and neck cancer is associated with internal carotid and common carotid artery occlusive disease. We now know that this incidence is approximately 37% for having at least a 30% stenosis. While it is tempting to suggest that critical stenosis in these patients be treated prophylactically, no evidence currently justifies such an approach. The difficulties of surgical management of such lesions, as well as the completely unknown natural history of carotid stents in these arteries, mandate that the initial treatment of significant stenoses in radiated carotid arteries be the administration of antiplatelet drugs. Intervention should be reserved for symptomatic patients.

G. L. Moneta, MD

Asymptomatic Carotid Arterial Disease in Young Patients Following Neck Radiation Therapy for Hodgkin Lymphoma

King LJ, Hasnain SN, Webb JAW, et al (St Bartholomew's Hosp, London)
Radiology 213:167-172, 1999   12–20

Objective.—Radiation therapy plays a role in the development of early and atypical carotid artery disease. The prevalence and severity of asymptomatic carotid artery disease in young patients after radiation therapy to the neck for lymphoma has not been studied by US. Such a study was performed and the results after radiotherapy alone were compared with those after radiotherapy and chemotherapy.

Methods.—Between November 1995 and March 1997, US was performed on 42 long-term Hodgkin disease survivors, aged 18 to 37 years, who received their diagnosis at ages 4 to 29 years, and were treated by radiation to the neck during childhood or early adulthood. US results were compared with those of 33 healthy volunteers, aged 23 to 36. Demographic data, cardiovascular risk factors, and smoking history were obtained. Intima-media thickness was measured on the posterior wall of the common carotid artery 3 times at each of 6 sites: the proximal, middle, and distal sections of both arteries.

Results.—Patients were treated at least 5 years prior to entering the study. The total radiation dose received varied from 2250 to 4000 cGy and was delivered in 15 to 25 fractions. The study group had significantly more abnormalities than did the control group (26% vs 3%). One (2%) patient had an abnormal biopsy classification of V, none had a classification of IV, 4 had a classification of III, 6 had a classification of II, and 31 had a classification of I. Ten patients had focal or generalized abnormalities. Patients treated with radiation alone or a combination of radiation and chemotherapy had similar numbers of abnormal scans. The median intimal thickness was similar for the 2 groups. The prevalence of abnormalities was significantly higher in patients aged 30 to 39 years than in patients aged 20 to 29 years.

Conclusion.—The prevalence of asymptomatic carotid artery disease is common in young patients treated with neck irradiation for lymphoma and is similar to that for patients treated with radiation and chemotherapy.

► This small but controlled study provides clear evidence of a relationship between early life cervical irradiation and increased thickness/stenosis of the cervical carotid arteries. As the authors fully acknowledge, it is not presently known nor addressed by their study whether this radiation-related abnormality is more or less likely to produce symptoms, occlusions, or both, than are carotid abnormalities resulting from atherosclerosis in patients with no history of radiation exposure.

L. M. Taylor, Jr, MD

Stroke

Immediate Reexploration for the Perioperative Neurologic Event After Carotid Endarterectomy: Is it Worthwhile?

Rockman CB, Jacobowitz GR, Lamparello PJ, et al (New York Univ)
J Vasc Surg 32:1062-1070, 2000   12–21

Background.—Debate over how to manage a patient who has a new neurologic deficit after carotid endarterectomy (CEA) continues. An important question is which of these perioperative neurologic events (PNEs) are likely to improve with surgical reexploration. A series of PNEs was analyzed to determine whether information on the timing and mechanisms of the event can predict the chances of improvement after reoperation.

Methods.—Using a prospective database, the investigators identified 2024 primary CEAs performed over a 12-year period. Thirty-eight patients had new neurologic deficits during the perioperative period, which yielded a rate of 1.9%. Causes were identified through clinical findings, reexploration, and imaging and other tests.

Results.—Causes of the PNEs included thromboembolic events in 63.2% of cases, ischemia related to intraoperative clamping in 13.2%, and intracerebral hemorrhaging in 13.2%. The new deficit was unrelated to the vessel operated on in CEA in 10.5% of cases. Eighty-eight percent of events occurring within the first 24 hours postoperatively were caused by thromboembolic events, whereas later deficits were more likely to result from other causes (Table 5). Immediate reexploration was performed in 18 of 25 patients with PNEs developing in the first 24 hours. Eighty-three percent of these explorations revealed intraluminal thrombi. Reexploration led to complete resolution or significant improvement in the new deficit in 12 of 18 cases.

Conclusions.—When new neurologic deficits occur after CEA, information on the timing and presentation of the PNE can aid in identifying patients likely to benefit from reexploration. Thromboembolic events are

TABLE 5.—Relationship Between Etiology and Timing of the PNEs Occurring in the Postoperative Period

	Thromboembolic	Other Cause	Total
Early PNE (< 24 h)	22 (88%)	3 (12%)	25
Late (> 24 h)	2 (25%)	6 (75%)	8
Total	24	9	33

Abbreviation: PNE, Perioperative neurologic event.
(Courtesy of Rockman CB, Jacobowitz GR, Lamparello PJ, et al: Immediate reexploration for the perioperative neurologic event after carotid endarterectomy: Is it worthwhile? *J Vasc Surg* 32:1062-1070, 2000.)

the likely cause of deficits occurring within 24 hours. In these cases, the authors recommend immediate reexploration to remove the source of the embolism and to correct any technical defects, unless another cause is identified. Such a strategy is likely to lead to improved neurologic outcomes.

▶ While this is a retrospective review, it encompasses a large number of patients and represents a very important contribution to the body of literature on management of carotid disease. The authors' conclusions completely support the position that those patients who develop neurologic deficits within 24 hours of CEA usually require immediate reexploration without imaging studies. Patients who develop deficits more than 24 hours after CEA should be considered for some type of imaging study before considering reexploration.

W. K. Williamson, MD

Five-Year Survival After First-Ever Stroke and Related Prognostic Factors in the Perth Community Stroke Study

Hankey GJ, Jamrozik K, Broadhurst RJ, et al (Royal Perth Hosp, Australia; Univ of Western Australia, Perth; Univ of Auckland, New Zealand)
Stroke 31:2080-2086, 2000
12–22

Background.—There is little community-based data on the long-term outcomes and prognostic factors for patients experiencing their first acute stroke. The Perth Community Stroke Study assessed 5-year survival and independent prognostic factors among patients with their first-ever stroke.

Methods.—The study included all patients in Perth, Western Australia, with suspected acute stroke or transient ischemic attack over an 18-month period from 1989 to 1990. All identified patients underwent a standard assessment and follow-up for up to 5 years after the index event. Absolute and relative survival and independent risk factors for death were assessed among all patients and all patients who survived for the first 30 days after stroke.

Results.—A total of 370 patients with initial stroke were entered into the study. Five-year follow-up data were available on 362 patients, 58% of whom died during follow-up. The risk of death was highest (36.5%) in the first year after stroke. This represented a 10-fold increase over the expected mortality rate for the age- and sex-matched population. Sixty-four percent of deaths were caused by the index stroke. For from 1 to 5 years, the annual mortality rate was about 10%, about 2-fold higher than expected. Forty-one percent of these deaths resulted from cardiovascular disease. For 30-day survivors, baseline factors that were independent predictors of death within 5 years were intermittent claudication (hazard ratio, [HR] 1.9), urinary incontinence (HR, 2.0), previous transient ischemic attack (HR, 2.4), and baseline Barthel Index of less than 20/20 (HR, 2.0).

Conclusion.—Most patients experiencing a first-ever acute stroke will die of stroke within the first year. For the second through fifth years, the mortality rate is about 10%, or twice as high as expected. Because most of these deaths are from cardiovascular disease, late mortality after stroke may be reduced by early implementation of effective strategies to lower the risk of cardiovascular events.

▶ This article provides important descriptive data for the outcome of patients after a first cerebrovascular accident. The increased death rate in those patients with cerebrovascular accident speaks to more virulent systemic vasculopathy. This article is an important contribution to our understanding of the natural history of stroke and cerebrovascular disease.

W. K. Williamson, MD

Hemispheric Stroke Following Cardiac Surgery: A Case-Control Estimate of the Risk Resulting From Ipsilateral Asymptomatic Carotid Artery Stenosis
Hill AB, Obrand D, O'Rourke K, et al (McGill Univ, Montreal)
Ann Vasc Surg 14:200-209, 2000   12–23

Background.—The case-control method offers an alternative to prospective cohort studies and is both efficient and inexpensive. Case-control studies are observational in nature work backward from the disease to the potential cause. Whether asymptomatic carotid artery stenosis (ACS) is independently associated with ipsilateral hemispheric stroke development after cardiac surgery was evaluated with a case–control study design.

Methods.—The 3069 patients reviewed for this study had undergone cardiac surgery between 1989 and 1994. The patients chosen from this population included 31 patients who had hemispheric strokes within 30 days after the surgery and 69 patients who had no hemispheric strokes, who served as control subjects.

Results.—Patients with postoperative hemispheric strokes were significantly more likely to have ipsilateral ACS than those not having strokes. A 5.2-fold increase in the odds ratio of a stroke accompanied an ACS of 50% to 99%. Patients who had an ACS of 80% to 99% at surgery had a 24.3-fold increase in the odds ratio over those who did not have an ACS of this degree. A significantly increased risk of a stroke was also associated with age 65 years or older, peripheral vascular disease, hypertension, and female sex. Factors not related to increased risk included smoking, diabetes mellitus, hyperlipidemia, atrial fibrillation, and valvular surgery. A conservative evaluation for missing data showed a significant association for ACS of 80% to 90% only, but this association remained even after multivariate adjustment using propensity score stratification.

Conclusions.—An ACS of 80% to 90% was linked independently with the risk of an ipsilateral hemispheric stroke after cardiac surgery, although no cause-and-effect relationship has been proven. Thus, no clear justification has been offered for the use of simultaneous carotid endarterectomy during cardiac surgery to manage ACS.

▶ Carotid stenosis of greater than 80% is associated with an increased risk of stroke after cardiac surgery. OK fine. But just what is the magnitude of this problem? The authors could identify only 31 strokes in more than 3000 cardiac operations (1%). If we believe the recent findings of the NASCET investigators that only about one half of strokes can be traced to carotid disease, you cut the incidence to about 0.5%. To me it seems futile to chase after such a small number of patients, especially since the stroke risk with carotid surgery in the best of series is about 2%. This article presents us with an observation that one could probably have guessed intuitively, but, as the authors correctly point out, it should not be used to guide therapy. A randomized, prospective trial comparing stroke rates in patients with asymptomatic high-grade lesions treated with and without carotid endarterectomy before or concomitantly with cardiac surgery would be nice, but with such small numbers of the primary outcome measure (ie, stroke), this would likely take a huge number of patients to find any difference.

G. J. Landry, MD

Ischemic Stroke Subtypes: A Population-Based Study of Functional Outcome, Survival, and Recurrence

Petty GW, Brown RD Jr, Whisnant JP, et al (Mayo Clinic and Mayo Found, Rochester, Minn)
Stroke 31:1062-1068, 2000   12–24

Background.—Despite the many reports of survival and recurrence rates after stroke, there are few population-based data on patient outcomes after specific subtypes of ischemic stroke. The functional outcome, survival, and recurrence rates after various ischemic stroke subtypes were assessed.

Methods.—Using the population-based Rochester Epidemiology Project medical records linkage system, the investigators identified all Rochester, Minn, residents experiencing an initial ischemic stroke from 1985 to 1989. On the basis of medical records and imaging studies, the patients' ischemic stroke subtype was classified as defined by the National Institute of Neu-

TABLE 2.—Kaplan-Meier Estimates of Probabilities of Recurrent Stroke After First Ischemic Stroke for Common Ischemic Stroke Subtypes, 1985-1989

Time After First Stroke	Percent With Recurrent Stroke (95% CI) Among Each Ischemic Stroke Subtype			
	Atherosclerosis With Stenosis	Cardioembolic	Lacunar	Ischemic Stroke of Uncertain Cause
7 d	8.5 (2.0-14.9)	2.4 (0.0-5.2)	1.4 (0.0-4.1)	1.9 (0.0-4.1)
30 d	18.5 (9.4-27.5)	5.3 (1.2-9.6)	1.4 (0.0-4.1)	3.3 (0.4-6.2)
90 d	21.4 (11.8-31.0)	8.6 (3.2-14.2)	1.4 (0.0-4.1)	4.8 (1.3-8.2)
6 mo	22.9 (13.0-32.8)	9.9 (4.0-15.8)	5.7 (0.3-11.1)	9.3 (4.4-14.1)
1 yr	24.4 (14.3-34.5)	13.7 (6.6-21.0)	7.1 (1.1-13.2)	13.2 (7.5-18.9)
2 yr	29.3 (18.4-40.1)	16.8 (8.8-25.1)	11.6 (4.0-19.2)	20.6 (13.6-27.7)
5 y	40.2 (27.9-55.0)	31.7 (18.2-47.3)	24.8 (14.1-39.3)	33.2 (24.2-42.3)

Note: Thirty-day recurrence rates were significantly different among subtypes (log rank, $P < .0001$) but long-term recurrence rates were not (log rank, $P = .12$).

(Courtesy of Petty GW, Brown RD Jr, Whisnant JP, et al: Ischemic stroke subtypes: A population-based study of functional outcome, survival, and recurrence. *Stroke* 31:1062-1068, 2000. Reproduced with permission of *Stroke*, copyright 2000, American Heart Association.)

rologic Diseases and Stroke Data Bank. Seventy-four patients had large-vessel cervical or intracranial atherosclerosis with stenosis (ATH), 132 had cardioembolic (CE) stroke, 72 had lacunar (LAC) stroke, and 164 had infarct of uncertain cause (IUC). Functional outcomes were assessed by means of the Rankin disability score. Survival and recurrence rates were compared among groups, and predictive factors were identified.

Results.—Significant variation was observed in Rankin disability scores among the various types of stroke, with LAC patients having milder deficits initially and at follow-up. The overall mean follow-up was 3 years. Estimated 30-day recurrence rates was 18.5% in the ATH group, 5.3% in the CE group, 1.4% in the LAC group, and 3.3% in the IUC group. The adjusted risk ratio for recurrence within 30 days for ATH patients was 3.3, compared with CE patients. Infarct subtype was not a significant predictor of long-term recurrence rate (Table 2). Of the 25 recurrent strokes occurring within 30 days, 4 were procedure related, all in the ATH group.

The 5-year mortality rate was 32.2% in the ATH group, 80.4% in the CE group, 35.1% in the LAC group, and 48.6% in the IUC group. The adjusted risk ratio for long-term survival for ATH patients was 0.47, compared with CE patients. However, stroke subtype was not a significant predictor of 30-day survival rate.

Conclusions.—Outcomes vary significantly for patients with different subtypes of ischemic stroke. Those with ATH stroke have the highest rates of recurrence within 30 days, with some of these recurrences being iatrogenic. Functional outcomes are better for patients with LAC infarction than those with other types of stroke. Patients with CE stroke have the poorest survival rate.

▶ Did you know that strokes caused by atherosclerotic stenosis of large cervical or intracranial vessels are more likely to have recurrences than ischemic strokes of other causes, and that a significant number of these recurrences are in fact iatrogenic in origin? This and other information is all here in this Rochester, Minnesota, population-based study. It's worth reading in detail.

L. M. Taylor, Jr, MD

13 Grafts and Graft Complications

Infection

Value of Bone Scintiscan for Diagnosis of Arterial Prosthesis Infection: Preliminary Results

Lehalle B, Lercher MN, David N, et al (CHU de Nancy, France)
Ann Vasc Surg 14:484-489, 2000   13–1

Background.—Confirming the diagnosis of an arterial prosthetic infection is often difficult. Lower extremity hypertrophic osteoarthropathy (HOA) has been associated with arterial prosthetic infection in several articles. Bone and joint abnormalities may be early signs of HOA. Thus, the diagnostic value of routine bone scintiscans in patients hospitalized for suspected arterial prosthesis infections was investigated.

Methods.—Seventeen patients with suspected infections admitted to 1 center between 1995 and 1997 were included in this prospective study. Bone scintiscans were obtained before surgery in all patients. In addition, bone scinticans were obtained in a control group of 8 patients with arterial prostheses but no clinical or laboratory signs of infection.

Findings.—Scintiscan results were normal in the control group and in a subgroup of patients in whom surgical findings discounted an arterial prosthesis infection. Among the 13 patients with surgically confirmed arterial prosthesis infections, 8 had positive scintiscan findings, and 5 had negative findings. Scintiscan findings were positive in both patients with clinical signs of HOA. Scintiscan abnormalities typical of HOA were seen distal to the infected prosthesis. Among patients with abdominal arterial prostheses, abnormalities occurred on the femur and tibia of 1 or both lower extremities. The shaft of the femur was normal in all patients with infected above-knee femoropopliteal bypasses. The femur and the shaft of the proximal tibia were normal in patients with infected femorotibial bypasses (Fig 3).

Conclusions.—Detecting scintiscan abnormalities suggesting HOA distal to an arterial prosthesis is a valuable diagnostic sign in patients with suspected infections. Additional research is needed to determine the underlying cause of HOA, as well as the indications for a bone scintiscan.

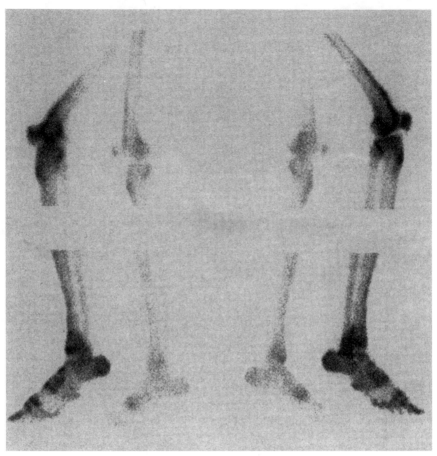

FIGURE 3.—Stationary scintiscans showing periostitis on the right lower extremity distal to an above-knee femoropopliteal bypass. (Courtesy of Lehalle B, Lercher MN, David N, et al: Value of bone scintiscan for diagnosis of arterial prosthesis infection: Preliminary results. *Ann Vasc Surg* 14:484-489, 2000.)

▶ The authors present a small comparative trial examining the use of bone scintiscan and the findings of secondary hypertrophic osteoarthropathy in limbs distal to a bypass graft in detecting prosthetic graft infection. With a total of 25 patients in the 2 groups, these are clearly only preliminary data. For what it's worth, a finding of hypertrophic osteoarthropathy (increased tracer uptake consistent with periosteal new bone or joint inflammation) was limited to cases with confirmed graft infection. Thus, in this study, a positive study result was clinically helpful, but a negative finding was not. Although this may be useful in selected cases of graft infection, I am skeptical.

M. R. Nehler, MD

Use of Cryopreserved Arterial Homografts for Management of Infected Prosthetic Grafts: A Multicentric Study

Verhelst R, Lacroix V, Vraux H, et al (Saint Luke's Univ Clinics, Brussels, Belgium; Univ Hosp Ctr, Liege, Belgium; Catholic Univ, Leuven, Belgium; et al)

Ann Vasc Surg 14:602-607, 2000   13–2

Objective.—The incidence of prosthetic graft infection after vascular surgery is 1% to 3%. The mortality rate is high in these patients. Because conventional surgical treatment followed by extra-anatomic bypass can lead to low patency, in situ reconstruction has been attempted. The experience of 6 European centers using cryopreserved arterial homografts (CAHs) for management of infected prosthetic grafts is presented.

Methods.—From October 1992 to July 1998, 90 patients (84 men), aged 25 to 78, received a CAH for prosthetic graft infection. The time to replacement after the primary procedure was less than 31 days in the early group (n = 15, 17%) and averaged 34 months in the late group (n = 75, 83%). The primary procedure was performed at a nonparticipating institution in 43 patients. The aorta was reconstructed in 66 patients (73%). The primary procedure was performed for aneurysm in 30 patients and for occlusive arterial disease in 60 patients. The infection was extra-abdominal in 49 patients and intra-abdominal in 41. Part of the graft that was not contaminated was left in place in 19 patients (21%). Bacterial cultures were positive in 75% of patients, and 42% had more than 1 microorganism. All homografts were obtained from the European Homograft Bank.

Results.—There were no intraoperative deaths, but 16 patients died within 1 month (Table 5). Patients having emergency surgery, profound infection, or enteroprosthetic fistulas (EPFs) had significantly higher mortality rates. Among the 74 patients followed for an average of 36 months, 14 died, 10 of causes unrelated to homograft implantation or infection. Seven patients experienced significant dilatation of the homograft. Fourteen (83%) of 17 patients with EPFs died. Five patients required surgical revision of homograft obstruction, and 1 required amputation.

Conclusion.—Patients with EPFs accounted for almost all the ruptures and most deaths. Fresh homografts have better resistance for unknown

TABLE 5.—Predictors of Early Mortality

	n	Mortality (%)	p
Emergency surgery	11/34	32	
Elective surgery	5/56	9	<0.05
Intraabdominal infection	13/64	20	
Extraabdominal infection	0/26	0	<0.03
Enteroprosthetic fistula	11/17	65	
No enteroprosthetic fistula	5/73	6.8	<0.01

reasons. Long-term complications included dilatation, stenosis, and thrombosis. CAH is a promising technique for managing infected prosthetic grafts.

▶ The treatment of patients with infected prosthetic vascular grafts continues to be a difficult problem. Most of the treatment options that exist have shortcomings. The authors report here their experience with CAH in 90 patients. One of the unique aspects of this report is that the grafts were supplied by the European Homograft Bank. In this series, tissue or blood compatibility was not a prerequisite in the use of these homographs. Ninety patients had implants; 16 died in the first 30 days, 40 patients had subsequent complications requiring reintervention, and 34 patients had no need for reintervention. The results reported in this series are quite respectable, and I believe that the use of this type of graft can play a role in the treatment of these very difficult patients. The authors point out that patients with EPFs had very poor results. They suggest that they may not use this material in the future in these patients. There was a high early mortality rate of 65% and a significant late mortality rate of 18%. In addition, a number of these grafts ruptured. Removal of the 17 patients with EPFs results in a significant improvement in the overall results. CAH for patients with infected prosthetic grafts needs to be added to the armamentarium of a vascular surgeon.

J. O. Menzoian, MD

Long-term Outcome After Treatment of Aortic Graft Infection With Staged Extra-anatomic Bypass Grafting and Aortic Graft Removal
Seeger JM, Pretus HA, Welborn MB, et al (Univ of Florida, Gainesville)
J Vasc Surg 32:451-461, 2000   13–3

Background.—The use of externally supported prosthetic grafts appears to improve the long-term patency of axillofemoral bypass grafts in the treatment of aortoiliac occlusive disease and for revascularization in the treatment of aortic sepsis. The initial and long-term outcomes of aortic graft infection treatment with staged extra-anatomic bypass grafting and aortic graft removal were analyzed.

Methods.—Thirty-six patients at 1 center underwent extra-anatomic bypass grafting and aortic graft removal for aortic graft infections between 1989 and 1999. The type of extra-anatomic bypass graft was axillofemoral femoral in 5 patients, axillofemoral in 26 (bilateral in 20), axillopopliteal in 3 (bilateral in 1), and axillofemoral/axillopopliteal in 2 (Table). The mean follow-up was 32.3 months.

Findings.—Four patients died in the postoperative period, which yielded a mortality rate of 11%. Two patients died during follow-up as a direct result of treatment. Another patient died 72 months after failure of a subsequent aortic reconstruction. Thus, the overall treatment-related mortality rate was 19%. The overall 5-year survival rate by life table analysis was 56%. None of the patients needed amputations in the postoperative

TABLE.—Configuration of Extra-anatomic Bypass Grafts Used for
Revascularization in Patients With Aortic Graft Infections

Axillofemoral femoral	5
Bilateral axillofemoral	20
Unilateral axillofemoral	6
Bilateral axillopopliteal	1
Unilateral axillopopliteal	2
Axillofemoral/axillopopliteal	2

(Courtesy of Seeger JM, Pretus HA, Welborn MB, et al: Long-term outcome after treatment of aortic graft infection with staged extra-anatomic bypass grafting and aortic graft removal. *J Vasc Surg* 32:451-461, 2000.)

period, although 4 required amputations during follow-up. In addition, 35% of the patients had extra-anatomic bypass graft failures during follow-up. Secondary aortic reconstructions were needed in 6 patients. However, when patients undergoing axillopopliteal grafting were excluded, only 7 (25%) had extra-anatomic bypass graft failures, and only 2 needed amputations. According to life table analysis, primary and secondary patency rates were 75% and 100%, respectively, at 41 months for axillofemoral femoral grafts and 64% and 100%, respectively, at 60 months for axillofemoral grafts (Fig 1).

Conclusions.—The initial and long-term results of staged extra-anatomic bypass grafting and aortic graft removal are acceptable in patients

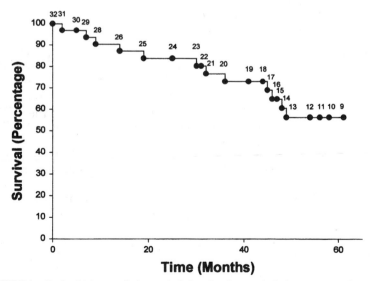

FIGURE 1.—Kaplan-Meier cumulative survival plot of patient survival after treatment of aortic graft infection. Survival SEs are less than 10% through 60 months. (Courtesy of Seeger JM, Pretus HA, Welborn MB, et al: Long-term outcome after treatment of aortic graft infection with staged extra-anatomic bypass grafting and aortic graft removal. *J Vasc Surg* 32:451-461, 2000.)

with aortic graft infections. Thus, this treatment should remain the primary approach in selected patients with this grave condition.

▶ There are numerous procedures that one can employ for treatment of an aortic graft infection. The gold standard has been staged extra-anatomic bypass grafting and aortic graft removal. Dr Seeger's group from Florida documents, in a moderately large series, that this procedure is safe and reasonably effective. The major problem with this approach, as shown in the present article, is a relatively high long-term failure rate associated with the extra-anatomic bypass. In our experience, if the extra-anatomic bypass has failed remotely from its placement and the infection is completely resolved, one can consider doing a secondary aortic reconstruction, either a supraceliac or thoracofemoral bypass.[1]

J. L. Mills, Sr, MD

Reference

1. 1993 YEAR BOOK OF VASCULAR SURGERY, pp 203-204.

Prosthetic Grafts

Tibial Bypass for Limb Salvage Using Polytetrafluoroethylene and a Distal Vein Patch

Neville RF, Tempesta B, Sidway AN (Georgetown Univ, Washington, DC; VA Med Ctr, Washington, DC)
J Vasc Surg 33:266-272, 2001   13–4

Objective.—Alternative conduits are available for tibial bypass grafting when the saphenous vein is not available. These include the lesser saphenous vein, arm vein, composite veins, composite vein with polytetrafluoroethylene (PTFE), and PTFE with or without a distal arteriovenous fistula. Unfortunately many prosthetic grafts to tibial arteries have failed, leading some to advocate primary amputation in certain patients. Others have used venous tissue at the distal anastomosis in the form of cuffs, collars, and boots to improve results. Long-term results of the use of PTFE grafts with a distal vein patch (DVP) in limb-threatened patients were reported.

Methods.—Between July 1993 and July 1999, 514 tibial artery bypass grafts were performed for limb salvage. Eighty (16%) bypass grafts were performed in 79 patients (39 men; average age, 67 years) with PTFE/DVP as the graft conduit (Fig 2). All patients underwent complete arteriography. Underlying diseases included diabetes in 42 (53%) patients, renal failure in 16 (20%), and Eagle's criteria perioperative cardiac risk in 48 (60%). All patients had limb-threatening ischemia, with rest pain in 39 (49%) and gangrene or nonhealing ulceration in 41 (51%). Lower extremity bypass grafting had failed in 47 (59%) patients, 21 (26%) had had previous coronary bypass grafting, 8 (10%) had unsuitable vein quality as a result of size of thrombosis, and 4 (5%) had had varicose vein stripping.

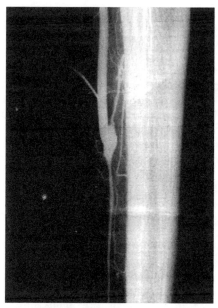

FIGURE 2.—Completion arteriogram after PTFE/DVP bypass graft to a posterior tibial artery. (Courtesy of Neville RF, Tempesta B, Sidway AN: Tibial bypass for limb salvage using polytetrafluoroethylene and a distal vein patch. *J Vasc Surg* 33:266-272, 2001.)

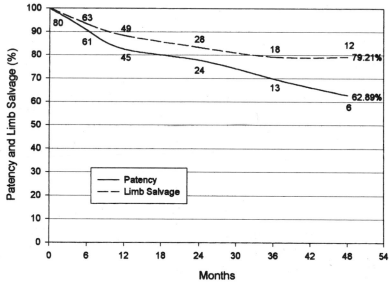

FIGURE 3.—Primary patency and limb salvage rates. Numbers on graph represent grafts at risk at beginning of specific time interval. (Courtesy of Neville RF, Tempesta B, Sidway AN: Tibial bypass for limb salvage using polytetrafluoroethylene and a distal vein patch. *J Vasc Surg* 33:266-272, 2001.)

Results.—Bypass grafts originated from the common femoral artery (50%), the external iliac artery (43%), and the superficial femoral artery (8%). Recipient arteries included the peroneal artery (44%), the posterior tibial artery (35%), and the anterior tibial artery (21%). Patients were followed up for from 30 days to 4 years. Life table analyses were performed on patency and limb salvage (Fig 3). Limb salvage and secondary patency were the same at all time points. After 48 months, there were 6 grafts at risk. Three failed, resulting in 3 amputations. There was 1 (1.25%) perioperative death, and there was a 24% mortality rate after 4 years. Seven grafts failed immediately, resulting in 5 amputations. A total of 17 grafts failed during the 48-month follow-up, resulting in 11 amputations.

Conclusion.—Tibial bypass grafting with PTFE/DVP should be considered for patients with limb-threatening ischemia but without a saphenous vein.

▶ Four-year limb patency with limb salvage results in a relatively small number of threatened limbs, comparable to contemporary but much larger series of arm-vein bypasses performed by Logerfo and associates.[1] Apparently Neville and colleagues no longer consider arm vein a suitable alternative conduit. In our own experience, arm vein, when available and of adequate caliber, is greatly preferable to tibial PTFE anastomosis, with or without interposition venous patches, hoods, or collars. Certainly, the simplicity of the venous patching technique described in this article makes it an attractive alternative when prosthetic conduit must be used, and the results presented suggest an outcome equivalent to more cumbersome collar and hood techniques in this limited single-center series. Compared with our experience with the modified Bard/Impra Distaflow prosthesis for tibial bypass grafting, the vein patch modification of standard externally supported 6 mm PTFE tibial bypass grafting is clearly preferable with regard to both clinical outcome and cost issues.

R. L. Dalman, MD

Reference

1. Faries PL, Logerfo FW, Arora S, et al: Arm vein conduit is superior to composite prosthetic-autogenous grafts in lower extremity revascularization. *J Vasc Surg* 31:1119-1127, 2000.

The Consequences of a Failed Femoropopliteal Bypass Grafting: Comparison of Saphenous Vein and PTFE Grafts
Jackson MR, Belott TP, Dickason T, et al (Univ of Texas, Dallas; William Beaumont Army Med Ctr, Ft Bliss, Tex)
J Vasc Surg 32:498-505, 2000   13–5

Objective.—The best patency rates after infrainguinal revascularization are obtained by means of the autologous saphenous vein (SV). Polytet-

TABLE 6.—Percentage of Graft Occlusion Resulting in Limb-Threatening
Ischemia (Grade II): Influence of Site of Distal Anastomosis

Graft	Distal Anastomosis	Grade II Ischemia
SV		
	Above-knee	11% (1/7)*
	Below-knee	30% (3/10)†
PTFE		
	Above-knee	79% (22/28)*
	Below-knee	78% (7/9)†

*P = .001.
†P = .029.
(Courtesy of Jackson MR, Belott TP, Dickason T, et al: The consequences of a failed femoropopliteal
bypass grafting: Comparison of saphenous vein and PTFE grafts. *J Vasc Surg* 32:498-505, 2000.)

rafluoroethylene (PTFE) grafts give acceptable patency rates. Little information is available on the ischemic consequences after occlusion of vein and PTFE grafts. The outcome of failed SV bypass grafts was compared retrospectively with that of PTFE femoropopliteal bypass grafts with a specific emphasis on the degree of ischemia caused by graft occlusion.

Methods.—Between 1991 and 1997, 189 femoropopliteal bypass grafts were performed using 108 SVs and 81 PTFE grafts. Acute limb ischemia was classified according to Society for Vascular Surgery/International Society for Cardiovascular Surgery (SVS/ISCVS) reporting standards as viable (I), threatened (II), or irreversible (III). Primary graft patency and limb salvage rates at 48 months were calculated by the Kaplan-Meier method. Differences between groups were analyzed by the log-rank test.

Results.—Patients were followed up for a mean of 20.2 months. All patients were smokers or had a history of smoking. More than 40% of both groups had diabetes. Indication for surgery was chronic critical ischemia in both the SV (82%) and PTFE (80%) groups. Significantly more SV than PTFE patients had distal anastomosis performed below the knee (60% vs 16%). Compared with SV patients, PTFE patients had a signifi-

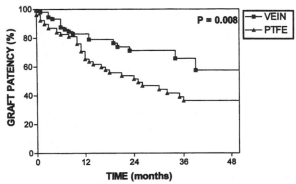

FIGURE 1.—Primary patency of vein and PTFE grafts. (Courtesy of Jackson MR, Belott TP, Dickason T, et al: The consequences of a failed femoropopliteal bypass grafting: Comparison of saphenous vein and PTFE grafts. *J Vasc Surg* 32:498-505, 2000.)

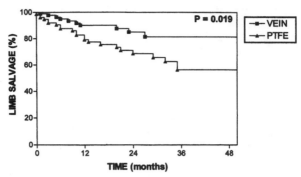

FIGURE 2.—Limb salvage with vein and PTFE grafts. (Courtesy of Jackson MR, Belott TP, Dickason T, et al: The consequences of a failed femoropopliteal bypass grafting: Comparison of saphenous vein and PTFE grafts. *J Vasc Surg* 32:498-505, 2000.)

cantly higher incidence of grade II ischemia (78% vs 21%), emergency revascularization (28% vs 3%), and major limb amputations (28% vs 10%), and a significantly lower incidence of primary patency at 48 months (58% vs 32%) and limb salvage at 48 months (81% vs 56%) (Table 6, Fig 1, and Fig 2).

Conclusion.—Patients receiving PTFE grafts for femoropopliteal bypass grafts are at higher risk for ischemic complications, including emergency limb revascularization and amputation.

▶ For years, many have had the clinical impression that a patient who has prosthetic graft material with subsequent occlusion presents with a severely ischemic limb more frequently than the patient who has undergone a saphenous vein bypass graft with subsequent graft occlusion. This well-written report seems to confirm this clinical prejudice. One of the very nice features of this article is the reporting of the run-off score in the various groups of patients. It seems clear that patients who underwent PTFE bypass grafts not only have less favorable patency but also, when the graft occluded, these patients were more likely to present with critical limb ischemia than patients with saphenous vein bypass grafts. A criticism of this article is that it is a retrospective review and thus is subject to differences in the groups of patients. An example of this is clearly pointed out in the variable sizes of PTFE grafts used in the patients. In spite of the retrospective nature of this article, I believe that the study provides more evidence against the routine use of PTFE bypass grafts for infrainguinal arterial reconstruction. In addition, a contemporary prospectively randomized study would include some of the newer adjuvant support methods of synthetic bypass grafts, such as anticoagulation and vein patch techniques.

J. O. Menzoian, MD

A Prospective Randomized Trial Comparing Vein With Polytetrafluoro-ethylene in Above-Knee Femoropopliteal Bypass Grafting

Burger DHC, Kappetein AP, van Bockel JH, et al (Leiden Univ, The Netherlands; Rode Kruis Ziekenhuis, The Hague, The Netherlands)

J Vasc Surg 32:278-283, 2000   13–6

Background.—For patients undergoing femoropopliteal reconstruction proximal to the knee, the relative advantages of the use of vein versus polytetrafluoroethylene (PTFE) are unclear. Good early results have been achieved with the use of thin-walled, stretched PTFE for suprageniculate bypass grafts. A randomized trial of PTFE versus reversed saphenous vein for above-knee arterial reconstruction is reported.

Methods.—The 3-year trial included a total of 151 above-knee femoropopliteal bypass graft procedures in 136 patients. One hundred twenty reconstructions were done for severe claudication, 20 for rest pain, and 11 for ulceration. Reversed saphenous veins were used in 75 procedures, and PTFE was used in 76. Risk factors included diabetes in 24% of cases, history of myocardial infarction in 23%, and current smoking in 74%. In-hospital mortality was nil, although there was a 5% rate of minor complications. The 2 groups were analyzed for differences in cumulative patency rates at 2 years' follow-up.

Results.—The 2-year primary patency rate was 83% for saphenous vein grafts versus 67% for PTFE grafts (Fig 1); secondary patency rates were 83% and 77%, respectively. These differences were nonsignificant, and no risk factors for occlusion were identified in either group.

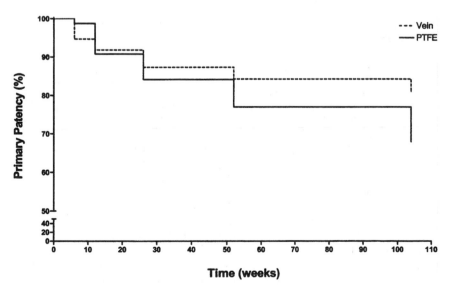

FIGURE 1.—Primary patency over time. *Abbreviation: PTFE,* Polytetrafluoroethylene. (Courtesy of Burger DHC, Kappetein AP, van Bockel JH, et al: A prospective randomized trial comparing vein with polytetrafluoroethylene in above-knee femoropopliteal bypass grafting. *J Vasc Surg* 32:278-283, 2000.)

Conclusions.—This short-term follow-up study shows equivalent performance with either saphenous veins or PTFE for above-knee femoropopliteal bypass grafting. The results suggest that PTFE is an acceptable alternative graft material. Other differences between the 2 materials may become apparent at a planned 5-year follow-up.

▶ Despite the authors' attempt to perform a randomized prospective trial, there are many faults with this study. First and foremost, the authors did not perform graft surveillance for their vein bypasses. Life tables show that the majority of veins occluded in the first 2 years because of initimal hyperplasia. Modern comparison should be between assisted primary patency of vein versus primary or secondary patency of PTFE. I suspect that, if the authors had performed graft surveillance for their veins, the majority of their early occlusions would have been prevented and the assisted primary patency would have been well above 83%. Nevertheless, primary patency of vein continues to be superior to that of PTFE. I will take a *P* value equal to .065 at 2 years as "quasi" significant. Also exemplified in this article was the fact that none of the patients needed vein for coronary bypass procedures, and only 3 veins were used after 31 occluded bypass grafts. Why not give the patient the best operation, that being a vein to limit the problems with thrombosis and overall substandard patency rates? It continues to amaze me that many vascular surgeons cling to PTFE for above-the-knee bypass grafting when, clearly, the data continue to show that it is substandard. I look forward to the 5-year results of this study.

R. B. McLafferty, MD

Interposition Vein Cuff Anastomosis Alters Wall Shear Stress Distribution in the Recipient Artery
How TV, Rowe CS, Gilling-Smith GL, et al (Univ of Liverpool, England)
J Vasc Surg 31:1008-1017, 2000   13–7

Background.—The patency rates of prosthetic infrainguinal bypass grafts can be improved by interposing a vein cuff between the graft and the recipient infrageniculate artery. This may result from redistribution of myointimal hyperplasia (MIH) away from critical heel and toe areas of the anastomosis. Low wall shear stress (WSS) is believed to play a key role in the development of MIH. The effects of an interposition vein cuff (IVC) on the magnitude and distribution of WSS, and thus on the redistribution of MIH were analyzed.

Methods.—The investigators created life-size models of conventional end-to-side (ETS) and IVC anastomoses. Using laser Doppler flow anemometry, they made detailed measurements of flow velocity in both models under conditions of pulsatile flow. Near-wall velocity measurements on the arterial floor and upper wall were used to estimate variation in WSS.

Findings.—The ETS anastomosis was associated with separation of flow at the graft hood, along with strong radial velocity at the heel and a stagnation point on the arterial floor, which moved slightly during the flow cycle. In contrast, the IVC anastomosis showed a coherent vortex occupying most of the cuff volume, from the systolic deceleration phase to end-diastole (Fig 4). A stagnation point was observed on the floor of the IVC anastomosis that oscillated by approximately 4 mm. Critical regions of low mean WSS were noted at the heel and floor of the ETS anastomosis.

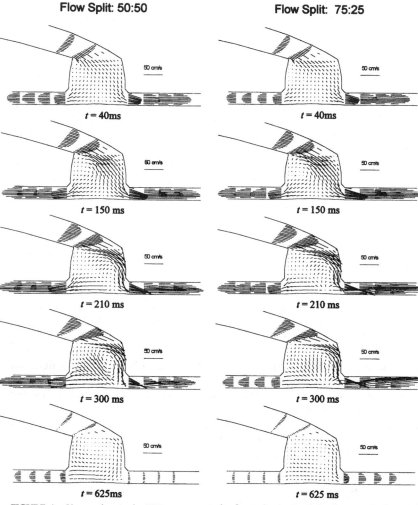

FIGURE 4.—Vector plots in the IVC anastomosis for flow splits (ratio of distal to proximal arterial outflow) of 50:50 and 75:25 at various times during the flow cycle. *Abbreviation: IVC*, Interposition vein cuff. (Courtesy of How TV, Rowe CS, Gilling-Smith GL, et al: Interposition vein cuff anastomosis alters wall shear stress distribution in the recipient artery. *J Vasc Surg* 31:1008-1017, 2000.)

The IVC anastomosis showed such critical regions only on the floor and of lesser magnitude.

Conclusions.—In prosthetic infrainguinal bypass grafting, an IVC anastomosis alters the mean distribution of WSS within the recipient artery. In IVC anastomoses, low mean WSS is limited to the floor of the anastomosis, removing an area of low WSS at the heel. These findings may account for the redistribution of MIH observed with IVC anastomoses.

▶ This interesting article represents the preliminary work by Peter Harris and his group, which led to the development of the Bard/Impra Distaflow bypass graft, which is now commercially available. Whether or not one understands wall shear stress (WSS), this work suggests that variance of anastomotic architecture can influence hemodynamic circumstances so that myointimal hyperplasia distribution may be altered. This group believes that mechanical forces, such as the anastomotic shape of the interposition vein cuff, alter specifically the magnitude and distribution of WSS, and that these forces explain the redistribution of myointimal hyperplasia in prosthetic bypass grafts that use a vein cuff anastomosis to a recipient artery. The Bard/Impra Distaflow bypass graft has a distal cuff of prosthetic material, which mimics the idealized shape of a distal anastomosis based on this work. Others believe that the protective effect of a vein-cuffed anastomosis is humoral and related to factors elaborated by the venous endothelium.[1] It is clear that adjunctive distal vein patches or vein cuffs will improve primary and secondary patencies of PTFE bypass grafts to infrageniculate targets. It remains to be determined whether a prosthetic distal cuff will enjoy similar success for distal bypass procedures.

E. J. Harris, Jr, MD

Reference

1. Norberto JJ, Sidawy AN, Trad KS, et al: The protective effect of vein cuffed anastomoses is not mechanical in origin. *J Vasc Surg* 21:558-566, 1995.

A Comparative Evaluation of Polytetrafluoroethylene, Umbilical Vein, and Saphenous Vein Bypass Grafts for Femoral-Popliteal Above-Knee Revascularization: A Prospective Randomized Department of Veterans Affairs Cooperative Study
Johnson WC, and Members of the Department of Veterans Affairs COOP Study 141 (Boston Veteran Affairs Med Ctr; et al)
J Vasc Surg 32:268-277, 2000   13–8

Background.—For a femoral-popliteal above-knee arterial bypass graft, the choice is currently left to the surgeon's preference because of inconclusive information regarding comparative evaluations of different graft materials. The Department of Veterans Affairs Cooperative Study 141 was designed to determine whether patency is improved with different bypass graft materials in patients who undergo femoral-popliteal above-knee bypass grafts.

Methods.—From June 1983 to June 1988, 752 patients at 20 Veterans Affairs medical centers throughout the United States were randomly assigned to receipt of externally supported polytetrafluoroethylene (PTFE) graft (265 patients), human umbilical vein (HUV) graft (261 patients), or saphenous vein (226 patients). Limb salvage was the indication for bypass grafting in 67.5% of the patients. Follow-up evaluation of the patients was performed every 3 months for the first year and every 6 months thereafter. All patients were told to take aspirin for the duration of the study. Doppler-derived ankle-brachial index (ABI) was determined preoperatively and postoperatively. A graft was considered patent if the postoperative Doppler-derived ABI was significantly improved (more than 0.15 units higher than the preoperative value) and additional data, such as angiographic data or operations, did not contradict the Doppler-derived ABI data. Bypass grafts that were removed because of infection or aneurysmal degeneration were also considered patency failures. The Kaplan-Meier life table analysis was used to determine patency rates.

Results.—A statistical similarity was found in the cumulative assisted primary patency rates among the different conduit types at 2 years (Fig 1). However, after 5 years the above-knee saphenous vein graft had a signifi-

FEMORAL-POPLITEAL
ABOVE KNEE BYPASSES

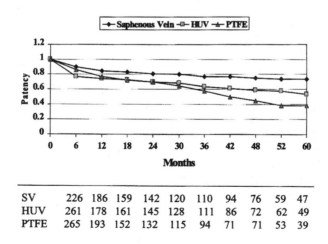

SV	226	186	159	142	120	110	94	76	59	47
HUV	261	178	161	145	128	111	86	72	62	49
PTFE	265	193	152	132	115	94	71	71	53	39

patients

FIGURE 1.—Life table analysis for the patency of saphenous vein (*V*), human umbilical vein (*H*), and PTFE (*P*). N represents the number of bypass grafts being observed for patency at that time. (Courtesy of Johnson WC, and Members of the Department of Veterans Affairs COOP Study 141: A comparative evaluation of polytetrafluoroethylene, umbilical vein, and saphenous vein bypass grafts for femoral-popliteal above-knee revascularization: A prospective randomized Department of Veterans Affairs cooperative study. *J Vasc Surg* 32:268-277, 2000.)

cantly better patency rate (73%) than HUV grafts (53%) and PTFE grafts (39%). The rate of limb salvage was slightly worse with PTFE grafts than with the other 2 types of conduits. Patients who received the HUV graft had the highest number of bypass graft thromboses and major amputations within the first 30 days.

Conclusions.—Overall, these results suggest that the saphenous vein bypass graft should be considered the bypass graft of choice for patients undergoing femoral-popliteal above-knee reconstruction. When a prosthetic bypass graft is used, the HUV graft should be considered as an alternative to the PTFE graft.

▶ Not surprisingly, saphenous vein proved to have the best 5-year assisted-primary patency (73% vs HUV 53%, PTFE 39%). Despite a higher early failure rate, HUV still had better long-term patency than PTFE. Very few aneurysms were detected in the HUV group, a finding that probably reflects the lack of duplex follow-up. HUV was compared with 6-mm PTFE, but perhaps 8-mm PTFE would have fared better. HUV continues to be an interesting choice of prosthetic. When a prosthetic is used in the above-knee position, HUV may offer some advantage over PTFE, but, on the whole, the choice of HUV versus PTFE remains more personal than scientific. Why did it take 9 years to publish this study, which was completed in 1991?

A. M. Abou-Zamzam Jr, MD

Heparin-Bonded Dacron or Polytetrafluoroethylene for Femoropopliteal Bypass Grafting: A Multicenter Trial
McCollum C, for the North West Femoro-Popliteal Trial Participants (South Manchester Univ, England)
J Vasc Surg 33:533-539, 2001   13–9

Objective.—Because of the relatively high failure rate of femoropopliteal reconstructions, any improvement in graft materials is desirable. The patency, and factors leading to graft occlusion, of collagen-coated heparin-bonded Dacron (HBD) were compared with those of polytetrafluoroethylene (PTFE).

Methods.—Patients, aged 32.9 to 86 years, having femoropopliteal bypass grafting (180 above the knee [AK] and 29 below the knee [BK]) were randomly allocated to receive HBD (n = 106) or PTFE (n = 103). Indications for surgery were claudication (31.3% and 35.9%) or critical ischemia (68.9% and 64.1%). Patients received aspirin before and after surgery as long as they could tolerate it. Kaplan-Meier life-table analysis and the log-rank test were used to compare the difference in patency between the 2 groups.

Results.—Patients were studied for an average of 42 months. There were 2 postoperative deaths and 38 deaths during follow-up. Fifteen patients died with patent grafts (11 HBD and 4 PTFE). Morbidity, mortality, and graft survival were similar for the 2 groups. A total of 106 grafts (46 HBD

FIGURE 1

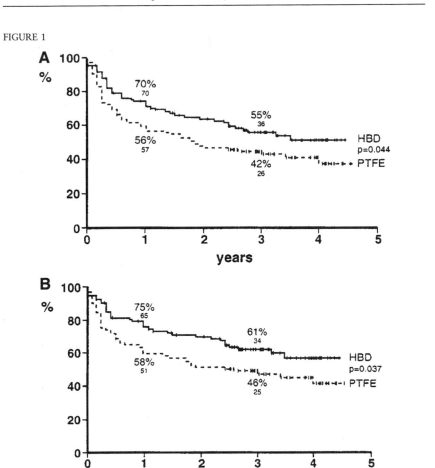

(Continued)

and 60 PTFE) occluded, 75 of them (71%) during the first 12 months. Patencies at 1, 2, and 3 years for AK grafts were higher for HBD than for PTFE grafts (Fig 1). The results for BK grafts were equally poor for both materials. At 3 years, there were 106 occlusions, with 29 patients treated conservatively, 20 with graft replacement, 9 with amputation, and 48 with 67 secondary procedures. Of the latter group, only 3 patients obtained long-term patency. Secondary patency rates were 74%, 64%, and 56% for HBD and 60%, 49%, and 45% for PTFE. Arterial disease risk factors had no influence on patency. There were a total of 23 amputations, 16 AK (5 HBD and 11 PTFE) and 7 BK (1 HBD and 6 PTFE).

FIGURE 1 (cont.)

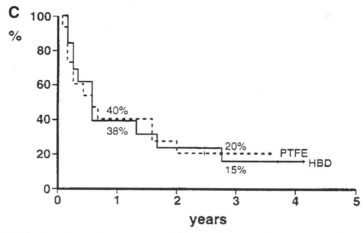

FIGURE 1.—Cumulative primary patency with life table is compared between HBD and PTFE. **A,** All 209 randomized grafts; **B,** 180 grafts to AK popliteal artery; and **C,** 29 grafts for BK popliteal artery. Larger percentage numbers refer to cumulative patency at 1 and 3 years; smaller numbers are the number of patent grafts still being followed at these times. (Courtesy of McCollum C, for the North West Femoro-Popliteal Trial Participants: Heparin-bonded Dacron or polytetrafluoroethylene for femoropopliteal bypass grafting: A multicenter trial. *J Vasc Surg* 33:533-539, 2001.)

Conclusion.—Compared with HBD graft, PTFE grafts have lower patency rates and increase the risk of amputation, possibly via distal embolization.

▶ This is one of those articles that make you go "Hmmm." Even if you concede the authors their conclusion that HBD is superior to PTFE, the fact of the matter is that neither outperforms autogenous conduit. Saying that Dacron is better than PTFE is like saying that poultices are better than incantations. Since neither of them works, who cares?

G. J. Landry, MD

Vein Grafts

Arm Vein Conduit Is Superior to Composite Prosthetic-Autogenous Grafts in Lower Extremity Revascularization

Faries PL, LoGerfo FW, Arora S, et al (Harvard Med School, Boston)
J Vasc Surg 31:1119-1127, 2000   13–10

Introduction.—Several alternative conduits have been used for lower-extremity revascularization when an adequate ipsilateral greater saphenous vein is not available. The effectiveness of all-autogenous multisegment arm vein bypass grafts was compared with that of composite grafts made up of combined prosthetic and autogenous conduits.

Methods.—The study included 153 lower-extremity revascularization procedures performed between 1990 and 1998 that were followed up

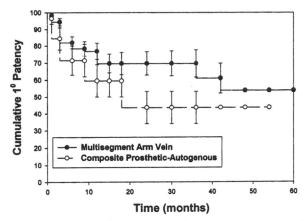

Time (months)

FIGURE 1.—Life-table analysis of the variation in primary patency rates categorized by type of conduit. Multisegment arm vein grafts (*solid line/solid circles*) demonstrate significantly higher patency rates at all time points after 30 days compared with composite grafts (*dashed line/open circles*). (Courtesy of Faires PL, LoGerfo FW, Arora S, et al: Arm vein conduit is superior to composite prosthetic-autogenous grafts in lower extremity revascularization. *J Vasc Surg* 31:1119-1127, 2000.)

prospectively via a computerized vascular registry. The grafts were made up of spliced arm vein segments with venovenostomy in 122 patients and of composite prosthetic-autogenous conduit in 31 patients. Arm vein conduit was prepared using intraoperative angioscopy for valve lysis and identification of luminal abnormalities in 47.7% of patients.

Results.—Bypass graft configurations were as follows: femoropopliteal (12 arm vein, 2 composite); femorotibial (75 arm vein, 23 composite); femoropedal (14 arm vein, 6 composite), and popliteo-tibial/pedal (21 arm vein, 0 composite). Indications for arm surgery were limb salvage and disabling claudication in 98% and 2% of patients, respectively. The mean follow-up was 25.1 months (range, 1 month to 7.9 years). The overall survival was 51% at 4 years after surgery. The overall mean patency and limb salvage rates were as follows (all values given are significant): primary patency for arm vein 1 year, 76.9%; composite, 59.5%; at 3 years, 70.0%; composite, 43.7%; and at 5 years, 53.8%; composite, 0%. Secondary patency for arm vein at 1 year, 77.5%; composite, 59.8%; at 3 years, 70.7%; composite, 44.9%; at 5 years, 57.7%, composite 0%. Limb salvage for arm vein at 1 year, 89.3%; composite, 73.9%; at 3 years, 80.5%; composite, 49.6%; and at 5 years, 76.3%; composite, 0% (Fig 1).

Conclusion.—Multisegment autogenous arm vein was used successfully in several lower-extremity revascularization procedures. Good long-term patency and limb salvage rates were observed that were well in excess of those observed with composite prosthetic-autogenous grafts. The superior durability of arm vein makes it the alternative conduit of choice when an adequate greater saphenous vein is not available.

▶ In case you need convincing, this study shows conclusively that autogenous conduits (even when splicing of multiple segments is required) are a superior alternative to combined autogenous/prosthetic grafts. Indeed, there seems no rational reason to ever create a composite conduit. If you must use prosthetic, you might as well use it for the entire conduit.

L. M. Taylor, Jr, MD

Preimplant Vein Intimal Thickness Is Not a Predictor of Bypass Graft Stenosis

James DC, Durrani T, Wixon CL, et al (Univ of Arizona, Tucson)
J Surg Res 96:1-5, 2001   13–11

Background.—Preimplant vein morphology is reportedly a risk factor for subsequent vein graft failure. Whether microscopic intimal thickening in random saphenous vein biopsy specimens is correlated with an increased risk of graft failure has not been determined. The incidence of preexisting intimal thickening in a macroscopically normal, preimplant vein was investigated.

Methods.—Samples of preimplant veins were obtained at primary leg bypass in 14 patients needing revision for severe graft stenosis or graft occlusion. Results of the analysis were compared with those of 13 preimplant vein specimens from patients with patent, stenosis-free grafts. The 2 groups were identical in preoperative risk factors.

Findings.—Overall, nearly half the specimens had marked intimal thickening. The mean preimplant intimal thickness was 0.108 mm in the stenosis group and 0.100 mm in the control group (Table 3).

Conclusion.—Grossly normal preimplant veins often contain prominent microscopic intimal thickening. However, preimplant vein intimal thickness determined from a random saphenous vein biopsy at primary leg bypass does not predict subsequent development of vein graft stenosis.

TABLE 3.—Intimal Thickness

	Stenosis Group	Control Group	P value
Mean thickness	0.108 ± 0.155 mm	0.100 ± 0.064 mm	NS ($P = 0.866$)
Range	0.003 – 0.609 mm	0.011 – 0.222 mm	
Observer correlation	0.989	0.900	
Marked thickening (>0.08 mm)	42.9% (6/14)	53.8% (7/13)	

(Courtesy of James DC, Durrani T, Wixon CL, et al: Preimplant vein intimal thickness is not a predictor of bypass graft stenosis. *J Surg Res* 96:1-5, 2001.)

A Comparative Study of Alternative Conduits for Lower Extremity Revascularization: All-Autogenous Conduit Versus Prosthetic Grafts

Faries PL, LoGerfo FW, Arora S, et al (Mount Sinai School of Medicine, New York; Harvard Med School, Boston)
J Vasc Surg 32:1080-1090, 2000   13–12

Objective.—Infrainguinal revascularization in patients without a useable greater saphenous vein presents a problem because the effectiveness of below-knee prosthetic grafts is inferior to autogenous conduits. Various modifications have been attempted to try to improve graft patency. The effects of autogenous arm vein grafts on the outcome of infrainguinal arterial reconstructive procedures were retrospectively compared with prosthetic conduits composed of polytetrafluoroethylene or knitted polyester.

Methods.—Between January 1991 and November 1999, 3128 consecutive infrainguinal arterial reconstructions were performed, including 740 lower extremity procedures. Bypass grafts included 126 femoro-above-knee-popliteal (26 arm vein, 100 prosthetic), 67 femoro-below-knee-popliteal (38 arm vein, 29 prosthetic), 229 femorotibial (174 arm vein, 55 prosthetic), 25 femoropedal (23 arm vein, 2 prosthetic), 102 popliteotibial/pedal (101 arm vein, 1 prosthetic); and 191 extension "jump" grafts (144 arm vein, 47 prosthetic) grafts. Most revascularization procedures were performed for limb salvage, and 2% of arm vein procedures and

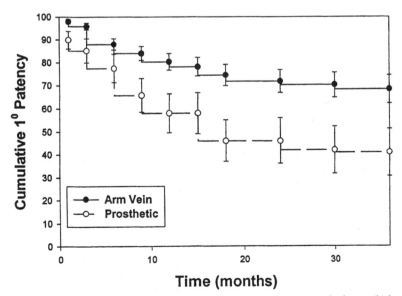

Time (months)

FIGURE 1.—Life table analysis of variation in cumulative primary patency rates for femorotibial grafts categorized by type of conduit. Arm vein grafts (*solid line/solid circle*) demonstrated significantly higher patency rates at all time points compared with prosthetic grafts (*dashed line/open circle*). (Courtesy of Faries PL, LoGerfo FW, Arora S, et al: A comparative study of alternative conduits for lower extremity revascularization: All-autogenous conduit versus prosthetic grafts. *J Vasc Surg* 32:1080-1090, 2000.)

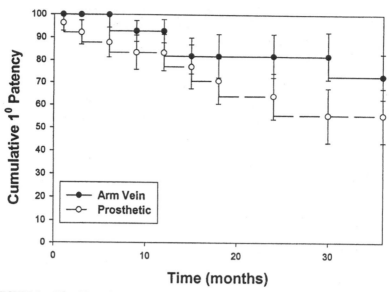

FIGURE 2.—Life table analysis of variation in cumulative primary patency rates for femoro-below-knee grafts categorized by type of conduit. Arm vein grafts (*solid line/solid circle*) achieved significantly higher patency rates compared with prosthetic grafts (*dashed line/open circle*). (Courtesy of Faries PL, LoGerfo FW, Arora S, et al: A comparative study of alternative conduits for lower extremity revascularization: All-autogenous conduit versus prosthetic grafts. *J Vasc Surg* 32:1080-1090, 2000.)

10.3% of prosthetic procedures were performed for disabling claudication. Patients were followed up every 3 months for the first year and every 6 months thereafter. Patency, limb salvage, and survival rates were tracked with life table analysis.

Results.—Respective arm vein and prosthetic perioperative systemic morbidities were 3.6% and 3.8%, perioperative local complication rates were 5.6% and 6.3%, and mortality rates were 1.4% and 1.2%. The morbidity rate from arm vein harvest was 1.8%. Patency and limb salvage rates were higher for arm vein conduits than for prosthetic conduits in the femorotibial and femoro-below-knee-popliteal configurations (Fig 1, Fig 2, and Fig 3A).

Conclusion.—Arm vein grafts are clinically superior to prosthetic grafts when extended below the knee.

▶ This nonrandomized study concludes that autogenous arm vein grafts provide better patency and limb salvage than prosthetic grafts in lower extremity revascularization procedures. Given the expertise of the Beth Israel Deaconess group in autogenous bypass grafting, this result is not unexpected. We continue also to believe that autogenous bypass grafting is to be preferred under almost all circumstances. For surgeons with appropriate interest and technical skills, there is no doubt that veins work better than prosthetic material. However, as the authors point out, prosthetic grafting to even infrageniculate vessels is a reasonable alternative when no autogenous

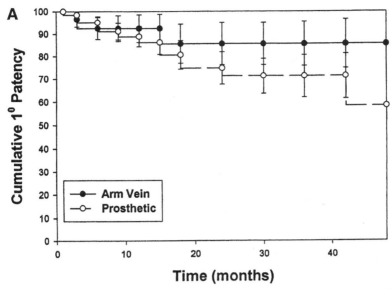

FIGURE 3.—A, Life table analysis of variation in cumulative primary patency rates for femoro-above-knee grafts categorized by type of conduit. Although arm vein grafts (*solid line/solid circle*) demonstrated a trend toward increased patency over prosthetic grafts (*dashed line/open circle*), this trend did not achieve statistical significance. (Courtesy of Faries PL, LoGerfo FW, Arora S, et al: A comparative study of alternative conduits for lower extremity revascularization: All-autogenous conduit versus prosthetic grafts. *J Vasc Surg* 32:1080-1090, 2000.)

conduit is available. What constitutes "available" is, of course, in the eye of the beholder. If one pursues a policy of using all available arm veins, including lesser saphenous veins, and exhibits a willingness to perform veno-venostomies, prosthetic grafts should be necessary in fewer than 10% of infrainguinal revascularizations.

G. L. Moneta, MD

Cellular Repopulation of Human Vein Allograft Bypass Grafts
Johnson TR, Tomaszewski JE, Carpenter JP (Univ of Pennsylvania, Philadelphia)
J Vasc Surg 31:994-1002, 2000   13–13

Background.—Autogenous vein grafts are the universally accepted conduits of choice for bypass grafts in the lower extremities; however, these veins are often unavailable either because they have been used in a prior graft or because they were removed by stripping, creating the need for an alternative. Synthetic materials have been used, but the results have been disappointing. Allograft and xenograft veins would be attractive substitutes because they are readily accessible and have the advantage of a human endothelium–lined biological conduit. A strong cell-mediated immune response to venous allografts in humans was demonstrated in an earlier report.

Because endothelial cells have been shown to play several essential roles in the survival of the vessel, the capacity for development of a neoendothelium is a potential advantage of allografts over other nonautogenous grafts. Repopulation by endothelial cells, which has not previously been demonstrated in humans, was investigated.

Methods.—In a prospective trial, 40 patients (20 men and 20 women) underwent bypass procedures for limb salvage by cryopreserved saphenous vein. All of the grafts were sampled at implantation. The follow-up interval was 31 months, during which time 22 allografts were explanted at the time of revision or subsequent surgical procedure. Intact endothelium was found at implantation and explantation in all 22 allografts. Histologic and immnofluorescent analyses were performed on 17 biopsy samples from 16 patients. The explant samples were stained with hematoxylin-eosin and immunohistochemical markers to enable quantitation of rejection. The samples were also subjected to fluorescence in situ hybridization, with probes for X and Y chromosomes and counterstaining for nuclear envelope. Cells were counted as XX, XY, XO, YO, or unstained. The analysis of the endothelium and vessel walls for origin of cells was based on sex-mismatched transplants, with sex-matched transplants used as controls.

Results.—All of the explanted allografts showed evidence of cellular damage, with moderate or severe rejection noted in 6 explanted samples (29%). Intact complete or partial endothelium was found in all of the allografts at implantation and explantation. As expected, sex-matched (male-male) control explants demonstrated only male cells, while male donor–female recipient transplants demonstrated complete repopulation with recipient (female) cells in 9 of 10 patients (90%). One patient had partial repopulation with a mosaic of male and female cells. Slides were unreadable for 1 patient. These findings in cells of the allograft were identical to findings in cells of the endothelium. Complete absence of donor cells was noted as soon as 1 week after implantation, although in 1 patient, mosaicism was demonstrated 3 months after the grafting. No relationship was observed between repopulation and time, quantity of rejection, or age of the donor.

Conclusion.—Both the endothelial lining and the vessel wall of venous allografts are repopulated with recipient cells, which results in either a completely new cellular composition or a mosaic of host and donor cells. However, the loss of donor cells may be mediated by rejection or apoptosis, and at present the rate of migration of repopulating host cells is unknown. Further investigation of the functional status of the neoendothelium and repopulated vessel wall is needed, as well as their role in maintaining the patency of the allograft.

▶ Enthusiasm for cyropreserved conduits continues. While this article provides some promising evidence for host endothelial repopulation, I am concerned that nearly 60% of the patients had explantation of all or part of their grafts at just over 2 years. More investigation is required before widespread use of cyropreserved grafts is indicated.

W. K. Williamson, MD

The Natural History of Intermediate and Critical Vein Graft Stenosis: Recommendations for Continued Surveillance or Repair
Mills JL Sr, Wixon CL, James DC, et al (Univ of Arizona, Tucson)
J Vasc Surg 33:273-280, 2001   13–14

Background.—There is debate as to the role of duplex US surveillance (DUS) in patients with autogenous lower extremity bypass grafts, particularly as to the criteria necessitating graft revision. Arteriography with selective repair has been recommended for grafts with intermediate stenosis, with revision for grafts with critical stenosis. The natural history of unrepaired vein graft stenoses was evaluated, including the risk of graft occlusion.

Methods.—The study included follow-up data on a total of 156 autogenous infrainguinal vein grafts in 142 patients. Based on the initial lesion detected by DUS, the grafts were classified as normal (a peak systolic velocity of less than 200 cm/s and a velocity ratio [V_r] of less than 2); intermediate stenosis (a PSV between 200 and 300 cm/s and a V_r of 2 to 4); or critical stenosis (a PSV of greater than 300 cm/s and V_r of greater than 4). The authors' department performed repair in grafts with critical

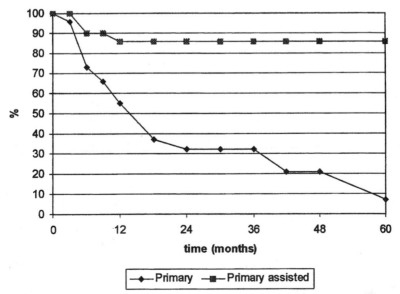

FIGURE 2.—Life-table and assisted-primary patency for 32 grafts in which intermediate stenosis was detected. SE measurements are less than 10% out to 24 months. (Courtesy of Mills JL Sr, Wixon CL, James DC, et al: The natural history of intermediate and critical vein graft stenosis: Recommendations for continued surveillance or repair. *J Vasc Surg* 33:273-280, 2001.)

lesions while monitoring all others. The 3 groups were compared for their risks of progressive stenosis, graft revision, and graft thrombosis.

Results.—Sixty-four percent of grafts had normal findings on serial DUS. At a mean follow-up of 27.5 months, the normal group had a 3% incidence of graft thrombosis. In 20% of grafts, intermediate lesions developed, indicating follow-up. At a mean follow-up of 26 months, 63% of these grafts progressed to critical stenosis requiring revision while 32% resolved or stabilized. For grafts with intermediate lesions, the incidence of graft occlusion was only 1.5%/y (Fig 2). Of 25 grafts with critical stenosis, 16 remained patent after successful repair. The remaining 9 grafts with critical stenosis remained unrepaired; 78% became occluded, all within 4 months after the DUS-detected index lesion.

Conclusion.—The findings support a policy of serial DUS for autogenous infrainguinal vein grafts with intermediate stenoses. The occlusion rate for these patients is similar to that of grafts without stenosis; unless they progress from intermediate to critical stenosis, arteriography is not required. When critical stenosis is present, the short-term risk of occlusion is very high, indicating the need for graft revision.

▶ The Arizona group has made great strides in stratifying the risk of graft occlusion based on duplex surveillance findings. Everyone agrees that no revisions should be performed if no lesion is present and that revisions should be performed in the face of critical stenoses. This article focuses on the intermediate group, with a focal PSV of 200 to 300 cm/sec, or a pre-stenotic to intrastenotic velocity ratio of 2:4. It appears that these lesions can be safely watched, with only 1.5% progressing to occlusion. However, most of these lesions (63%) will ultimately progress to critical lesions and require revision.

In Oregon, we have been very aggressive about vein graft revision. It has been our philosophy to return all stray sheep to the flock. In younger patients who are good surgical risks, we will likely continue to recommend repair of intermediate lesions. However, in the higher-risk patient groups, we will feel more comfortable following intermediate lesions based on the data from this article.

G. J. Landry, MD

Long-term Effects on Clinical Outcomes of Aggressive Lowering of Low-Density Lipoprotein Cholesterol Levels and Low-Dose Anticoagulation in the Post Coronary Artery Bypass Graft Trial

Knatterud GL, and Post CABG Investigators (Maryland Med Research Inst, Baltimore; NHLBI, Bethesda, Md; Montreal Heart Inst; et al)
Circulation 102:157-165, 2000   13–15

Background.—The multicenter Post Coronary Artery Bypass Graft (Post CABG) Trial found that patients who followed an aggressive lipid-reducing regimen—lowering low-density lipoprotein cholesterol (LDL-C)

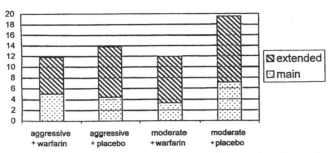

FIGURE 1.—Percent dead by treatment group. Percent dead during trial are shown at *bottom of each bar (stippled)*, and percent dead during period of extended follow-up at *top of each bar (hatched)*. (Courtesy of Knatterud GL, and Post CABG Investigators: Long-term effects on clinical outcomes of aggressive lowering of low-density lipoprotein cholesterol levels and low-dose anticoagulation in the Post Coronary Artery Bypass Trial. *Circulation* 102:157-165, 2000.)

to less than 100 mg/dL, compared with 132 to 136 mg/dL with moderate regimens—limited atherosclerotic progression in saphenous vein grafts. Low-dose anticoagulation had no effect on progression. A follow-up study was performed to assess the long-term outcomes of the various treatment strategies.

Methods.—The analysis included a total of 1351 patients from the Post CABG Trial. It included an additional 3 years of follow-up, in addition to the average 4-year follow-up in the main study. Cardiovascular events and procedures were assessed by telephone interview, and vital status from the National Death Index.

Results.—Aggressive lipid-lowering treatment reduced the long-term risk of revascularization by 30%, compared with moderate lipid reduction. Aggressive lipid reduction was also associated with a 24% reduction in a composite clinical end point. However, the 2 lipid strategies were not significantly different in terms of death during the trial or during extended follow-up. Low-dose anticoagulation reduced mortality by 35% and reduced the risk of mortality or myocardial infarction by 31% compared with placebo (Fig 1).

Conclusions.—Extended follow-up confirms the long-term benefit of an aggressive lipid-reduction strategy in patients who have undergone CABG. These benefits are supported by the angiographic evidence of delayed atherosclerotic progression in the vein grafts of patients assigned to aggressive lipid reduction. The findings support recent recommendations that LDL-C should be reduced to less than 100 mg/dL in patients with coronary artery disease. The late clinical benefit of low-dose anticoagulation was unexpected and remains to be explained.

▶ Another trial that underscores the importance of lipid-lowering therapy in patients with vascular disease. This article appears to support mounting evidence that lipid metabolism is one of the most powerful of many risk factors for atherosclerosis. The effect of warfarin is interesting and worthy of further research.

W. K. Williamson, MD

14 Vascular Trauma

Subclavian-Vertebral

Six-Year Experience With Management of Subclavian Artery Injuries
Kalakuntla V, Patel V, Tagoe A, et al (Morehouse School of Medicine, Atlanta, Ga)
Am Surg 66:927-931, 2000   14–1

Background.—Penetrating injuries of the subclavian artery are uncommon. However, when they occur they carry potentially high rates of morbidity and mortality. An experience of 25 patients with penetrating subclavian artery injuries is presented.

Methods.—The patients were seen over a 6-year period in one emergency department. For 65% of patients, the diagnosis was made on clinical grounds, followed by expedient surgical exploration. Twenty-seven percent were in unstable hemodynamic condition at presentation, leading to immediate surgery. The remaining patients were in hemodynamically stable condition with hard evidence of vascular injury; after appropriate evaluation and resuscitation, they were taken to surgery expediently. Thirty-five percent of patients were in sufficiently stable condition for angiographic evaluation. These preoperative studies helped in localizing the injury, planning the surgical approach, and achieving vascular control.

Results.—Three patients required subclavian artery ligation. Otherwise, subclavian flow was successfully re-established in all operated patients (Table 1). All limbs were successfully salvaged; 1 patient died of an associated gunshot wound to the liver. The morbidity rate varied with the patients' initial hemodynamic condition and associated injuries.

TABLE 1.—Repair Techniques

	Right	Left
Ligation of subclavian artery	2	1
Graft repair	4	2
Saphenous vein graft	2	0
Primary repair	7	3
Percutaneous intraluminal stent	0	1
Shunt	1	0

(Courtesy of Kalahuntla V, Patel V, Tagoe A, et al: Six-year experience with management of subclavian artery injuries. *Am Surg* 66:927-931, 2000.)

Conclusions.—The authors' approach to this uncommon presentation included aggressive resuscitation, early surgery, and selective preoperative angiography in hemodynamically stable patients. Following this strategy, they have achieved low morbidity and mortality rates.

▶ Another compelling indication for fluoroscopically guided, catheter-based operative intervention: (1) a percutaneously placed occlusion balloon will control bleeding and stabilize the patient, (2) catheter-directed imaging will determine the nature and location of injury, (3) subsequent stent-graft versus open arterial repair can be selected, depending on the size, significance, and location of the injury. Clearly, when OR-based imaging facilities and suitably trained surgeons are available, the angiography suite should be bypassed entirely in favor of definitive image-based operative management. More evidence that vascular surgery today depends less on historical surgical precepts (which incision to make? should patient have pre-operative angiography?) and more on catheter-based imaging, assessment, and (frequently) definitive intervention.

R. L. Dalman, MD

The Devastating Potential of Blunt Vertebral Arterial Injuries

Biffl WL, Moore EE, Elliott JP, et al (Denver Health Med Ctr; Univ of Colorado, Denver)

Ann Surg 231:672-681, 2000   14–2

Background.—Blunt vertebral arterial injury (BVI) has traditionally been thought of as an uncommon event of little significance. The literature abounds with case reports of BVI-associated cerebrovascular accidents, both ischemic and hemorrhagic; however, the clinical series regarding vertebral arteries that have been reported have primarily involved penetrating injuries. Screening for BVI has been recommended, particularly in patients with cervical injuries, but the appropriate therapy for these patients is controversial. The authors' experience with BVI was analyzed in an effort to develop a rational diagnostic and therapeutic approach to these patients.

Methods.—In 1996, the authors adopted an aggressive screening protocol for blunt carotid arterial injuries. Four-vessel cerebral arteriography was used in the identification of a significant number of BVIs as well as blunt carotid injury. A prospective database was maintained for all screened patients, and data regarding analysis of injury mechanisms and patterns, BVI grades, treatment, and outcomes were evaluated.

Results.—There were 38 patients with 47 BVIs during a 3½-year period, a rate of 0.53% of blunt trauma admissions. The most common mechanism of injury was automobile accident, and these patients commonly had associated injuries. Cervical spine injuries were prevalent, occurring in 71% of patients with BVI. However, there appeared to be no predilection for cervical vertebral level and no fracture pattern. The incidence of posterior circulation stroke among these patients was 24%, and the rate of death attributable to BVI was 8%. Stroke incidence and neurologic outcome were found to be independent of BVI injury grade. There were fewer poor outcomes overall among patients treated with systemic heparin, and fewer poor outcomes after stroke among patients treated with systemic heparin. Several trends were associated with heparin therapy, including fewer injuries progressing to a higher injury grade, fewer patients in whom stroke developed, and fewer patients who deteriorated neurologically between diagnosis and discharge.

Conclusion.—In this study, the incidence of BVI was higher than had been previously reported. Screening of patients based on injury mechanisms and patterns allowed the diagnosis of asymptomatic injuries, which enables therapy to be instituted before stroke. It appeared that systemic anticoagulation is effective therapy and was associated with improved neurologic outcome in patients both with and without stroke. It also appeared that systemic anticoagulation can prevent progression to a higher injury grade, stroke, and a decline in neurologic status.

▶ An interesting extension of work previously reported by this group on blunt carotid artery injury. The salient points in this article are that BVI is more frequent than expected and, although asymptomatic initially, may become symptomatic without treatment. In contrast to carotid arterial blunt injury, occlusive injuries are less likely to cause symptoms than nonocclusive injuries in BVI. Low-dose heparin therapy in BVIs is effective in preventing progression to stroke or deteriorating neurologic status. The aggressive arteriographic screening protocol used in this study may become obsolete as better techniques of MRA and CT angiography emerge, which may allow an even more aggressive screening protocol, and benefit an even larger number of blunt trauma victims.

E. J. Harris, Jr, MD

Subclavian Artery Disruption Resulting From Endovascular Intervention: Treatment Options

Lin PH, Bush RL, Weiss VJ, et al (Emory Univ, Atlanta, Ga)
J Vasc Surg 32:607-611, 2000   14–3

Background.—Endovascular intervention is a common treatment for subclavian artery stenosis. As the use of catheter-based interventions continues to increase, complications will undoubtedly occur. Two patients with subclavian artery disruption associated with endovascular interventions were reported.

Case 1.—Woman, 74, had contrast extravasation after a balloon-expandable stent was deployed in a stenotic subclavian artery (Fig 2). The arterial injury was treated successfully with a balloon tamponade.

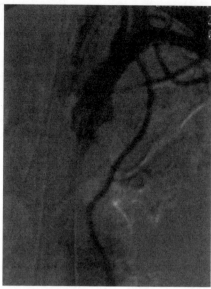

FIGURE 2.—After the placement of a balloon-expandable stent, completion angiogram demonstrated contrast extravasation in the subclavian artery. (Courtesy of Lin PH, Bush RL, Weiss VJ, et al: Subclavian artery disruption resulting from endovascular intervention: Treatment options. *J Vasc Surg* 32:607-611, 2000.)

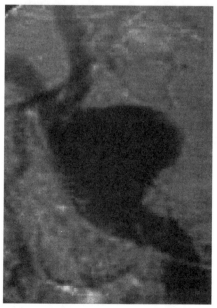

FIGURE 4.—A large pseudoaneurysm (5 × 6 cm²) was found in the proximal right subclavian artery 4 months after a balloon-expandable stent placement. (Courtesy of Lin PH, Bush RL, Weiss VJ, et al: Subclavian artery disruption resulting from endovascular intervention: Treatment options. *J Vasc Surg* 32:607-611, 2000.)

Case 2.—Man, 68, had a large subclavian pseudoaneurysm found 4 months after a balloon-expandable stent was placed (Fig 4). Arterial reconstruction with a prosthetic bypass graft resulted in successful repair.

Conclusions.—Subclavian artery disruption can result from an endovascular intervention with balloon angioplasty or stenting. Completion angiography is required to ensure satisfactory results and to document the vascular integrity of the artery after the endovascular intervention. Contrast extravasation can be treated with a balloon angioplasty for an extended time to tamponade and seal the arterial disruption. Follow-up chest CT should be done to exclude delayed pseudoaneurysm formation. In a patient with a large or symptomatic pseudoaneuyrsm after an endovascular intervention, direct operative repair is indicated to prevent life- or limb-threatening complications.

▶ There is no free lunch.

G. L. Moneta, MD

Thoracic Aorta

Repair of Traumatic Aortic Rupture: A 25-Year Experience
Razzouk AJ, Gundry SR, Wang N, et al (Loma Linda Univ, Calif)
Arch Surg 135:913-918, 2000   14–4

Background.—Acute rupture of the thoracic aorta after blunt trauma is a potentially fatal injury that often requires urgent surgical intervention. Emergency repair of aortic disruption in a trauma patient continues to be associated with a high mortality rate, despite improvements in resuscitation, transport, and critical care. In addition, paraplegia is a potential complication of traumatic aortic rupture (TAR). A number of surgical techniques have been described for the management of this potentially fatal injury, but the optimal method of repair (primary anastomosis vs interposition graft) continues to be debated. There is also debate as to whether distal aortic perfusion modifies patients' outcomes. The hypothesis that the outcome of patients who undergo repair of TAR is not dependent on the repair technique used was tested retrospectively.

Methods.—A retrospective review of 115 patients was conducted at a tertiary care teaching hospital and a level 1 regional trauma center. All the patients were victims of blunt chest trauma and had sustained an aortic tear. The patients ranged in age from 5 to 81 years and were seen between January 1, 1974 and June 30, 1999. Two groups of patients were evaluated: those who underwent surgical repair of TAR with distal aortic perfusion (group 1), and those who underwent surgical repair of TAR without distal aortic perfusion (group 2). Prehospital data, operative findings, and outcome were assessed from medical records. A paired two-tailed t test was used for statistical comparison.

Results.—Group 1 comprised 32 patients, 18 with TAR repair using active bypass and 14 using a Gott shunt. In the 83 patients in group 2, the clamp-and-sew technique was used. Primary repair was performed in 14 patients (44%) in group 1 and 69 patients (83%) in group 2. The average aortic cross-clamp time for group 1 was 48 minutes, and for group 2, 20 minutes. No significant difference was observed between groups 1 and 2 in hospital mortality or incidence of paraplegia. In the last 15 years, 78 patients (73 in group 2) underwent surgical repair of TAR with an operative mortality of 19.2%.

Conclusions.—Acute TAR continues to be a highly life-threatening injury. During the past 25 years there has been no change in prognosis. In most patients, repair of TAR with simple aortic cross-clamping alone is feasible without the risk of increased mortality or spinal cord injury.

▶ The most interesting information from this article regarding repair of TAR is that no significant difference in mortality rate between early and late eras and between those patients having distal perfusion during repair and those undergoing the clamp-and-sew technique was observed. Despite the incredible advances in intensive care medicine and anesthesia, TAR continues to have high mortality and morbidity rates. Although the magic clamp time of 30 minutes was not applied to the data in this study, other studies have shown that aortic cross-clamp times greater than 30 minutes do have significantly higher rates of paraplegia. In the hands of surgeons who routinely take care of this problem at very busy trauma centers, the clamp-and-sew technique is perfectly acceptable. In those centers in which an occasional patient arrives with aortic rupture and requires emergent or urgent surgical repair, a distal shunt may be indicated because the skill of the surgeon does not allow for keeping clamp time less than 30 minutes. Therefore, the only caveat I would add to the authors' conclusions is that clamping alone is feasible in the majority of patients if the surgeons performing the surgery can do it in an expeditious manner.

R. B. McLafferty, MD

Surgical Outcome of Traumatic Rupture of the Thoracic Aorta
Tatou E, Steinmetz E, Jazayeri S, et al (Hôpital du Bocage, Dijon, France)
Ann Thorac Surg 69:70-73, 2000   14–5

Background.—Surgical treatment of traumatic rupture of the thoracic aorta is challenging because it is not easily diagnosed, mortality is high, and morbidity is tragic. The mortality rate of traumatic rupture of the thoracic aorta is related to the seriousness of the lesions, the multiple traumatic injuries that may be associated, and the immediate operation. The morbidity is related to the difficult challenge of protecting the spinal cord, leading to paraplegia in young patients. The results of various techniques of spinal cord protection in patients with traumatic thoracic aorta (TTA) treated surgically were presented.

TABLE 2.—Mortality as Related to Age, Cross-Clamp Time, Hemothorax, and Type of Aortic Tear

Variable	Dead	Alive	p
Age (y)	41.6 (± 17.8)	31.2 (± 12.5)	0.003
Cross-clamp time (min)	35 (± 11.9)	29 (± 13.6)	0.003
Hemothorax (n)			
Yes	21	60	
No	12	81	0.02
Aortic tear (n)			
Partial	11	67	
Total	18	69	0.05
Complex	4	5	

(Reprinted with permission from the Society of Thoracic Surgeons, from Tatou E, Steinmetz E, Jazayeri S, et al: Surgical outcome of traumatic rupture of the thoracic aorta. *Ann Thorac Surg* 69:70-73, 2000.)

Methods.—The multicentric study involved 174 patients with aortic isthmus disruption. The mean age of the patient group was 32.3 ± 14.29 years, and the group comprised 126 men and 48 women. Most of the patients (136) had TTA as a result of vehicle accidents, and polytraumatism was common. In 94.8% of the patients, a standard chest radiograph led to a diagnosis that was confirmed with aortography. Surgical repair of visceral lesions was accomplished in 52 of 174 patients (29.9%) for traumatic injury to the spleen, liver, diaphragm, mesentery, and gut. These procedures were performed before aortic repair in 21.3% of patients and after aortic repair in 8.6% of patients. The mortality rate was 19% (33 patients) and morbidity was 5.2% (9 patients). The clamp-and-sew technique was used in 69 patients (group 1), various types of extracorporeal circulation were used in 93 patients (group 2), and a Gott shunt was used in 12 patients (group 3). No differences were observed among the groups in mortality and paraplegia; however, the sex ratio, age, visceral lesions, craniocerebral lesions, type of aortic repair, and cross-clamp time were discriminative among the 3 groups.

Results.—Risk factors for death according to univariate analysis were age, cross-clamp time, hemothorax, and anatomic type of aortic injury (Table 2). Multivariate analysis confirmed these findings.

Conclusions.—TTA is a serious injury with a bad prognosis. However, surgical management has improved. The main obstacles to lowering the high mortality and morbidity rates in surgery for TTA are immediate operation and medullary protection. For some patients, surgery can be delayed, but the surgeon needs to take care of hemodynamic instability. In this situation, repair of serious associated lesions is required first, or quick performance of a thoracotomy is required for ruptured aorta. One question that remains is whether it is better to protect the spinal cord with the lower aortic perfusion and avoid the simple cross-clamp. Studies have yet to answer this question.

▶ This article describes a current, state-of-the-art surgical treatment of traumatic thoracic aortic dissection. The surgical mortality rate in this series was only 20%, which appears commendable, but these patients may represent a highly select group of survivors who made it to the treatment hospital. It is my personal opinion that many of these patients in the future will be treated with endovascular techniques, which have the potential for being simpler and reducing some of the rates of morbidity and death associated with open repair.

J. L. Mills, Sr, MD

Endovascular Treatment of Penetrating Thoracic Outlet Arterial Injuries
du Toit DF, Strauss DC, Blaszczyk M, et al (Tygerburg Hosp, South Africa; Univ of Stellenbosch, Tygerberg, South Africa)
Eur J Vasc Endovasc Surg 19:489-495, 2000   14–6

Background.—The achievement of surgical access to arterial injuries of the thoracic outlet is difficult, and conventional approaches to treating these injuries are associated with high morbidity. An experience with the endovascular stent-graft treatment of pseudoaneurysm and arteriovenous fistula of the thoracic outlet was described.

Methods.—Over a 10-month period, 41 patients with penetrating injuries to the carotid, subclavian, and proximal axillary arteries were considered for endovascular management. Twenty-six patients were excluded because they required urgent surgery for active bleeding or acute occlusion. The remaining 15 patients underwent arteriography to assess their suitability for stent-graft treatment. Five patients were excluded because their lesion could not be transversed by guidewire or because there was a large proximal/distal lumen discrepancy. Thus, 10 patients (7 men and 3 women; mean age, 27 years) underwent endovascular stent-grafting of the subclavian (7 patients), carotid (2 patients), or axillary (1 patient) arteries.

Arteriovenous fistulas were present in 7 patients, and pseudoaneurysms were present in 3. During the procedure, arterial branches that could participate in complex lesions were embolized to prevent endoleak; neurologic complications were avoided by checking vertebral artery cross-flow before embolization. Stents were initially placed under the guidance of image masking, but subsequently angiography was used for stent positioning. A routine completion angiogram was obtained after stent deployment. Patients were followed up clinically and sonographically at 1 month and every 3 months thereafter for a mean of 7 months.

Results.—Stent-grafting successfully excluded the lesion in all 10 patients, with no endoleaks (Fig 3). None of the patients required conversion to open repair or experienced procedure-related complications, including

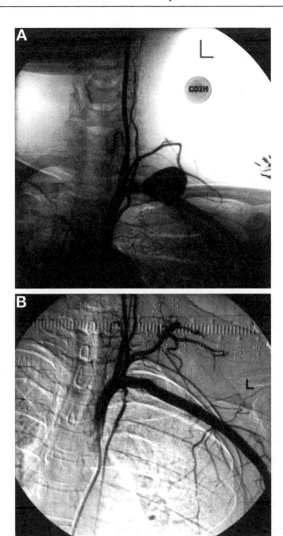

FIGURE 3.—Treatment of a pseudoaneurysm of the left subclavian artery. **A,** Selective left subclavian artery arteriogram demonstrating the pseudoaneurysm; **B,** complete exclusion of the lesion after stent-graft deployment. (Reprinted from the *European Journal of Vascular and Endovascular Surgery* courtesy of du Toit DF, Strauss DC, Blaszczyk M, et al: Endovascular treatment of penetrating thoracic outlet arterial injuries. *Eur J Vasc Endovasc Surg* 19:489-495, 2000. Copyright 2000, by permission of the publisher, W B Saunders Company Limited London.)

neurologic deterioration. Furthermore, none of the patients have died or lost a limb, nor do they have evidence of graft stenosis or occlusion to date.

Conclusion.—Endovascular stent-graft treatment was successful in managing the thoracic outlet arterial injuries in these selected patients. The procedure was safe and patients suffered no complications, although thrombosis, late stenosis, and occlusion caused by neointimal hyperplasia remain potential disadvantages of all stent-graft repairs. Given the inaccessibility of these injuries to standard surgical repair, more research is warranted to determine whether endovascular stent-grafting is a superior method for treating arterial injuries of the thoracic outlet.

▶ This well-written and -illustrated case series uses endovascular methods to treat hemodynamically stable patients with arterial injuries to the thoracic outlet (either pseudoaneurysms or arteriovenous fistula). This application of endovascular therapy is clearly a dramatic improvement over open surgical techniques. These lesions are anatomically difficult to access. The authors make their case with excellent short-term results.

M. R. Nehler, MD

Contrast-Enhanced Helical Computerised Tomography in the Investigation of Thoracic Aortic Injury

Beese RC, Allan R, Treasure T (St George's Hosp, London)
Ann R Coll Surg Engl 83:10-13, 2001   14-7

Background.—Aortic angiography is the gold standard in the diagnosis of traumatic thoracic aortic injury, but it is not routinely available at all hospitals in the United Kingdom. In contrast, the availability of contrast-enhanced helical CT (CEHCT) is increasing rapidly, especially in district general hospitals. Some studies have shown that CEHCT is as sensitive and specific as angiography in detecting aortic trauma. Four patients whose thoracic aortic injury was diagnosed by CEHCT were described.

Methods.—The subjects were 4 men 26 to 42 years of age who had sustained multiple injuries during traffic accidents. The 4 patients were admitted to different hospitals and underwent chest radiography at presentation. In all cases, the thoracic aortic injury was diagnosed by CEHCT (although imaging techniques varied slightly). In preparation for CEHCT, the patient's arms were elevated above his head. All potential sources of artifact in the field of view were removed, including electrocardiographic leads and nasogastric tubing (which was pulled back above the aortic arch).

CEHCT is best performed by using 7-mm slices with 7-mm table movements and a pitch of 1. An IV bolus of 100 mL of nonionic contrast (300 mg of iodine/mL) was administered via a pump injector at a rate of 2 mL/sec, then scanning began 20 seconds later. With the patient holding his breath, scanning was performed from the base of the neck to the diaphragm. Surgery was performed at 1 of 2 hospitals, and findings at surgery were compared with those at diagnostic CEHCT.

Results.—In all 4 cases, the chest radiograph showed evidence of mediastinal hematoma (Fig 1). This was confirmed by CEHCT, which also showed signs of aortic pseudoaneurysm at the level of the aortic isthmus (3 patients) or the left atrium (1 patient). Findings at surgery correlated with the type and site of aortic injury as shown by CEHCT. All patients survived and were alive at their 6-month follow-up evaluations.

FIGURE 1

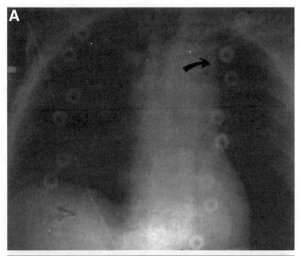

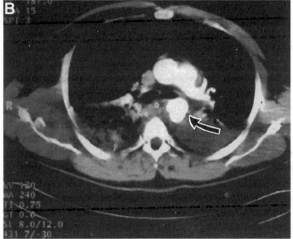

(*Continued*)

Conclusions.—CEHCT can accurately diagnose thoracic aortic injuries. Its use will likely improve the management of patients with thoracic trauma, enabling faster diagnosis at the referring hospital and more rapid transfer to regional cardiothoracic centers. CEHCT is noninvasive, and can identify thoracic injuries other than aortic disruption as well. CEHCT has many advantages over conventional CT in the evaluation of thoracic aortic injury. First, it can image the entire chest during 1 breath-hold. Thus, contrast can be injected and scanning timed to occur during optimal opacification of the aorta.

FIGURE 1 (cont.)

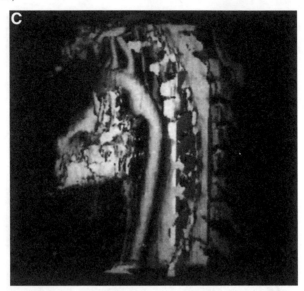

FIGURE 1.—A, Supine chest radiograph demonstrating a widened upper mediastinum with loss of the normal aortic contour and depression of the left main stem bronchus. The left paraspinal line is widened and extends above the aortic arch, indicating the presence of a posterior mediastinal hematoma (*arrow*). B, Contrast-enhanced CT of the same patient at the level of the isthmus demonstrating a mediastinal hematoma with an abnormal contour of the thoracic aorta diagnostic of a pseudoaneurysm (*arrow*). C, Subsequent 3-dimensional reconstruction demonstrates the abnormal contour of the thoracic aorta at the level of the isthmus. (Courtesy of Beese RC, Allan R, Treasure T: Contrast-enhanced helical computerised tomography in the investigation of thoracic aortic injury. *Ann R Coll Surg Engl* 83:10-13, 2001.)

Optimal contrast opacification of the aorta also facilitates subsequent 3-dimensional reconstruction and CT angiography. Furthermore, acquiring the CEHCT imaging during 1 breath-hold avoids loss of information caused by erratic breath movements. On CEHCT, aortic disruption is indicated by the presence of abnormal material in the mediastinum surrounding the aorta, and this matter is generally adjacent to the site of vascular injury. Large areas of altered contour of the thoracic aorta indicate pseudoaneurysm, while small irregularities in the contour indicate intimal tears. Filling defects within the aortic lumen indicate intimal flaps.

▶ In this 4-patient study of CEHCT scans for the diagnosis of traumatic thoracic aortic injury, the authors found that a clearly positive scan could be used as the basis for surgical repair. CEHCT scanning appears to be a significant improvement over traditional CT scanning primarily because motion and averaging artifacts are often eliminated. The authors' suggestion that aortography be reserved for situations in which CEHCT scanning is not available or is equivocal seems reasonable. However, it may well be premature, and further study should be undertaken.

J. M. Edwards, MD

Miscellaneous

Angiographic Embolization of Bilateral Internal Iliac Arteries to Control Life-Threatening Hemorrhage After Blunt Trauma to the Pelvis

Velmahos GC, Chahwan S, Hanks SE, et al (Univ of Southern California, Los Angeles)

Am Surg 66:858-862, 2000   14–8

Objective.—Mortality and morbidity rates are high for pelvic fractures after blunt trauma, mainly as a result of uncontrolled retroperitoneal bleeding. Temporary angiographic embolization of bilateral internal iliac arteries (TAEBIIA) is increasingly being used as an alternative to subselective embolization. The indications, safety, and efficacy of TAEBIIA associated with complex pelvic fractures were reported.

Methods.—Between November 1991 and March 1998, 30 consecutive patients (12 females) (average age, 43 years) with an average Injury Severity Score of 25 were treated with TAEBIIA because of continued fluid and blood transfusion requirements despite apparently successful subselective embolization. Angiography revealed multiple bleeding sites. Demographics; injury characteristics; time from admission to TAEBIIA; duration of TAEBIIA; hemodynamic parameters before, during, and after TAEBIIA; hospital course; and outcome were evaluated.

Results.—Thirteen patients had exploratory laparotomy. Three, who continued to bleed, received TAEBIIA. Seventeen patients were treated with TAEBIIA primarily. Angiographically proven bleeding in 28 (93%) patients was controlled by TAEBIIA in 25 (89%). Two patients with no angiographic evidence of bleeding had bilateral embolization, followed by TAEBIIA when pelvic bleeding could not be excluded. TAEBIIA controlled bleeding in 90% of patients. Two of the 3 patients who continued to bleed were treated with repeat embolization and repeat TAEBIIA to control bleeding. The third, who demonstrated initial angiographic control by TAEBIIA, died as a result of continued hemodynamic instability. There was no severe in-hospital morbidity. Nonexpanding hematomas developed in 2 patients and were treated by local measures. Ten patients died, 1 as a result of uncontrolled bleeding and 9 from non–TAEBIIA-related causes. No patients had ischemia of surrounding soft tissues or pelvic organs.

Conclusion.—TAEBIIA is a safe and effective alternative technique for control of severe pelvic bleeding not staunched by selective embolization.

▶ Selective angiographic embolization of pelvic arteries now plays an essential role in the management of hemorrhage associated with blunt pelvic trauma. The group at USC reports on 30 patients in whom hemorrhage did not respond to selective embolization. These patients underwent "temporary" bilateral internal iliac artery embolization as a last-ditch effort to control hemorrhage. This technique was successful in 97% of the patients, with no significant ischemic complications. This is clearly a technique that should be considered in these difficult patients. While the authors describe this as "temporary" embolization, there were no follow-up studies to determine recanalization of the iliac vessels. Embolization of internal iliac arteries does appear to have long-term consequences of hip and buttock claudication, as we are learning from the stent-graft arena.[1] Long-term sequelae are unknown in these trauma patients; however, faced with "life with claudication versus exsanguination," most would choose life.

A. M. Abou-Zamzam, Jr, MD

Reference

1. Lee WA, O'Dorisio J, Wolf YG, et al: Outcome after unilateral hypogastric artery occlusion during endovascular aneurysm repair. *J Vasc Surg* 33:921-926, 2001.

Arteriovenous Fistulae Complicating Cardiac Pacemaker Lead Extraction: Recognition, Evaluation, and Management
Kumins NH, Tober JC, Love CJ, et al (Ohio State Univ, Columbus)
J Vasc Surg 32:1225-1228, 2000   14–9

Objective.—Removal of chronically implanted pacemaker leads is complicated when they are encased in fibrotic tissue. Two cases of arteriovenous fistula between aortic arch branches and the left brachiocephalic vein that occurred after pacing lead removal with the excimer laser are described.

Case 1.—Woman, 49, who had removal of 3 pacemaker leads placed through the left subclavian vein and replacement with a single ventricular lead, showed bright red bleeding around the sheath and became cyanotic and hypotensive. Because her oxygen saturation was 93% and she had no pericardial effusion or cardiac insufficiency, she was treated for superior vena cava syndrome. Although she improved, a chest radiograph at 6 hours revealed pulmonary edema, a widened mediastinum and a large pleural effusion. An arteriogram, performed the next day for a continuous murmur, revealed a communication between the innominate artery and the left brachiocephalic vein and a tight stenosis at the junction of the superior vena cava to the atrium (Fig 1). The patient died of cardiopulmonary arrest.

Case 2.—Woman, 68, with a dual-chamber pacemaker and bipolar leads through the subclavian vein and who had a failed standard lead extraction, had an attempted extraction with the excimer laser. Arterial blood began to escape around the sheath. The sheath was removed, the blood flow was stanched, and the procedure was terminated. When the patient had back and chest pain, an arteriogram was performed. An arteriovenous fistula was revealed connecting the left common carotid artery and the left brachiocephalic vein. She also had early filling of the brachiocepha-

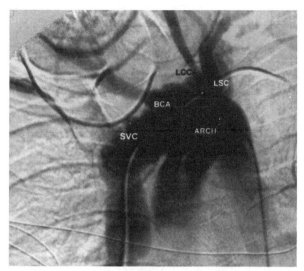

FIGURE 1.—An arteriogram demonstrating brisk filling of the superior vena cava (SVC) through the left brachiocephalic vein during an arch injection. The newly placed pacing lead can be seen coursing through the left brachiocephalic vein and the SVC. *Abbreviations: BCA*, Brachiocephalic artery (innominate artery); *LCCA*, left common carotid artery; *LSC*, left subclavian artery. (Courtesy of Kumins NH, Tober JC, Love CJ, et al: Arteriovenous fistulae complicating cardiac pacemaker lead extraction: Recognition, evaluation, and management. *J Vasc Surg* 32:1225-1228, 2000.)

lic vein. She became hypotensive while awaiting surgery and showed a hyperdynamic response with cardiac outputs in excess of 10 L/min. A median sternotomy was performed, and the brachiocephalic vein, which had a large tear, was ligated. Tears in the left common carotid artery and the innominate artery were repaired and an ascending aorta to the left common carotid artery bypass was constructed. The patient recovered without sequelae.

Conclusion.—Arteriovenous fistula, although rare, can be fatal. Chest or back pain, persistent or copious bleeding, hypotension, anemia, or signs of heart failure require immediate arteriography and percutaneous or surgical intervention.

▶ I hope this complication never occurs when I'm on call, but if it does, this article will be of some help to me. Unlike arteriovenous fistulas associated with pacemaker insertion, which are more common and have a generally benign clinical course, those associated with pacemaker lead extraction are fortunately rare but potentially lethal. Like any traumatic injury to the great vessels, these acute arteriovenous fistulas require immediate arteriography and interventions with either percutaneous techniques or open surgery.

R. A. Yeager, MD

Prolonged Use of Intraluminal Arterial Shunts Without Systemic Anticoagulation

Granchi T, Schmittling Z, Vasquez J Jr, et al (Baylor College of Medicine, Houston; Ben Taub Gen Hosp, Houston)
Am J Surg 180:493-497, 2000   14–10

Background.—The first use of temporary arterial shunts in the management of arterial injuries was reported in 1971. With the development of damage control surgery, the use of temporary arterial shunts has been expanded to include maintenance of distal limb perfusion while life-threatening abdominal or thoracic injuries are treated. The duration of patency and the need for systemic anticoagulation have been unresolved questions and were the focus of this investigation.

Methods.—A chart review was conducted of all patients who underwent placement of intraluminal arterial shunts in the Trauma Service at the Baylor College of Medicine and the Harris County Hospital District from January 1993 to December 1998. Data were collected on mechanism of injury, artery injured, shunt time, blood loss and transfusions, injury severity score, mangled extremity severity score, and anticoagulation.

Results.—A total of 19 patients were identified for this review. Of these patients, 10 received shunts for damage control (group 1), and 9 received shunts for treatment of orthopedic/vascular injuries (group 2) (Fig 1).

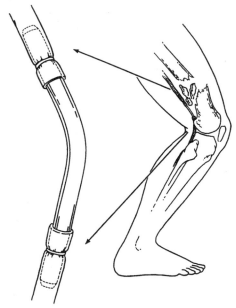

FIGURE 1.—The Argyle shunt is placed in the arterial lumen and secured with soft rubber vessel loops. The shunt is flexible but resists kinking. Shunts are not oversized. (Reprinted from the *American Journal of Surgery* courtesy of Granchi T, Schmittling Z, Vasquez J Jr, et al: Prolonged use of intraluminal arterial shunts without systemic anticoagulation. *Am J Surg* 180:493-497, 2000. Copyright 2001, with permission from Excerpta Medica Inc.)

Shunt times, mortality, injury severity score, and mangled extremity severity score were all significantly higher in group 1 compared with group 2. Shunt time ranged from 47 minutes to 52 hours. Amputations were required for 1 patient in each group.

Conclusion.—Temporary shunts can be used effectively for damage control and for treatment of combined orthopedic and vascular injuries. In this study, shunts remained open for as long as 52 hours without systemic anticoagulation.

▶ While most vascular surgeons know that vascular surgery can be performed safely without anticoagulation, we routinely use it except in situations such as massive trauma where the risk of anticoagulation to the patient outweighs the risk of failed reconstruction. This report extends our knowledge on withholding anticoagulation to situations in which temporary arterial shunts are placed either for patients with life-threatening injuries that preclude immediate arterial repair or while associated orthopedic injuries are being addressed. Shunts were left in place for prolonged periods of time, even days, without anticoagulation in a small number of patients without an apparent increase in complications. While it is not something I would routinely use or recommend, it is useful to know what the limits of the use of prosthetic shunts are for those rare cases in which the alternatives are limited.

J. M. Edwards, MD

Operative Management and Outcome of 302 Abdominal Vascular Injuries
Asensio JA, Chahwan S, Hanpeter D, et al (Univ of Southern California, Los Angeles; Los Angeles County–Univ of Southern California Med Ctr, Los Angeles)
Am J Surg 180:528-534, 2000   14–11

Background.—High mortality rates are associated with abdominal vascular injuries. Institutional experience with these injuries and the additive effect of multiple vessel injuries on mortality were reviewed. Investigators also sought to determine the mortality of combined arterial and venous injuries and to correlate mortality with American Association for the Surgery of Trauma–Organ Injury Scale (AAST-OIS) for abdominal vascular injury.

Methods.—In a retrospective 6-year study at an urban level I trauma center, the survival of patients with abdominal vascular injuries was evaluated.

Results.—A total of 302 patients were identified. They had a mean age of 28 years and a mean Injury Severity Score (ISS) of 25 (range, 4-75). The mechanism of injury was penetrating trauma in 266 (88%) patients and blunt trauma in 36 (12%) patients. Forty-three of 302 (14%) patients required thoracotomy in the emergency department. A total of 504 vessels

TABLE 2.—Multiple-Vessel Injuries Versus Mortality

Number of Patients	Number of Vessels Injured	Mortality (Died)	Percent
160	1	72	45%
102	2	61	60.0%
33	3	24	73.0%
2	4	2	100%
2	5	2	100%
1	6	1	100%

(Reprinted from the *American Journal of Surgery* courtesy of Asensio JA, Chahwan S, Hanpeter D, et al: Operative management and outcome of 302 abdominal vascular injuries. *Am J Surg* 180:528-534, 2000. Copyright 2000, with permission from Excerpta Medica Inc.)

were injured, including 238 arteries and 266 veins. Surgical management involved ligation in 245 vessels, primary repair in 141 vessels, prosthetic interposition grafts in 24 vessels, and autogenous grafts in 2 vessels. The overall mortality rate was 54% (162 of 302 patients). The mortality in terms of multiple vessels injured was as follows: 1 vessel, 45%; 2 vessels, 60%; 3 vessels, 73%; more than 4 vessels, 100% (Table 2). The mortality rate in terms of arterial injuries was as follows: isolated injury of the aorta, 78%; isolated aorta combined with other arterial injuries, 82.4%; superior mesenteric artery alone, 47.6%; superior mesenteric artery combined with other arterial injuries, 71.4%; iliac artery alone, 53%; iliac artery combined with other arterial injuries, 72.7%; renal artery alone, 37.5%; and renal artery combined with other arterial injuries, 66.7%. In terms of venous injuries, those of the inferior vena cava when isolated was 70%, compared with 77.7% when combined with other venous injuries; those of the superior mesenteric vein alone was 52.7%, compared with 65% when combined with other venous injuries; and those of the inferior mesenteric vein was 16% alone, compared with 50% in combination with other venous injuries. The specific mortality rate expressed as a combination of arterial and venous injuries was as follows: aorta plus inferior vena cava, 93%; superior mesenteric artery plus superior mesenteric vein, 43%; and iliac artery and vein, 45.5%. When mortality was compared with the AAST-OIS scale, the mortality rate for grade II was 25%; for grade III, 32%; for grade IV, 65%; and for grade V, 88%.

Conclusion.—Abdominal vascular injuries are extremely life threatening, and the risk for mortality increases with multiple arterial and venous injuries. Mortality in these injuries was found to be correlated with the AAST-OIS for abdominal vascular injury.

▶ Abdominal vascular injuries continue to be highly lethal. The trauma group at Los Angeles County unfortunately encounters on average 1 of these cases per week at their center. The overall mortality rate of 54% is sobering when one considers that these are modern-day results at an urban trauma center that is well equipped and staffed to manage these injuries. Improved outcomes may not be linked to better surgical management but, rather, to societal changes resulting in prevention of these devastating injuries.

R. A. Yeager, MD

15 Venous Thrombosis and Pulmonary Embolism

Drug Prophylaxis/Treatment

Subcutaneous Enoxaparin Once or Twice Daily Compared With Intravenous Unfractionated Heparin for Treatment of Venous Thromboembolic Disease

Spiro TE, for the Enoxaparin Clinical Trial Group (Thomas Jefferson Univ, Philadelphia; et al)

Ann Intern Med 134:191-202, 2001   15–1

Objective.—Unfractionated heparin is being replaced by low molecular weight heparins as the treatment of choice for acute venous thromboembolic disease. Because low molecular weight heparins differ in their physicochemical and pharmacologic properties, it is difficult to compare results among studies. Whether enoxaparin, administered subcutaneously once or twice daily, is as effective as continuously infused unfractionated heparin for patients with acute, symptomatic venous thromboembolic disease was investigated in a parallel-group, randomized, partially blinded, international, multicenter clinical trial.

Methods.—Patients were randomly assigned to receive dose-adjusted intravenous unfractionated heparin (n = 290), 1.0 mg/kg body weight subcutaneous enoxaparin twice daily (n = 312), or 1.5 mg/kg body weight once daily (n = 298) for at least 5 days, followed by warfarin administration within 72 hours of initiation of 1 of the treatments for at least 3 months. Prothrombin time was measured daily. Efficacy and safety were assessed in all patients.

Results.—Venous thromboembolism recurred in 4.1% of the heparin group, in 4.4% of the once-daily enoxaparin group, and in 2.9% of the twice-daily enoxaparin group. Cancer (odds ratio [OR], 3.7) and symptomatic pulmonary embolism (OR, 3.4) were risk factors for recurrence in all groups. Obesity (OR, 4.0) was a significant risk factor in the enoxaparin groups (Figure). The numbers of deaths and hemorrhages were similar in all groups.

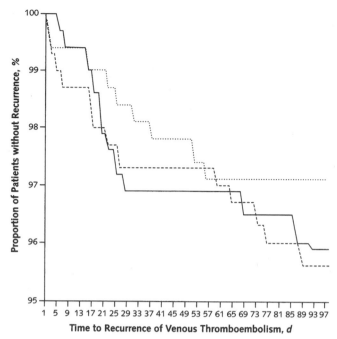

FIGURE.—Product-limit analysis of time to first recurrence of a venous thromboembolic event among all treated patients. *Dotted line* represents twice-daily enoxaparin; *solid line* represents unfractionated heparin; *dashed line* represents once-daily enoxaparin. (Courtesy of Spiro TE, for the Enoxaparin Clinical Trial Group: Subcutaneous enoxaparin once or twice daily compared with intravenous unfractionated heparin for treatment of venous thromboembolic disease. *Ann Intern Med* 134:191-202, 2001.)

Conclusion.—Enoxaparin administered once or twice daily is as safe and effective as continuously infused unfractionated heparin for the treatment of venous thromboembolic disease.

▶ The treatment of venous thromboembolic disease (deep venous thrombosis and pulmonary embolism) continues to evolve. In this large, randomized, multicenter study, treatment of DVT and PE with once- and twice-daily administration of enoxaparin was found to be equivalent to treatment with intravenous unfractionated heparin with respect to recurrent thromboembolic episodes, hemorrhagic complications, and death. A similar study last year[1] reported equivalence of once- and twice-daily dosing of the LMWH nadroparin. Certainly, there are a number of hospitalized patients with DVT and PE to whom this does not apply, not to mention the issues of patient compliance. However, for selected patients, it appears as though outpatient therapy for DVT and, as this study boldly suggests, PE may become the standard of care.

G. J. Landry, MD

Reference

1. 2001 Year Book of Vascular Surgery, p 455.

A Synthetic Pentasaccharide for the Prevention of Deep-Vein Thrombosis After Total Hip Replacement

Turpie AGG, for the Pentasaccharide Investigators (McMaster Univ, Hamilton, Ont, Canada; et al)
N Engl J Med 344:619-625, 2001   15–2

Background.—A reduction in the incidence of venous thromboembolism after hip replacement surgery continues to present a challenge to clinicians. Current prophylactic treatments for this potentially fatal but preventable disease include the use of low–molecular-weight heparins, adjusted-dose subcutaneous heparin, and warfarin. Standard heparin and the low–molecular-weight heparins are heterogenous compounds that are derived from animals, and, as such, have the potential for induction of antiplatelet antibodies and impairment of hemostasis through complex effects on platelet function.

A new class of synthetic antithrombotic agents has been developed. The first of them, Org31540/SR90107A, is a highly selective, indirect inhibitor of activated factor X (Fig 1). This study investigated the optimal dose of this compound for phase 3 studies by means of a double-blind dose-ranging study in which Org31540/SR90107A was compared with a low–

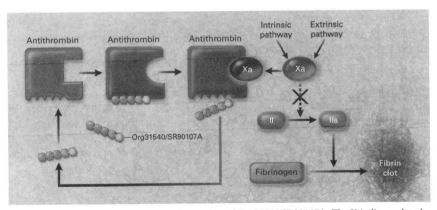

FIGURE 1.—Mechanism of anticoagulant action of Org31540/SR90107A. The X indicates that the inhibition of activated factor X leads to interruption of the coagulation cascade by preventing the activation of factor II (prothrombin) to factor IIa (thrombin). Org31540/SR90107A binds with high affinity to the pentasaccharide binding site on antithrombin, producing an irreversible conformational change in antithrombin; an arginine residue is exposed, which binds to and inhibits activated factor X, a key factor in the activation of coagulation. Org31540/SR90107A is then released and made available to bind to other antithrombin molecules. (Reproduced by permission of *The New England Journal of Medicine* courtesy of Turpie AGG, for the Pentasaccharide Investigators: A synthetic pentasaccharide for the prevention of deep-vein thrombosis after total hip replacement. *N Engl J Med* 344:619-625, 2001. Copyright 2001, Massachusetts Medical Society. All rights reserved.)

molecular-weight heparin, enoxaparin, in patients undergoing total hip replacement.

Methods.—Patients were randomly assigned to postoperative administration of 1 of 5 daily doses of Org31540/SR90107A, given once daily, or enoxaparin, 30 mg, given every 12 hours. Treatment continued for 10 days or until performance of bilateral venography after a minimum of 5 days. A total of 933 patients were treated; 593 were eligible for the efficacy analysis.

Results.—A dose effect was observed with Org31540/SR90107A, with venous thromboembolism occurring at rates of 11.8%, 6.7%, 1.7%, 4.4%, and 0% for the groups assigned to 0.75 mg, 1.5 mg, 3.0 mg, 6.0 mg, and 8.0 mg of the drug, respectively. This compared with a rate of 9.4% in the enoxaparin group. The reduction in risk for venous thromboembolism was 82% for the group that received 3.0 mg of Org31540/SR90107A and 29% for the group that received 1.5 mg of the drug. Bleeding complications prompted discontinuance of enrollment in the 6.0 mg and 8.0 mg Org31540/SR90107A groups. Major bleeding occurred 3.5% less frequently in the 0.75-mg group and 3% less frequently in the 1.5-mg group compared with the enoxaparin group, which had a rate of major bleeding similar to that of the 3.0-mg group.

Conclusion.—The synthetic pentasaccharide Org31540/SR90107A has the potential to significantly improve the risk-benefit ratio for the prevention of thromboembolism, compared with low–molecular-weight heparin.

▶ This article provides important information on a new class of anticoagulants of synthetic oligosaccharides, which I believe will have great clinical application in the near future. The agent studied is particularly attractive in that it is given once daily and yields reliable dose-response effects in a varied population. I anxiously await further studies on this compound in prophylaxis and treatment.

W. K. Williamson, MD

Effects of a Low-Molecular-Weight Heparin on Thrombus Regression and Recurrent Thromboembolism in Patients With Deep-Vein Thrombosis

Breddin HK, for the CORTES Investigators (Internatl Inst of Thrombosis and Vascular Diseases, Frankfurt, Germany; et al)
N Engl J Med 344:626-631, 2001   15–3

Background.—The treatment of choice for deep-vein thrombosis or pulmonary embolism has been immediate anticoagulation, usually with unfractionated heparin. In randomized controlled trials, treatment of deep-vein thrombosis and pulmonary embolism with low molecular weight heparins has been shown to be at least as effective and safe as unfractionated heparin. Venous thromboembolism is frequently treated with low molecular weight heparin, but there has been a need for further definition of optimal dosing regimens and clinical outcomes.

Methods.—A multicenter, open-label study with blinded adjudication of end points was conducted. Patients with acute deep-vein thrombosis were randomly assigned to 1 of 3 treatment regimens: IV administration of unfractionated heparin, subcutaneous administration of low molecular weight heparin (reviparin, twice daily for 1 week), or subcutaneous reviparin once daily for 4 weeks. The primary end point was evidence of regression of the thrombus on venography on day 21. The secondary end points were recurrent venous thromboembolism, major bleeding within 90 days after enrollment, and death.

Results.—A total of 321 patients received unfractionated heparin, of whom 129 (40.2%) had thrombus regression, compared with 53.4% of patients (175 of 328) receiving reviparin twice daily and 53.5% of patients (167 of 312) receiving reviparin once daily (Fig 1). In terms of thrombus regression, reviparin twice daily and reviparin once daily were both significantly more effective than unfractionated heparin. Mortality and the incidence of major bleeding were similar for all 3 groups.

Conclusion.—Reviparin regimens were found to be more effective than unfractionated heparin in reducing the size of the thrombus in patients

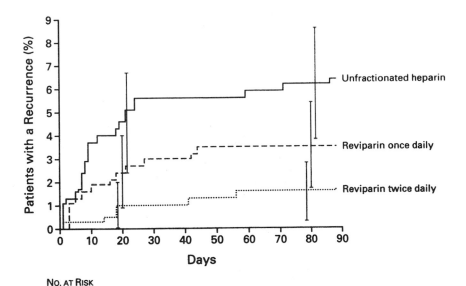

FIGURE 1.—Kaplan-Meier analysis of the time to the recurrence of thromboembolic events over a period of 90 days in the 3 treatment groups. *I bars* represent 95% of confidence intervals at 20 and 80 days. (Reprinted by permission of *The New England Journal of Medicine* courtesy of Breddin HK, for the CORTES Investigators: Effects of a low-molecular-weight heparin on thrombus regression and recurrent thromboembolism in patients with deep-vein thrombosis. *N Engl J Med* 344:626-631, 2001. Copyright 2001, Massachusetts Medical Society. All rights reserved.)

with acute deep-vein thrombosis. Reviparin was also found to be as safe as and more effective than unfractionated heparin in the prevention of recurrent thromboembolism.

▶ The study is well designed and demonstrates that the use of a low molecular weight heparin subcutaneously supplemented by vitamin K inhibition can be more effective than the standard intravenous unfractionated heparin treatment supplemented by vitamin K inhibition. Greater venographic improvement, less recurrence, and fewer bleeding complications are all desirable and were observed with the low–molecular-weight heparin regimen. Clearly, logistical and cost issues remain to be sorted out because outpatient therapy is still not covered by some insurers.

M. A. Golden, MD

Low Molecular Weight Heparin Versus Oral Anticoagulants in the Long-term Treatment of Deep Venous Thrombosis

López-Beret P, Orgaz A, Fontcuberta J, et al (Hosp Virgen de la Salud, Toledo, Spain)

J Vasc Surg 33:77-90, 2001   15–4

Introduction.—The long-term administration of low molecular weight heparins (LMWHs) for secondary prophylaxis of thromboembolic events has been used in patients with high risk of bleeding, those with complications from oral anticoagulants (OAs), and those with OA therapy that cannot be easily monitored. The effectiveness of LMWH therapy raises the question of whether LMWH may be used in the long-term treatment of all patients with deep vein thrombosis (DVT). One hundred fifty-eight patients with symptomatic DVT of the lower extremities were evaluated to determine whether LMWH is equal to or more effective than conventional OAs in the long-term treatment of DVT.

Methods.—All patients had DVT confirmed by duplex ultrasound scan. Patients were randomly assigned to 3 to 6 months of treatment with either nadroparine calcium or acenocoumarol. Quantitative and qualitative duplex scan scoring systems were used to examine the evolution of thrombosis in both groups at 1, 3, 6, and 12 months.

Results.—During the 12-month evaluation period, 2 of 81 patients (2.5%) who received LMWH and 7 of 77 (9%) who received OAs experienced recurrent DVTs (*P* = NS). There was no incidence of major bleeding in the LMWH group, compared with 4 patients in the OA group (*P* = NS). Mortality rates were 11.1% and 7.8%, respectively, in the LMWH and OA groups (*P* = NS) (Fig 1). The quantitative mean duplex scan score dropped in both groups during follow-up. This reached significance after long-term LMWH treatment for iliofemoral DVT (1, 3, 6, and 12 months), femoropopliteal DVT (1-3 months), and infrapopliteal DVT (first month). Duplex scan examination revealed that the rate of venous recanalization significantly rose in the common femoral vein at 6 and 12

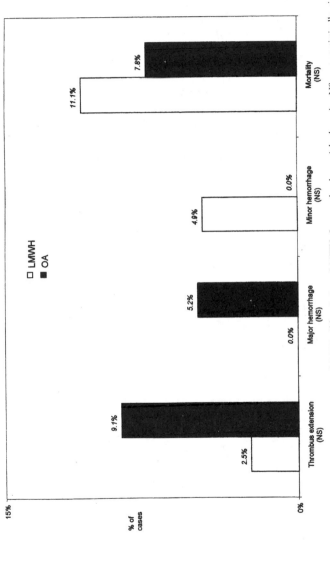

FIGURE 1.—Complications after long-term treatment of DVT. *Abbreviations: LMWH,* Low molecular weight heparin; *NS,* not statistically significant; *OA,* oral anticoagulants. (Courtesy of López-Beret P, Orgaz A, Fontcuberta J, et al: Low molecular weight heparin versus oral anticoagulants in the long-term treatment of deep venous thrombosis. *J Vasc Surg* 33:77-90, 2001.)

months and during each follow-up time point in the superficial and popliteal veins in the LMWH group. Reflux was significantly less common in communicating veins after LMWH treatment vs OA treatment (17.9% vs 32.2%). The reflux rates in the superficial (22.4%, LMWH; 30.6%, OA) and deep (13.4% vs 17.7%) venous systems revealed no significant differences between groups.

Conclusion.—The unmonitored subcutaneous administration of nadroparine in fixed daily doses was more effective than oral acenocoumarol with laboratory control adjustment in accomplishing recanalization of leg thrombi. Less late valvular communicating vein insufficiency was observed with nadroparine; it was at least as efficacious and safe as OAs after long-term administration. LMWHs may offer a real therapeutic advantage in the long-term management of DVT.

▶ Another article adding to the ongoing debate of LMWH versus oral anticoagulation in the long-term treatment of DVT. Previous studies have returned mixed data on bleeding complications between the 2 treatment regimens; however, treatment efficacy seems to be in favor of LMWH, as is seen in this study. Our own practice is to reserve the use of LMWH for those patients in whom oral anticoagulant therapy is clearly unsuccessful, a practice that is due in large part to the much higher cost of LMWH. As costs fall, I am sure there will be a greater trend to the use of LMWH for not only DVT but also pulmonary emboli.

W. K. Williamson, MD

Phlegmasia Cerulea Dolens of the Upper Extremity
Bolitho DG, Elwood ET, Roberts F (Emory Univ, Atlanta, Ga)
Ann Plast Surg 45:644-646, 2000   15–5

Introduction.—Phlegmasia cerulea dolens (PCD) is a severe form of peripheral venous thrombosis that is well described in the lower extremity. Its occurrence in the upper extremity is rare. Reported is a patient with PCD of the upper extremity who underwent amputation because of disease that was refractory to thrombolytic therapy.

> *Case Report.*—Man, 72, was hospitalized for diarrhea and vomiting. Past medical history included hypertension and chronic obstructive airway disease complicated by cor pulmonale and iron deficiency anemia. His stools were guaiac-positive and became positive for *Clostridium difficile* during hospitalization. A peripherally inserted central catheter had been placed in the right antecubital fossa during an earlier admission. Some swelling was noted in the ipsilateral extremity. The catheter was removed after administration of antibiotics. Within 2 days of removal, the patient developed severe pain associated with additional swelling and ecchymosis of the extremity distal to the midforearm (Fig 1A). On initial

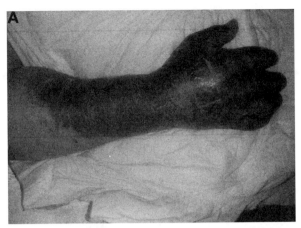

FIGURE 1.—A, The patient's arm at initial consultation. (Courtesy of Bolitho DG, Elwood ET, Roberts F: Phlegmasia cerulea dolens of the upper extremity. *Ann Plast Surg* 45:644-646, 2000.)

clinical examination, arterial pulsation was noted at the wrist, and sensation was noted in the distribution of the radial, median, and ulnar nerves. The patient had no clinical evidence of compartment syndrome. The capillary refill in the nailbed was preserved yet brisk, indicating venous congestion. After a diagnosis of PCD, urgent venography was performed via an antecubital vein. Complete occlusion of the brachial vein and thrombus extended to within the subclavian vein. Thrombolytic therapy was initiated, and an indwelling catheter was placed in an antecubital vein. Tissue plasminogen activator (tPA) was infused in an antegrade manner. Circulating fibrinogen levels, partial thrombin time, and the prothrombin index were assessed periodically. A trial of 36-hour thrombolytic therapy was administered using tPA in a dose of 1 to 2 mg/h. The patient experienced progressive loss of capillary refill with progression to frank venous gangrene. When it was determined that thrombolytic therapy had failed, anticoagulation therapy was started. Heparin was used to decrease the risk of proximal thromboembolism. The patient's mental status and renal function declined. There was marked deterioration of the viability of the skin with full-thickness necrosis. The involved extremity was amputated at the right midforearm immediately proximal to the level of venous staining. All veins transected at surgery contained organized thrombus. The patient required mechanical ventilation because of his precarious pulmonary status. His condition remained grave for the next 5 days, necessitating inotropic support. Additional active intervention was withheld as his family requested, and he died shortly thereafter.

Conclusion.—Upper extremity PCD was described in an elderly man with a complex medical history, complicated clinical course, and poor outcome, which is usual for this rare condition.

▶ PCD is bad. It does not happen very frequently in the upper extremity, but when it does it is bad there too. I wonder whether the increasing use of peripherally inserted central catheters (PICC lines), as was used in the patient in this report, will lead to an increased occurrence of this condition. We have avoided PICC lines in our patients because of the increased thrombotic risk. In vascular surgical patients, in whom usable peripheral vein is at a premium, it seems wise to stick with the internal jugular vein for long-term intravenous access when needed.

G. J. Landry, MD

A Comparison of the Safety and Efficacy of Oral Anticoagulation for the Treatment of Venous Thromboembolic Disease in Patients With or Without Malignancy

Palareti G, Legnani C, Lee A, et al (Univ Hosp S Orsola-Malpighi, Bologna, Italy; McMaster Univ, Hamilton, Ontario; Ospedale Regionale, Parma, Italy; et al)

Thromb Haemost 84:805-810, 2000   15–6

Objective.—The best treatment for acute venous thromboembolism (VTE) in cancer patients is controversial because of frequent monitoring requirements and excessive bleeding. The safety and effectiveness of oral anticoagulation therapy for the long-term treatment of acute VTE was prospectively examined in an inception cohort of patients with and without malignancy.

Methods.—From May 1993 to October 1994, 95 cancer patients (48 men), aged 29 to 86 years, and 733 patients (387 women), aged 14 to 93 years, without cancer were given oral anticoagulation therapy for acute leg deep vein thrombosis and/or pulmonary embolism. Bleeding incidence and episodes, thrombosis recurrence, and deaths were recorded. Differences between groups were analyzed statistically.

Results.—Compared with patients without cancer, cancer patients had significantly higher incidences of major bleeding (5.4% vs 0.9%), minor bleeding (16.2% vs 3.6%), and total bleeding (21.6% vs 4.5%) episodes. Patients without cancer were significantly more likely to complete anticoagulation therapy than cancer patients were (61.9% vs 39.0%). Compared with patients without cancer, cancer patients had a significantly higher death rate (32.6% vs 2.5%) and a significantly higher bleeding rate (4.2% vs 0.7%; relative risk factor [RR], 6.2). Cancer patients tended to have a higher thrombotic complication rate (6.8% vs 2.5%; RR, 2.5). Cancer patients had consistently high bleeding rates at all international normalized ratio (INR) levels. Patients without cancer had increased bleeding rates only at INR values higher than 4.5. Thrombosis recurrence was significantly higher in both the cancer and cancer-free groups at INR values lower than 2.0 (RR, 5.2 vs 3.0).

Conclusion.—Oral anticoagulation was associated with significantly more bleeding complications in cancer patients than in patients without cancer. There were also significantly more deaths among cancer patients, significantly more bleeding independent of the intensity of anticoagulation achieved, and a trend toward more venous thrombotic recurrences.

▶ The study confirms the clinical observation of many that bleeding and perhaps recurrent thrombosis are more frequent in patients with cancer. Granted, we need better therapy for this patient group. I wish this or some other study would give us a hint as to what it should be.

L. M. Taylor, Jr, MD

Postmenopausal Hormone Therapy Increases Risk for Venous Thromboembolic Disease: The Heart and Estrogen/progestin Replacement Study
Grady D, for the Heart and Estrogen/progestin Replacement Study Research Group (Univ of California, San Francisco; Emory Univ, Atlanta, Ga; Wake Forest Univ, Winston-Salem, NC; et al)
Ann Intern Med 132:689-696, 2000   15–7

Background.—Oral contraceptive use is known to increase the risk for venous thromboembolism, but limited data are available on the effect of postmenopausal hormone treatment. The effects of estrogen plus progestin therapy on the risk for venous thromboembolic events in postmenopausal women were investigated.

Methods.—Twenty clinical centers in the United States enrolled 2763 postmenopausal women in the randomized, double-blind, placebo-controlled study. All women were younger than 80 years and had coronary heart disease but no history of venous thromboembolism. None had had a hysterectomy. The women were assigned to conjugated equine estrogens, 0.625 mg, plus medroxyprogesterone acetate, 2.5 mg, or placebo. The mean follow-up was 4.1 years.

Findings.—Venous thromboembolic events occurred in 34 hormone treatment recipients and in 13 placebo recipients. The relative hazard ratio was 2.7. Multivariate analysis showed that the risk for venous thromboembolism was increased in women with lower-extremity fractures, the relative hazard being 18.1, or cancer, the relative hazard being 3.9. The risk was also increased for 90 days after inpatient surgery (relative hazard, 4.9) or nonsurgical hospitalization (relative hazard, 5.7). Aspirin and statin use reduced the risk.

Conclusion.—Estrogen plus progestin treatment in postmenopausal women with coronary heart disease increases the risk for venous thromboembolism. Clinicians need to consider this when weighing the risks and benefits of such therapy.

▶ In this very important article from the Heart and Estrogen/progestin Replacement Study, the investigators present the first randomized, prospective study to demonstrate an increased risk of venous thromboembolic events from postmenopausal hormone therapy. While subjects received combination therapy with conjugated estrogen and medroxyprogesterone, estrogen is believed to be primarily responsible for the increased thromboembolic risk. So what do we tell our postmenopausal vascular patients when they come into the clinic asking if it is safe for them to be on hormone replacement? First, it is important to examine the scope of the problem. After a mean follow-up of 4 years, the incidence of thromboembolic events was 2.4% in subjects receiving hormone replacement therapy versus 0.9% in those receiving placebo, for a relative hazard of 2.7. Furthermore, subjects at increased risk of thromboembolic events were those who had other significant risks, namely, lower extremity fractures, cancer, or prolonged periods of immobility. Therefore, it appears as though the average postmenopausal woman without other significant risk factors for thromboembolic events can safely undergo hormonal replacement therapy.

G. J. Landry, MD

Low-Molecular-Weight Heparin Prophylaxis Using Dalteparin in Close Proximity to Surgery vs Warfarin in Hip Arthroplasty Patients: A Double-blind, Randomized Comparison
Hull RD, for the North American Fragmin Trial Investigators (Univ of Calgary, Alberta, Canada; Calgary Gen Hosp, Alberta, Canada; Foothills Med Ctr, Calgary, Alberta, Canada; et al)
Arch Intern Med 160:2199-2207, 2000   15–8

Background.—Both perioperative and postoperative venous thrombosis occur commonly among high-risk patients who are having surgery. Of those receiving hip implants, 40% to 60% have venous thrombosis, so prophylactic medications are used, generally warfarin sodium and subcutaneous low molecular weight heparin. The timing of prophylaxis was reviewed for its effect on the efficacy of therapy.

Methods.—The 1472 patients studied received either subcutaneous dalteparin sodium (given once daily) administered immediately before or early after surgery or warfarin sodium given postoperatively. Contrast venography was performed to assess whether deep vein thrombosis occurred postoperatively.

Results.—Four hundred ninety-six patients received preoperative dalteparin, 487 received postoperative dalteparin, and 489 received warfarin. The frequencies of deep vein thrombosis for patients were 36 (10%) for preoperative dalteparin, 44 (13.1%) for postoperative dalteparin, and 81 (24%) for warfarin. Proximal deep vein thrombosis occurred at frequencies of 3 patients (0.8%) for preoperative dalteparin, 3 (0.8%) for postoperative dalteparin, and 11 (3.0%) for warfarin. Relative risk reductions ranged from 45% to 72% among the dalteparin groups and the warfarin group. The preoperative group had fewer instances of symptomatic thrombi than those receiving warfarin, but serious bleeding occurred with similar frequencies. Patients who received preoperative dalteparin had increased major bleeding at the surgical site when compared with those receiving warfarin.

Conclusions.—Substantial risk reductions for deep vein thrombosis were noted when dalteparin was given in close proximity to surgery. Postoperative warfarin therapy did not produce equivalent reductions. Comparison of the use of low molecular weight heparin either 12 hours preoperatively or 12 to 24 hours postoperatively with oral anticoagulants has not shown these findings. Patients who received the preoperative dalteparin had increased major bleeding, but it was not serious. Overall, dalteparin given just before the operation or just after the operation was more effective in preventing deep vein thrombosis than warfarin among this population of patients undergoing hip arthroplasty.

▶ This well-conducted clinical trial represents a true advance in prophylaxis for deep vein thrombosis (DVT) in total hip arthroplasty patients. "Just in time" prophylaxis with a low molecular weight heparin (LMWH), dalteparin, allows more freedom in choice of anesthetic, because patients will not be anticoagulated at surgery, and regional anesthesia can be used. This "just in time" strategy allows for equivalent prophylaxis against DVT with decreased bleeding complications when compared with standard perioperative warfarin or LMWH regimens. And, as we all know, any advance that will decrease the cognitive requirements of orthopedic surgery will be greatly appreciated by orthopedic surgeons and by their referring internists as well.

E. J. Harris, Jr, MD

Greenfield Filter

Lessons Learned From a 6-Year Clinical Experience With Superior Vena Cava Greenfield Filters

Ascher E, Hingorani A, Tsemekhin B, et al (Maimonides Med Ctr, Brooklyn, NY)
J Vasc Surg 32:881–887, 2000   15–9

Background.—In the face of ongoing debate, the authors' center favors an aggressive approach to the treatment of upper extremity deep vein thrombosis (UEDVT). For patients with contraindications to anticoagulation or with pulmonary embolism despite anticoagulation, placement of a superior vena cava (SVC) filter may be beneficial. An experience with Greenfield SVC filter placement for prevention of pulmonary embolism in patients with UEDVT is reported.

Methods.—The 6.5-year experience included 72 patients (47 women and 25 men; mean age, 74 years) with UEDVT who underwent Greenfield

TABLE 3.—Comparison of SVC and IVC Filters

	SVC Filter ($n = 72$)	IVC Filter ($n = 72$)	P Value
Mean follow-up ± SEM (mo)	7.8 ± 2	10 ± 1.9	.25
In-hospital death (%)	47	12.5	< .001
Posthospital death (%)	6	43	< .001
Mean time to death ± SEM (mo)	0.7 ± 0.2	4.6 ± 0.8	< .001

Abbreviations: SVC, Superior vena cava; *IVC*, inferior vena cava.
(Courtesy of Ascher E, Hingorani A, Tsemekhin B, et al: Lessons learned from a 6-year clinical experience with superior vena cava Greenfield filters. *J Vasc Surg* 32:881-887, 2000.)

SVC filter placement. Anticoagulation was contraindicated in 67 patients and ineffective in preventing recurrent pulmonary embolism or thrombus extension in 5. The patients were followed up for a mean of 7.8 months after filter placement.

Results.—Subsequent chest radiographs in 26 patients, obtained for reasons other than follow-up of the SVC filter, showed no evidence of filter migration or displacement. In-hospital deaths occurred in 34 patients, a mean of 20 days after filter placement, from causes unrelated to the SVC filter or to recurrent thromboembolism. After a mean follow-up of 22 months, none of the survivors had any signs of pulmonary embolism. One patient had a filter incorrectly placed in the innominate vein, which remained patent at 2 months' follow-up.

Conclusions.—This experience supports placement of Greenfield SVC filters for prevention of recurrent thromboembolic events in patients with UEDVT, in cases in which anticoagulation is contraindicated or ineffective. Comparative data on patients with SVC versus inferior vena cava filters (Table 3) are included. Further study is needed to confirm the safety and efficacy of Greenfield SVC filter placement.

▶ The authors of this article have a great deal of experience with vena cava filter placement. Not only am I surprised by the number of patients enrolled in this series, I am equally surprised by the number of patients who had DVT of the lower extremity and required filter placement. In 30% of the patients with lower extremity DVT, an inferior vena cave filter was placed. This difference, compared with our own experience, must be due to referral patterns because the indications stated in this article are similar to our own. It is important to note that PE was diagnosed in 5 (7%) of the patients and that 32% of the patients in this series also had lower extremity DVT. What the authors don't state is whether these 5 patients also had concomitant lower extremity DVT. Further follow-up of these 5 patients with PE would have been helpful in discerning the efficacy of a filter in the SVC. Were the patients in whom PE was diagnosed the most sick and those who subsequently died, or were the patients with PE among the 26 remaining survivors who were discharged from the hospital? I am surprised that migration was not more common in this series because the SVC seems to be more mobile in its relationship to the right atrium. Perhaps the mean follow-up by chest radiograph, obtained in this series for other reasons, is a bit short. Given this worry, I would be more inclined to obtain a chest film every 3 months for the first year to observe for filter migration. Finally, a removable filter may be appropriate in the SVC for select patients. To my knowledge, the Food and Drug Administration has not approved removal of removable filters but, rather, only placement of them.

R. B. McLafferty, MD

Prognosis of Cancers Associated With Venous Thromboembolism
Sørensen HT, Mellemkjær L, Olsen JH, et al (Aarhus Univ, Denmark; Inst of Cancer Epidemiology, Copenhagen; Dartmouth Med School, Hanover, NH)
N Engl J Med 343:1846-1850, 2000   15–10

Background.—The prognosis of cancer found during or after an episode of venous thromboembolism is a recognized risk but whether the relationship has implications for the clinical course of the cancer remains unclear. Population-based data were analyzed to determine the association between a history of venous thromboembolism and extent of disease at the time of cancer diagnosis.

Methods.—The Danish National Registry of Patients, the Danish Cancer Registry, and the Danish Mortality Files were linked to obtain data on the survival of patients given a diagnosis of cancer at the same time as or

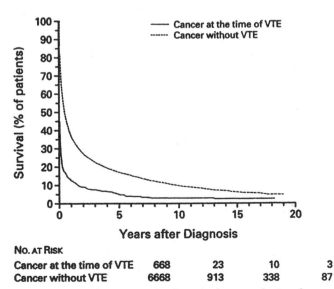

FIGURE 1.—Survival curves for patients with a diagnosis of cancer at the time of venous thromboembolism (*VTE*) and matched control patients with cancer. The control patients, who did not have VTE, were matched with the patients who had VTE according to cancer type, sex, age, and year of diagnosis. *P* < .001 for the overall curves, by the log-rank test. (Reprinted by permission of *The New England Journal of Medicine* from Sørensen HT, Mellemkjær L, Olsen JH, et al: Prognosis of cancers associated with venous thromboembolism. *N Engl J Med* 343:1846-1850, 2000. Copyright 2000, Massachusetts Medical Society. All rights reserved.)

after an episode of venous thromboembolism. Six hundred eighty-eight such patients were matched by type of cancer, age, sex, and year of diagnosis to a control group of 5371 patients with cancer but no venous thromboembolism.

Findings.—Forty-four percent of the patient group and 35.1% of the control group had distant metastasis. Survival at 1 year was 12% in the patient group and 36% in the control group (Fig 1). The mortality ratio for the whole follow-up period was 2.20. Patients with a diagnosis of cancer within 1 year after venous thromboembolism had a slightly increased risk for distant metastasis at the time of diagnosis and a somewhat lower rate of survival at 1 year.

Conclusion.—Cancer diagnosed at the same time as or within 1 year of an episode of venous thromboembolism carries a poor prognosis. The stage of cancer in such patients tends to be advanced.

▶ In a group of more than 600 patients with known cancer at the time of their venous thromboembolism, the 1-year survival rate was only 12%. Data such as these may have implications on how aggressively we should treat patients with advanced cancer and thromboembolism in view of the fact that their prognosis is poor.[1]

J. L. Mills, Sr, MD

Reference

1. 2000 YEAR BOOK OF VASCULAR SURGERY, p 460.

Clinical Outcome and Cost of Hospital vs Home Treatment of Proximal Deep Vein Thrombosis With a Low-Molecular-Weight Heparin: The Vascular Midi-Pyrenees Study
Boccalon H, for the Vascular Midi-Pyrenees Network Group (Centre Hospitalier Universitaire, Toulouse, France)
Arch Intern Med 160:1769-1773, 2000   15–11

Objective.—Care of patients with deep venous thrombosis (DVT) is expensive. The introduction of low molecular weight heparins (LMWH), with their improved bioavailability, longer plasma half-life, and better efficacy-safety ratio, has opened up the possibility of outpatient treatment for proximal DVT. Clinical outcomes and costs of DVT treatment were compared for outpatient and inpatient settings in a randomized, comparative, multicenter trial.

Methods.—From September 1993 to April 1997, LMWH were administered to DVT patients for 10 days in the hospital and then at home (n = 102) or at home only (n = 99). The primary end point was the incidence of DVT recurrence, pulmonary embolism, or major bleeding. An economic analysis compared the cost of treating complications and the direct medical costs of inpatient versus outpatient care during the first 10 days. The number of days of treatment, the number of nursing visits, and the number of biochemical analyses were collected prospectively. Patients' status was followed for 6 months.

Results.—Of the screened patients, 11.8% were eligible and gave informed consent. There were 38 patients (18.9%) who did not complete follow-up. Almost twice as many hospitalized patients as home patients were withdrawn from the study, most by patient request. Four hospitalized patients and 3 home patients were withdrawn because of DVT extensions (n = 3) and major hemorrhage (n = 4). Two hospitalized patients died of their underlying diseases. Minor bleeding was reported in 11 inpatients and 17 outpatients. The costs of the initial 10-day hospital treatment for outpatients versus inpatients were Fr 9230 versus Fr 20932. Outpatient management decreased costs by 56%.

Conclusion.—Costs of outpatient care are significantly lower than the costs of inpatient care for patient with DVT, while complication rates are comparable.

▶ This well-designed trial demonstrates similar efficacy and reduced cost (56%) for LMWH outpatient treatment compared with inpatient treatment of proximal (iliac, femoral, or popliteal) DVT. However, before we (and, more important, the third-party payers) conclude that DVT is now an outpatient disease, it is important to note a few details from this important trial. Only 12% of the total patients with proximal DVT screened during the trial were eligible for randomization. Of those excluded, 60% were excluded because their DVT occurred while they were inpatients for another cause, but 40% were excluded for other reasons, including inappropriateness for outpatient therapy. In addition, although 75% of the outpatient arm in the trial had hospitalizations of less than 24 hours, 9% stayed more than 2 days.

These observations are important because, as similar data accumulate, DVT will be considered an exclusively outpatient disease. We all have had situations in which medical director for an HMO has denied payment for a hospitalization because, in his or her opinion (remote from the clinical situation), the intravenous antibiotics should have been delivered in an outpatient setting, despite patient/clinical circumstances that would have made this suboptimal. I am certain that similar arguments will be used in the future against the inpatient treatment of DVT.

M. R. Nehler, MD

A Population-Based Study of the Effectiveness of Inferior Vena Cava Filter Use Among Patients With Venous Thromboembolism
White RH, Zhou H, Kim J, et al (Univ of California-Davis)
Arch Intern Med 160:2033-2041, 2000   15–12

Background.—Generally an inferior vena cava (IVC) filter is inserted if anticoagulant therapy has failed or a strict contraindication to the use of anticoagulant therapy is present, but these indications have been relaxed.

It has been suggested that the filter alone may achieve the desired therapeutic result as well as combining the use of the filter with heparin sodium plus warfarin sodium treatment; in addition, the incidence of adverse outcomes may be the same as or less than that shown with use of combined treatment. The 1-year cumulative incidence of venous thrombosis or pulmonary embolism (PE) requiring hospitalization in patients with thromboembolism who received a vena cava filter was compared with the incidence seen in a control group of patients with thromboembolism.

Methods.—A retrospective analysis was performed covering 3632 patients who had filter treatment and 64,333 control patients admitted to the hospital with a primary diagnosis of venous thromboembolism.

Results.—Patients who were treated with filters had significantly increased comorbidity. Findings included more instances of previous pulmonary embolism, recent major bleeding episodes, malignant neoplasms, and strokes. Patients hospitalized for PE had a significantly greater likelihood of being readmitted for the same diagnosis when compared with patients whose initial diagnosis was venous thrombosis only, regardless of treatment. Placement of a filter carried a significantly higher relative risk for rehospitalization for venous thrombosis if the patient initially had PE than when the patient had venous thrombosis. No significant difference was shown between those receiving filters and control subjects with respect to the relative hazard of rehospitalization for PE.

Conclusions.—At 1 year, the incidence of rehospitalization for PE was not significantly reduced by the insertion of a vena cava filter. Patients who initially had PE had a higher incidence of rehospitalization for venous thrombosis; those who did not initially have PE did not show this association.

▶ The authors use a cumbersome, population-based retrospective analysis of linked hospital discharge abstracts in California over a 5-year period. By analyzing patients with venous thromboembolism treated with and without IVC filters, the authors conclude that an IVC filter does not significantly reduce rehospitalization for PE at 1 year and may be associated with increased rehospitalization for venous thrombosis. With no information on the concurrent use of anticoagulation, and no standard indication for IVC filter placement, it is hard to make sense of the data. A recent randomized, controlled trial reported by Decousus et al[1] concluded that the initial beneficial effect of IVC filters for the prevention of PE in patients with proximal DVT was counterbalanced by an excess rate of recurrent DVT in these patients with no difference in mortality rate at 2 years. The results of Decousus, et al are much easier to interpret and avoid the pitfalls of this retrospective study based on hospital discharge diagnosis. Vena cava filters should be reserved for those patients who have failed anticoagulation, or have true contraindications to anticoagulation.

A. M. Abou-Zamzam, Jr, MD

Reference

1. Decousus H, Leizorovicz A, Parent F, et al: A clinical trial of vena caval filters in the prevention of pulmonary embolism in patients with proximal deep vein thrombosis. *N Engl J Med* 338:409-415, 1998.

Inferior Vena Caval Filters: Review of a 26-Year Single-Center Clinical Experience
Athanasoulis CA, Kaufman JA, Halpern EF, et al (Harvard Med School, Boston)
Radiology 216:54-66, 2000   15–13

Background.—The standard approach to the management of venous thromboembolism is anticoagulant therapy. In patients for whom there are contraindications to the use of anticoagulants, other management methods may be used to prevent the passage of large emboli to the lungs. Until the early 1970s, surgical ligation, plication, or clipping of the inferior vena cava were the methods of choice. However, substantial morbidity was associated with surgical caval interruption. In the late 1960s, an early umbrella type of filter was introduced, but an unacceptably high incidence of caval thrombosis was associated with this filter and ultimately led to its demise. Further technological advances culminated in the Greenfield stainless steel device, which eventually became the standard caval filter. The first true percutaneous filter, the Bird's Nest device, was introduced in 1983 and released for clinical use in 1987. A single center's 26-year experience with inferior vena caval filters was evaluated.

Methods.—From 1973 to 1998, 1765 filters were implanted in 1731 patients (Fig 5). Medical records for each patient were reviewed, and data regarding indications, safety, effectiveness, numbers, and types of caval filters were collected. The primary outcome was the occurrence of fatal postfilter pulmonary embolism (PE). Secondary outcomes were morbidity and mortality, and survival and morbidity-free survival curves were calculated.

Results.—Observed postfilter PE had a prevalence of 5.6%. For 3.7% of patients, the postfilter PE was fatal. Fatal PE occurred at a median of 4 days after insertion in most patients. Major complications occurred in 0.3% of procedures. Observed postfilter caval thrombosis had a prevalence of 2.7%. The overall mortality rate at 30 days was 17%, and was higher among patients with neoplasms (19.5%) than among those without neoplasms (14.3%). For 46 patients with suprarenal filters, filter efficacy and associated morbidity were not different. The overall rate of filters placed for prophylaxis was 4.7%, which increased to 16.4% in 1998. Caval filter implantation increased fivefold from 1980 to 1998. In more recent years, more filters were implanted in younger patients.

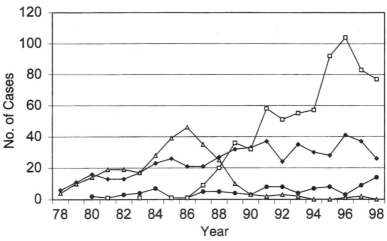

FIGURE 5.—Graph shows types of imaging examinations used to confirm venous thromboembolism: *filled diamond*, pulmonary angiography, *open squares*, venous US, *triangle*, conventional venography, and *filled circle*, ventilation-perfusion lung scans. (Courtesy of Athanasoulis CA, Kaufman JA, Halpern EF, et al: Inferior vena caval filters: Review of a 26-year single-center clinical experience. *Radiology* 216:54-66, 2000, Radiological Society of North America.)

Conclusions.—Inferior vena caval filters were shown to be effective in protecting patients from life-threatening PE. Morbidity associated with the use of these filters was minimal.

▶ This observational retrospective review of a 26-year experience with inferior vena caval filters at Massachusetts General Hospital provides some worthwhile information. While the authors used inferior vena caval filters to protect against PE, they identified an unfortunate, residual incidence of PE after filter placement (5.6% overall, 3.6% fatal). The morbidity of filter placement was low, with only a 2.7% incidence of caval thrombosis after exclusion of the outdated Mobin-Uddin filter. The placement of a suprarenal filter, when necessary, was not associated with increased risk. There was a significant increased use of caval filters in young trauma patients, and the authors predict that development of a temporary, retrievable filter device will have broad application in the future.

R. A. Yeager, MD

Duodenocaval Fistula: A Life-Threatening Condition of Various Origins
Guillem PG, Binot D, Dupuy-Cuny J, et al (Hôpital Huriez, Lille, France; Clinique de la Côte d'Opale, Boulogne, France; Ctr Hosp de Valenciennes, France)
J Vasc Surg 33:643-645, 2001   15–14

Introduction.—Duodenocaval fistulas are rare. The etiology, clinical diagnosis, and management of 2 cases and a literature review are presented.

Case 1.—Man, 73, with fever, chills, and weight loss for 3 weeks, and with right nephrectomy and radiotherapy 20 months earlier, had an elevated white cell count, microcytic anemia, and several digestive tract bacteria. Endoscopy revealed a congested duodenum with leakage into the inferior vena cava on contrast swallow radiograph. CT confirmed a duodenocaval fistula. Dense retroperitoneal fibrosis was dissected, the duodenum was mobilized, and the fistula was sutured. Duodenal exclusion was performed by gastroenterostomy and antral stapling, vagotomy, and epiploic patch interposition. Postoperatively, the patient had cardiorespiratory failure. A subhepatic abscess was surgically drained. The duodenal leakage progressively dried up, and the patient was discharged in 37 days. His symptoms disappeared in 6 months, and he was able to eat a regular diet.

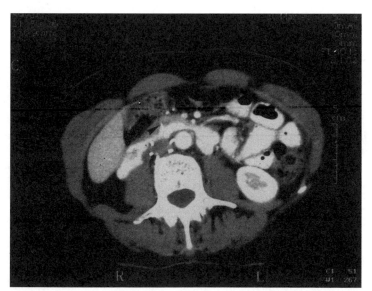

FIGURE 2.—Transverse abdominal CT scan showing protrusion of caval filter's strut into duodenal lumen (*arrowhead*). (Courtesy of Guillem PG, Binot D, Dupuy-Cuny J, et al: Duodenocaval fistula: A life-threatening condition of various origins. *J Vasc Surg* 33:643-645, 2001.)

Case 2.—Woman, 60, had abdominal and lumbar pain for 3 months and a caval filter placed earlier for thrombophlebitis and recurrent pulmonary infarction. An abdominal US was normal except for a slight choledochal dilatation. Endoscopy revealed a metallic strut protruding into the lumen of the duodenum, resulting in a fistula (Fig 2). The fistula was dissected using laparotomy, and the filter was removed. The inferior vena cava was sutured with a prosthetic patch. The patient required reoperation for bleeding on day 3 to ligate a disrupted venous collateral branch. At 6 months, she was doing well.

Conclusion.—Duodenocaval fistulas are life-threatening with high mortality for all etiologies except migrating caval filters. With the latter, the prognosis is improved, probably because of early diagnosis. The fistula is repaired surgically, and the procedures include measures to prevent recurrence, particularly where ulcers can result.

▶ While the chance of a vascular surgeon in practice encountering a duodenocaval fistula is small, it is worth considering the diagnosis and management of this condition, however briefly. Migration of vena caval filters, tumor resection and radiation therapy, peptic duodenal ulcers, and ingested foreign bodies were the most likely causes. Patients presented with gastrointestinal bleeding, sepsis, or both. The group of patients with migration of vena caval filters as the cause of the fistula had a mortality rate of only 10% as opposed to a 60% mortality rate for other causes.

J. M. Edwards, MD

Pulmonary Embolism

Balloon Pulmonary Angioplasty for Treatment of Chronic Thromboembolic Pulmonary Hypertension
Feinstein JA, Goldhaber SZ, Lock JE, et al (Harvard Med School, Boston)
Circulation 103:10-13, 2001   15–15

Objective.—Not all patients with chronic thromboembolic pulmonary hypertension (CTEPH) are candidates for pulmonary thromboendarterectomy. An alternative interventional strategy of balloon pulmonary angioplasty (BPA) is described.

Methods.—Between October 1994 and February 1999, BPA was performed in 18 patients with CTEPH aged 14 to 75 years (Fig 1).

Technique.—The pulmonary artery segment selected for dilatation had to be completely occluded, have a filling defect, or have signs of intravascular webs. Segments were sequentially dilatated. Balloons were inflated by hand under fluoroscopic guidance, and dilatation was repeated if there was less than 50% increase ob-

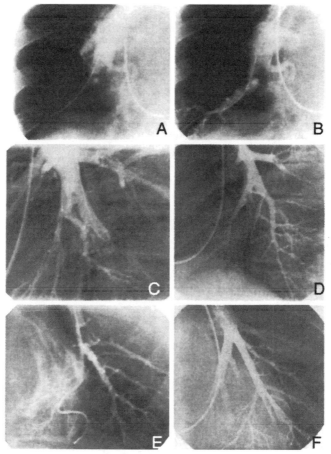

FIGURE 1.—Angiographic appearance of occluded (**A, C**), and stenotic (**E**) lower lobe pulmonary artery segmental branches that were deemed surgically inaccessible. They are horizontally paired with angiograms performed immediately after successful BPA (**B, D,** and **F**). (Courtesy of Feinstein JA, Goldhaber SZ, Lock JE, et al: Balloon pulmonary angioplasty for treatment of chronic thromboembolic pulmonary hypertension. *Circulation* 103:10-13, 2001.)

served on angiography. Patients were observed for 2 days, and catheterization was repeated after 6 to 12 weeks.

Results.—One patient died 7 days after the procedure of right ventricular failure. The remaining patients were followed up for an average of 35.9 months. New York Heart Association class and 6-minute walk distances improved significantly (Fig 2). Reperfusion pulmonary edema developed in 11 patients, 3 required mechanical ventilation, and 1 died.

A

New York Heart Association Classification

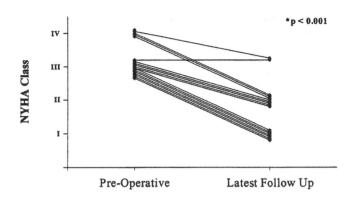

B **Six Minute Walk Capacity**

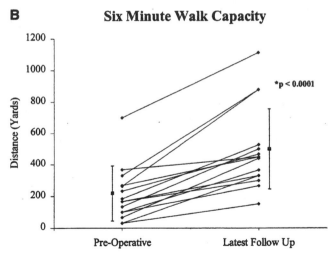

FIGURE 2.—NYHA classification (A) and 6-minute walk capacity (B) before BPA and at latest follow up. (Courtesy of Feinstein JA, Goldhaber SZ, Lock JE, et al: Balloon pulmonary angioplasty for treatment of chronic thromboembolic pulmonary hypertension. *Circulation* 103:10-13, 2001.)

Conclusion.—Extending BPA to patients with CTEPH is promising but expensive and labor intensive. Controlled randomized trials are needed to validate the use of BPA with maximal medical therapy.

▶ The authors describe their use of pulmonary balloon angioplasty in the treatment of patients with chronic thromboembolic pulmonary hypertension who are not surgical candidates because of surgical risk or inaccessibility of the thrombus. At a mean of 3 years after treatment, patients demonstrated continued clinical improvement. The treatment was not without risk because two thirds of the patients had postprocedure pulmonary edema and 1 died. The results are promising enough that the authors call for a randomized trial of angioplasty versus medical therapy in patients who are not surgical candidates.

J. M. Edwards, MD

Low-Molecular-Weight Heparin vs Heparin in the Treatment of Patients With Pulmonary Embolism
Hull RD, for the American-Canadian Thrombosis Study Group (Univ of Calgary, Alberta, Canada; Univ of Oklahoma, Oklahoma City; Univ of Utah, Salt Lake City; et al)
Arch Intern Med 160:229-236, 2000   15–16

Background.—Fifty percent of patients who have proximal deep vein thrombosis (DVT) also have pulmonary embolism (PE). The treatment of DVT with low molecular weight heparin is both effective and safe, which indicates that it may also be useful in treating PE. The effectiveness of low molecular weight heparin was compared with that of IV heparin in the treatment of patients with PE and underlying proximal DVT in a double-blind study.

Methods.—A fixed dose of subcutaneous low molecular weight heparin was given once a day to 213 patients, and an additional 219 patients received dose-adjusted IV heparin given by continuous infusion. The presence of PE was documented by high-probability lung scans.

Results.—Four hundred nineteen patients had lung scans; 200 had high-probability findings, 183 had nondiagnostic patterns, and 36 had normal results. One hundred three of the 219 who received IV heparin and 97 of those receiving subcutaneous heparin had high-probability scan findings. More elderly patients were in the low molecular weight heparin treatment group, but no effect of age was noted. None of the 97 receiving subcutaneous heparin had new episodes of venous thromboembolism; seven of the 103 receiving IV heparin did. One patient given subcutaneous heparin and 2 given IV heparin had major bleeding episodes.

Conclusions.—In the prevention of recurrent venous thromboembolism in patients with PE and associated DVT, the use of low molecular weight heparin given subcutaneously once daily was at least as effective and perhaps more so than the use of IV heparin.

▶ Evidence continues to mount favoring low molecular weight heparin in the treatment of venous thromboembolism. The American-Canadian Thrombosis Study Group compares low molecular weight and IV heparin in this prospective, randomized, double-blind trial of patients with proximal DVT and high-probability perfusion lung scans. Initially 432 consecutive patients with proximal DVT were enrolled in the study, of whom 419 patients underwent lung scanning. Altogether, 200 (47.7%) of these patients had high-probability scans consistent with PE. Of note is that only 14% of these patients had clinical symptoms of PE. The 200 patients with high-probability scans were randomly chosen to receive either standard IV heparin or low molecular weight heparin. Significantly more patients treated with standard IV heparin experienced new episodes of venous thromboembolism (6.8%) compared with patients treated with low molecular weight heparin (0%). Bleeding complications were the same in both groups.

R. A. Yeager, MD

Decreasing Mortality From Pulmonary Embolism in the United States, 1979–1996
Lilienfeld DE (Bristol-Myers Squibb Corp, Princeton, NJ)
Int J Epidemiol 29:465-469, 2000   15–17

Background.—Previous research had shown that mortality from pulmonary embolism (PE) declined between the early 1960s and the middle 1980s. Such decreases have also been reported in the Medicare beneficiary population between 1984 and 1991. Because the US health care delivery system has changed dramatically since 1991, trends in mortality from PE were investigated between 1979 and 1996.

Methods and Findings.—Data on annual age-specific and age-adjusted PE mortality among US residents between 1979 and 1996 were obtained from the US National Center for Health Statistics. Age-adjusted mortality declined in all racial groups and in both sexes during that period (Fig 1).

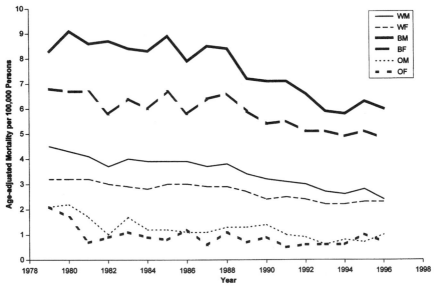

FIGURE 1.—Annual age-adjusted pulmonary embolism mortality in the United States, by race and sex, 1979-1996. (Courtesy of Lilienfeld DE: Decreasing mortality from pulmonary embolism in the United States, 1979–1996. *Int J Epidemiol* 29:465-469, 2000. Reproduced by permission of Oxford University Press.)

The greatest rate of decrease occurred among black men, followed by black women, white men, other men, white women, and other women (in descending order). Despite these declines, blacks still had the highest mortality rate from PE, followed by whites and others. In addition, rates of death from PE were greater among men than women. The mortality rate increased during the life span (ie, the risk doubled with each decade of life). The annual age-adjusted rates of death from PE in 1996 were 2.4 per 100,000 white men, 2.3 per 100,000 white women, 6 per 100,000 black men, 4.8 per 100,00 black women, 1 per 100,000 men of other races, and 0.7 per 100,000 women of other races.

Conclusions.—Between 1979 and 1996, mortality from PE among US residents declined significantly. Differences in such mortality among racial groups and between men and women persist.

▶ This article from epidemiology documents a decrease in United States mortality rates for pulmonary embolism between the years 1979 and 1996. The source for this data is death certificate information. Because of the reduction in autopsy data in the United States, death certificate information has become the sole source for cause of death in epidemiologic studies. As any clinician knows, the accuracy of death certificate data ranges greatly, particularly with a clinical entity such as pulmonary embolism, which can be difficult to diagnose. It is encouraging that these findings are mirrored by a previous UK study, which demonstrated a reduction in prevalence of pulmonary embolism at autopsy, which is noted in the discussion. The obvious conclusion is that mortality reduction is due to improved DVT prophylaxis and changes in clinical practice.

M. R. Nehler, MD

Short-term Clinical Outcome of Patients With Acute Pulmonary Embolism, Normal Blood Pressure, and Echocardiographic Right Ventricular Dysfunction
Grifoni S, Olivotto I, Cecchini P, et al (Univ of Perugia, Italy; Azienda Ospedaliera Careggi, Florence, Italy)
Circulation 101:2817-2822, 2000   15–18

Introduction.—The prognostic value of right ventricular (RV) dysfunction in patients with pulmonary embolism (PE) and normal blood pressure (BP) has not been addressed specifically. The prevalence and short-term prognosis of patients with objectively confirmed PE, normal BP, and echocardiographic RV dysfunction were prospectively assessed in 209 consecutive patients.

Methods.—The mean age of 84 men and 125 women was 65 years (range, 18-90 years). Patients were considered to have RV dysfunction if they had one or more of the following: (1) RV dilatation (end-diastolic diameter greater than 30 mm or RV/left ventricular end-diastolic diameter ratio greater than 1 in 4-chamber view), (2) paradox septal systolic motion, and (3) pulmonary hypertension. When PE was suspected, patients received IV heparin. A bolus dose of 80 IU/kg was followed by an 18-IU·kg^{-1}·h^{-1} infusion rate, which was later adjusted to maintain the activated partial thromboplastin time between 60 and 90 seconds in patients with a confirmed diagnosis. Thrombolytic treatment was started in patients with confirmed PE and hemodynamic impairment as appropriate. Four different patient profiles were used for prognostic assessment: (1) patients with shock or cardiac failure, (2) patients who were hypotensive without shock, (3) normotensive patients with RV dysfunction, and (4) normotensive patients without RV dysfunction. Hypotension was defined as a systolic BP below 100 mm Hg, and normotension was defined as a systolic BP of 100 mm Hg or above.

Results.—Diagnosis of PE was made on the basis of a high-probability lung scan in 145 patients (69%), a positive CT scan in 31 (15%), and a positive pulmonary angiography in 29 patients (14%). Of 209 patients, 162 (78%) were clinically stable and normotensive, and 47 (22%) had a systolic BP of less than 100 mm Hg. Of the latter, 28 were in shock. All except 2 patients with cardiac arrest underwent echocardiographic examination. Patients were categorized as (1) presenting with shock or cardiac arrest (n = 28, 13%), (2) hypotensive without shock (n = 19, 9%), (3) normotensive with RV dysfunction (n = 65, 31%), and (4) normotensive without RV dysfunction (n = 97, 47%). Thirty-one patients (15%) underwent initial administration of thrombolytic treatment, and 3 patients were treated with recombinant tissue-type plasminogen activator (rtPA) or urokinase. Two thrombolytic-treated patients had severe complications. There were 17 deaths (18%) during admission; 13 were directly related to PE. Echocardiography showed a 100% negative predictive value for death related to PE, although it had a low positive predictive value. Of 65 patients with RV dysfunction who were normotensive on initial evaluation, 6 (10%) had clinical deterioration and developed shock, despite heparin treatment. Three of these patients died shortly after the event, and 3 were successfully treated with urgent thrombolysis started at the time of clinical deterioration. The following variables were correlated with short-term clinical worsening or PE-related death among the 65 patients who were normotensive and had RV dysfunction: advanced age, recent trauma or orthopedic treatment, and lower systolic BP and dizziness on initial evaluation.

Conclusion.—Thirty-one percent of patients with acute PE who were normotensive had RV dysfunction. These patients with latent hemodynamic impairment had a 10% rate of PE-related shock and a 95% in-hospital mortality rate. They may need aggressive therapeutic approaches. Patients who are normotensive without RV dysfunction tend to have a benign short-term prognosis. Early detection of echographic RV dysfunction is highly important in the risk stratification of normotensive patients with acute PE.

▶ The clinical manifestations of pulmonary embolism range from no symptoms to complete cardiovascular collapse. When patients have hemodynamic compromise, aggressive treatment is clearly indicated. There are, however, a large number of patients who present with pulmonary embolus and normal blood pressure. These authors used echocardiography to examine patients with PE and normal blood pressure and found that 40% had evidence of RV dysfunction. Of the patients with RV dysfunction, 10% subsequently developed shock and 5% died. In the group of 97 patients with normal blood pressure and no evidence of RV dysfunction, there were no episodes of PE-related shock or death. This suggests that an early echocardiogram may be very useful in risk stratification of patients presenting with acute PE. Perhaps those with no evidence of RV dysfunction can undergo outpatient therapy with LMWH, and greater consideration should be given to early thrombolysis in patients with RV dysfunction. Further prospective, randomized studies will be needed to validate treatment options stratified by echo findings. These authors were able to obtain echos within 1 hour of admission. Clearly, this is not a widespread phenomenon.

A. M. Abou-Zamzam, Jr, MD

Prevention of Pulmonary Embolism and Deep Vein Thrombosis With Low Dose Aspirin: Pulmonary Embolism Prevention (PEP) Trial
Rodgers A, for the Pulmonary Embolism Prevention (PEP) Trial Collaborative Group (Univ of Auckland, New Zealand; et al)
Lancet 355:1295-1302, 2000   15–19

Introduction.—Earlier trials of antiplatelet therapy for prevention of venous thromboembolism (VTE) have been inconclusive. A meta-analysis of their findings shows decreases in the risks of deep-vein thrombosis and pulmonary embolism in various high-risk groups. A randomized placebo-controlled Pulmonary Embolism Prevention (PEP) trial of low-dose aspirin was performed to verify or refute its benefits in patients at increased risk of VTE and to determine the effects on perioperative bleeding.

Methods.—Between 1992 and 1994, 148 hospitals in Australia, New Zealand, South Africa, and the United Kingdom randomly assigned 13,356 patients undergoing surgery for hip fractures; 22 hospitals in New Zealand randomly assigned an additional 4088 patients undergoing elective arthroplasty. Patients received 160 mg daily of either aspirin or placebo, initiated preoperatively and continued for 35 days. Patients were allowed to receive any other thromboprophylaxis deemed necessary and were followed up for mortality data and in-hospital morbidity data up to day 35.

Results.—Patients in the aspirin group had significant proportional decreases in pulmonary embolism (PE) of 43% and of symptomatic deep-vein thrombosis of 29% (Table 1). A diagnosis of PE or deep-vein thrombosis was significantly verified in 105 (1.6%) of 6679 patients in the aspirin group, compared with 165 (2.5%) of 6677 patients in the placebo group. This represents an absolute decrease of 9 per 1000 patients and a proportional reduction of 36%. Similar proportional effects were ob-

TABLE 1.—Effects of Aspirin on Nonfatal Vascular Events and Deaths in Hip-Fracture Patients up to Day 35

Event	Aspirin (n=6679)	Placebo (n=6677)	Hazard Ratio (95% CI)*
Non-fatal vascular events			
Deep-vein thrombosis	69	97	0·71 (0·52-0·97)
Pulmonary embolism	28	38	0·74 (0·45-1·21)
Venous thromboembolism†	87	122	0·71 (0·54-0·94)
Myocardial infarction	36	23	1·57 (0·93-2·65)
Stroke	34	30	1·13 (0·69-1·85)
Vascular death			
Pulmonary embolism	18	43	0·42 (0·24-0·73)
Ischaemic heart disease	69	56	1·23 (0·87-1·75)
Stroke	20	19	1·05 (0·56-1·97)
Heart failure	66	55	1·20 (0·84-1·72)
Other vascular cause	16	31	0·52 (0·28-0·94)
Unknown cause‡	46	48	0·96 (0·64-1·44)
All vascular deaths	235	252	0·93 (0·78-1·11)
Non-vascular death			
Pneumonia or bronchitis	114	126	0·90 (0·70-1·17)
Other non-vascular cause	98	83	1·18 (0·88-1·58)
All non-vascular deaths	212	209	1·01 (0·84-1·23)
All deaths up to day 35§	447	461	0·97 (0·85-1·10)

*Proportional reductions in risk and 95% confidence index (CI) are derived as 100 (1-hazard ratio).

†Deep-vein thrombosis, pulmonary embolism, or both (without death due to pulmonary embolism).

‡Deaths reported but not confirmed as pulmonary embolism (14 vs 13), ischaemic heart disease (14 vs 19), and stroke (14 vs 14), and deaths with no ascribed cause (4 vs 3).

§Deaths during days 36-365: 271 vs 291.

(Courtesy of Rodgers A, for the Pulmonary Embolism Prevention (PEP) Trial Collaborative Group: Prevention of pulmonary embolism and deep-vein thrombosis with low-dose aspirin: Pulmonary embolism prevention (PEP) trial. *Lancet* 355:1295-1302, 2000, copyright by The Lancet Ltd, 2000.)

served in all major subgroups, including patients receiving subcutaneous heparin. Aspirin prevented 4 fatal PEs per 1000 patients (18 aspirin vs 43 placebo deaths). This represented a significant proportional decrease of 58%, with no apparent effect on deaths from any other vascular or nonvascular cause. Deaths caused by bleeding were rare (13 with aspirin vs 15 with placebo). There was a significant excess of 6 postoperative transfused bleeding episodes per 1000 patients in the aspirin group. For patients with elective arthroplasty, the rates of VTE were lower. The proportional effects of aspirin were compatible with those in patients with hip fracture.

Conclusion.—These findings, together with those of the earlier meta-analysis, reveal that aspirin decreases the risk of PE and deep-vein thrombosis by at least a third during a period of increased risk. These data provide good evidence for considering aspirin routinely in a wide range of surgical and medical patient groups at high risk for VTE.

▶ Most investigators, according to a large number of studies done in the 70s and 80s, have believed that aspirin was relatively ineffective for the prevention of venous thromboembolism in high-risk groups. This large study of more than 13,000 patients undergoing surgery for hip fractures suggests that aspirin may be effective in the prevention of postoperative deep vein thrombosis. One major flaw, however, is that patients also received "any other form of thromboprophylaxis thought necessary." I would regard this article as interesting but not definitive. Anticoagulation and intermittent compression appear to be the best forms of prophylaxis for deep vein thrombosis. Aspirin prophylaxis, however, may warrant another look.

J. L. Mills, Sr, MD

Suspected Pulmonary Embolism: Prevalence and Anatomic Distribution in 487 Consecutive Patients
de Monyé W, for the Advances in New Technologies Evaluating the Localisation of Pulmonary Embolism (ANTELOPE) Group (Leiden Univ, The Netherlands; et al)
Radiology 215:184-188, 2000   15–20

Introduction.—The size and location of the embolus in patients with pulmonary embolism (PE) may influence the accuracy of various diagnostic modalities. Data regarding the frequency distribution of lobar, segmental, and isolated subsegmental PE are needed to determine the appropriate role of the imaging modalities in the diagnostic workup. The prevalence and anatomical distribution of PE was analyzed in 487 patients suspected of having PE.

Methods.—All patients underwent ventilation-perfusion (V-P) scintigraphy. Diagnosis of PE was excluded when perfusion was normal. After all abnormal scintigram result, ventilation scintigraphy, spiral CT angiography, or digital subtraction pulmonary angiography was performed, according to a strict diagnostic protocol. Three experienced nuclear physicians examined all the V-P scans and used consensus with standardized criteria. Findings were classified as either normal, nondiagnostic, or high probability. Complete digitally subtracted pulmonary angiograms were analyzed by 2 experienced radiologists. Patients were classified according to the largest pulmonary vessel in which PE could be observed: central (main pulmonary stem, left or right main pulmonary branch), lobar, segmental, or subsegmental artery.

Results.—Of 983 eligible patients, written confirmed consent was obtained from 627 (64%). A conclusive diagnosis was established in 487 (78%) patients. Of these, 130 (27%) had PE. A clot was observed in the main pulmonary trunk in 10 (7.7%) patients, in the left or right pulmonary branch in 19 (14.6%), in the lobar pulmonary artery in 37 (28.5%), in a segmental artery in 35 (26.9%), and in an isolated subsegmental arterial branch in 29 (22.3%) (Table 3). No correlation was found between a high-probability V-P scan and the largest pulmonary arterial branch with PE. A high-probability V-P scan did not indicate a large embolus. Nondiagnostic V-P scans usually corresponded with relatively smaller emboli.

Conclusion.—No firm conclusion may be made regarding the size of PE on the basis of a high-probability V-P scan result alone. The largest

TABLE 3.—Distribution of Largest Pulmonary Artery Involved, Stratified According to
V-P-Based Diagnosis

Vessel	High-Probability	Non-diagnostic*	Normal*	Not Available†	Total‡
Main pulmonary stem	10	0	0	0	10 (7.7)
Left or right pulmonary branch	19	0	0	0	19 (14.6)
Lobar artery	30	4	0	3	37 (28.5)
Segmental artery	24	9	2	0	35 (26.9)
Subsegmental artery	23	5	1	0	29 (22.3)
Total	106	18	3	3	130

*Diagnosis of PE established with pulmonary angiography.
†In these patients, no V-P examination was performed owing to logistic reasons, and the diagnosis of PE was established with pulmonary angiography.
‡The numbers in parentheses are the percentage.
Abbreviations: V-P, Ventilation-perfusion; *PE,* pulmonary embolism.
(Courtesy of de Monyé W, for the Advances in New Technologies Evaluating the Localisation of Pulmonary Embolism (ANTELOPE) Group: Suspected pulmonary embolism: Prevalence and anatomic distribution in 487 consecutive patients. *Radiology* 215:184-188. Copyright 2000, Radiological Society of North America.)

pulmonary arterial branch with PE was central or lobar, segmental, and isolated subsegmental in 66 (51%), 35 (27%), and 29 (22%) patients, respectively.

▶ In this amazing study, which is part of the ANTELOPE trial, 27% of the patients who underwent the full workup for pulmonary embolism were positive for PE. This extraordinarily high number continues to confirm the incredible prevalence of PE. Moreover, this prospective study validated by many radiologists along the protocol trail shows PE to be relatively evenly distributed from the main pulmonary stem to the subsegmental artery. What is not clearly stated in the study, but is blatantly obvious to the intuitive reader, is the conclusion as to which study to obtain to make the diagnosis of PE. In those patients with high-probability V-Q scans, 15% had a CT scan that did not correspond to the V-Q scan, thus necessitating a pulmonary angiogram. In addition, 20% of the V-Q scans were either nondiagnostic or normal. Considering the seriousness of PE, and the overall reliability of V-Q scanning, it seems wise to again advise abandonment of V-Q scanning and assure the diagnosis by pulmonary arteriography. I am impressed by the number of spiral CT scans that were not confirmatory of the diagnosis of PE compared with the number of high-probability V-Q scans in patients who indeed did have a PE as diagnosed by pulmonary arteriography.

R. B. McLafferty, MD

Pulmonary Embolism Revealed on Helical CT Angiography: Comparison With Ventilation–Perfusion Radionuclide Lung Scanning

Blachere H, Latrabe V, Montaudon M, et al (Hôpital Cardiologique Haut-Lévêque, Pessac, France)
AJR 174:1041-1047, 2000   15–21

Introduction.—Many institutions are reluctant to use pulmonary angiography in the diagnosis of pulmonary embolism (PE) because of its invasive nature and associated morbidity and mortality. Large differences (25%-30%) in interpretation of ventilation-perfusion (V-P) radionuclide lung scanning have been reported, particularly in the classification of low probability or intermediate probability scans. Helical CT angiography and V-P radionuclide lung scanning as initial tests were prospectively compared in the diagnosis of acute PE.

Methods.—Two hundred sixteen consecutive patients with clinically suspected acute PE underwent helical CT angiography, V-P radionuclide lung scanning, and Doppler US of the veins of the legs. Based on concordance of the results of V-P radionuclide lung scanning and helical CT angiography and on the degree of clinical suspicion, selected patients underwent pulmonary angiography. Patients without PE on initial examination in whom no treatment was started was followed up for at least 3 months to ascertain the potential recurrence of thromboembolic disease.

Results.—Of 216 patients who entered the protocol, the final group comprised 179 patients. Of these, clinical suspicion of PE was high in 49 (27.4%), intermediate in 56 (31.3%), and low in 74 (41.3%). Of these, 137 (76.5%) were inpatients, 28 (15.6%) were outpatients, and 14 (7.8%) were from the ICU. Sixty-eight patients (37.9%) had a final diagnosis of PE based on pulmonary angiography in 12 patients and outcome in 56 patients. There were 3 false-positive helical CT angiography results; 5 results were interpreted as indeterminate (Table 2). Significant differences

TABLE 2.—First Interpretation Accuracy of Helical CT Angiography and Ventilation-Perfusion Radionuclide Lung Scanning for Diagnosis of Pulmonary Embolism

| | Pulmonary Embolism | |
| | Present | Absent |
Technique	($n = 68$)	($n = 111$)
Helical CT angiography		
Positive	64	3
Indeterminate	1	4
Negative	3	104
Ventilation-perfusion scanning		
High probability	55	17
Intermediate probability	6	12
Low probability	6	64
Normal	1	18

(Courtesy of Blachere H, Latrabe V, Montaudon M, et al: Pulmonary embolism revealed on helical CT angiography: Comparison with ventilation–perfusion radionuclide lung scanning. *AJR* 174:1041-1047, 2000.)

were observed ($P < .05$) between sensitivity, specificity, positive predictive value, and negative predictive value for helical CT angiography and V-P radionuclide scanning (94.1% vs 80.8%; 93.6% vs 73.8%; 95.5% vs 82%; and 96.2% vs 75.9%, respectively). Interobserver agreement was rated excellent and moderate, respectively, for helical CT angiography and V-P radionuclide lung scanning.

Conclusion.—Helical CT angiography may be a better initial imaging modality than V-P radionuclide lung scanning. When helical CT angiography findings are negative and clinical suspicion remains high, pulmonary angiography is still recommended.

▶ I, like my mentor Dr Porter, always enjoy reading an article that supports my bias. I believe that CT angiography is the study of choice in 2002 to confirm clinically significant pulmonary thromboembolism. Unfortunately, the data from this article do not convincingly support this position. CT angiography is compared with V-P scanning, but only 13% of the study patients underwent the gold-standard procedure, pulmonary angiography. Weak end points of concordance of initial positive tests and event-free 3-month survival without anticoagulation are not very convincing, especially when the interobserver agreement was only moderate ($\kappa = 0.22$) for the V-P scanning in this series.

E. J. Harris, Jr, MD

Subclavian Vein

Claviculectomy for Subclavian Venous Repair: Long-term Functional Results
Green RM, Waldman D, Ouriel K, et al (Univ of Rochester, NY)
J Vasc Surg 32:315-321, 2000   15–22

Background.—In the acute setting, the preferred treatment of axillo-subclavian venous thrombosis resulting from thoracic outlet compression is catheter-directed thrombolysis. If treatment is successful, an underlying abnormality is often found in or near the vein at the costoclavicular space. If the lesion is extrinsic (ie, the venous abnormality is only produced with abduction of the shoulder), then a first rib resection through either the axilla or the neck with external venolysis as needed is usually sufficient. This procedure can be performed in the same hospital setting or at a later date. However, controversy surrounds both the treatment and the timing of treatment of intrinsic lesions (ie, the abnormality is within the vein itself). Among the options for treatment of intrinsic lesions are anticoagulation and delayed outlet decompression, depending on the level of symptoms; outlet decompression with external venolysis; outlet decompression followed by angioplasty and stenting; and outlet decompression with venous reconstruction. The long-term functional results were evaluated after medial claviculectomy and venous patch angioplasty or bypass grafting using internal jugular vein after incomplete thrombolysis of the subclavian vein.

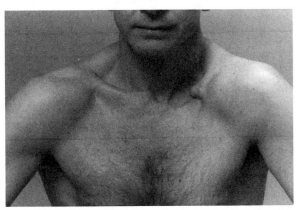

FIGURE 7.—Appearance of cut end of distal clavicle after shoulder abduction and internal rotation. One patient complained of a clicking sensation with shoulder movement but no associated pain. (Courtesy of Green RM, Waldman D, Ouriel K, et al: Claviculectomy for subclavian venous repair: Long-term functional results. *J Vasc Surg* 32:315-321, 2000.)

Methods.—In a retrospective review, the records of 11 patients with effort thrombosis, who were treated over 9 years were evaluated. These patients have been followed up for 3 to 9 years at 6-month intervals by means of duplex imaging and contrast venography (when indicated). All the patients have received an orthopedic evaluation of their shoulder function.

Results.—At the most recent follow-up, all the reconstructed veins were patent, with only one patient complaining of arm swelling after prolonged use. This patient is 1 of 3 patients with postphlebitic changes at the repair site, and she has similar findings in her basilic vein. All the patients have been able to return to their prethrombosis work without limitations. Four patients perform work in which significant physical labor is required. None of the patients has described any limitations in shoulder function, although one patient, who works as a diesel mechanic, has complained of pain in the shoulder with overuse with repetitive pulling (Fig 7). Upper extremity paresthesias when lying on the operated side have been described by 3 patients. Two patients are bothered by the large scar and indentation at the incision site; however, every patient has reported that they consider the overall result completely successful from a functional standpoint.

Conclusions.—Early subclavian venous repair performed through a medial claviculectomy is an effective procedure that provides excellent long-term functional results. Minor but significant symptoms were reported in half of the patients, but all were able to return to normal function.

▶ Despite the upbeat outcome assessment provided in the abstract, a review of the manuscript (especially Table 1) reveals that 7 of 11 patients experienced significant cosmetic, positional or functional limitations after medial claviculectomy and axillo-subclavian venoplasty and/or jugular-venous turndown. Since these procedures were performed immediately following thrombolysis and partial recanalization, one cannot help but wonder whether the cosmetic, positional and functional outcome of each patient would have been further impaired or perhaps improved by reserving surgery for patients who symptomatically failed a trial of anticoagulation alone after thrombolysis prior to surgery.[1] Despite the uniformly adequate technical results (as determined by long-term vein/graft patency) achieved in this series, the optimal timing and patient selection for surgical decompression to maximize symptomatic improvement remains undetermined.

R. L. Dalman, MD

Reference

1. Lee WA, Hill BB, Harris EJ Jr, et al: Surgical intervention is not required for all patients with subclavian vein thrombosis. *J Vasc Surg* 32: 57-67, 2000.

Surgical Intervention Is Not Required for All Patients With Subclavian Vein Thrombosis
Lee WA, Hill BB, Harris EJ Jr, et al (Stanford Univ, Calif)
J Vasc Surg 32:57-67, 2000   15–23

Objective.—The indications and the timing of surgical thoracic outlet decompression for the treatment of primary axillary–subclavian vein thrombosis is controversial. The efficacy of a treatment algorithm for the management of primary subclavian vein thrombosis, deferring the decision for surgical intervention for 1 month, to determine the patient's response to conservative therapy was studied.

Methods.—Color-flow venous duplex US scans and catheter-directed thrombolysis with heparin were performed between June 1996 and June 1999 in 22 patients (9 women), aged 18 to 47 years, with suspected primary deep venous thrombosis. Patients were discharged, given warfarin to take, and observed for 1 month. The effectiveness of thrombolysis was assessed by serial venograms. Those who remained asymptomatic continued taking warfarin for an additional 2 months and stopped taking it if there were no adverse findings on the venograms. Those who did not respond had thoracic outlet decompression and were given warfarin for 1 month and observed. Those who responded were given warfarin therapy for another 2 months and then had therapy discontinued if there were no adverse findings on the venograms. Those whose conditions failed to improve received balloon angioplasty.

Results.—Of 18 patients who underwent thrombolysis, 8 (44%) had complete and 10 (56%) had partial clot lysis. Rethrombosis occurred in 2 patients with complete lysis 2 weeks and 1 year after warfarin was discontinued. Of the 9 patients (41%) treated conservatively, 8 had minimal symptoms and 1 had moderate, subjective symptoms of early arm fatigue with exercise. Among the 13 patients who had surgery, 5 had minimal symptoms, 6 had moderate, and 2 had severe symptoms (Table 1). One patient who had an acute, symptomatic rethrombosis underwent an urgent

TABLE 1.—Summary of Results

	Surgical	Nonsurgical
Total	13	9
Sex (male/female)	7/6	6/3
Side (right/left)	9/4	6/3
Lytic therapy	11 (85%)	7 (78%)
Angioplasty	8 of 11	4 of 7
Postlysis result (complete/partial)	4/7	4/3
Symptom: at last follow-up	10 minimal/3 moderate*	9 minimal†
ASCV patency by means of duplex at last follow-up	13 (100%)	9 (100%)

*Includes 1 patient whose symptoms improved from a preoperative severe level to postoperative moderate level. The other 2 patients' symptoms did not significantly improve postoperatively compared with preoperative levels.
†Includes 1 patient who had persistent moderate symptoms despite lack of objective findings but who, at last follow-up, at 18 months from the initial event, had significant improvement.
Abbreviation: ASCV, Axillary–subclavian vein.
(Courtesy of Lee WA, Hill BB, Harris EJ Jr, et al: Surgical intervention is not required for all patients with subclavian vein thrombosis. *J Vasc Surg* 32:57-67, 2000.)

second lysis and surgery. Eleven of 13 patients (85%) who underwent thoracic outlet decompression had significant or partial symptom resolution. The remaining 2 had moderate symptoms. All patients who underwent surgery maintained patency on subsequent duplex scans.

Conclusion.—The treatment algorithm is effective in identifying patients with subclavian vein thrombosis who can be treated nonsurgically. Patients with persistent symptoms can be treated with thoracic outlet decompression. None of these patients requires long-term anticoagulation.

▶ Having taken the first step toward conservative management of this largely benign condition, the authors have reached the richly justified conclusion that nonoperative management suffices for many patients. I wonder if they are ready to ask the logical follow-up question: Is surgical intervention required in any patients with subclavian vein thrombosis? I predict the answer will prove to be "no," at least in the acute setting.

L. M. Taylor, Jr, MD

Venous Thrombosis

Compression and Walking Versus Bed Rest in the Treatment of Proximal Deep Venous Thrombosis With Low Molecular Weight Heparin

Partsch H, Blättler W (Wilhelminenspital, Vienna; Angio Bellaria, Zurich, Switzerland)
J Vasc Surg 32:861-869, 2000   15–24

Objective.—Observation has established that patients with deep vein thrombosis (DVT) recover much faster when they are encouraged to walk with firm compression bandages, yet evidence-based data are lacking. Preliminary results of a 9-day, randomized, unblinded, controlled trial comparing bed rest with walking exercises and compression are reported.

Methods.—Consecutive mobile patients with proximal DVT were divided into 3 groups: Group A (n = 15) was treated with inelastic Unna boot bandages and walking exercises, group B (n = 15) received elastic compression stockings and walking exercises, and group C (n = 15) had bed rest and no compression. All patients had dalteparin injections (200 IU/kg/body weight) every 24 hours for at least 6 days and oral anticoagulants with doses adjusted to reach international normalized ratio values of 2.0 to 3.0. Outcome measures included daily walking distance measurements, pain levels, and the bilateral Lowenberg test. Clinical scores and leg circumferences were measured on days 0, 3, 6, and 9. Compression sonography and ventilation-perfusion lung scans were performed on days 0 and 9.

Results.—Average walking distances improved from day 0 to day 9 in group A from 1793.0 to 4048.5 meters, in group B from 2058.0 to 3659.9 meters, and in group C from 66.0 to 179.3 meters. The differences between groups A and B and group C are significant. Pain levels were significantly reduced in groups A and B beginning on day 1. Pain levels in group C were lower on day 5. Lowenberg scores were significantly lower on day 2 for groups A and B. There was no significant difference in Lowenberg scores for group C up to day 9. Swelling was reduced more in the compression groups than in the bed rest group on day 9. The frequency of new pulmonary emboli and thrombus diameter were similar for all groups, although the longest extension of the thrombi was found in the bed rest group.

Conclusion.—Patients with acute proximal DVT who walk with compression bandages or compression stockings have significantly less pain and swelling and no increased risk of pulmonary emboli compared with bed rest patients.

▶ Inpatient therapy of patients with DVT receives yet another blow. It appears from this report that not only is early ambulation and compression therapy safe in patients with DVT; they actually do better. Pain and swelling are reduced more quickly than in patients subjected to bed rest. This is a small study, with only 15 patients randomly assigned to each treatment group. Nonetheless, the results are encouraging. The groups from Vienna and Zurich continue to randomly assign patients in this protocol. We look forward to future reports.

G. J. Landry, MD

Recurrent Venous Thromboembolism After Deep Vein Thrombosis: Incidence and Risk Factors
Hansson P-O, Sörbo J, Eriksson H (Sahlgrenska Univ, Göteborg, Sweden)
Arch Intern Med 160:769-774, 2000   15–25

Background.—Deep vein thrombosis (DVT) is a common occurrence in most medical disciplines. The estimated incidence of symptomatic DVT in the lower extremities is 0.5 to 1.6 per 1000 urban residents each year. However, this estimate is probably understated because many venous thromboembolic events (VTEs) are asymptomatic. The short-term outcome for patients with acute DVT of the leg has been well investigated, but less is known about the long-term clinical course. In recent studies, there have been indications of a high incidence rate for VTEs after a first DVT. Preventive actions are vital because a recurrence of DVT, particularly in the ipsilateral leg, may increase the risk of a postthrombotic syndrome as well as recurrent pulmonary embolism, which may be fatal. The cumulative incidence of recurrent VTEs after a first or second DVT was estimated, and possible risk factors for recurrent VTE were identified.

Methods.—The study group comprised 738 consecutive patients admitted to a single institution in Sweden for treatment of DVT between March 1988 and April 1993. These patients had objectively verified symptomatic DVT followed up for 3.7 to 8.8 years. Follow-up included a review of medical records and death certificates for all patients for recurrent DVT and pulmonary embolism.

Results.—Over the 5 years of the study, the cumulative incidence of recurrent DVTs was 21.5% after a first DVT and 27.9% after a second DVT. The 5-year cumulative incidence of fatal pulmonary embolism was 2.6% after a first DVT. Three independent predictors of increased risk of recurrent VTEs were identified by multivariate survival analysis: proximal DVT, a history of venous thromboembolism, and cancer. A small risk of recurrent VTE was associated with postoperative DVT and a long duration of oral anticoagulation therapy. Sex, age, initial thromboembolic therapy, or immobilization were not found to be associated with the risk of a recurrent event.

Conclusion.—There is a high rate of recurrence for venous thromboembolism after symptomatic DVT. Patients with proximal DVT, diagnosed cancer, a short duration of oral anticoagulation therapy, or history of thromboembolic events had a higher risk of recurrent VTEs, but patients with postoperative DVT had a lower recurrence rate. Awareness of the relative risk of these factors could aid in the identification of patients who might receive the most benefit from prolonged prophylactic treatment.

The Anatomy of Deep Venous Thrombosis of the Lower Extremity

Ouriel K, Green RM, Greenberg RK (Cleveland Clinic Found, Ohio; Univ of Rochester, NY)
J Vasc Surg 31:895-900, 2000   15–26

Introduction.—The diagnosis, treatment, and long-term sequelae of lower-extremity deep vein thrombosis (DVT) depend on the anatomical location and extent of the process. Protocols for managing patients with DVT are limited by a lack of fundamental knowledge. Lower-extremity venograms were examined to provide anatomical information on which to base therapeutic decisions in patients with lower-extremity DVTs.

Methods.—During the 10-year period ending in 1998, 2762 lower-extremity venograms were performed in 2541 patients. All venograms

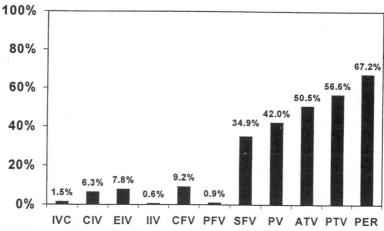

FIGURE 1.—Distribution of thrombus in venous segments. The frequency of thrombi in the hypogastric and profunda femoris veins may be underestimated by the venographic technique. (Courtesy of Ouriel K, Green RM, Greenberg RK: The anatomy of deep vein thrombus of the lower extremity. *J Vasc Surg* 31:895-900, 2000.)

with evidence of acute DVT were examined and the extent of the thrombotic process was noted and correlated with clinical findings. Thrombi were classified according to the venous segments involved, along with the thrombus isolation to 1 segment or multiple segments. The left-to-right ratio of the DVT was evaluated for various etiologic subgroups.

Results.—There were 885 (34.8%) documented instances of DVT. Of these 344 (39%) were idiopathic, 307 (35%) were postoperative, 84 (10%) occurred in the setting of malignancy, and 70 (8%) occurred as the result of trauma. Distal thrombi were observed more frequently than proximal thrombi; 734 patients (83%) had calf involvement, 470 (53%) had femoropopliteal involvement, and 75 (9%) had iliac involvement. The most frequent site of thrombus was the peroneal vein, which was involved in 595 patients (67%) (Fig 1). The ratio of left-to-right-sided DVT was 1.32:1 overall. It was higher for proximal thrombi, which had a ratio of 2.4:1 for iliac DVT versus 1.3:1 for infrainguinal DVT. The preponderance of left-sided DVT appeared to be associated with high-frequency, left common iliac vein involvement. The left-to-right ratio was much closer to equality (1.09:1) for patients with isolated infrainguinal DVT. A correlation was observed between the anatomical configuration of the DVTs and the etiologic subgroup. Postoperative DVTs were usually distal; DVTs developing in the setting of malignancy were more commonly proximal and frequently right sided. Proximal, left-sided DVTs were frequent in the idiopathic subgroup, most likely because of undiagnosed left iliac vein webs.

Conclusion.—The rate of distal vein involvement is considerably higher than that of proximal involvement in patients with DVTs. Proximal DVTs are more commonly left-sided; distal DVTs occur with a more equal left-to-right distribution. The anatomical extent of DVTs seems to depend on the cause of the process.

▶ This review provides interesting anatomic data on DVT categorized by etiology; however, the results may be affected by selection bias and faults of retrospective review. I think the significance of these results lies more with clarifying the pathophysiology of the disease than with clinical application. We rely on venous duplex to assess DVT and a combination of duplex and physical findings to direct treatment, such as thrombolysis.

W. K. Williamson, MD

Predictors of Recurrence After Deep Vein Thrombosis and Pulmonary Embolism: A Population-Based Cohort Study
Heit JA, Mohr DN, Silverstein MD, et al (Mayo Clinic and Mayo Found, Rochester, Minn)
Arch Intern Med 160:761-768, 2000   15–27

Background.—Anticoagulation is appropriate for preventing recurrent venous thromboembolism (VTE), but its optimal duration has not been determined. Factors accounting for varied duration include diagnostic uncertainty or misdiagnosis and failure to separate initial from recurrent episodes. Predictors of recurrence were identified, as was the rate of recurrent VTE.

Methods.—Medical records were evaluated for (1) patients whose first deep vein thrombosis or pulmonary embolism was diagnosed between 1966 and 1990 and (2) any recurrence of VTE.

Results.—Review of a total of 10,198 person-years of follow-up yielded 404 patients who had recurrent VTE. Recurrences were found most often in the first 6 to 12 months after the initial event, but the risk never dropped to 0. Among the factors deemed independent predictors of the first recurrence were increasing age and body mass index; neurologic diseases with paresis; malignant neoplasms, and neurosurgery performed between 1966 and 1980. The first probable/definite recurrence was independently predicted by the diagnostic certainty of the incident event and neurologic disease in patients whose VTE was acquired in the hospital. Malignant neoplasms increased the risk of recurrence, but the risk varied with respect to concomitant chemotherapy, patient age, patient sex, and study year.

Conclusions.—The incidence of recurrent VTE is especially high during the first 6 to 12 months after the initial event, but VTE may recur over a period of at least 10 years. An increase in risk is associated with concomitant neurologic diseases and paresis or a malignant neoplasm. When the identified risk factors are transient or reversible, risk decreases.

▶ The authors have provided important information that allows the clinician to determine duration of anticoagulation therapy after VTE. These data support other evidence that a minimum of 6 months of anticoagulation is of benefit and fit our bias that anticoagulation of longer duration is indicated in patients with malignant neoplasms or other hypercoagulable conditions.

W. K. Williamson, MD

Minor Events and the Risk of Deep Venous Thrombosis

Eekhoff EMW, Rosendaal FR, Vandenbroucke JP (Leiden Univ, The Netherlands)

Thromb Haemost 83:408-411, 2000   15–28

Introduction.—Many patients with deep vein thrombosis (DVT) have a history of minor events (short periods of immobilization, including prolonged travel; short illness; minor surgery; or injuries) before the onset of venous thrombosis. The influence of these minor events on the occurrence of DVT has rarely been evaluated. It is not known how a minor event could interact with the presence of genetic prothrombotic defects (factor V Leiden mutation, factor II mutation, protein C, S, and antithrombin deficiency). The role of minor events in DVT was assessed, along with their possible interaction with genetic prothrombotic defects.

Methods.—This study was an extension of the Leiden Thrombophilia Study, a population-based case-control trial on hereditary venous thrombosis conducted between 1988 and 1993. A follow-up period for a case-cross-over analysis of minor events as risk factors was added, along with a case-only analysis for the interaction with factor V Leiden. The study included 187 patients with first, objectively diagnosed venous thrombosis of the legs. No patients had any major acquired risk factors. A matched odds ratio was used for the analysis of minor events in the case-cross-over analysis. The multiplicative synergy index was used in the case-only analysis.

Results.—The only external risk factor in 32.6% of 187 patients with DVT was a history of minor events. The risk of thrombosis rose about 3-fold with such a history, as estimated in the case-cross-over analysis. In the case-only analysis, the synergy index between minor events and factor V Leiden mutation was 0.7.

Conclusion.—A history of minor events may have an important role in the development of deep venous thrombosis, particularly in the presence of genetic prothrombotic conditions.

▶ The hypothesis that minor events (eg, as travel, short-term immobilization, minor injuries, and minor surgery) are important in the etiology of DVT was tested by comparing how frequently these events occurred in the 2 weeks before an episode of DVT to how frequently these events occurred in a later and nearly randomly selected 2-week period for the same patients. A positive relationship was demonstrated, especially if factor V Leiden was present. I have my doubts. Recording of the minor events at the time of the DVT was retrospective, based on medical records, whereas the later period was examined contemporaneously and in standardized fashion. Minor events may be related to DVT, but it will take more than this to convince me.

L. M. Taylor, Jr, MD

16 Chronic Venous and Lymphatic Disease

Chronic Venous Disease

The Venous Stasis Syndrome After Deep Venous Thrombosis or Pulmonary Embolism: A Population-Based Study

Mohr DN, Silverstein MD, Heit JA, et al (Mayo Clinic, Rochester, Minn)
Mayo Clin Proc 75:1249-1256, 2000   16–1

Background.—Patients with venous stasis syndrome usually experience lower leg pain and swelling in the dependent position, which may progress to stasis pigmentation, stasis dermatitis, lipodermatosclerosis, indurated cellulitis, and venous ulceration. Venous stasis has been estimated to affect 2% of the population in Sweden. Extrapolation of data from a Michigan study has suggested that 6 to 7 million persons in the United States have dermatologic changes in their legs, and that about half a million of these persons have or have had venous ulcers. The high prevalence of lower extremity venous stasis syndrome makes it important to gain an epidemiologic understanding of this disease. The incidence of venous stasis syndrome and venous ulcers after deep venous thrombosis and pulmonary embolism was estimated in a population-based retrospective study. Predictors of venous stasis syndrome and venous ulcers were identified.

Methods.—The medical records of 1527 patients with incident deep venous thrombosis or pulmonary embolism between 1966 and 1990 were reviewed. Investigators recorded baseline characteristics, event type (whether deep venous thrombosis with or without pulmonary embolism or pulmonary embolism alone), leg side and site of deep venous thrombosis (proximal with or without distal deep venous thrombosis vs distal deep venous thrombosis alone), and venous stasis syndrome and venous ulcer.

Results.—Venous stasis syndrome occurred in 245 of 1527 patients. Cumulative incidence rates were 7.3% for 1 year, 14.3% for 5 years, 19.7% for 10 years, and 26.8% for 20 years (Fig 3). The cumulative incidence rate of venous ulcers by 20 years was 3.7%. In patients with deep venous thrombosis, venous stasis syndrome was 2.4 times more likely to develop compared with patients with pulmonary embolism and no diagnosis of deep venous thrombosis. In patients who were 40 years of age

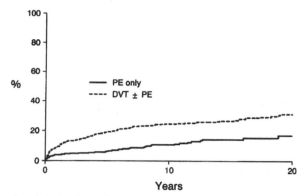

FIGURE 3.—Cumulative incidence of venous stasis syndrome after incident venous thromboembolism conditional on surviving 7 days by type of initial event (deep venous thrombosis with or without pulmonary embolism [*DVT ± PE*] vs *PE* only) among residents of Olmsted County, Minnesota. Time to venous stasis syndrome in years is tracked on the x-axis. (Courtesy of Mohr DN, Silverstein MD, Heit JA, et al: The venous stasis syndrome after deep venous thrombosis or pulmonary embolism: A population-based study. *Mayo Clin Proc* 75:1249-1256, 2000.)

or younger with proximal versus distal-only deep venous thrombosis, venous stasis was three times more likely. Venous stasis syndrome usually developed in the concordant leg of patients with unilateral leg deep venous thrombosis. The risk for venous ulcer increased 30% per decade of age at the incident venous thromboembolism.

Conclusion.—There is a continual increase in the cumulative incidence of venous stasis syndrome for 20 years after venous thromboembolism. Pulmonary embolism alone was found to be less likely to cause venous stasis syndrome.

▶ Perhaps no group of persons have had their health history dissected and laid out on the table as thoroughly as the good people of Olmsted County. Several interesting nuggets are presented here. Interestingly, the risk of development of venous stasis syndrome (VSS) after deep venous thrombosis (DVT) does not plateau but, rather, continues to increase out to at least 20 years. Proximal DVT leads to an increased risk of VSS, regardless of age, but in patients over the age of 40, the risk of VSS is essentially the same in patients with both calf and proximal DVT. VSS occurs occasionally in the contralateral limb in which DVT had not been diagnosed, most likely indicating that asymptomatic DVT occurs at a rate yet undefined, but probably higher than is appreciated.

This study is retrospective, and there is no uniformity in diagnosis or treatment. Be that as it may, the sheer number of subjects examined gives it a certain credibility. We typically encourage patients with DVT to wear compression stockings indefinitely after DVT. The fact that the rate of development of VSS continues to rise up to at least 20 years and possibly beyond lends support to this recommendation, particularly in all patients with proximal DVT and patients older than 40 with calf vein DVT.

G. J. Landry, MD

Differences in Pressures of the Popliteal, Long Saphenous, and Dorsal Foot Veins
Neglén P, Raju S (River Oaks Hosp, Jackson, Miss)
J Vasc Surg 32:894-901, 2000   16–2

Objective.—Popliteal, tibial, and dorsal foot vein pressures vary differently during calf exercise. The relationship among pressures obtained simultaneously in the popliteal/posterior tibial, long saphenous, and dorsal foot veins were examined.

Methods.—During toe stands, venous pressures were measured simultaneously in the legs of 8 patients, at the knee joint level, at the middle third of the calf, and 5 to 7 cm above the ankle (Fig 3). One patient had deep reflux, and 2 patients had undergone stripping of the long saphenous vein above the knee, Millar probes were inserted into the long saphenous vein and posterior tibial veins, and an external transducer was connected to the cannula in the dorsal foot vein.

Results.—For 7 patients, venous pressure dropped in all veins at the knee level. Patient 8 had an increase in deep venous pressure and a decrease in both saphenous and dorsal foot vein pressures at all calf levels. The dorsal foot venous pressure decrease was significantly larger than the long saphenous and deep vein pressure decreases. The recovery times were shortest for the deep vein, significantly longer for the long saphenous vein, and longer still for the dorsal foot vein. The pattern was similar for legs with long saphenous vein incompetence and veins with no reflux.

Conclusion.—Postexercise pressure, percentage pressure drop, and recovery times vary widely in the 3 veins, indicating different hydraulic behavior in response to calf exercise.

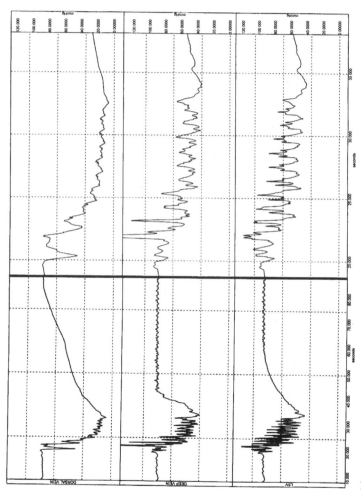

FIGURE 3.—The dorsal foot (top), popliteal (middle), and long saphenous (bottom) venous pressure tracings simultaneously recorded 5 to 7 cm above the ankles during 10 toe stands in 1 patient with no reflux or obstruction. Right set of curves are a magnification of the left set. (Courtesy of Neglén P, Raju S: Differences in pressures of the popliteal, long saphenous, and dorsal foot veins. *J Vasc Surg* 32:894-901, 2000.)

Ambulatory Venous Pressure Revisited

Neglen P, Raju S (River Oaks Hosp, Jackson, Miss)
J Vasc Surg 31:1206-1213, 2000   16–3

Background.—The overall hemodynamic impact of altered venous function is believed to be detectable by measuring dorsal foot vein pressure. However, signs and symptoms of obstruction to venous outflow or of improving hemodynamic function may not be reflected accurately. To document that regional hemodynamic changes occurring in the deep or superficial hemodynamic system may not be detected by measuring dorsal foot vein pressure, investigators evaluated an alternative method, involving simultaneous measurement of pressure in the deep venous system and dorsal vein pressure while the patient performs toe stands.

Methods.—For 45 patients with indications of chronic venous insufficiency, the posterior tibial vein was cannulated, as was the dorsal foot vein, then a catheter with a pressure tranducer in the tip was inserted via the posterior tibial vein to the knee joint level. Simultaneous pressure recordings were made at both sites while the patient did toe stands and then were repeated with the probe located in the upper, middle, and lower calf.

Results.—With use of duplex Doppler scanning and ascending and descending venography, saphenous vein incompetence was noted in 11 lower extremities; incompetent perforators were seen in 11 extremities, 8 of which also had saphenous vein incompetence; 28 extremities had marked compression of the popliteal vein with plantar flexion. Neither the duplex Doppler examination nor the descending venography detected significant deep axial reflux, nor was morphological outflow obstruction noted. During toe stands, the mean deep pressure at the knee joint decreased 15% and the mean dorsal foot vein pressure fell 75%. All patients had a decrease in exercise pressure measured in the dorsal foot vein, but popliteal vein pressure rose in 9 limbs, fell only marginally in 15 limbs, and declined markedly in 21 limbs (from 22% to 65%). Dorsal vein measurements indicated longer deep vein recovery times than did the other measurements. Limbs with superficial incompetence had recovery times in the deep system that were significantly shorter in a comparison of limbs with and without superficial reflux.

Conclusions.—Dorsal foot vein pressure measurements may remain normal even when deep venous pressure has fallen or risen. Thus, ambulatory dorsal foot vein pressure does not reliably reflect pressure changes in the tibial and popliteal veins.

The Relationship Between the Number, Competence, and Diameter of Medial Calf Perforating Veins and the Clinical Status in Healthy Subjects and Patients With Lower-Limb Venous Disease

Stuart WP, Adam DJ, Allan PL, et al (Royal Infirmary, Edinburgh, Scotland)
J Vasc Surg 32:138-143, 2000   16–4

Background.—Uncontrolled data from some studies have suggested that the eradication of superficial venous reflux in patient with normal deep veins results in augmentation of the healing process and reduction of the recurrence of chronic venous ulceration. However, the benefits of venous surgery are much less certain in patients with deep venous disease. In particular, the value of interruption of incompetent perforating veins (IPVs) on the medial aspect of the calf in an effort to protect the skin of the gaiter area from excessively high deep venous pressures is unproved. Open perforator ligation has for the most part been abandoned because of the high incidence of wound-related complications, despite some evidence that this procedure may benefit patients with popliteal vein reflux who have a poor prognosis. The relationship between abnormal medial calf perforating vein structure and function and the clinical severity of chronic venous insufficiency was examined.

Methods.—Duplex ultrasound was used in determination of number, flow characteristics, and diameter of medial calf perforating veins, and the presence of deep and superficial main stem reflux or occlusion in 50 limbs with no clinical or duplex evidence of venous disease (as determined by clinical, etiologic, anatomical, and pathologic [CEAP] grade 0), 95 limbs with varicose veins only (CEAP 2/3), 58 limbs affected by lipodermatosclerosis but not ulcer (CEAP 4), and 108 limbs affected by healed or open venous ulcer (CEAP 5/6).

Results.—The proportion of limbs in which any perforating veins and IPVs were demonstrated increased significantly as clinical status deteriorated. Similarly, there was an increase with deteriorating CEAP grade in the total number of perforators, the total number of IPVs, and the median diameter of perforators.

Conclusions.—Deterioration of the CEAP grade of chronic venous insufficiency was associated with increases in both the number and diameter of medial calf perforating veins, particularly those that permit bidirectional flow.

Pericapillary Fibrin Deposits and Skin Hypoxia Precede the Changes of Lipodermatosclerosis in Limbs at Increased Risk of Developing a Venous Ulcer

Stacey MC, Burnand KG, Bhogal BS, et al (St Thomas' Hosp, London; St John's Inst of Dermatology, London; Fremantle Hosp, Western Australia)

Cardiovasc Surg 8:372-380, 2000   16–5

Introduction.—The skin changes of lipodermatosclerosis (pigmentation, induration, and inflammation in the skin of the gaiter region of the leg) may precede or coincide with the development of venous ulceration. There is a possibility that pericapillary fibrin deposition, located in calf skin of patients with venous ulceration and lipodermatosclerosis, may already be

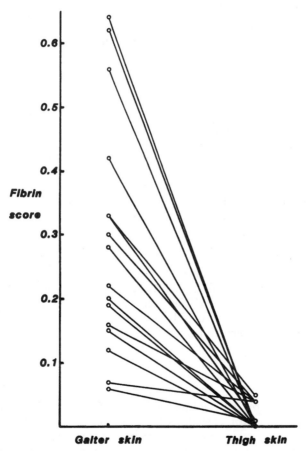

FIGURE 2.—Fibrin scores for biopsy specimens of skin from the gaiter region of the lower leg and the thigh (Statistically significant difference, *P* < .01, Wilcoxon signed rank test). (Courtesy of Stacey MC, Burnand KG, Bhogal BS: Pericapillary fibrin deposits and skin hypoxia precede the changes of lipodermatosclerosis in limbs at increased risk of developing a venous ulcer. *Cardiovasc Surg* 8:372-380, 2000. Reproduced with permission of *Cardiovascular Surgery*. Copyright 2000 by Elsevier Science Inc.)

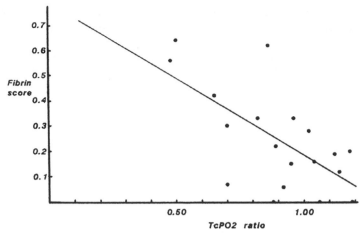

FIGURE 3.—Correlation between the transcutaneous oxygen ratio and the fibrin score from the skin of the gaiter region of the lower leg. (Spearman rank correlation coefficient −0.62, $P < 0.01$). (Courtesy of Stacey MC, Burnand KG, Bhogal BS: Pericapillary fibrin deposits and skin hypoxia precede the changes of lipodermatosclerosis in limbs at increased risk of developing a venous ulcer. *Cardiovasc Surg* 8:372-380, 2000. Reproduced with permission of *Cardiovascular Surgery*. Copyright 2000 by Elsevier Science Inc.)

present in the dermis of the gaiter area of apparently healthy appendages before any skin changes are visible. The apparently healthy limbs of 19 consecutive patients with a healed venous ulcer on 1 leg and no history of ulceration or clinical evidence of lipodermatosclerosis on the opposite calf were examined.

Methods.—All limbs were examined by bipedal ascending phlebography and foot volume plethysmography. Systemic fibrinolytic activity and fibrinogen levels were determined. Transcutaneous oxygen determinations were expressed as a ratio of levels from a fixed position in the gaiter skin over a control site on the arm. Biopsy specimens of a standard site in the gaiter skin and thigh were examined for the presence of laminin, fibrinogen, and fibronectin with the use of immunofluorescent microscopy. A ratio of the number of capillaries with deposits divided by the total number of capillaries staining with laminin (fibrin and fibronectin scores) was used to express the extent of pericapillary fluorescence.

Results.—Pericapillary fibrin deposits were seen in the dermis in 16 biopsy specimens of the gaiter region (median score, 0.20) and in 8 biopsy specimens of the thigh (median score, 0.0) ($P < .01$) (Fig 2). There was a negative correlation between the transcutaneous oxygen ratio and the fibrin score (−0.62; $P < .01$) (Fig 3). A weak negative correlation was observed between the half-volume refilling time on foot volume plethysmography (an indicator of venous reflux) and the fibrin score (−0.47; $P < .05$). No such correlation was seen between the fibrin score and the indicators of calf pump function, the euglobulin clot lysis time, or the plasma fibrinogen.

Conclusion.—The presence of significant numbers of pericapillary fibrin deposits within the dermis of the gaiter skin was observed before any evidence of clinical lipodermatosclerosis in 84% of this cohort of patients with at-risk limbs.

▶ The authors performed skin biopsies and measured transcutaneous oxygen levels in the skin of apparently normal ankles in patients with healed venous ulcers on the contralateral side. The skin of apparently healthy ankles had increased pericapillary fibrin and decreased transcutaneous oxygen levels. This study demonstrates for the first time that pericapillary fibrin deposits precede the development of clinical disease. While this finding supports the hypothesis that the pericapillary fibrin cuff may impede oxygen diffusion to the skin, the authors point out that the role of white cell trapping remains to be determined. The authors' suggestion that skin biopsy might be used to determine which patients should be treated with compression will likely be the object of a further study from this group. I will continue to recommend compression on both legs of patients with deep venous insufficiency, even if 1 side appears normal.

J. M. Edwards, MD

Deep Venous Thrombosis and Superficial Venous Reflux

Meissner MH, Caps MT, Zierler BK, et al (Univ of Washington, Seattle)
J Vasc Surg 32:48-56, 2000   16–6

Objective.—Postthrombotic syndrome is the most important long-term complication of acute deep vein thrombosis (DVT). The mechanism of superficial venous thrombosis and its contribution to the development of postthrombotic syndrome has not been investigated. The frequency of superficial venous incompetence after an episode of acute DVT was evaluated, and the factors important to its development were examined.

Methods.—Patients (n = 66, 32 men; average age, 48 years), with confirmed acute DVT in 69 legs participated in a longitudinal study involving venous duplex US scanning to evaluate the natural history of the condition at 1 and 7 days, 1 month, every 3 months thereafter for 1 year, and annually thereafter for an average of 48 months. Valvular reflux was assessed with distal pneumatic cuff deflation in the greater saphenous vein (GSV) above the knee and in the lesser saphenous vein (LSV) with the patient standing.

Results.—The incidence of DVT was significantly higher in limbs with GSV thrombosis than in limbs without GSV thrombosis and increased with time (Fig 1). With GSV reflux, the relative risk was 1.4 for DVT without GSV thrombosis, 8.7 for DVT with GSV thrombosis, 3.7 for every 10-point increase in the thrombus score, and 1.5 for female sex (compared with male sex). With LSV reflux, the relative risk was 3.2 for DVT (compared with extremities without DVT), 1.4 for every 10-year increase in age, and 1.7 for female sex (compared with male sex). Reflux, unrelated to thrombosis, also tends to develop in uninvolved limbs. The thrombosis score was a significant predictor of reflux in GSV and LSV.

Months	DVT / GSV Thrombosis		DVT / No GSV Thrombosis		Uninvolved Limb	
	Percent Reflux	S.E.	Percent Reflux	S.E.	Percent Reflux	S.E.
12	47%	0.06	2%	0.02	7%	0.03
36	62%	0.13	14%	0.06	12%	0.04
60	77%	0.11	29%	0.09	15%	0.05
96	77%	0.11	29%	0.09	15%	0.05

FIGURE 1.—Cumulative incidence of reflux in the GSV among extremities with DVT and GSV thrombosis (N = 15), DVT without GSV thrombosis (N = 50), and without DVT (N = 61). The incidence and SE at selected intervals are shown in the table at the bottom of the figure. Differences between groups are statistically significant ($P < .0001$; log-rank test). However, in comparison with uninvolved limbs, the relative risk of reflux is significantly greater only for limbs with GSV thrombosis ($P < .001$). *Abbreviations: DVT*, Deep venous thrombosis; *GSV*, greater saphenous vein. (Courtesy of Meissner MH, Caps MT, Zierler BK, et al: Deep venous thrombosis and superficial venous reflux. *J Vasc Surg* 32:48-56, 2000.)

Conclusion.—The origin of superficial venous reflux appears to be related to superficial venous thrombosis and to independent processes taking place in uninvolved limbs. Superficial venous thrombosis and DVT frequently occur together.

▶ While the finding of a 20% incidence of superficial thrombophlebitis in combination with DVT is not a new finding, the long-term findings regarding the high incidence of superficial venous incompetence are new. The authors suggest that there are 2 mechanisms responsible for the development of superficial incompetence, 1 related to the initial DVT with thrombosis of the superficial system and the other related to degeneration of the superficial system. Both of these mechanisms contribute to the high incidence of superficial incompetence, which, in combination with deep venous incompetence, leads to the most severe cases of postthrombotic syndrome.

J. M. Edwards, MD

Venous Disease Treatment

Treatment of Primary Venous Insufficiency by Endovenous Saphenous Vein Obliteration

Chandler JG, Pichot O, Sessa C, et al (Univ of Colorado, Denver; Univ of Grenoble, France; Univ of Graz, Austria; et al)
Vasc Surg 34:201-214, 2000   16–7

Introduction.—Greater saphenous vein reflux is usually observed with primary venous insufficiency and is frequently treated by surgically stripping the saphenous vein from the groin to just below the knee. The effectiveness of the treatment of primary venous insufficiency by endovenous saphenous vein obliteration was investigated in 301 limbs.

Methods.—The mean Clinical-Etiology-Anatomic-Pathophysiologic (CEAP) Clinical Class was 2.4 in 206 females and 67 males. Treated limbs represented the spectrum of venous reflux disease. The mean patient age was 47 years.

Endovenous Technology.—The Closure System is made up of a dedicated, computer-controlled bipolar generator and 1.7-mm (5F) and 2.7-mm (8F) catheters with sheathable electrodes (Fig 1). The catheter is passed through a venipuncture sheath many times with proper positioning determined by ultrasonic imaging. Base-of-toes-to-groin Esmarch wrapping and head-down patient position are used while exsanguinating the entire superficial venous network, directing flow into the deep veins. Supplemental direct manual

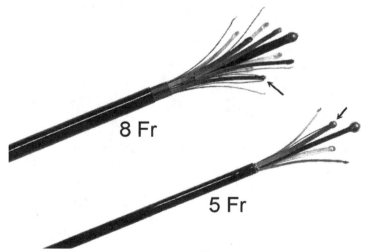

FIGURE 1.—Closure catheters (1.7- and 2.7-mm shaft diameters) with electrodes unsheathed. Electrodes are insulated except at their cupped tips. *Arrows* indicate microthermocouples. (Courtesy of Chandler JG, Pichot O, Sessa C, et al: Treatment of primary venous insufficiency by endovenous saphenous vein obliteration. *Vasc Surg* 34:201-214, 2000.)

compression is commonly used to clear blood from the saphenofemoral junction, because the wrap tends to curl back upon itself as it gets closer to the groin. An infusion of heparinized saline is administered through the central lumen to reduce thrombus formation on the electrodes. The treatment circuit is activated, and the wall temperature is allowed to equilibrate to the temperature set point for 15 seconds, at which time the catheter is withdrawn at a rate of about 3 cm/min, keeping the wall temperature within ±3°C of the set temperature and the wattage display below 4 watts to ensure the 12- to 16-second exposure necessary for the maximal wall contraction (Fig 2). After treatment, duplex imaging is used over the entire treated length to show absence of reflux or flow and noncompressibility.

Results.—Endovascular obliteration was combined with high ligation and with stab avulsion phlebotomy in 67 limbs (22%) and 290 limbs (96%), respectively. Paresthesias occurred in 15% of treatments confined to the thigh and upper leg; 30% of limbs were significantly affected when treatment extended to the ankle. There were 8 potentially preventable thermal skin injuries. Of these, 5 were in particularly superficial venous

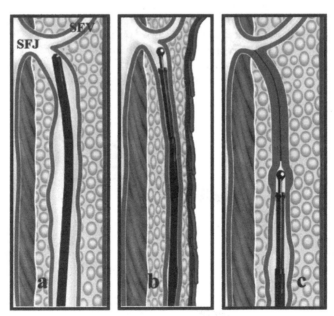

FIGURE 2.—Endovenous obliteration treatment sequence: a, introduction with electrodes sheathed, b, unsheathed electrodes in compressed saphenous vein positioned near SFJ; c, treatment in progress, with maximal vein wall contraction, as catheter is slowly withdrawn along the vein length to be treated (compression wrap omitted to show undistorted posttreatment anatomy). *Abbreviations: SFJ*, Saphenofemoral junction; *SEV*, superficial epigastric vein. (Courtesy of Chandler JG, Pichot O, Sessa C, et al: Treatment of primary venous insufficiency by endovenous saphenous vein obliteration. *Vasc Surg* 34:201-214, 2000.)

segments; 4 of 5 occurred in male patients. At a mean follow-up of 4.9 months, 21 (7.2%) of successfully treated veins had partially (19) or totally (2) recanalized. Only 11 of 290 (3.8%) had Doppler-detectable reflux. The 91 patients followed up for 6 months to 1 year had significant improvement in CEAP class and progressive relief from clinical symptoms. At the latest follow-up, 94% rated themselves as being symptom-free or markedly improved.

Conclusion.—The treatment results of endovenous obliteration in patients with primary varicose veins indicate that this approach may be as effective as surgical stripping in eradicating greater saphenous vein reflux and delaying the appearance of new varicose veins. Simple procedural modifications, including not treating to the ankle, prophylactic infiltration about superficially placed veins, and early duplex surveillance should decrease the complications observed in this early experience.

▶ Perhaps I am missing something here, but I fail to see the advantage of this technique over saphenous vein stripping other than its marketing potential. (Perhaps we need an alternative word to *stripping* to make it more palatable. Getting something stripped sounds horrible.) Is this really less invasive when incisions are still frequently required to place the device, stab avulsions (another unfortunate term) are still required to remove tributaries, and thermal injuries to skin and nerves are not infrequent? As for the improvement in CEAP clinical classification, I would hope that patients with varicose veins would no longer have varicose veins after treatment. With a mean follow-up of only 4 months, the authors can hardly make claims about its long-term efficacy, and, to their credit, they do not. Nonetheless, I do believe that technology and innovation are wonderful things. I just think that this one needs a little more work before it can be crowned victorious.

G. J. Landry, MD

Defining the Role of Extended Saphenofemoral Junction Ligation: A Prospective Comparative Study

Chandler JG, Pichot O, Sessa C, et al (Univ of Colorado, Boulder; Univ of Grenoble, France; Univ of Graz, Austria; et al)
J Vasc Surg 32:941-953, 2000   16–8

Objective.—Studies of recurrent reflux around the saphenofemoral junction (SFJ) support the need for removal of the thigh portion of the greater saphenous vein (GSV). Whether extended SFJ ligation is merited when the thigh portion of the GSV has been eliminated, and whether such ligation would interfere with the venous drainage of lower abdominal and pudendal tissues, which may be an important stimulus to new vessel formation, were investigated in a prospective, comparative, nonrandomized study.

Methods.—In a study of patients (77% female; age 19-78 years) selected from an ongoing multicenter trial of endovenous obliteration in Europe,

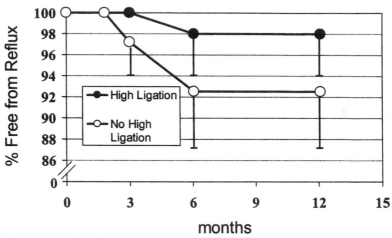

FIGURE 7.—Freedom from recurrent reflux after endovenous obliteration with (*filled circles*) and without (*open circles*) high ligation. *Range bars* indicate lower 95% confidence limits. (Courtesy of Chandler JG, Pichot O, Sessa C, et al: Defining the role of extended saphenofemoral junction ligation: A prospective comparative study. *J Vasc Surg* 32:941-953, 2000.)

the United States, and Australia, 60 limbs were treated with high ligation and 120 were treated without high ligation. Patients' status was followed at 1 week and at 3, 6, and 12 months.

Results.—Five high ligation limbs and 7 without high ligation had partial patency at less than 6 weeks. At 6 months, symptoms were significantly reduced in 86% to 88% of limbs in both groups. The improvement was sustained at 12 months in 26 and 31 limbs, respectively. Complications included 1 case (0.8%) of femoral-vein thrombus propagation in the group without high ligation, 15 cases (25%) of paresthesia in the high ligation group and 19 (16%) in the group without high ligation, 9 cases (15%) of perivenous or dermal inflammation in the high ligation group and 4 (3%) in the group without high ligation, and 2 skin burns (3%) in the high ligation group and 4 (3%) in the group without high ligation. There was recurrence at 6 months in 3 high-ligation limbs and 4 limbs that did not have high ligation, and at 12 months in 1 additional high ligation limb and in 2 limbs without high ligation. Recurrent GSV reflux was diagnosed in 1 high ligation limb and in 8 without high ligation at 6 months (Fig 7).

Conclusion.—Extended SFJ ligation does not appear to enhance the benefits of GSV obliteration.

▶ The authors attempt to determine the added effect of extended SFJ ligation when the GSV is eliminated by means of endovenous obliteration. Their preliminary results indicate that SFJ ligation with branch excision may not be necessary to achieve the therapeutic benefit of removing the thigh portion of the GSV. However, in the authors' own words, "These are relatively early negative findings in a nonrandomized observational study, lacking sufficient statistical power to exclude possible between-group differences. . . ." Of note is that, even when extended SFJ ligation was not performed, only 35% of the limbs studied were found to have patent SFJ tributaries. In addition, only 32% of the limbs studied were followed up for at least 12 months. We will await more definitive word from these authors after a longer period of follow-up.

R. A. Yeager, MD

A Comparison of Multilayer Bandage Systems During Rest, Exercise, and Over 2 Days of Wear Time
Hafner J, Botonakis I, Burg G (Univ Hosp of Zurich, Switzerland)
Arch Dermatol 136:857-863, 2000   16–9

Background.—The 3 types of compression bandages are short stretch, with less than 70% extensibility; medium stretch, with a 70% to 140% extensibility; and long stretch, with more than 140% extensibility. The interface pressures between the leg and 8 different multilayer bandage systems were studied during postural changes, during walking, and during 2 days of wear.

Methods.—Ten healthy volunteers, aged 26 to 65 years, participated in the study. Measures included pressure changes from the standing position to the sitting position to the supine position at rest; pressure amplitude during a 200-m treadmill walk at 3.2 m/s, at a 0° incline; and pressure decrease during 2 days of wear time.

Findings.—Compared with medium and long stretch bandage systems, short and medium stretch multilayer bandages had greater pressure decreases when the research subject was supine. Most multilayer bandage systems were similar in the amplitude of pressure waves during walking. Pressure loss over time was lowest for elastic bandages compared with short stretch bandages.

Conclusions.—Highly elastic multilayer bandage systems have the smallest pressure loss over several days of wear, but the small pressure decrease occurring while the patient is supine makes these bandages potentially hazardous to those with arterial occlusive disease. Short stretch bandages and the Unna boot with an inelastic zinc plaster bandage produce large pressure waves during walking and also have a marked pressure decrease when the patient is supine, but these systems lose much of their pressure in the first hours of wear. Multilayer systems that consist of short stretch and cohesive medium stretch bandages are a good compromise.

▶ Compression therapy remains the cornerstone of treatment for venous ulcers. A variety of compression dressings are available, and this article examines the changes in interface pressures on lower extremities treated with 8 different compression bandages. The merits of short-, medium-, and long-stretch bandages are delineated. However, this experiment included only normal legs, calling into question the clinical relevance of the findings. A leg that has significant variations in edema with activity and position will clearly affect the pressure interface, regardless of the type of dressing. Perhaps a dressing that allows a greater pressure decrease in the supine position may be beneficial in patients with arterial insufficiency, but this is speculative. The choice of optimal dressings is ultimately based on healing rates, not pressure differentials. Interestingly, not included in this study is the mainstay of our armamentarium—the graded compression stocking.

A. M. Abou-Zamzam, Jr, MD

Prognostic Indicators in Venous Ulcers

Phillips TJ, Machado F, Trout R, et al (Boston Univ; Convatec Inc, Princeton, NJ; Oregon Health Sciences Univ, Portland; et al)
J Am Acad Dermatol 43:627-630, 2000   16–10

Background.—Many new treatments have been proposed for the difficult problem of venous ulcers. Prognostic factors for healing remain uncertain. Data from a large trial of treatment for venous ulcers were analyzed to identify factors associated with ulcer healing.

Methods.—Data were retrospectively analyzed from a large, randomized trial of ifetroban versus placebo for the treatment of venous ulcers. Both groups received optimal local wound care, including a moisture-retentive dressing and graduated compression using a paste bandage and self-adherent wrap. Local treatments were applied daily for 12 weeks, in addition to the assigned systemic therapy. Analysis of prognostic factors was based on 165 patients who completed the full course of treatment.

Results.—As reported previously, outcomes were similar between the ifetroban and placebo groups. However, with consistent local treatment, a 55% healing rate was achieved. This was despite the ulcers' large size (mean area, 15.9 cm^2) and long duration (mean, 27 months). The initial size and duration of the ulcer were important predictors of outcome. The early response to treatment was also an important indicator: whether an ulcer had healed at least 40% by 3 weeks correctly predicted the final outcome in more than 70% of cases.

Conclusions.—For patients with venous ulcers, the most important prognostic factors for complete healing are the initial size and duration of the ulcer and the extent of healing within the first 3 weeks of treatment. A good healing response is unlikely in large, long-standing ulcers with a slow response to treatment. Patients with such ulcers might be targeted for alternative forms of treatment.

▶ A useful technique in clinical research is to pool the results from a negative randomized trial and attempt to ask some important natural history questions. The present report used a negative trial of an oral medication for the treatment of venous ulcers for this purpose. The authors found that smaller ulcers of shorter duration in compliant patients healed faster and were more likely to have healed completely at the end of the 12-week treatment period. I do not believe that any vascular surgeons caring for patients with venous ulcers would find this earth-shattering news. However, it does provide me with an opportunity to make a few personal observations about venous ulcer care. As I survey the types of patients in my general vascular practice at a University and VA setting, I find that the patients with venous ulcers are often on the lower end of the socioeconomic spectrum. This frequently complicates their outpatient care, because the majority of compression therapy other than an Unna boot is not covered financially. In addition, obesity is a frequent problem in this patient group, further complicating compliance. Until some of these issues are addressed, venous ulcer care will continue to be a frustrating clinical problem.

M. R. Nehler, MD

Randomised Double-blind Placebo Controlled Trial of Topical Autologous Platelet Lysate in Venous Ulcer Healing

Stacey MC, Mata SD, Trengove NJ, et al (Fremantle Hosp, Western Australia, Australia)

Eur J Vasc Endovasc Surg 20:296-301, 2000   16–11

Background.—Topical application of platelet-derived growth factors, collected as either a releasate or a lysate, has been proposed as a treatment for chronic venous ulcers. Most clinical trials of this approach have included only small numbers of patients with venous ulcers. Topical autologous platelet lysate for the treatment of chronic venous ulcers was evaluated in a randomized, controlled trial.

Methods.—The study included 86 patients (50 women and 36 men; median age, 70 years) with confirmed chronic venous ulcers. The patients were randomized in double-blind fashion to receive treatment with autologous platelet lysate or placebo buffer solution, in concert with standard compression bandaging. The treatment was applied twice weekly for up to 9 months. Venous ulcer healing was compared between groups.

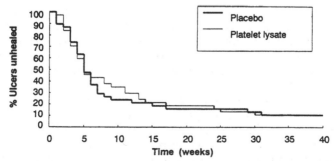

FIGURE 2.—Life table graph showing healing of ulcers over time for both the control group (placebo) and the treatment group (platelet lysate). (Courtesy of Stacey MC, Mata SD, Trengove NJ, et al: Randomised double-blind placebo controlled trial of topical autologous platelet lysate in venous ulcer healing. *Eur J Vasc Endovasc Surg* 20:296-301, 2000. Reprinted by permission of the publisher W B Saunders Company Limited London.)

Results.—The 2 groups were comparable in their baseline characteristics, including ulcer size and duration. Differences in outcome were not significant between groups (Fig 2). On Cox regression analysis, ulcer size was the only factor significantly affecting total healing time. In both groups, more than three fourths of patients had complete ulcer healing by 3 months.

Conclusions.—At least as prepared and applied in this study, autologous platelet lysate does not improve healing of chronic venous ulcers. These findings, in addition to measurements of cytokines in platelet preparations and chronic wound fluid, do not support the use of platelet solutions in patients with chronic venous ulcers.

▶ This study and a previous well-constructed one by Krupski and associates[1] demonstrate that platelet-derived "wound goop" (autologous platelet lysate) is of no benefit in the healing of lower extremity venous ulcers. Numerous wound care clinics use this agent, or some similar platelet growth factor derivative, to entice patients to their wound care center. It would appear that the clinical benefit of these lysates is minimal.

J. L. Mills, Sr, MD

Reference

1. Krupski WR, Reilly LM, Perez S, et al: A prospective randomized trial of autologous platelet derived wound healing factors for the treatment of chronic, nonhealing wounds: A preliminary report. *J Vasc Surg* 14:526-536, 1991.

Graduated Compression Stockings: Knee Length or Thigh Length
Benkö T, Cooke EA, McNally MA, et al (Semmelweis Univ, Budapest, Hungary; Queen Univ of Belfast, Northern Ireland; John Radcliffe Hosp, Oxford, England)
Clin Orthop 383:197-203, 2001   16–12

Background.—Both knee-length and thigh-length graduated compression stockings prevent deep venous thrombosis (DVT) after orthopedic surgery. However, little information is available comparing the effects of these 2 stocking lengths on blood flow. Differences in patient attitudes between knee-length and thigh-length graduated compression stockings were compared.

Methods.—The subjects were 200 patients (55% women; mean age, 60.4 years) scheduled to undergo orthopedic surgery (primarily total hip replacement or total knee replacement). None of the patients had a history of previous DVT or pulmonary embolism. Patients were randomly assigned in equal numbers to 1 of 5 groups. All measurements were made before the patient underwent surgery. Patients in groups A and B wore 1 of 2 different types of thigh-length graduated compression stockings on both legs. Patients in groups AK and BK wore the corresponding types of knee-length graduated compression stockings. Patients in the fifth group wore no compression stockings and served as controls.

Venous capacitance and outflow were measured by computerized strain-gauge plethysmography before and after patients applied the stockings. All measurements were made after 20 minutes of bed rest. After the repeat measurements, patients were allowed to move freely for 40 minutes. At that time, they were asked how comfortable they found the stockings, and assistants recorded whether the stockings had significant wrinkles and whether the patient could manage the stockings independently.

Results.—Venous capacitance and venous outflow in the control group did not differ between the first and second measurements. However, in all 4 groups wearing graduated compression stockings, venous capacitance and venous outflow increased significantly between the first measurement and the measurement after the patient had worn the stockings for 20 minutes. The mean percentage changes in venous capacitance did not differ significantly between groups A, B, AK, or BK. However, the mean percentage change in venous outflow was significantly less with 1 type of knee-length graduated compression stocking (group BK) compared with the other 3 active treatment groups (Fig 2). After 1 hour of wearing the graduated compression stockings, patients wearing the thigh-length versions were significantly more likely than those wearing the knee-length versions to have wrinkles and to report discomfort. Finally, 38% of patients wearing thigh-length stockings and 44% of those wearing knee-

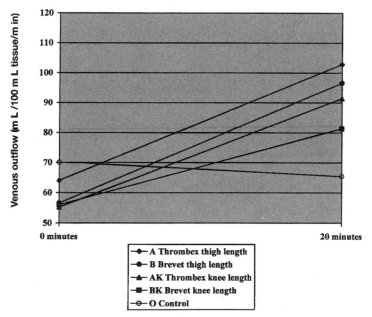

FIGURE 2.—The effect of graduated compression stockings on the venous outflow. (Courtesy of Benkö T, Cooke EA, McNally MA, et al: Graduated compression stockings: Knee length or thigh length. *Clin Orthop* 383:197-203, 2001.)

length stockings reported them to be difficult to use (between-group difference was not significant).

Conclusion.—Both thigh-length and knee-length graduated compression stockings significantly decrease venous stasis in the lower limb. The mean percentage change in venous capacitance did not differ significantly between the shorter and longer versions, but 1 of the knee-length stockings was significantly less efficient in increasing venous outflow. However, subjects reported that the knee-length stockings were more comfortable, and these versions also wrinkled less. Furthermore, knee-length stockings are less expensive than the longer versions. Thus, the use of knee-length graduated compression stockings, either alone or in combination with other prophylactic measures, is recommended to prevent DVT in patients undergoing orthopedic surgery.

▶ I am impressed by the authors' diligence to determine whether an above-knee or a below-knee graduated compression stocking provides better prophylaxis for venous thromboembolism. The authors should be commended on their methods. Compared with controls, above- and below-knee stockings show significantly increased percentage change in venous outflow, whereas the below-knee compression stockings were not quite as efficient in regard to percentage change in venous capacitance. What is more interesting is that, despite the fact that stockings show a 50% to 105% change in venous outflow, graduated compression stockings alone are not sufficient for DVT prophylaxis during and after surgery. Anticoagulation with either low molecular weight heparin or warfarin is further required to minimize risk. Interestingly, the authors did look at the fit of the stockings and whether the above- or below-knee stockings were uncomfortable. As expected, the thigh-length stockings had more wrinkles and were more uncomfortable than below-knee stockings, but both types of stockings were equally difficult to put on. We know from our own experience that below-knee compression stockings are no worse than above knee compression stockings for healing a venous stasis ulcer, and these data support the reason that is so. It would be interesting to repeat venous capacitance and outflow testing in groups of patients with venous insufficiency, comparing above- and below-knee stockings.

R. B. McLafferty, MD

Venous/Lymphatic Malformations

Surgical Treatment of Venous Malformations in Klippel-Trénaunay Syndrome

Noel AA, Gloviczki P, Cherry KJ Jr, et al (Mayo Clinic and Found, Rochester, Minn)
J Vasc Surg 32:840-847, 2000   16–13

Background.—Patients with the congenital anomaly Klippel-Trénaunay syndrome (KTS) have varicosities and venous malformations of the extremities, in addition to port-wine stains and hypertrophy of the bone and soft tissues. Many patients with KTS have venous drainage abnormalities. An updated surgical experience with KTS is reported.

Methods.—The authors performed surgery for venous malformations in 20 patients with KTS over a 12.5-year period, which accounted for 7% of the total number of patients with KTS seen during that time. The patients (28 males and 8 females; mean age, 23 years) underwent a total of 30 vascular operations in 21 lower limbs. Varicose veins and venous malformations were present in all patients; in addition, 90% had limb hypertrophy and 65% had port-wine stains. Eighty percent complained of pain, and 75% had swelling, 40% had bleeding, and 15% had superficial thrombophlebitis and cellulitis. The deep veins were patent in 18 patients, and 4 had large persistent sciatic veins, among other findings (Table 2). Eighty-five percent of patients had a CEAP clinical classification of C-3, whereas 5% had a C-4 and 10% had a C-6 classification.

For each affected limb, surgery included stripping of the large lateral veins and avulsion and excision of varicosities or venous malformations. Staged resections were carried out in 3 patients. Other procedures in individual patients included release of entrapped popliteal veins, popliteal–saphenous bypass, excision of a persistent sciatic vein, and open or endoscopic ligation of a perforator vein. Hematomas were evacuated in 2 patients. No vena caval filters were placed, and there were no thromboembolic events.

Results.—Surgery brought initial improvement in all patients. During a mean follow-up of 64 months, 50% of patients had some recurrent varicosities. There was 1 case of a nonhealing ulcer and 1 new ulcer at 8 years' follow-up. Three patients underwent additional surgery to manage recurrent varicosities. At follow-up, the CEAP scores were C-2 in 50% of patients, C-3 in 30%, C-4 and C-5 in 5% each, and C-6 in 10%. The mean clinical score decreased from 4.3 to 3.1.

Conclusions.—Most patients with KTS are managed nonoperatively, but patients with patent deep veins may benefit from excision of varicose veins and venous malformations, if symptomatic. Surgery is associated

TABLE 2.—Preoperative Contrast Phlebography Findings in 20 Patients With KTS

Anatomic Feature	No. of Patients (%)
Large lateral embryonic vein	20 (100)
Medial varicosities	13 (65)
Band-like narrowing of popliteal vein	9 (45)
Incompetent perforating veins	6 (30)
Hypoplastic SFV	5 (25)
Popliteal vein aneurysm	4 (20)
SFV ectasia	4 (20)
PSV	4 (20)
Entrapped popliteal veins	1 (5)

Abbreviations: KTS, Klippel-Trénaunay syndrome; *SFV,* superficial femoral vein; *PSV,* persistent sciatic vein.
(Courtesy of Noel AA, Gloviczki P, Cherry KJ Jr, et al: Surgical treatment of venous malformations in Klippel-Trénaunay syndrome. *J Vasc Surg* 32:840-847, 2000.)

with good clinical improvement, although recurrences are frequent; surgery may be repeated if necessary. Patients with KTS require specialized, multidisciplinary care at a vascular center.

▶ KTS is a rare congenital anomaly that is characterized by an atretic or absent deep venous system and significant venous varicosities or venous malformations, which arise from embryonic veins or superficial veins acting as collateral pathways. Most busy vascular surgeons will see 1 or 2 such patients a year. Therefore, this report from the Mayo Clinic, with 290 patients evaluated over a 12.5-year period, or 23 patients per year, is significant for the volume alone. My own experience with this syndrome is limited to 10 to 15 patients, all of whom have absent or atretic deep venous systems. Their varicosities and edema have been managed with compression therapy alone. A motivated patient with KTS can be quite functional with a well-fitted compression garment. Although this report documents a surgical experience with KTS patients, the obvious message is that fewer than 10% of the patients with KTS will require surgery. Candidates for surgery in this series were those patients with symptoms who had a patent deep venous system, with or without hypoplasia. One could argue that these are not classic KTS patients, but the true definition of KTS remains elusive. Therefore, when one is considering superficial venous or perforator vein surgery on a patient who fits the general description of KTS, I believe it is imperative to document a patent deep venous system. Without a deep venous system, KTS patients are best managed conservatively with compression.

E. J. Harris, Jr, MD

Prevalence of Deep Venous Anomalies in Congenital Vascular Malformations of Venous Predominance
Eifert S, Villavicencio JL, Kao T-C, et al (Uniformed Services Univ of the Health Sciences, Bethesda, Md)
J Vasc Surg 31:462-471, 2000   16–14

Background.—About two thirds of congenital vascular malformations are of venous predominance. Malformations of the deep venous trunks are sometimes associated with large superficial compensatory varices. When aplasia or hypoplasia of the deep venous trunks is present, excision of the enlarged superficial veins may have harmful effects. The prevalence and characteristics of deep venous anomalies associated with congenital vascular malformations were assessed.

Methods.—By reviewing the medical literature of the past 35 years, 7 series that contained data on the presence of deep venous anomalies in patients with congenital vascular malformations were identified. In addition, data from 392 patients with congenital vascular malformations seen at 2 hospitals from 1963 to 1998 were analyzed. Two hundred fifty-seven of these patients had malformations of venous predominance. The prevalence of various types of deep venous anomalies, as diagnosed by a wide range of imaging studies, was assessed.

Results.—In the 7 series of patients, 47% of malformations of venous predominance were associated with 1 or more anomalies of the deep venous system. Phlebectasia accounted for 36% of these anomalies, and 8% were aplasia or hypoplasia of the deep venous trunks. Eight percent of cases were associated with venous aneurysms and 7% with avalvulia.

Conclusions.—Nearly one half of patients with congenital vascular malformations of venous predominance are associated with anomalies of the deep venous system. The most common deep venous anomaly is phlebectasia. Aplasia/hypoplasia, venous aneurysms, and avalvulia are less common, but their recognition has important implications for treatment.

▶ Although most deep venous abnormalities detected in this series and in the literature at large were relatively benign phlebectasias, the point still stands: aplasia, hypoplasia, and avalvulia occur with predictable frequency in these patients. Superficial venous surgery should not be performed in patients with congenital vascular malformations of venous predominance before comprehensive anatomic and physiologic analysis of the deep system.

R. L. Dalman, MD

Sclerosing Treatment of Lymphangiomas With OK-432
Luzzatto C, Midrio P, Tchaprassian Z, et al (Divisione di Chirurgia Pediatrica, Padova, Italy)
Arch Dis Child 82:316-318, 2000   16–15

Introduction.—The surgical treatment of lymphangiomas is challenging because of the high incidence of recurrence and local nerve damage. Alternative modes of treatment are needed. Treatment of lymphangiomas with OK-432 has been proposed as the first line of treatment in Japan. The drug is difficult to obtain outside of Japan. An experience of 15 patients with lymphangiomas treated with OK-432 between 1992 and 1998 is discussed.

Methods.—The age of the patients was from birth to 15 years (median age, 22 months). All patients received a minimum of 3 injections. Ten patients received OK-432 as a first-line treatment, and 5 received OK-432 after surgery (3 had a residual lymphangioma after incomplete removal, and 2 had a late recurrence).

Results.—The OK-432 was effective in primitive and recurrent lymphangiomas. Complete regression was observed in all 7 patients with macrocystic disease. For 5 patients with microcystic disease, 2 had more than 50% regression and 3 had less than 50% regression. Three patients had mixed disease, with both large and microscopic cysts; 1 had more than 50% regression and 2 had less than 50% regression. The last 2 patients required surgery after receiving sclerosing treatment. The outcome was excellent in 100% of patients with macroscopic disease, and a shrinkage in size was seen in all patients with microcystic disease.

Conclusion.—Treatment with OK-432 is safe and easy in the treatment of lymphangiomas, with the exception of patients in whom the airway is involved and for whom a multidisciplinary approach must be considered.

▶ Fifteen children with lymphangiomas, some of whom also had surgical therapy, appeared to have a favorable response to injection of this sclerosing agent directly into the tumors. This extends and confirms a larger and also favorable experience reported previously by Ogita.[1] Certainly, this approach to treatment should be familiar to all who undertake the care of these children.

L. M. Taylor, Jr, MD

Reference

1. Ogita S: OK-432 therapy in 64 patients with lymphangioma. *J Pediatr Surg* 29:784-785, 1994.

17 Portal Hypertension

Imaging

Detection of Thrombosis in the Portal Venous System: Comparison of Contrast-Enhanced MR Angiography With Intraarterial Digital Subtraction Angiography

Kreft B, Strunk H, Flacke S, et al (Univ of Bonn, Germany)
Radiology 216:86-92, 2000   17–1

Background.—The treatment of patients with portal hypertension requires accurate assessment of the portal venous system, which is necessary to differentiate the increased portal blood pressure and plan adequate therapy. When the patients also have variceal bleeding, it is necessary to determine whether the portal hypertension has pre-, intra-, or posthepatic causes. The portal venous system in patients with elevated portal pressure is usually assessed with Doppler US. However, a more exact diagnostic method covering the entire portal venous system is needed for patients who are candidates for portosystemic shunt procedures. Traditionally, this has been accomplished with intra-arterial splenoportal and mesenterico-portal angiography. Recently, MR angiography (MRA) with gadopentetate dimeglumine or time-of-flight or phase-contrast techniques has shown promise as a noninvasive method for assessing of the portal venous system. The question of whether intra-arterial digital subtraction angiography (DSA) can be replaced with contrast-enhanced MRA in assessing patency or thrombosis of the portal venous system in patients with portal hypertension was investigated.

Methods.—The 2 techniques were used to assess the portal venous system in 36 patients with portal hypertension. The images were then evaluated for vessel patency or thrombosis of the portal, splenic, or superior mesenteric vein (Fig 2).

Results.—Thrombosis was seen in 42 of 101 vessels evaluated. For MRA, the overall sensitivity, specificity, and accuracy for detection of thrombosis were 100%, 98%, and 99%, respectively. For DSA, the overall sensitivity, specificity, and accuracy for detection of thrombosis were 91%, 100%, and 96%, respectively. The differences observed between the 2 systems were not found to be statistically significant. There were discordant findings between the 2 modalities for 6 vessels (6%).

523

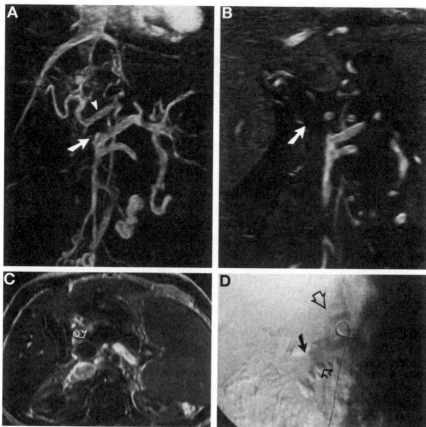

FIGURE 2.—Images obtained in a 30-year-old man with alcohol-induced hepatic cirrhosis who was suspected of having acute portal vein thrombosis on the basis of color Doppler US findings. (A) Coronal maximum intensity projection image from the portal venous phase of contrast-enhanced 3-dimensional T1-weighted fast-field-echo MRA (4.7/1.4, 40° flip angle), (B) coronal single section from the portal venous phase of contrast-enhanced dynamic 3-dimensional T1-weighted fast-field-echo MRA (4.7/1.4, 40° flip angle), (C) transverse T1-weighted gradient-echo MR image (220/4.5, 100° flip angle) obtained after gadopentetate dimeglumine administration, and (D) anteroposterior intra-arterial DSA splenoportographic image. In A and B, the thrombosis (*arrow*) of the main portal vein is clearly seen; however, the extent of the thrombosis is better appreciated in B because of the signal void. The thrombus (*arrow*) is also clearly seen in C. In A, there is prolonged contrast medium enhancement of the hepatic artery (*arrowhead*), which was confirmed on the hepatic arterial phase image (not shown). D also shows complete thrombosis of the portal vein and a splenic vein up to a point just proximal to the portal confluence (*solid arrow*). The inferior mesenteric vein filling is retrograde (*small open arrow*), and gastroesophageal varices are filled (*large open arrow*). In comparison with the angiographic images, the MR images show the whole portal venous system better. The portal vein thrombosis was surgically verified during liver transplantation. (Courtesy of Kreft B, Strunk H, Flacke S, et al: Detection of thrombosis in the portal venous system: Comparison of contrast-enhanced MR angiography with intraarterial digital subtraction angiography. *Radiology* 216:86-92, 2000, Radiological Society of North America.)

Conclusions.—Noninvasive contrast-enhanced MR angiography demonstrated the sensitivity, specificity, and accuracy to be considered a potential replacement for intra-arterial DSA as the standard technique for assessing of the whole portal venous system.

▶ The image quality obtained via gadolinium-enhanced, portal-venous phase dynamic MRA in this series compares very favorably with DSA. CT angiography of the portal venous system is also quick, reliable and well tolerated. Duplex US alone (augmented with UR contrast[1]) is probably the best single test to exclude splenic or hepatic vein thrombosis, since most US patients with recalcitrant variceal bleeding are referred for DSA-guided transjugular intrahepatic portosystemic shunting and may not require comprehensive preprocedural MRA imaging.

R. L. Dalman, MD

Reference

1. Sidhu PS, Marshall MM, Ryan SM, et al: Clinical use of Levovist, an ultrasound contrast agent, in the imaging of liver transplantation: Assessment of the pre- and post-transplant patient. *Eur Radiol* 10:1114-1126, 2000.

Comparison of Portal Vein Velocity and the Hepatic Venous Pressure Gradient in Assessing the Acute Portal Hemodynamic Response to Propranolol in Patients With Cirrhosis
Schepke M, Raab P, Hoppe A, et al (Univ of Bonn, Germany)
Am J Gastroenterol 95:2905-2909, 2000   17–2

Objective.—To determine the effectiveness of propranolol treatment for portal hypertension, portal hemodynamics must be assessed directly. Although quantitative Doppler sonography has been evaluated as a noninvasive method for such monitoring, no studies have investigated the temporal relationship between invasive and noninvasive portal hemodynamic parameters. Whether Doppler changes in the portal vein velocity (PVV) reliably reflect the effect of propranolol on the hepatic venous pressure gradient (HVPG) and whether the PVV can be used in clinical practice to distinguish propranolol responders from nonresponders were evaluated in a blinded, prospective study.

Methods.—PVV and HVPG were measured every 30 minutes for 4 hours in 11 patients (9 men) with liver cirrhosis and portal hypertension who ingested a 40-mg tablet of propranolol. Effect versus time profiles of the HVPG and PVV reductions were calculated. Prediction of HVPG response by Doppler sonography was calculated for responders and nonresponders.

Results.—After 2.5 hours, maximal reductions in HVPG and PVV compared with baseline values were 24.8% and 23.3%, respectively (Fig 1). Averaged results clearly distinguished 7 (65%) responders (HVPG reduction range 22.8%-37.9%) and 4 (35%) nonresponders (HVPG reduction

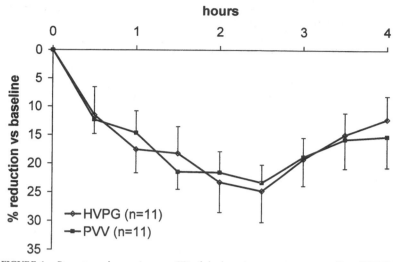

FIGURE 1.—Percentage changes (mean ± SE) of the hepatic venous pressure gradient (HVPG) and portal vein velocity (PVV) after 40 mg propranolol *p.o.* HVPG and PVV were assessed simultaneously and independently by 2 observers each blinded for the results of the other method. (Courtesy of Schepke M, Raab P, Hoppe A, et al: Comparison of portal vein velocity and the hepatic venous pressure gradient in assessing the acute portal hemodynamic response to propranolol in patients with cirrhosis. *Am J Gastroenterol* 95:2905-2909, 2000. Copyright 2000 by Elsevier Science Inc.)

range -5.7% to 4.6%). A threshold of 20% PVV reduction 2 hours after drug administration distinguished between responders and nonresponders with a sensitivity of 1.0, a specificity of 0.86, and a positive predictive value of 0.9.

Conclusion.—Doppler sonography distinguished between responders and nonresponders to propranolol.

▶ Duplex US has become increasingly important in the management of patients with chronic liver failure. Duplex US is quite useful in following TIPS procedures and for detecting early stenoses. This interesting article tests the usefulness of Doppler sonography, or PVV measurements specifically, to identify propranolol responders in patients with portal hypertension. Nonresponders were identified with excellent sensitivity, specificity, and positive predictive value when compared with standard invasive hepatic venous pressure measurements. As with any Duplex US study, the absolute numbers will vary from laboratory to laboratory, but the key finding is that a drop of more than 20% in PVV 2 hours after propranolol will identify responders to this treatment and potentially will decrease variceal bleeding.

E. J. Harris, Jr, MD

Sclerotherapy

A Comparative Study of the Elective Treatment of Variceal Hemorrhage With β-Blockers, Transendoscopic Sclerotherapy, and Surgery: A Prospective, Controlled, and Randomized Trial During 10 Years
Orozco H, Mercado MA, Chan C, et al (Instituto Nacional de la Nutrición, "Salvador Zubirán," Mexico City)
Ann Surg 232:216–219, 2000   17–3

Background.—The most feared complication of portal hypertension is variceal bleeding, which leads to a significant number of deaths and complications worldwide. No single therapeutic modality is effective for all patients. Variceal bleeding recurs in two thirds of patients. Several long-term treatment alternatives are available for patients who survive the bleeding episode, including pharmacotherapy, transendoscopic sclerotherapy and ligamentation, transjugular intrahepatic portosystemic shunts, surgical shunts, devascularization, and liver transplantation. Several studies have compared these alternatives, with varying short- and long-term results. Three options for elective treatment of portal hypertension—β-blockers, transendoscopic sclerotherapy, and surgery—were evaluated in this report.

Methods.—This prospective, controlled, randomized trial included 119 patients between the ages of 18 and 76 years. All the patients had a history of bleeding portal hypertension and had undergone no previous treatment. The patients were randomly assigned to receive propanolol (n = 40), sclerotherapy (n = 46), or surgery (n = 33). There were no differences among the 3 groups in terms of age, Child-Pugh classification, or cause of liver disease.

Results.—The rate of rebleeding was significantly lower in the surgical group than in the other 2 groups. In the Child A surgical group, the rebleeding rate was only 5%, compared with 715 in the sclerotherapy group and 68% in the pharmacotherapy group. Low-risk patients had a better chance of survival in all 3 groups, but no significant differences in survival were found when the 3 options were compared.

Conclusions.—Among low-risk patients undergoing elective surgery, portal blood flow–preserving procedures resulted in the lowest rebleeding rates.

► This study should be commended for its patient accrual in the randomization process for the complex disease of variceal bleeding from portal hypertension. Two thirds of the patients underwent the Sugiura-Futagawa operation, and in this group only 16.7% of the patients had rebleeding. The large majority of patients were Child A group, and the Sugiura-Futagawa operation may be the operation of choice for these patients, who are obviously the best surgical candidates. Classically, the Sugiura-Futagawa operation is performed through a thoracoabdominal approach and includes the devascularization of the perforating veins draining the esophageal varices and preserving the paraesophageal plexus of veins that connect the coronary venous system to the azygos system. In addition, splenectomy and devascularization of the abdominal esophagus are carried out with selective vagotomy and pyloroplasty. Interestingly, patients undergoing sclerotherapy or β-blocker therapy had very high rebleeding rates ranging from 63% to 77.5%, respectively. These were significantly higher than in the surgery group. As expected, there was no significant difference in long-term survival between groups. Another question that arises is whether patients who undergo surgery should be continued on β-blocker therapy and whether this will further reduce the incidence of rebleeding. These authors conclude that electively performed portal blood flow–preserving procedure gives better results in preventing variceal bleeding.

R. B. McLafferty, MD

Prophylactic Sclerotherapy in Children With Esophageal Varices: Long-term Results of a Controlled Prospective Randomized Trial
Gonçalves MEP, Cardoso SR, Maksoud JG (Univ of São Paulo, Brazil)
J Pediatr Surg 35:401-405, 2000   17–4

Background.—Previous reports of prophylactic sclerotherapy (PS) after an initial episode of bleeding esophageal varices have been limited to adults, and have shown conflicting results. No randomized, controlled trials of PS in children with portal hypertension have been reported. The effectiveness of PS to prevent bleeding of esophageal varices in a group of patients is investigated.

Methods.—The randomized trial included 100 consecutive children (median age, 4.3 years) with PH of various causes. Most children had Pugh-Child class A liver function. The patients were randomized to either undergo or not to undergo PS. Those who did not undergo PS (control group) received clinical and endoscopic follow-up only. All patients were followed up for at least 18 months after the end of sclerotherapy sessions; the median follow-up was 4.5 years.

Results.—The 2 groups were similar in their baseline clinical characteristics. Although PS eliminated esophageal varices in 94% of treated patients, only 76% remained free from upper-gastrointestinal (GI) hemorrhage. Twenty-four percent of patients in the PS group had upper-GI bleeding before the varices were eliminated. Gastric varices occurred in 6 (12%) patients, with bleeding in 3 of these 6 cases. The rate of congestive hypertensive gastropathy was 16%, with 4 of these 8 patients having bleeding episodes. Two patients had bleeding of unknown cause.

Fifty-eight percent of children in the control group were free of bleeding from esophageal varices, and 52% were free of any upper-GI bleeding. Ten percent of patients developed gastric varices, and 6% developed congestive hypertensive gastropathy. None of these patients had bleeding episodes. Survival rates were not significantly different between the 2 groups (Table 3).

TABLE 3.—Effects of Prophylactic Sclerotherapy in Prevention of the First Episode of Esophageal Variceal Bleeding, Upper GI Bleeding, Development of Gastric Varices, Congestive Hypertensive Gastropathy, and Mortality Rate

	PS (n = 50)	Control (n = 50)	P Value
No esophageal variceal bleeding (%)	47 (94)	29 (58)	<.05
No upper GI bleeding (%)	38 (76)	26 (52)	<.05
Gastric varices (%)	6 (12)	5 (10)	Not significant
CHG (%)	8 (16)	3 (6)	<.05
Mortality rate (%)	9 (18)	8 (16)	Not significant

(Courtesy of Gonçalves MEP, Cardoso SR, Maksoud JG: Prophylactic sclerotherapy in children with esophageal varices: Long-term results of a controlled prospective randomized trial. *J Pediatr Surg* 35:401-405, 2000.)

Conclusions.—For children with portal hypertension, PS reduces the risk of bleeding esophageal varices, eliminating the varices completely in most cases. Untreated children have a higher rate of bleeding from varices, but those undergoing sclerotherapy are more likely to bleed from the stomach. The complication rate of PS is low. This procedure has no effect on the incidence of gastric varices, but it increases the risk of congestive hypertensive gastropathy. It has no effect on survival rates in children with portal hypertension.

▶ In adults with esophageal varices, prophylactic sclerotherapy has not been shown to be beneficial. In this large study of prophylactic sclerotherapy in children with esophageal varices with a mean follow-up of nearly 5 years, although prophylactic sclerotherapy eliminated esophageal varices in 90% of the patients, it did not reduce the risk of bleeding (caused by gastric varices and congestive hypertensive gastropathy) and did not alter patient survival rate. Thus, prophylactic sclerotherapy would appear to be of no benefit.

J. L. Mills, Sr, MD

Shunt

Transjugular Intrahepatic Portasystemic Shunt vs Surgical Shunt in Good-Risk Cirrhotic Patients: A Case-Control Comparison

Helton WS, Maves R, Wicks K, et al (Univ of Washington, Seattle)

Arch Surg 136:17-20, 2001   17–5

Background.—For patients with variceal bleeding undergoing portal decompression judged to be at good risk, surgical shunt may be more effective and durable, as well as less costly, than angiographic shunt. Clinical and resource allocation outcomes were compared in good-risk cirrhotic patients with portal hypertensive bleeding undergoing transjugular intrahepatic portasystemic shunt (TIPS) or surgical portasystemic shunt (PSS).

Methods.—Twenty patients undergoing TIPS and 20 undergoing PSS were followed up for 385 and 456 patient-months, respectively. All patients had Child-Pugh class A or B cirrhosis.

Findings.—The mortality rate at 30 days was 20% in the TIPS group and 0 in the PSS group. Long-term mortality in the 2 groups was comparable. Compared with PSS, TIPS was associated with significantly more rebleeding episodes, rehospitalization, diagnostic studies of all types, and shunt revisions. In addition, TIPS resulted in significantly higher hospital, professional, and total charges.

Conclusion.—For this patient population, operative portal decompression was more effective, more durable, and less costly than TIPS. Surgical shunt should be the treatment of choice for good-risk patients with portal hypertensive bleeding.

▶ The article adds more fuel to the debate of TIPS versus surgical PSS. While Orloff has provided data in favor of surgical shunt, newer TIPS technology with covered stents is showing promising early outcomes with greater durability, perhaps permitting its use in Child B or A cirrhotic patients. Before surgical shunts can be widely recommended, further studies must be performed comparing newer TIPS technology with surgery.

W. K. Williamson, MD

Portal Venous Decompression With H-Type Mesocaval Shunt Using Autologous Vein Graft: A North American Experience

Sigalet DL, Mayer S, Blanchard H (Alberta Children's Hosp, Calgary, Canada; Hopital Sainte-Justine, Montreal)
J Pediatr Surg 36:91-96, 2001   17–6

Background.—When portal hypertension occurs in children, it is often the result of prehepatic venous obstruction or intrahepatic fibrosis without cirrhosis. Treatment with shunts is particularly helpful in these cases, and European centers have reported success with this approach. The effectiveness of an H-type mesocaval shunt with the use of autologous vein grafts was determined after use by 3 North American centers.

Methods.—The charts of 20 patients who had been treated with the use of shunt procedures for decompression of the portal system from 1980 to 1999 were reviewed retrospectively. The cause of the portal hypertension, details of the diagnostic workup, preoperative management, operative details and outcome (Fig 1), shunt patency postoperatively, patient well-being, and whether liver transplantation was eventually needed were recorded.

Results.—Patients received diagnoses at a median age of 3.7 years and had undergone an extensive period of follow-up before referral for surgery, often with several attempts at sclerotherapy and through multiple episodes of bleeding. Esophageal varices were found in all patients, and 15 also had gastric varices. Eleven had portal venous thrombosis or cavernous trans-

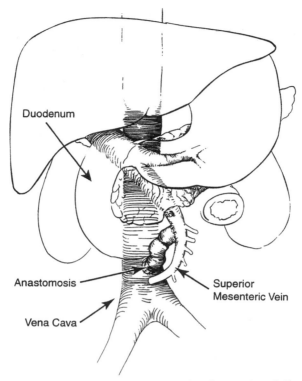

FIGURE 1.—Diagram of shunt placement. (Courtesy of Sigalet DL, Mayer S, Blanchard H: Portal venous decompression with H-type mesocaval shunt using autologous vein graft: A North American experience. *J Pediatr Surg* 36:91-96, 2001.)

formation, and 3 of these had umbilical catheter placement neonatally. American-Indian cirrhosis was found in 5 children, congenital hepatic fibrosis was found in 1, and hepatic fibrosis with polycystic kidney disease was found in 3. At the time of the operations, the average age was 8 years and the average weight was 30 kg; the requirement for blood perioperatively was 200 mL. The postoperative course was generally good; 2 patients required a reoperation for lymphatic leakage, 2 had transient encephalopathy, 1 had severe pancreatitis, and 1 died as a result of a leaking G-tube (not related to the shunt). Shunt patency was achieved in all cases, no further bleeding occurred, and functioning was normal. An algorithm outlining the appropriate steps for investigating and treating gastrointestinal bleeding in pediatric patients was formulated.

Conclusions.—The H-type mesocaval shunt with the use of an autologous vein graft was associated with good results in these pediatric patients with portal hypertension from prehepatic causes. The algorithm presented could serve as a guide for future approaches.

▶ The optimal treatment for portal hypertension in children remains unknown. H-type mesocaval shunts using an internal jugular vein graft proved safe (5% mortality), durable (no autogenous graft thromboses), and effective (no patient with prehepatic portal hypertension required liver transplantation during a mean follow-up of 4.3 years). The favorable results call into question the repeated efforts at sclerotherapy often employed, which may lead to esophageal strictures and other complications. The authors argue for an earlier role of surgical intervention. Unfortunately, the proper controlled trial will likely never be performed because of the small numbers of these patients encountered.

A. M. Abou-Zamzam, Jr, MD

Subject Index

A

Abciximab
  plus coronary stenting *vs.* alteplase in
    myocardial infarction, 273
Abdominal
  aorta (*see* Aorta, abdominal)
  ischemic manifestations of
    antiphospholipid antibody
    syndrome, 51
  surgery, external pneumatic compression
    and fibrinolysis in, 45
  thrombotic manifestations of
    antiphospholipid antibody
    syndrome, 51
  vascular injuries, operative management
    and outcome, 451
Acenocoumarol
  vs. nadroparine in long-term treatment
    of deep venous thrombosis, 460
Acetylcysteine
  prevents radiographic contrast
    agent-induced reductions in renal
    function, 214
Activator protein 1
  in vascular smooth muscle, effect of
    Chlamydia pneumoniae on, 29
Activity
  physical (*see* Exercise)
Adenosine
  and hypothermic saline, retrograde
    venous perfusion for protection of
    ischemic spinal cord with (in pig),
    95
Adrenergic
  vasoconstriction of resistance arteries,
    effect of elevated homocysteine
    levels on, 62
Age
  as predictor of death in patients with
    claudication, 333
Alcohol, 1
  consumption
    cholesterol levels raised by, HDL, 3
    claudication and, intermittent, 256
    moderate, beneficial effect on
      myocardial infarction, and genetic
      variation in alcohol dehydrogenase,
      4
  dehydrogenase, genetic variation in, and
    beneficial effect of moderate
    alcohol intake on myocardial
    infarction, 4
  type, effect on mortality from all causes,
    coronary heart disease, and cancer,
    1

Allograft
  bypass grafts, vein, cellular repopulation
    of, 429
Alteplase
  vs. coronary stenting plus platelet
    glycoprotein IIb/IIIa blockade in
    myocardial infarction, 273
Anastomosis
  interposition vein cuff, effect on wall
    shear stress distribution in recipient
    artery, 418
  technique, new distal, in femorodistal
    PTFE bypass grafting for severe
    limb ischemia, 330
  venous anastomosis Tyrell vein collar,
    effect on primary patency of
    arteriovenous hemodialysis grafts,
    360
Anatomical
  distribution of suspected pulmonary
    embolism, 485
  risk factors for proximal perigraft
    endoleak and graft migration after
    endovascular repair of abdominal
    aortic aneurysms, 121
Anatomy
  of deep venous thrombosis of lower
    extremity, 493
AneuRx stent graft
  endovascular repair using, aneurysm
    rupture after, 135
  percutaneous placement, 141
Aneurysm
  aortic, 287
    abdominal (*see below*)
    management, 292
    screening for, 287
    in Takayasu's arteritis, CT of, 240
    thoracic, endovascular self-expanding
      stent grafts for, 195
    thoracic, mycotic, anatomic and
      extra-anatomic repair, 281
    thoracoabdominal, ruptured, repair
      technique with minimal aortic
      occlusion time and continuous
      visceral perfusion, 275
  aortic, abdominal
    Chlamydia pneumoniae detection in,
      viable, 26
    collagen increase in, type III pN-, 104
    femoral and popliteal artery
      aneurysms and, incidence of, 300
    hyperhomocysteinemia and, mild, 55
    mycotic, anatomic and
      extra-anatomic repair, 281

Author Index